Diseases of the Salivary Glands

Diseases of the Salivary Glands

Editor

Margherita Sisto

MDPI • Basel • Beijing • Wuhan • Barcelona • Belgrade • Manchester • Tokyo • Cluj • Tianjin

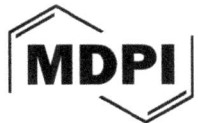

Editor
Margherita Sisto
University of Bari Medical
School
Italy

Editorial Office
MDPI
St. Alban-Anlage 66
4052 Basel, Switzerland

This is a reprint of articles from the Special Issue published online in the open access journal *Journal of Clinical Medicine* (ISSN 2077-0383) (available at: https://www.mdpi.com/journal/jcm/special_issues/Salivary_Glands).

For citation purposes, cite each article independently as indicated on the article page online and as indicated below:

LastName, A.A.; LastName, B.B.; LastName, C.C. Article Title. *Journal Name* **Year**, *Volume Number*, Page Range.

ISBN 978-3-0365-0272-4 (Hbk)
ISBN 978-3-0365-0273-1 (PDF)

Cover image courtesy of Margherita Sisto.

© 2021 by the authors. Articles in this book are Open Access and distributed under the Creative Commons Attribution (CC BY) license, which allows users to download, copy and build upon published articles, as long as the author and publisher are properly credited, which ensures maximum dissemination and a wider impact of our publications.
The book as a whole is distributed by MDPI under the terms and conditions of the Creative Commons license CC BY-NC-ND.

Contents

About the Editor vii

Margherita Sisto
Special Issue—"Diseases of the Salivary Glands"
Reprinted from: *J. Clin. Med.* **2020**, *9*, 3886, doi:10.3390/jcm9123886 1

Giuseppe Ingravallo, Eugenio Maiorano, Marco Moschetta, Luisa Limongelli, Mauro Giuseppe Mastropasqua, Gisella Franca Agazzino, Vincenzo De Ruvo, Paola Tarantino, Gianfranco Favia and Saverio Capodiferro
Primary Breast Extranodal Marginal Zone Lymphoma in Primary Sjögren Syndrome: Case Presentation and Relevant Literature
Reprinted from: *J. Clin. Med.* **2020**, *9*, 3997, doi:10.3390/jcm9123997 5

Braxton D. Noll, Alexandre Grdzelishvili, Michael T. Brennan, Farah Bahrani Mougeot and Jean-Luc C. Mougeot
Immortalization of Salivary Gland Epithelial Cells of Xerostomic Patients: Establishment and Characterization of Novel Cell Lines
Reprinted from: *J. Clin. Med.* **2020**, *9*, 3820, doi:10.3390/jcm9123820 13

Tatsurou Tanaka, Masafumi Oda, Nao Wakasugi-Sato, Takaaki Joujima, Yuichi Miyamura, Manabu Habu, Masaaki Kodama, Osamu Takahashi, Teppei Sago, Shinobu Matsumoto-Takeda, Ikuko Nishida, Hiroki Tsurushima, Yasushi Otani, Daigo Yoshiga, Masaaki Sasaguri and Yasuhiro Morimoto
First Report of Sublingual Gland Ducts: Visualization by Dynamic MR Sialography and Its Clinical Application
Reprinted from: *J. Clin. Med.* **2020**, *9*, 3676, doi:10.3390/jcm9113676 37

Katarzyna Morawska, Mateusz Maciejczyk, Łukasz Popławski, Anna Popławska-Kita, Adam Krętowski and Anna Zalewska
Enhanced Salivary and General Oxidative Stress in Hashimoto's Thyroiditis Women in Euthyreosis
Reprinted from: *J. Clin. Med.* **2020**, *9*, 2102, doi:10.3390/jcm9072102 47

Mateusz Maciejczyk, Julita Szulimowska, Katarzyna Taranta-Janusz, Anna Wasilewska and Anna Zalewska
Salivary Gland Dysfunction, Protein Glycooxidation and Nitrosative Stress in Children with Chronic Kidney Disease
Reprinted from: *J. Clin. Med.* **2020**, *9*, 1285, doi:10.3390/jcm9051285 65

Saverio Capodiferro, Giuseppe Ingravallo, Luisa Limongelli, Mauro Giuseppe Mastropasqua, Angela Tempesta, Gianfranco Favia and Eugenio Maiorano
Intra-Cystic (In Situ) Mucoepidermoid Carcinoma: A Clinico-Pathological Study of 14 Cases
Reprinted from: *J. Clin. Med.* **2020**, *9*, 1157, doi:10.3390/jcm9041157 83

Hideki Nakamura, Toshimasa Shimizu and Atsushi Kawakami
Role of Viral Infections in the Pathogenesis of Sjögren's Syndrome: Different Characteristics of Epstein-Barr Virus and HTLV-1
Reprinted from: *J. Clin. Med.* **2020**, *9*, 1459, doi:10.3390/jcm9051459 93

Dorian Parisis, Clara Chivasso, Jason Perret, Muhammad Shahnawaz Soyfoo and Christine Delporte
Current State of Knowledge on Primary Sjögren's Syndrome, an Autoimmune Exocrinopathy
Reprinted from: *J. Clin. Med.* **2020**, *9*, 2299, doi:10.3390/jcm9072299 . . . . **119**

Margherita Sisto, Domenico Ribatti and Sabrina Lisi
Understanding the Complexity of Sjögren's Syndrome: Remarkable Progress in Elucidating NF-κB Mechanisms
Reprinted from: *J. Clin. Med.* **2020**, *9*, 2821, doi:10.3390/jcm9092821 . . . . **181**

Richard Witas, Shivai Gupta and Cuong Q. Nguyen
Contributions of Major Cell Populations to Sjögren's Syndrome
Reprinted from: *J. Clin. Med.* **2020**, *9*, 3057, doi:10.3390/jcm9093057 . . . . **199**

Martha S. van Ginkel, Andor W.J.M. Glaudemans, Bert van der Vegt, Esther Mossel, Frans G.M. Kroese, Hendrika Bootsma and Arjan Vissink
Imaging in Primary Sjögren's Syndrome
Reprinted from: *J. Clin. Med.* **2020**, *9*, 2492, doi:10.3390/jcm9082492 . . . . **225**

Kimberly J. Jasmer, Kristy E. Gilman, Kevin Muñoz Forti, Gary A. Weisman and Kirsten H. Limesand
Radiation-Induced Salivary Gland Dysfunction: Mechanisms, Therapeutics and Future Directions
Reprinted from: *J. Clin. Med.* **2020**, *9*, 4095, doi:10.3390/jcm9124095 . . . . **247**

Soo-Min Ok, Donald Ho, Tyler Lynd, Yong-Woo Ahn, Hye-Min Ju, Sung-Hee Jeong and Kyounga Cheon
Candida Infection Associated with Salivary Gland—A Narrative Review
Reprinted from: *J. Clin. Med.* **2021**, *10*, 97, doi:10.3390/jcm10010097 . . . . **285**

About the Editor

Margherita Sisto is a Professor of Human Anatomy at the Faculty of Medicine, University of Bari, Italy, with a Biological Degree *cum laude* and a Ph.D. in "Human and Experimental Morphology (macroscopic, microscopic, and ultrastructural)", also from the University of Bari, Italy. Professor Sisto's research interests are primarily in the area of pathophysiology and molecular immunology applied to immunological research lines, with emphasis on the elucidation of molecular processes underlying the interaction between receptors of the immune response, inflammation, and the characterization of new anti-inflammatory molecules. Her particle research has involved in vitro analysis of dysregulated immunological responses during the pathogenesis of chronic inflammatory diseases such as the autoimmune Sjogren's syndrome. Professor Sisto's innovative research has been highlighted in a number of prestigious, peer-reviewed journals.

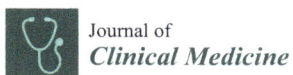

Editorial

Special Issue—"Diseases of the Salivary Glands"

Margherita Sisto

Department of Basic Medical Sciences, Neurosciences and Sense Organs, Section of Human Anatomy and Histology, Laboratory of Cell Biology, University of Bari Medical School, 70124 Bari, Italy; margherita.sisto@uniba.it

Received: 26 November 2020; Accepted: 27 November 2020; Published: 30 November 2020

Editorial

Salivary glands (SGs) are of the utmost importance for maintaining the health of the oral cavity and carrying out physiological functions such as mastication, protection of teeth, perception of food taste, and speech. SGs may be affected by a number of diseases—local and systemic—and the prevalence of SG diseases depends on various etiological factors. The glands can be blocked by small stones that form in the gland ducts, which may cause painful swelling. The glands may become infected by viral, bacterial, or (rarely) fungal agents, or they may be the targets of autoimmune attacks that affect their functions. Management of salivary disorders encompasses a broad array of diseases—both benign and malignant. To better demonstrate the evolution of this field, the present Special Issue in the *Journal of Clinical Medicine* aims to cover recent and novel advancements as well as future trends in the field of research evaluating diagnostic and therapeutic treatment of SG diseases, reflecting the diverse nature of SG anatomy, physiology, and dysfunction in various states of disease.

Several interesting findings are derived from this collective body of work. Firstly, in alignment with the most advanced diagnostic techniques for the identification of pathologies affecting the SGs, Tanaka et al. [1] reported the effective application of MR sialography and dynamic MR sialography to visualize the sublingual gland ducts, demonstrating, successfully, that MR sialography can be more useful in the diagnosis of patients with lesions of sublingual gland ducts. Van Ginkel and colleagues [2] enriched the Special Issue by contributing a descriptive review discussing imaging techniques that are used in the identification and characterization of primary Sjögren's syndrome (pSS) with a focus on the SGs. Primary Sjögren's syndrome (pSS) is a systemic autoimmune disease characterized by dysfunction and lymphocytic infiltration of the salivary and lacrimal glands, with unknown etiology. The review emphasizes the contribution of innovative techniques to the diagnosis of pSS and the monitoring of the progression of the disease, underlining the contribution to diagnosis and staging of pSS-associated lymphomas. Several of the papers published in this Special Issue provide insights into the etiology of pSS, highlighting aspects that contribute to the pathophysiology of the disease and exploring treatment options that target different mediators of the pSS pathogenesis. An important experimental contribution is given by the development of a pSS experimental model represented by immortalized SG epithelial cells derived from labial salivary gland biopsies of pSS patients [3]; these cells represent a viable model for salivary research due to their passaging capacity and maintenance of acinar cell characteristics. The etiology of pSS remains poorly understood, but recent findings highlight the involvement of both immune system cells and various types of glandular cells that cooperate in the perpetuation of chronic inflammatory conditions that characterize pSS. Witas et al. [4] summarized the evidence for participation in disease pathogenesis by both various classes of immune cells and glandular epithelial cells in an interesting review collecting data from both preclinical mouse models and human patients. Relatedly, my research group [5] collected from the literature the most recent findings concerning the involvement of the transcription factor nuclear factor κ (kappa)-light-chain-enhancer of activated B cells (NF-κB) in the chronic inflammatory mechanisms implicated in the pathogenesis of pSS. To enrich this panorama of possible mechanisms underlying the pSS disease, Paris and colleagues [6] contributed a comprehensive review which addresses the clinical presentation, diagnosis, and complications of the disease, focusing on the fundamental role played by epithelial cells in autoimmune mechanisms and on the genetic, environmental, and hormonal features that represent risk factors for the disease. The important article by Nakamura et al. [7], which suggests and explains a viral etiology at the basis of pSS, fits well into this scenario. Nakamura delved into the role played by various viruses such as Epstein–Barr virus (EBV) or human T-cell leukemia virus type 1 (HTLV-1) that, regardless of the different cellular targets that they have, are involved in pathological immune modifications in pSS.

Finally, a part of the Special Issue is dedicated to the analysis of interesting case reports related to primary or secondary diseases of the SGs. The research group of Drs. Ingravallo and Capodiferro reported a clinical study conducted on a series of intraoral mucoepidermoid carcinomas showing exclusive intracystic growth [8] and a rare case of primary breast lymphoma occurring in a woman with long-standing pSS [9]. Morawska and colleagues performed a study on women with Hashimoto's thyroiditis (HT) that evaluated the redox homeostasis of the SGs; data collected demonstrate that salivary secretion is impaired in patients with HT, and the release of oxidant molecules was found to be significantly higher in patients with HT than in healthy controls [10]. From the same research group, Maciejczyk et al. evaluated protein glycooxidation products, lipid oxidative damage, and nitrosative stress in chronic kidney disease (CKD) condition. Interestingly, their analysis indicates that children with CKD suffer from SG dysfunction that increases with CKD progression [11].

Given these diverse contributions, it is evident that research on SG diseases will continue to flourish. There are still many fundamental questions that remain unanswered, promising a great future for this field. As the Guest Editor, I would like to give special thanks to the reviewers for their timely and professional comments and to the members of the *JCM* Editorial Office for their robust support. Finally, I sincerely thank all the authors for their valuable contributions. I believe the readers of this Special Issue will find them very useful.

Conflicts of Interest: The authors declare no conflict of interest.

References

1. Tanaka, T.; Oda, M.; Wakasugi-Sato, N.; Joujima, T.; Miyamura, Y.; Habu, M.; Kodama, M.; Takahashi, O.; Sago, T.; Matsumoto-Takeda, S.; et al. First Report of Sublingual Gland Ducts: Visualization by Dynamic MR Sialography and Its Clinical Application. *J. Clin. Med.* **2020**, *9*, 3676. [CrossRef] [PubMed]
2. Van Ginkel, M.S.; Glaudemans, A.W.; van der Vegt, B.; Mossel, E.; Kroese, F.G.; Bootsma, H.; Vissink, A. Imaging in Primary Sjögren's Syndrome. *J. Clin. Med.* **2020**, *9*, 2492. [CrossRef] [PubMed]
3. Noll, B.D.; Grdzelishvili, A.; Brennan, M.T.; Mougeot, F.B.; Mougeot, J.-L.C. Immortalization of Salivary Gland Epithelial Cells of Xerostomic Patients: Establishment and Characterization of Novel Cell Lines. *J. Clin. Med.* **2020**, *9*, 3820. [CrossRef]
4. Witas, R.; Gupta, S.; Nguyen, C.Q. Contributions of Major Cell Populations to Sjögren's Syndrome. *J. Clin. Med.* **2020**, *9*, 3057. [CrossRef] [PubMed]
5. Sisto, M.; Ribatti, D.; Lisi, S. Understanding the Complexity of Sjögren's Syndrome: Remarkable Progress in Elucidating NF-κB Mechanisms. *J. Clin. Med.* **2020**, *9*, 2821. [CrossRef] [PubMed]
6. Parisis, D.; Chivasso, C.; Perret, J.; Soyfoo, M.S.; Delporte, C. Current State of Knowledge on Primary Sjögren's Syndrome, an Autoimmune Exocrinopathy. *J. Clin. Med.* **2020**, *9*, 2299. [CrossRef] [PubMed]
7. Nakamura, H.; Shimizu, T.; Kawakami, A. Role of Viral Infections in the Pathogenesis of Sjögren's Syndrome: Different Characteristics of Epstein-Barr Virus and HTLV-1. *J. Clin. Med.* **2020**, *9*, 1459. [CrossRef] [PubMed]
8. Capodiferro, S.; Ingravallo, G.; Limongelli, L.; Mastropasqua, M.G.; Tempesta, A.; Favia, G.; Maiorano, E. Intra-Cystic (In Situ) Mucoepidermoid Carcinoma: A Clinico-Pathological Study of 14 Cases. *J. Clin. Med.* **2020**, *9*, 1157. [CrossRef] [PubMed]
9. Ingravallo, G.; Capodiferro, S.; Moschetta, M.; Favia, G.; Maiorano, E. Primary Sjögren Syndrome Complicated by Late Onset of Extranodal Marginal Zone Lymphoma in the Breast. *J. Clin. Med.* **2020**. under review.

10. Morawska, K.; Maciejczyk, M.; Popławski, Ł.; Popławska-Kita, A.; Krętowski, A.; Zalewska, A. Enhanced Salivary and General Oxidative Stress in Hashimoto's Thyroiditis Women in Euthyreosis. *J. Clin. Med.* **2020**, *9*, 2102. [CrossRef] [PubMed]
11. Maciejczyk, M.; Szulimowska, J.; Taranta-Janusz, K.; Wasilewska, A.; Zalewska, A. Salivary Gland Dysfunction, Protein Glycooxidation and Nitrosative Stress in Children with Chronic Kidney Disease. *J. Clin. Med.* **2020**, *9*, 1285. [CrossRef] [PubMed]

Publisher's Note: MDPI stays neutral with regard to jurisdictional claims in published maps and institutional affiliations.

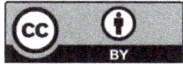

© 2020 by the author. Licensee MDPI, Basel, Switzerland. This article is an open access article distributed under the terms and conditions of the Creative Commons Attribution (CC BY) license (http://creativecommons.org/licenses/by/4.0/).

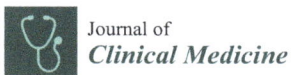 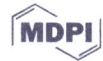

Article

Primary Breast Extranodal Marginal Zone Lymphoma in Primary Sjögren Syndrome: Case Presentation and Relevant Literature

Giuseppe Ingravallo [1,*], Eugenio Maiorano [1], Marco Moschetta [2], Luisa Limongelli [3], Mauro Giuseppe Mastropasqua [1], Gisella Franca Agazzino [1], Vincenzo De Ruvo [2], Paola Tarantino [1], Gianfranco Favia [3] and Saverio Capodiferro [3]

1. Department of Emergency and Organ Transplantation—Section of Pathology, University of Bari Aldo Moro, Piazza G. Cesare, 11, 70124 Bari, Italy; eugenio.maiorano@uniba.it (E.M.); mauro.mastropasqua@uniba.it (M.G.M.); gisella.agazzino@libero.it (G.F.A.); tarpa80@gmail.com (P.T.)
2. Department of Emergency and Organ Transplantation—Breast Unit, University of Bari Aldo Moro, Piazza G. Cesare, 11, 70124 Bari, Italy; marco.moschetta@uniba.it (M.M.); vincenzo.deruvo@yahoo.it (V.D.R.)
3. Department of Interdisciplinary Medicine—Section of Odontostomatology, University of Bari Aldo Moro, Piazza G. Cesare, 11, 70124 Bari, Italy; lululimongelli@gmail.com (L.L.); gianfranco.favia@uniba.it (G.F.); capodiferro.saverio@gmail.com (S.C.)
* Correspondence: giuseppe.ingravallo@uniba.it

Received: 14 November 2020; Accepted: 7 December 2020; Published: 10 December 2020

Abstract: The association between autoimmune diseases, mostly rheumatoid arthritis, systemic lupus erythematosus, celiac disease and Sjögren syndrome, and lymphoma, has been widely demonstrated by several epidemiologic studies. By a mechanism which has not yet been entirely elucidated, chronic activation/stimulation of the immune system, along with the administration of specific treatments, may lead to the onset of different types of lymphoma in such patients. Specifically, patients affected by Sjögren syndrome may develop lymphomas many years after the original diagnosis. Several epidemiologic, hematologic, and histological features may anticipate the progression from Sjögren syndrome into lymphoma but, to the best of our knowledge, a definite pathogenetic mechanism for such progression is still missing. In fact, while the association between Sjögren syndrome and non-Hodgkin lymphoma, mostly extranodal marginal zone lymphomas and, less often, diffuse large B-cell, is well established, many other variables, such as time of onset, gender predilection, sites of occurrence, subtype of lymphoma, and predictive factors, still remain unclear. We report on a rare case of primary breast lymphoma occurring three years after the diagnosis of Sjögren syndrome in a 57-year-old patient. The diagnostic work-up, including radiograms, core needle biopsy, and histological examination, is discussed, along with emerging data from the recent literature, thus highlighting the usefulness of breast surveillance in Sjögren syndrome patients.

Keywords: autoimmune diseases; Sjögren syndrome; minor salivary glands; B-cell lymphoma; extranodal marginal zone lymphoma; MALT lymphoma; primary breast lymphoma

1. Introduction

Sjögren's syndrome (SS) is the second most common autoimmune disease; it is usually classified as primary or secondary to rheumatoid arthritis and other autoimmune diseases, such as lupus erythematosus, sclerodermia, vasculitis, etc., mainly involves the exocrine glands (salivary and lacrimal glands) and is characterized by progressive infiltration of T-and B-lymphocytes [1,2]. The common detectability of hyper-gamma-globulinemia and different autoantibodies (such as rheumatoid factor, anti-Sjögren's syndrome A and B antibodies) in the blood of SS patients underlines the relevance of B-cell hyperactivity in the pathogenesis [2,3]. Common clinical findings in SS patients are kerato-conjunctivitis sicca, xerostomia, angular cheilitis, and additional symptoms related to the qualitative/quantitative reduction of exocrine secretions [3]. Along with dryness, SS patients may show disabling symptoms, such as fatigue and pain, but also develop systemic manifestations in up to 30–50% of cases, including renal, lung, or neurological disorders [4,5]. In addition, SS patients have an increased risk of lymphoma, such as marginal zone lymphoma (MZL) or mucosal-associated lymphoid tissue (MALT) lymphoma [6–10]. The World Health Organization in 2016 classified MZLs into three distinct types, according to the involved sites: extranodal MZL of MALT (generally termed as MALT lymphoma), nodal MZL, and splenic MZL [11].

The worldwide incidence of SS is difficult to assess as many cases remain undiagnosed for years [12,13]. Overall, extranodal MALT lymphomas more frequently affect the stomach, spleen, thyroid, ocular adnexal tissues, and salivary glands, while they are rare in the breast (1.7–2.2% of primary breast lymphomas), possibly due to the anecdotic presence of MALT tissue at this site [14,15].

Moreover, SS patients may be affected by non-Hodgkin lymphomas (NHL) over the course of the disease; less than 20% are diffuse B-cell lymphomas while the most frequent are of the MALT type (up to 60%), the latter more commonly involving the minor and major salivary glands, pharynx, stomach, small intestine, and thyroid, with an incidence 10–44 times higher than in the general population [4,5,8–10,16,17].

We report on a case of an extranodal marginal zone lymphoma of MALT, occurring in the breast of a Caucasian woman, with a three-year history of Sjögren's syndrome; also, data from the literature on this topic have been collected and reviewed.

2. Case Presentation

A 57-year-old Caucasian female was referred to the breast care unit of the Policlinic Hospital of the University of Bari Aldo Moro for a small mass in her right breast. The patient had been suffering from persistent and severe dry eyes and moderate dry mouth for several years. Three years earlier, a biopsy of the minor salivary glands, along with the presence of anti-Sjögren's syndrome A and B (anti-SSA/SSB) antibodies, lead to the diagnosis of primary SS, in the absence of other autoimmune diseases, as detected by clinical examination and serological tests. The revision of the original histopathological preparations confirmed the diagnosis of lymphocytic sialadenitis with a focus score >1/4 mm^2, grade 4 according to Chisholm and Mason (Figure 1A,B).

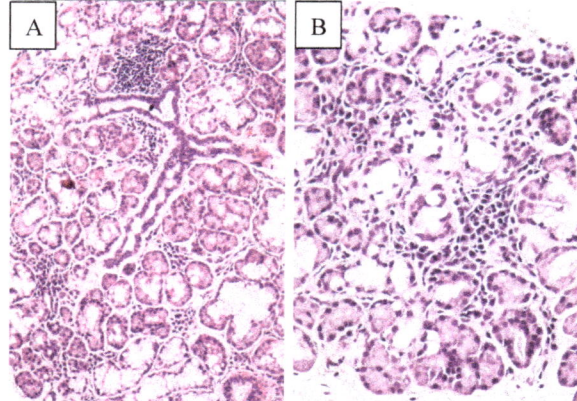

Figure 1. Low power magnification of minor salivary gland biopsy ((**A**): hematoxylin and eosin, original magnification 100×); at higher magnification, small lymphocyte and plasma cell aggregates (i.e., more than one lymphocytic focus) associated with mildly collagenized stroma are detectable ((**B**): hematoxylin and eosin, original magnification 200×).

The patient reported that, immediately after the diagnosis of SS, she received methotrexate and prednisone for a few months; currently, she still is only undergoing antihypertensive and hydroxychloroquine therapy and shows no relevant signs of SS (e.g., parotid enlargement or eye/mouth dryness). Routine laboratory tests were within normal limits. As to the breast lesion, a painless swelling of small size was detected on palpation; conventional mammography showed a small radiolucency with regular and well-defined margins of the lower inner quadrant (Figure 2), while ultrasound examination highlighted a round opacity with regular edges (Figure 3A–D).

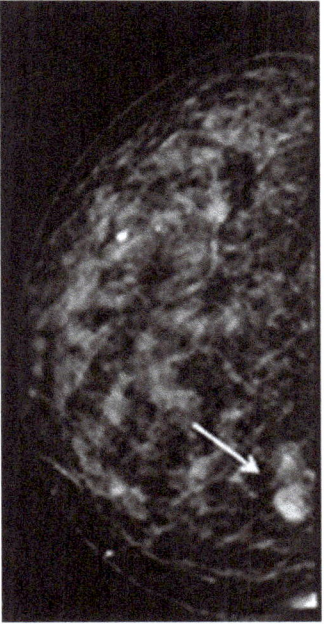

Figure 2. Digital cranio-caudal mammographic view: the lesion appears as a round opacity with regular edges located in the lower inner quadrant of the right breast (arrow).

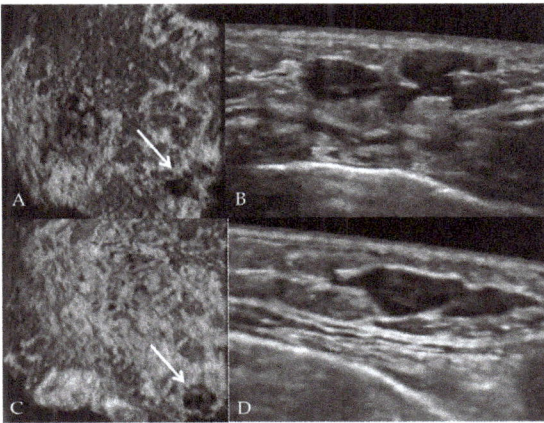

Figure 3. Automated breast ultrasound scan on coronal (**A,C**) and axial planes (**B,D**). The lesion appears as an oval hypoechoic nodule with regular edges, mimicking duct ectasia (arrows).

Regardless of the benign appearance on both imaging investigations, a US-guided core needle biopsy of the lesion was performed; unexpectedly, the subsequent histopathological examination showed diffuse proliferation of small to medium-sized lymphoid cells, with slightly hyperchromatic nuclei, without plasmacytic differentiation, accompanied by stromal sclerosis and residual atrophic ducts.

Complimentary immunohistochemical investigations were performed to confirm the purportedly monoclonal nature of the lymphoid proliferation, highlighting the vast majority of infiltrating lymphocytes being of the B phenotype, and distinctly immunoreactive for CD20, CD79a and bcl2, while no immunoreactivity for CD3, CD5, CD10, CD23, cyclin D1, bcl6 and LEF1 was detected in lymphoid neoplastic cells. Less than 10% tumor cells displayed nuclear anti-Ki 67 (MIB 1) positivity. MALT gene rearrangement, involving the MALT1 locus at chromosome 18q21, using a MALT FISH Split Signal DNA Probe, could not be demonstrated. All such findings pointed at the diagnosis of primary extranodal MZL of MALT (MALT lymphoma) (Figure 4A–D). No lymphadenopathy, spleen enlargement, bone marrow involvement or other localizations of the disease were detected. Peripheral blood tests revealed the persistence of anti-SS A and B (anti-SSA/SSB) antibodies, cryoglobulins and low levels of C4 and C3.

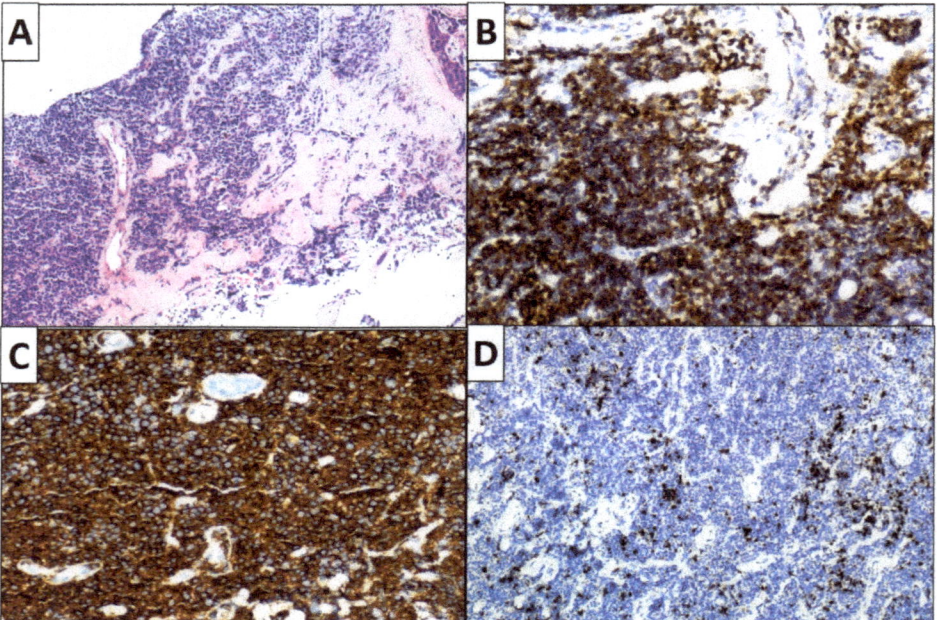

Figure 4. Primary breast marginal zone NHL is characterized by diffuse proliferation of small to medium-sized lymphoid cells and accompanied by stromal sclerosis and residual atrophic ducts ((**A**): hematoxylin and eosin, original magnification 40×). The neoplastic lymphocytes are strongly immunoreactive for bcl2 ((**B**): original magnification 200×) and CD20 ((**C**): original magnification 200×). The immunohistochemical stain for Ki67 shows a very low proliferative index, pointing at an "indolent" lymphoma ((**D**): original magnification 100×).

3. Discussion

Primary breast lymphomas (PBL) represent approximately 1% of all NHLs, 1.7–2.2% of all extra-nodal NHLs and 0.04–0.5% of all malignancies of the breast. [18–21] Around 9% of all primary breast lymphomas are MZLs of MALT and usually manifest an indolent clinical behavior [21–23].

It is generally accepted that chronic inflammatory diseases (such as SS, Hashimoto thyroiditis, *Borrelia Burgdorferi* dermatitis, Helicobacter pylori-associated chronic gastritis and HCV, HHV8, EBV and HTLV-1 infections) may play a role in lymphoma development, resulting in the transition from polyclonal B cell activation into monoclonal expansion of B-lymphocytes. The transition into B-cell NHL only affects a minority of the aforementioned patients harboring chronic inflammatory diseases and has been associated with increased overall disease mortality rate [5–9,11,24].

Bizjak et al. in 2015 [25] extensively reviewed the role of inflammation related to breast silicone implants and other silicone prostheses (such as cardiac pacemakers and defibrillators, cardiac valvular and testicular/penile prostheses) in lymphoma development. They assumed that chronic inflammation in predisposed individuals could evolve into severe scarring of peri-implant tissues and to persistent activation of the local/systemic immune system. Such a pathogenetic mechanism was demonstrated for a distinct type of NHL, namely breast implant-associated anaplastic large T-cell lymphoma (BI-ALCL).

Patients with autoimmune diseases represent 5% of NHL patients, and NHL surely is the most severe complication occurring during SS patients' follow-up; [5–10,24] nevertheless, the pathogenetic mechanism for such association has not been clarified [1–6,9–11,24,26].

As widely discussed by Vasaitis et al. in a recent population-based study [26], data available in the literature on NHL in SS patients are not at all uniform, and even basic data on gender preferences and overall lymphoma prevalence are not well established yet [26]. In view of the mostly indolent clinical behavior of NHL in SS patients, and in consideration of a median follow-up time that rarely exceeds 10 years in most reported studies, an accurate definition of epidemiologic data, including prevalence, can be hardly assessed. In addition, while several studies have reported on the occurrence of NHL in the breast, these were not focused on possible associations between breast NHL and SS [15,26–29].

In a recent update on prognostic markers of lymphoma development in SS patients, Retamozo et al. (2019) [30] stated that such patients show a seven-fold increased risk of lymphoma in comparison with systemic lupus erythematosus patients, four-fold with rheumatoid arthritis patients and globally >10-fold in comparison with the general population [5,30].

The same authors listed, point-to-point evaluated and discussed the different prognostic/predictive factors outlined in previously published studies, such as epidemiologic markers (age and sex), clinical markers (parotid enlargement, dry mouth and eyes, arthralgias, splenomegaly, lymphadenopathy, skin purpura/vasculitis), laboratory markers (systemic activity, hypergamma/raised IgG, CD4/CD8 ≤ 0.8, raised beta2-microglobulin, raised B-cell activating factors, anemia, leukopenia, lymphopenia, neutropenia, ANA, rheumatoid factor, Anti-Ro/La, low C4, C3 and CH 50 levels, cryoglobulins, mIgs) and histologic markers (focus score and ectopic primary or secondary follicle). They concluded that, although the association of more risk factors surely increases the risk of NHL, such prediction still remains imperfect; therefore, SS patients surely deserve closer follow-up, with attentive evaluation of the aforementioned risk factors, including cryoglobulin-related markers and increased EULAR SS disease activity index (ESSDAI), to more accurately identify patients at higher risk for SS-associated NHL [30,31].

As to primary breast lymphomas (PBLs), they are usually detected as palpable masses, associated or not with axillary lymph node enlargement, thus mimicking breast carcinoma or other breast neoplasms [32]. Furthermore, notwithstanding several attempts, no specific clinical or imaging patterns have been reported for breast lymphomas [33–36]. Radiologically, as for the case reported herein, PBL more commonly resembles inflammatory lesions, such as lymphocytic mastitis [37], IgG4-related sclerosing mastitis [38] and cutaneous lymphoid hyperplasia [39].

Consequently, the diagnosis of breast MZL of MALT usually is based on morphologic examinations. At this regard, fine needle aspiration cytology, a minimally invasive procedure, was proven effective to accurately diagnose the most common non-neoplastic (e.g., fibrocystic disease) and neoplastic (e.g., fibroadenoma and carcinoma) breast lesions at a pre-operative stage; nevertheless, such a diagnostic procedure may be of limited value when dealing with lymphoid proliferations, which may not show unequivocal morphologic features or may require extensive immunohistochemical investigations to achieve the final diagnosis. Consequently, histological preparations are more frequently adopted in such cases, which may allow proper morphologic evaluation of the lymphoid populations, appropriate immunohistochemical characterization, along with the possible detection of genetic alterations by in situ hybridization techniques, whenever deemed necessary. In the current case, all necessary morphologic and ancillary procedures could be carried out, even if dealing with small tissue fragments, thus highlighting the appropriateness of core needle biopsy as a diagnostic tool for PBL.

Based on the data available in the literature about PBL-SS association [40–44], and the current theories about lymphoma prevalence at immune-privileged sites [45], we can assume that the diagnosis of SS-related lymphoid proliferations, especially when occurring in the breast, currently is very challenging and would probably benefit from wider studies including SS patients with prolonged follow-up (>10 years). Therefore, we may suggest more attentive monitoring for lymphoma development in those SS patients who display higher risk factors (such as palpable purpura, low C4, mixed monoclonal cryoglobulinemia) and to incorporate breast surveillance in such patients.

Author Contributions: Conceptualization, S.C., G.I., E.M., G.F.; methodology, G.F.A. and, P.T.; validation, M.M., M.G.M., S.C., E.M.; investigation, G.I., E.M., M.G.M., M.M.; resources, P.T. and G.F.A.; writing—original draft preparation, S.C. and G.I.; writing—review and editing, E.M. and G.F.; visualization, V.D.R., G.F., L.L.; supervision, G.I., S.C., E.M., G.F. All authors have read and agreed to the published version of the manuscript.

Funding: This research received no external funding.

Conflicts of Interest: The authors declare no conflict of interest.

References

1. Brito-Zeron, P.; Baldini, C.; Bootsma, H.; Bowman, S.J.; Jonsson, R.; Mariette, X.; Sivils, K.; Theander, E.; Tzioufas, A.; Ramos-Casals, M. Sjogren syndrome. *Nat. Rev. Dis. Primers* **2016**, *2*, 16047. [CrossRef]
2. Brito-Zeron, P.; Ramos-Casals, M.; EULAR-SS task force group. Advances in the understanding and treatment of systemic complications in Sjogren's syndrome. *Curr. Opin. Rheumatol.* **2014**, *26*, 520–527. [CrossRef]
3. Sisto, M.; Lorusso, L.; Tamma, R.; Ingravallo, G.; Ribatti, D.; Lisi, S. Interleukin-17 and -22 synergy linking inflammation and EMT-dependent fibrosis in Sjögren's syndrome. *Clin. Exp. Immunol.* **2019**, *198*, 261–272. [CrossRef] [PubMed]
4. Retamozo, S.; Brito-Zerón, P.; Ramos-Casals, M. Prognostic markers of lymphoma development in primary Sjögren syndrome. *Lupus* **2019**, *28*, 923–936. [CrossRef] [PubMed]
5. Nocturne, G.; Pontarini, E.; Bombardieri, M.; Mariette, X. Lymphomas complicating primary Sjögren's syndrome: From autoimmunity to lymphoma. *Rheumatology* **2019**, kez052. [CrossRef] [PubMed]
6. Tzioufas, A.G. B-cell lymphoproliferation in primary Sjögren's syndrome. *Clin. Exp. Rheumatol* **1996**, *14* (Suppl. 14), S65–S70. [PubMed]
7. Royer, B.; Cazals-Hatem, D.; Sibilia, J.; Agbalika, F.; Cayuela, J.M.; Soussi, T.; Maloisel, F.; Clauvel, J.P.; Brouet, J.C.; Mariette, X. Lymphomas in patients with Sjogren's syndrome are marginal zone B-cell neoplasms, arise in diverse extranodal and nodal sites, and are not associated with viruses. *Blood* **1997**, *90*, 766–775. [CrossRef]
8. Voulgarelis, M.; Dafni, U.G.; Isenberg, D.A.; Moutsopoulos, H.M. Malignant lymphoma in primary Sjogren's syndrome: A multicenter, retrospective, clinical study by the European Concerted Action on Sjogren's Syndrome. *Arthritis Rheum.* **1999**, *42*, 1765–1772. [CrossRef]
9. Baimpa, E.; Dahabreh, I.J.; Voulgarelis, M.; Moutsopoulos, H.M. Hematologic manifestations and predictors of lymphoma development in primary Sjogren syndrome: Clinical and pathophysiologic aspects. *Medicine* **2009**, *88*, 284–293. [CrossRef]
10. Nocturne, G.; Mariette, X. Sjögren syndrome-associated lymphomas: An update on pathogenesis and management. *Br. J. Haematol.* **2015**, *168*, 317–327. [CrossRef]
11. Swerdlow, S.; Campo, E.; Harris, N.; Jaffe, E.; Pileri, S.; Stein, H.; Thiele, J. *WHO Classification of Tumours of Haematopoietic and Lymphoid Tissues*; IARC Press: Lyon, France, 2017; ISBN 13-9789283244943-13.

12. Ramírez Sepúlveda, J.I.; Kvarnstrom, M.; Eriksson, P.; Mandl, T.; Braekke Norheim, K.; Joar Johnsen, S.; Hammenfors, D.; Jonsson, M.V.; Skarstein, K.; Brun, J.G.; et al. Long-term follow-up in primary Sjogren's syndrome reveals differences in clinical presentation between female and male patients. *Biol. Sex Differ.* **2017**, *8*, 25. [CrossRef] [PubMed]
13. Ramos-Casals, M.; Solans, R.; Rosas, J.; Camps, M.T.; Gil, A.; del Pino-Montes, J.; Calvo-Alen, J.; Jiménez-Alonso, J.; Micó, M.L.; Beltrán, J.; et al. Primary Sjogren's syndrome in men. *Scand. J. Rheumatol.* **2008**, *37*, 300–305.
14. Hissourou, M., III; Zia, S.Y.; Alqatari, M.; Strauchen, J.; Bakst, R.L. Primary MALT lymphoma of the breast treated with definitive radiation. *Case Rep. Hematol.* **2016**, *2016*, 1831792. [CrossRef] [PubMed]
15. Thomas, A.; Link, B.K.; Altekruse, S.; Romitti, P.A.; Schroeder, M.C. Primary Breast Lymphoma in the United States: 1975–2013. *J. Natl. Cancer Inst.* **2017**, *109*, djw294. [CrossRef] [PubMed]
16. Theander, E.; Henriksson, G.; Ljungberg, O.; Mandl, T.; Manthorpe, R.; Jacobsson, L.T.H. Lymphoma and other malignancies in primary Sjogren's syndrome: A cohort study on cancer incidence and lymphoma predictors. *Ann. Rheum. Dis.* **2006**, *65*, 796–803. [CrossRef] [PubMed]
17. Baldini, C.; Pepe, P.; Luciano, N.; Ferro, F.; Talarico, R.; Grossi, S.; Tavoni, A.; Bombardieri, S. A clinical prediction rule for lymphoma development in primary Sjögren's syndrome. *J. Rheumatol.* **2012**, *39*, 804–808. [CrossRef] [PubMed]
18. Ludmir, E.B.; Milgrom, S.A.; Pinnix, C.C.; Gunther, J.R.; Westin, J.; Fayad, L.E.; Khoury, J.D.; Medeiros, L.J.; Dabaja, B.S.; Nastoupil, L.J. Emerging Treatment Strategies for Primary Breast Extranodal Marginal Zone Lymphoma of Mucosa-associated Lymphoid Tissue. *Clin. Lymphoma Myeloma Leuk.* **2019**, *19*, 244–250. [CrossRef]
19. Koganti, S.B.; Lozada, A.; Curras, E.; Shah, A. Marginal zone lymphoma of the breast—A diminished role for surgery. *Int. J. Surg. Case Rep.* **2016**, *25*, 4–6. [CrossRef]
20. Wiseman, C.; Liao, K.T. Primary lymphoma of the breast. *Cancer* **1972**, *29*, 1705–1712. [CrossRef]
21. Kim, S.H.; Ezekiel, M.P.; Kim, R.Y. Primary lymphoma of the breast. *Am. J. Clin. Oncol.* **1999**, *22*, 381–383. [CrossRef]
22. Shapiro, C.M.; Mansur, D. Bilateral primary breast lymphoma. *Am. J. Clin. Oncol.* **2001**, *24*, 85–86. [CrossRef] [PubMed]
23. Martinelli, G.; Ryan, G.; Seymour, J.F.; Nassi, L.; Steffanoni, S.; Alietti, A.; Calabrese, L.; Pruneri, G.; Santoro, L.; Kuper-Hommel, M.; et al. Primary follicular and marginal-zone lymphoma of the breast: Clinical features, prognostic factors and outcome: A study by the International Extranodal Lymphoma Study Group. *Ann. Oncol.* **2009**, *20*, 1993–1999. [CrossRef]
24. Solimando, A.G.; Annese, T.; Tamma, R.; Ingravallo, G.; Maiorano, E.; Vacca, A.; Specchia, G.; Ribatti, D. New Insights into Diffuse Large B-Cell Lymphoma Pathobiology. *Cancers* **2020**, *12*, 1869. [CrossRef] [PubMed]
25. Bizjak, M.; Selmi, C.; Praprotnik, S.; Bruck, O.; Perricone, C.; Ehrenfeld, M.; Shoenfeld, Y. Silicone implants and lymphoma: The role of inflammation. *J. Autoimmun.* **2015**, *65*, 64–73. [CrossRef] [PubMed]
26. Vasaitis, L.; Nordmark, G.; Theander, E.; Backlin, C.; Smedby, K.E.; Askling, J.; Rönnblom, L.; Sundström, C.; Baecklund, E. Population-based study of patients with primary Sjögren's syndrome and lymphoma: Lymphoma subtypes, clinical characteristics, and gender differences. *Scand. J. Rheumatol.* **2020**, *49*, 225–232. [CrossRef] [PubMed]
27. Foo, M.Y.; Lee, W.P.; Seah, C.M.J.; Kam, C.; Tan, S.M. Primary breast lymphoma: A single-centre experience. *Cancer Rep. (Hoboken)* **2019**, *2*, e1140. [CrossRef] [PubMed]
28. Pérez, F.F.; Lavernia, J.; Aguiar-Bujanda, D.; Miramón, J.; Gumá, J.; Álvarez, R.; Gómez-Codina, J.; Arroyo, F.G.; Llanos, M.; Marin, M.; et al. Primary Breast Lymphoma: Analysis of 55 Cases of the Spanish Lymphoma Oncology Group. *Clin. Lymphoma Myeloma Leuk.* **2017**, *17*, 186–191. [CrossRef] [PubMed]
29. Avilés, A.; Delgado, S.; Nambo, M.J.; Neri, N.; Murillo, E.; Cleto, S. Primary breast lymphoma: Results of a controlled clinical trial. *Oncology* **2005**, *69*, 256–260. [CrossRef]
30. Shiboski, C.H.; Shiboski, S.C.; Seror, R.; Criswell, L.A.; Labetoulle, M.; Lietman, T.M.; Rasmussen, A.; Scofield, H.; Vitali, C.; Bowman, S.J.; et al. International Sjögren's Syndrome Criteria Working Group. 2016 American College of Rheumatology/European League Against Rheumatism classification criteria for primary Sjögren's syndrome: A consensus and data-driven methodology involving three international patient cohorts. *Ann. Rheum. Dis.* **2017**, *76*, 9–16. [CrossRef] [PubMed]

31. Zintzaras, E.; Voulgarelis, M.; Moutsopoulos, H.M. The risk of lymphoma development in autoimmune diseases: A meta-analysis. *Arch. Intern. Med.* **2005**, *165*, 2337–2344. [CrossRef]
32. Alsadi, A.; Lin, D.; Alnajar, H.; Brickman, A.; Martyn, C.; Gattuso, P. Hematologic Malignancies Discovered on Investigation of Breast Abnormalities. *South Med. J.* **2017**, *110*, 614–620. [CrossRef] [PubMed]
33. Lyou, C.Y.; Yang, S.K.; Choe, D.H.; Lee, B.H.; Kim, K.H. Mammographic and sonographic findings of primary breast lymphoma. *Clin. Imaging* **2007**, *31*, 234–238. [CrossRef] [PubMed]
34. Nicholas, S.; Richard, G.B. Sonoelastography of Breast Lymphoma. *Ultrasound Q.* **2016**, *32*, 208–211. [CrossRef]
35. Santra, A.; Kumar, R.; Reddy, R.; Halanaik, D.; Kumar, R.; Bal, C.S.; Malhotra, A. FDG PET-CT in the management of primary breast lymphoma. *Clin. Nucl. Med.* **2009**, *34*, 848–853. [CrossRef]
36. Hoang, J.T.; Yang, R.; Shah, Z.A.; Spigel, J.J.; Pippen, J.E. Clinico-radiologic features and management of hematological tumors in the breast: A case series. *Breast Cancer* **2019**, *26*, 244–248. [CrossRef] [PubMed]
37. Bilir, B.E.; Atile, N.S.; Bilir, B.; Guldiken, S.; Tuncbilek, N.; Puyan, F.O.; Sezer, A.; Coskun, I. A metabolic syndrome case presenting with lymphocytic mastitis. *Breast Care (Basel)* **2012**, *7*, 493–495. [CrossRef]
38. Chougule, A.; Bal, A.; Das, A.; Singh, G. IgG4 related sclerosing mastitis: Expanding the morphological spectrum of IgG4 related diseases. *Pathology* **2015**, *47*, 27–33. [CrossRef]
39. Boudova, L.; Kazakov, D.V.; Sima, R.; Vanecek, T.; Torlakovic, E.; Lamovec, J.; Kutzner, H.; Szepe, P.; Plank, L.; Bouda, J.; et al. Cutaneous lymphoid hyperplasia and other lymphoid infiltrates of the breast nipple: A retrospective clinicopathologic study of fifty-six patients. *Am. J. Dermatopathol.* **2005**, *27*, 375–386. [CrossRef]
40. De Vita, S.; Gandolfo, S. Predicting lymphoma development in patients with Sjögren's syndrome. *Expert Rev. Clin. Immunol.* **2019**, *15*, 929–938. [CrossRef]
41. Voulgarelis, M.; Skopouli, F.N. Clinical, immunologic, and molecular factors predicting lymphoma development in Sjogren's syndrome patients. *Clin. Rev. Allergy Immunol.* **2007**, *32*, 265–274. [CrossRef]
42. González López, A.; Del Riego, J.; Martín, A.; Rodríguez, A.; Javier Andreu, F.; Piernas, S.; Sentís, M. Bilateral MALT Lymphoma of the Breast. *Breast J.* **2017**, *23*, 471–473. [CrossRef] [PubMed]
43. Belfeki, N.; Bellefquih, S.; Bourgarit, A. Breast MALT lymphoma and AL amyloidosis complicating Sjögren's syndrome. *BMJ Case Rep.* **2019**, *12*, e227581. [CrossRef] [PubMed]
44. Kambouchner, M.; Godmer, P.; Guillevin, L.; Raphaël, M.; Droz, D.; Martin, A. Low grade marginal zone B cell lymphoma of the breast associated with localised amyloidosis and corpora amylacea in a woman with long standing primary Sjögren's syndrome. *J. Clin. Pathol.* **2003**, *56*, 74–77. [CrossRef] [PubMed]
45. King, R.L.; Goodlad, J.R.; Calaminici, M.; Dotlic, S.; Montes-Moreno, S.; Oschlies, I.; Ponzoni, M.; Traverse-Glehen, A.; Ott, G.; Ferry, J.A. Lymphomas arising in immune-privileged sites: Insights into biology, diagnosis, and pathogenesis. *Virchows Arch.* **2020**, *476*, 647–665. [CrossRef] [PubMed]

Publisher's Note: MDPI stays neutral with regard to jurisdictional claims in published maps and institutional affiliations.

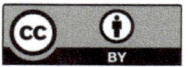

© 2020 by the authors. Licensee MDPI, Basel, Switzerland. This article is an open access article distributed under the terms and conditions of the Creative Commons Attribution (CC BY) license (http://creativecommons.org/licenses/by/4.0/).

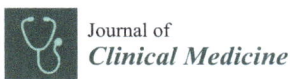

Article

Immortalization of Salivary Gland Epithelial Cells of Xerostomic Patients: Establishment and Characterization of Novel Cell Lines

Braxton D. Noll, Alexandre Grdzelishvili, Michael T. Brennan, Farah Bahrani Mougeot and Jean-Luc C. Mougeot *

Carolinas Medical Center-Atrium Health, Charlotte, NC 28203, USA; braxton.noll@atriumhealth.org (B.D.N.); alexandre.grdzelishvili@atriumhealth.org (A.G.); mike.brennan@atriumhealth.org (M.T.B.); farah.mougeot@atriumhealth.org (F.B.M.)
* Correspondence: jean-luc.mougeot@atriumhealth.org

Received: 30 September 2020; Accepted: 23 November 2020; Published: 25 November 2020

Abstract: Primary Sjögren's Syndrome (pSS) is an autoimmune disease mainly affecting salivary and lacrimal glands. Previous pSS studies have relied on primary cell culture models or cancer cell lines with limited relevance to the disease. Our objective was to generate and characterize immortalized salivary gland epithelial cells (iSGECs) derived from labial salivary gland (LSG) biopsies of pSS patients (focus score > 1) and non-Sjögren's Syndrome (nSS) xerostomic (i.e., sicca) female patients. To characterize iSGECs ($n = 3$), mRNA expression of specific epithelial and acinar cell markers was quantified by qRT-PCR. Protein expression of characterization markers was determined by immunocytochemistry and Western blot. Secretion of α-amylase by iSGECs was confirmed through colorimetric activity assay. Spheroid formation and associated alterations in expression markers were determined using matrigel-coated cell culture plates. Consistent mRNA and protein expressions of both epithelial and pro-acinar cell markers were observed in all three iSGEC lines. When cultured on matrigel medium, iSGECs formed spheroids, secreted α-amylase after β-adrenergic stimulation, and expressed multiple acinar cell markers at late passages. One iSGEC line retained adequate cell morphology without a loss of SV40Lt expression and proliferation potential after over 100 passages. In conclusion, our established iSGEC lines represent a viable model for salivary research due to their passaging capacity and maintenance of pro-acinar cell characteristics.

Keywords: Sjögren's syndrome; xerostomia; salivary gland; SGEC; immortalization; acinar; ductal; spheroid

1. Introduction

Development of restorative therapies for salivary gland dysfunction has been significantly hampered by a lack of accessible and pertinent cell culture models. Salivary glands are made of several cell types, including the saliva-producing acinar cells, ductal cells modifying the saliva as it travels through the lumen, and myoepithelial cells mediating acinus contraction. Acinar cells commonly fail to regenerate following high-dose radiation therapy, aging, or from autoimmune exocrinopathy such as primary Sjögren's syndrome (pSS) [1–3]. pSS is a chronic autoimmune disease characterized by a loss of salivary acinar cell function and a decline in acinar progenitor cell populations exacerbated by lymphocytic glandular infiltration.

Dysfunction of the salivary glands can lead to a reduction in salivary flow, thereby altering saliva composition, pH, and buffering capacity, causing the sensation of dry mouth (xerostomia) [2]. Cell culture models for pSS and xerostomia have been limited, leading researchers to rely on cancer cell lines or short-term cultures of primary salivary gland epithelial cells (SGECs) [4,5]. Moreover, the cell lines extensively used in salivary research (e.g., HSG, A253, NS-SV-AC) are of male origin [4,6–8]. These cell lines may not recapitulate the pathological processes occurring in pSS, a disease with a higher incidence in female patients [9].

Isolated SGECs have been shown to share ductal and pro-acinar characteristics and exhibit a moderate cell division capacity when grown in serum-free low-calcium media [5,10–13]. As with any primary cell culture model, their limited growth potential can impede reproducibility and applications including, but not limited to, high-throughput drug screening assays. In addition, pSS patient derived SGECs show a markedly reduced proliferation capacity in vitro [3]. The reduced growth capacity of pSS SGECs is mirrored in affected patients' salivary glands where narrowed pools of progenitor cells are found with markedly shortened telomeres [3]. Overall, suboptimal cell culture models combined with the reduced growth ability of pSS SGECs have proven to be major obstacles in salivary research.

Diagnosis of pSS may require a labial salivary gland (LSG) biopsy for histologic analysis of lymphocytic aggregates within the tissue [14]. LSG biopsy tissue is a common explant source for culturing SGECs, but due to limited availability based on clinical access, their potential as a universal model is restricted. Culture of SGECs is typically performed using a dual media approach, where the initial explant medium contains 2.5% fetal bovine serum and is replaced with a second serum-free media to sustain passaging and growth [5,11]. Minor differences in culture conditions, including FBS concentration and time spent in explant medium can have a profound effect on salisphere (i.e., 3D spheroid) formation and passage number, as previously shown for parotid gland progenitor cells isolated from mice [15].

Primary SGEC cultures are comprised of cells with pro-acinar and/or ductal cell-like features depending on the growth substrate, presence of serum in medium, and the specificity of characterization markers used [5,10–13]. The previous work of Fujita-Yoshigaki et al. demonstrated the dedifferentiation of primary parotid acinar cells occurs in culture, which could explain the variety of ductal and acinar cell features expressed [16,17]. In addition, Jang et al. revealed that primary SGECs (known as phmSG) of ductal origin exhibited trans-epithelial resistance, expressed several acinar and epithelial cell markers (i.e., AQP5, SLC12A2, AMY1A), and secreted α-amylase upon β-adrenergic stimulation [5]. Overall, SGECs represent a suitable cell culture model to investigate salivary gland dysfunction in vitro but lack the unlimited growth potential needed for widespread use.

To our knowledge no reliable immortalized human primary SGEC lines derived from female patient's LSG biopsies have been developed or made readily available to researchers. To address this gap, the objective of our study was to generate an in vitro cell culture model for the investigation of the pathophysiology of salivary gland disorders. Using an SV40 Large-T (SV40Lt) lentiviral vector, we generated and characterized immortalized SGECs isolated from LSG biopsies of pSS and xerostomic (sicca) patients. The SV40Lt antigen subunit inhibits both cell cycle regulators, pRB and p53, and prevent telomere shortening-induced cell senescence in some cell types [18,19]. We characterized immortalized SGECs (iSGEC) lines from two non-Sjögren's syndrome (nSS) female patients (referred to as iSGEC-nSS1 and iSGEC-nSS2) and one pSS (referred to as iSGEC-pSS1) female patient, based on the expression of pro-acinar and epithelial cell markers using various molecular methods. iSGECs were grown on matrigel-coated plates to determine three-dimensional (3D) spheroid forming ability, along with the extent to which spheroids recapitulated acinus characteristics, such as differentiated myoepithelial and acinar cells.

2. Materials and Methods

2.1. Culture of Salivary Gland Cell Lines (SGCLs) and HeLa Cells

Salivary gland cell lines, HSG and HSY, and HeLa cells were cultured in DMEM supplemented with 10% FBS (VWR, Radnor, PA, USA) (37 °C; 5% CO_2). A253 cells were cultured according to the provider's (ATCC, Manassas, VA, USA) recommendations [20]. HMC-3A cells were cultured according to the providers' recommendations [21]. Salivary gland cell lines (SGCLs) (HSG, HSY, A253, and HMC-3A) and HeLa cells were grown in T-75 tissue culture-treated flasks (Corning Life Sciences, Tewksbury, MA, USA) until 80–90% confluency. For experiments, SGCLs and HeLa cells were re-plated using 0.25% trypsin +0.053 mM EDTA (Corning Life Sciences, Tewksbury, MA, USA).

2.2. LSG Biopsies and Culture of Salivary Gland Epithelial Cells (SGECs)

Atrium Health institutional review board (Charlotte, NC, USA) approval (IRB Protocol #: 08-16-24E) was granted for this study and all patients gave informed consent.

Anti-Ro (SSA) serum-negative (-) xerostomic patients undergoing a LSG biopsy for the assessment of pSS according to the 2016 ACR/EULAR classification criteria were asked to participate in this study [6]. Xerostomic nSS and pSS patient clinical characteristics are listed in Table 1. Remaining LSG biopsy tissue was transported to the research laboratory in complete SGEC explant medium supplemented with 5x antibiotic/antimycotic solution (Gibco, Thermo Fisher Scientific, Waltham, MA, USA).

Table 1. Patient demographics and clinical features.

Demographics	iSGEC-pSS1	iSGEC-nSS1	iSGEC-nSS2
Age	70	57	47
Gender	Female	Female	Female
Race	C	C	C
Clinical Features	pSS	nSS	nSS
Focus Score	1.8	0.3	0.16
Anti-Ro (SSA)	(−)	(−)	(−)
Unstim. Salivary Flow (<1.5 mL/15 min)	0.66	0.66	0.06 *
Stimulated Salivary Flow (mL/min)	11.7	8.91	1.02 *
Schirmer's (+/−)	NA	NA	(−)
DMARDs	(−)	(−)	(−)

Labial salivary gland biopsies used in this study were collected from one pSS and two sicca patients (nSS). All patients were negative (−) for serum Anti-Ro (SSA) and were not taking disease-modifying anti-rheumatic drugs (DMARDs). * The patient with the lowest focus score had the lowest salivary flow rates (unstimulated/stimulated). NA: Schirmer's test was not performed due to patient objection or information not listed in electronic medical records.

SGEC cultures were established according to the methods outlined by Jang et al. and are briefly explained as follows [3]. LSG tissue was minced into 0.5–1 mm^2 fragments and placed in T-75 flask with 3.5 mL of complete SGEC explant medium supplemented with 1x antibiotic/antimycotic solution (Gibco, Thermo Fisher Scientific, Waltham, MA, USA) and grown (37 °C, 5% CO_2). Complete SGEC explant medium consisted of 1:3 Ham's F12 and DMEM supplemented with 2.5% FBS (VWR, Radnor, PA, USA), 20 μg/mL EGF (Gibco, Thermo Fisher Scientific, Waltham, MA, USA), 200 μg/mL insulin (MP Biomedicals, Santa Ana, CA, USA), 100 ng/mL hydrocortisone (Sigma-Aldrich, Saint Louis, MO, USA), and 1x antibiotic/antimycotic solution (Gibco, Thermo Fisher Scientific, Waltham, MA, USA). After 72 h, 5 mL of SGEC explant media was added. Cells at 80–90% confluency were split 1:3 into T-75 flasks with 0.05% trypsin +0.045 mM EDTA. Trypsin was neutralized by soybean trypsin inhibitor (Gibco, Thermo Fisher Scientific, Waltham, MA, USA) at a 1:1 ratio (v/v). For remaining passages, SGEC sub-culturing medium was used. SGEC sub-culturing medium consisted of Epi-life Basal^{TM} medium (0.06 mM Ca^{2+}) (Gibco, Thermo Fisher Scientific, Waltham, MA, USA, Catalogue# MEPI500CA) supplemented with 1x human keratinocyte growth supplement (HKGS) (Gibco, Thermo Fisher Scientific, Waltham, MA, USA, Catalogue# S0015). Fibroblasts were gradually removed from culture using a combination of 0.02% EDTA or 0.01% trypsin.

2.3. Transduction of SGECs by Lentiviral SV40Lt Particles

During passage number 2 (p-2), SGECs were spit into 6-well (VWR, Radnor, PA, USA) tissue culture-treated plates at a confluency of 60–70% and allowed to adhere for 24 h. Cell medium was removed and replaced with 1 mL SV40Lt lentiviral supernatant (ABMgood, Richmond, Canada, Catalogue# G258) diluted with 1 mL of SGEC sub-culturing medium (2 mL total) and polybrene

(Sigma-Aldrich, Saint Louis, MO, USA) at a final concentration of 4 μg/mL. After 48 h, SV40Lt lentiviral cell medium was replaced with SGEC sub-culturing medium and grown for 24 h. Medium was removed and cells were supplied with 1 mL SV40 lentiviral supernatant diluted with 1 mL of SGEC sub-culturing media (2 mL total) and polybrene at a final concentration of 4 μg/mL, for 48 h.

SV40Lt lentiviral cell medium was removed and replaced with SGEC sub-culturing medium and cells were grown to 80–90% confluency before being split into 6-well tissue culture-treated plates at a ratio of 1:6. For cell passages after SV40Lt lentiviral transfection, cells were split 1:6 up to passage 10. The remaining passages were split at 1:3 using T-75 (Corning Life Sciences, Tewksbury, MA, USA) tissue culture-treated flasks. To determine increased expression of pro-acinar markers in high Ca^{2+} supplemented medium, all iSGECs at early passage 14 (p-14) and only iSGEC-nSS2 at passage 80 (p-80) were subjected to 1.2 mM Ca^{2+} in SGEC medium for 72 h prior to experimentation [3].

2.4. RNA Extraction and cDNA Synthesis

RNA was extracted from iSGECs, SGCLs, and Hela cells in 6-well plates using the RNAeasy kit (Qiagen, Valencia, CA, USA) according to the manufacturer's protocol. RNA was quantified using a Nanodrop 1000 (Thermo Fisher Scientific, Waltham, MA, USA). A total of 500 ng RNA from each sample was used per cDNA synthesis reaction. cDNA synthesis was carried out using the SmartScribe reverse transcription kit (Takara Bio, Mountain View, CA, USA) with random hexamers (20 μg) (Promega, Madison, WI, USA) and dNTPs (10 mM final) (Promega, Madison, WI, USA) according to the manufacturer's protocol. After synthesis, the cDNA was diluted to a final volume of 200 μL.

2.5. Matrigel Induced 3D Spheroid Cultures

Matrigel (Corning Life Sciences, Tewksbury, MA, USA) diluted in 1.2 mM Ca^{2+} SGEC sub-culturing medium (2 mg/mL final concentration) was solidified in 8-well Nunc™ Lab-Tek™ II Chamber Slides™ (Thermo Fisher Scientific, Waltham, MA, USA) or 12-well tissue culture-treated plates (VWR, Radnor, PA, USA) and incubated for 1 h at 37 °C. Cells were seeded at 3×10^5 or 1×10^6 per well, respectively. Cell cultures on matrigel-coated plates were grown at 37 °C and 5% CO_2 for up to 7 days.

2.6. Real-Time Quantitative and Semi-Quantitative Polymerase Chain Reaction

All qRT-PCR and semi-qRT-PCR reactions were performed using a BioRad C1000 Touch Thermal Cycler (Biorad, Hercules, CA, USA) in 96-well qPCR plates. All qRT-PCR reactions were carried out in triplicate wells per plate using three separate plates and average cycle threshold (Ct) values were used for quantification. Relative expression was calculated applying the ΔCt method for iSGECs, SGCLs, and Hela cells normalized to the expression of GAPDH. Per well, 10 μL of RT2 SYBR Green Fast Master Mix (Qiagen, Valencia, CA, USA) was added to 2 μL of cDNA, 1 μL of forward and reverse primers (10 mM) (IDT, Newark, NJ, USA) and 7 μL of nuclease-free water. Primers are listed in Supplementary Table S1 along with their respective target for cell expression characterization purposes.

Semi-qRT-PCR was employed to detect the expression of the SV40Lt transcript at multiple passage numbers (Supplementary Figure S1). Products from semi-qRT-PCR reactions were run on a 1% agarose TAE gel alongside a 1 kb DNA ladder (New England Biolabs, Ipswich, MA, USA) for 35 min and visualized using a gel doc system (GE Healthcare Life Sciences, Chicago, IL, USA).

2.7. Expression of ZO-1, AQP5, and α-Amylase by Western Blot

iSGECs and SGCLs were plated at 80% confluency in 6-well tissue culture-treated plates and allowed to adhere for 48 h prior to experimentation. To generate whole-cell lysates, medium was removed from cells and the wells washed 3 times with DPBS. Protein was harvested from cells using M-PER buffer (Pierce, Thermo Fisher Scientific, Waltham, MA, USA) and briefly sonicated before centrifugation at $15,000 \times g$ for 10 min. The resulting insoluble pellet was discarded, and the supernatant was used for Western blotting of ZO-1, AQP5, and vinculin.

For the determination of α-amylase secretion, iSGECs were grown in SGEC sub-culturing media without HKGS for 24 h and then replaced with complete SGEC sub-culturing media supplemented with 10μM epinephrine (MP Biomedicals, Santa Ana, CA, USA). After 45 min, the cell culture media were harvested and centrifuged (4 °C, 1000× g) for 10 min to remove whole cells. The media were then spun in Millipore concentrator tubes with a 10 kDa size exclusion limit (Millipore, Burlington, MA, USA) for 30 min and an appropriate amount of 6x reducing Lameli buffer (Roche, Basel, Switzerland) added to the resulting concentrated supernatant. iSGECs adhered to the tissue culture plate were lysed and harvested using M-PER buffer. Protein samples in M-PER were briefly sonicated and centrifuged at 15,000× g for 10 min and the pellet discarded.

Samples were measured by Bradford assay (Pierce, Thermo Fisher Scientific, Waltham, MA, USA) and equal amounts of protein were loaded into each lane and subjected to electrophoresis on a 7–14% gradient pre-cast SDS–PAGE gel (Biorad, Hercules, CA, USA). Proteins were transferred onto nitrocellulose membranes (GE Healthcare Life Sciences, Chicago, IL, USA) and blotted (12 h, 4 °C) with selected antibodies at listed concentrations (Supplementary Table S2) followed by incubation (room temperature, 1 h) with HRP-conjugated anti-mouse secondary (Cell signaling Technology, Danvers, MA, USA).

Membranes were washed (3 times, 5 min) and developed using Super Signal West pico Chemiluminescent substrate kit (Pierce, Thermo Fisher Scientific, Waltham, MA, USA). Western blots were photographed using an ImageQuant LAS4000 (GE Healthcare Life Sciences, Chicago, IL, USA) system. Densitometry was performed using Image Studio V.5.2 software (LI-COR, Lincoln, NE, USA) and protein levels were normalized to vinculin in their corresponding whole-cell lysate.

2.8. β-. Adrenergic Stimulation and Measurement of α-Amylase Activity in Supernatant

iSGECs were plated at a density of 4×10^5 cells in either uncoated (2D) or coated (matrigel) tissue culture plates. Cells were grown in SGEC sub-culturing medium supplemented with 1.2 mM Ca^{2+} for 72 h or 5 days prior to experimentation. At the times indicated, medium supplemented with 10 μM epinephrine (MP Biomedicals, Santa Ana, CA, USA) was added. After 45 min, cell culture medium was collected and subjected to the colorimetric amylase activity assay (Biovision, Milpitas, CA, USA) as per the manufacturer's protocol.

2.9. Immunocytochemistry (ICC)

iSGECs and SGCLs were plated onto Coating Matrix (2D) (Gibco, Thermo Fisher Scientific, Waltham, MA, USA,) covered 8-well Nunc™ Lab-Tek™ II Chamber Slides™ (Thermo Fisher Scientific, Waltham, MA, USA). Antibodies and concentrations are listed in Supplementary Table S2. Cells were grown for 48–72 h, then fixed with ice-cold methanol (−20 °C, 10 min) and incubated with the following antibodies directed against them: KRT8, KRT18, KRT19, AQP5, ZO-1, α-SMA, Vimentin, and E-cadherin proteins. Cells were also fixed with 4% paraformaldehyde (room temperature, 15 min) to stain Ki-67 and α-amylase. Fixed cells were permeabilized with 0.25% Triton X-100 in TBS (room temperature, 10 min).

Cells were fixed then washed (3x) in TBS and incubated (room temperature, 5 min) in 3% H_2O_2 (v/v) TBS to block endogenous peroxidases. Next, cells were incubated in blocking buffer consisting of 1% BSA (w/v), 2% skim-milk (w/v), and 0.1% Tween-20 in TBS (room temperature, 1 h). Primary antibodies were diluted in TBS with 0.1% Tween-20 and 1% BSA. The fixed cells were incubated with the primary antibody (4 °C, 12 h) (Supplementary Table S2). Cells were washed with TBS (3 times, 5 min each) and incubated with anti-mouse secondary antibodies at different concentrations (Supplementary Table S2) and diluted in TBS with 0.1% Tween-20 (room temperature, 1–2 h). After incubation, cells were washed with TBS (3X).

Monolayer culture-fixed cells were incubated in diaminobenzidine (DAB) (Pierce, Thermo Fisher Scientific, Waltham, MA, USA) 1x solution (2–7 min). DAB was washed away using TBS to stop the reaction and the cells were counterstained with Gills II hematoxylin (Richard-Allan Scientific,

Kalamazoo, MI, USA) (diluted 1:5 *v/v* DPBS) for 30 s to highlight nuclei. Slides without primary antibody served as negative controls.

For immunocytochemistry (ICC)–immunofluorescence (IF) visualization of 3D spheroid cultures grown on matrigel, cells were fixed using 4% paraformaldehyde (room temperature, 25 min) and permeabilized with 0.25% triton X-100 in TBS (room temperature, 10 min). The same blocking and incubation procedure previously outlined was followed except 4′,6-diamidino-2-phenylindole (DAPI) (Abcam, Cambridge, UK) was used to highlight DNA. Slides without primary antibody served as negative controls.

Slides were observed using an Olympus BX51 fluorescence microscope (Shinjuku City, Tokyo, Japan) and photographed with an Olympus DP70 (Shinjuku City, Tokyo, Japan) mounted camera. Cells in culture plates were viewed by phase contrast on an Olympus IX-71 inverted fluorescence microscope and photographed using an Olympus DP70 mounted camera. Proliferation scores were determined based on Ki-67 protein detection, a nuclear protein expressed during several cell cycle phases (G1/S/G2/M), which is frequently employed as an indicator of actively proliferating cells [22]. Proliferation scores (%) were generated by selection of three random images for nuclei counting using Fiji-ImageJ software [23]. The total number of cell nuclei was divided by the total number of Ki-67 (+) nuclei and averaged among three images.

3. Data Analysis and Statistics

Data are presented as the mean +/−standard error of the mean (SEM) from a minimum of three separate experiments. Significant results were calculated using Student's *t*-test on GraphPad Prism 8 (San Diego, CA, USA). P-values were determined to be significant using the Holm–Šidák post hoc test for multiple comparisons with alpha = 0.05.

4. Results

4.1. Primary Isolation, Culture, and Growth of iSGECs

LSG biopsy fragments remained in SGEC explant medium for approximately 7–14 days to ensure sufficient cell outgrowth. Once the cells reached approximately 70–80% confluency, the culture medium was replaced with SGEC sub-culturing medium. Transitioning to the serum-free low calcium (0.06 mM) medium for 3–5 days prior to trypsinization reduced fibroblast contamination in later passages. Before SV40Lt transduction in all three cell lines, two separate populations of cells were observed and consisted of either larger cells with complex cytoplasm or smaller cells with reduced cytoplasm. The smaller cells were predominant during later passages in all three iSGEC lines. At late passages iSGEC-pSS1 gave rise to colonies appearing that were mixed in size, with polygonal or cobblestone-like cells with differing rates of cytoplasmic complexity (Figure 1A). iSGEC-nSS1 late passages demonstrated a mix of small polygonal and filiform-appearing cells (Figure 1B). Mixed morphology of iSGECs most likely indicates an inhomogeneous population (Table 2) (Figure 1A–D). Therefore, we selected iSGEC-nSS2 for late-passage outgrowth and in-depth characterization over iSGEC-pSS1 and -nSS1. Long term passaged iSGEC-nSS2 exhibited a stable, small cobblestone type of morphology and did not give rise to filiform-appearing cells (Figure 1C,D). iSGEC-nSS2 cultured in 1.2 mM Ca^{2+} acquired more complex appearing cytoplasm with granulations and formed tight clusters at both early and late passages (Figure 1E,F).

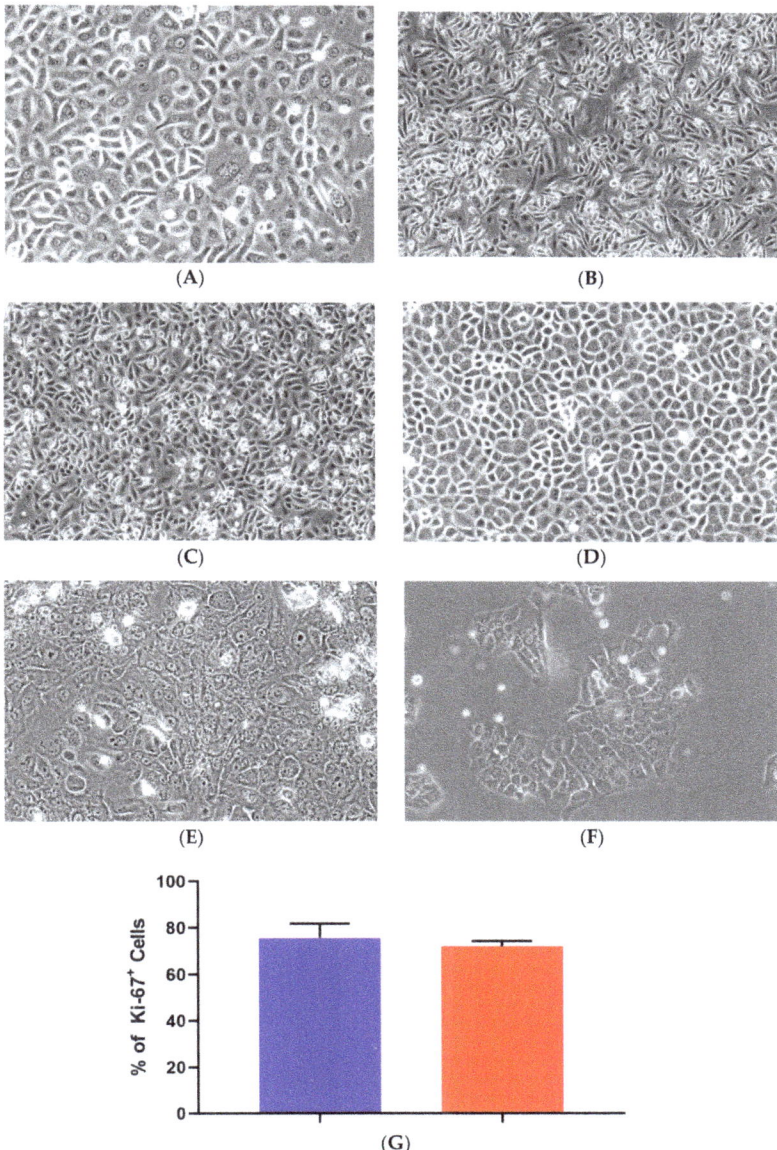

Figure 1. Morphology and proliferation of iSGECs. **Legend.** Representative images of early passage (p-14) monolayer culture (**A**) iSGEC-pSS1 (**B**) iSGEC-nSS1 (**C**) iSGEC-nSS2 and (**D**) late (p-80) iSGEC-nSS2. iSGEC-nSS2 "cobblestone-like" morphology was maintained across multiple passages when grown in SGEC sub-culturing media with low (0.06 mM) Ca^{2+}. Cell morphology changes in (**E**) iSGEC-nSS2 p-14 and (**F**) iSGEC-nSS2 p-80 are observed when medium is supplemented with 1.2 mM Ca^{2+} (final concentration) for 72 h. (**G**) Proliferation of iSGEC-nSS2 was assessed by the percentage (%) of Ki-67$^+$ cells using immunocytochemistry. No significant difference in the percentage of Ki-67$^+$ cells was detected between early (p-14) and late (p-80) iSGEC-nSS2 cultures. Student's t-test (* $p < 0.05$, NS = not significant). Data are means +/− SEM. Magnification ×20, scale bar = 200 μm.

Table 2. Immortalized salivary gland epithelial cells (iSGECs), salivary gland cell lines (SGCLs), and HeLa protein expression of characterization markers by immunocytochemistry (ICC).

Protein Target Cell Line	KRT8	K18	K19	ZO-1	E-Cadherin	AQP5	Vimentin	α-Amylase	α-SMA
iSGEC-pSS1	+	+	+	+	+	+	+	+	(−/+)
iSGEC-nSS1	+	+	+	(−/+)	+	+	+	+	(−/+)
iSGEC-nSS2	+	+	+	+	+	+	+	+	(−)
A253	+	+	+	(−/+)	+	(−/+)	+	+	+
HMC-3A	+	+	+	(−/+)	+	+	+	+	+
HSY	+	+	+	(−/+)	+	(−/+)	+	+	+
HSG	+	+	+	(−/+)	+	(−/+)	+	+	+
HeLa	+	+	+	(−/+)	(−)	(−/+)	+	(−/+)	+

Results of protein expression of characterization markers in iSGECs, SGCLs, and HeLa cells by ICC are shown. Cells were grown on type-1 collagen-coated coverslips for up to 72 h prior fixation. iSGECs were additionally plated on coverslips and grow in SGEC sub-culturing media supplemented with 1.2mM Ca^{2+} to determine changes in acinar cell marker expression. (+) indicates positive expression of protein. (+/−) indicates low or diffuse expression of protein. (−) indicates no protein expression was detected by methods outlined.

During later passages (iSGEC-nSS2, p-80), colony formations that were different in their overall shape arose from single-cell clonal outgrowths (Supplementary Figure S2A). However, these single-cell outgrowth populations quickly became incorporated into other colonies and were unremarkable at lower confluency.

Proliferation rates of iSGEC-nSS2 did not substantially waver across early (p-14) and late (p-80) passages, as indicated by Ki-67 staining percentage (Figure 1G). No decrease in the % of Ki-67 (+) cells was observed at later passages. Spheroid formation on matrigel was observed after 24 h in all three cell lines (Figure 2, Supplementary Figure S2B–G). iSGEC-nSS2 retained its spheroid formation ability into late passages (>p-80), which could be observed after 24 h of plating. At three days in matrigel, spheroids measured roughly ~75–200 μm in all iSGECs.

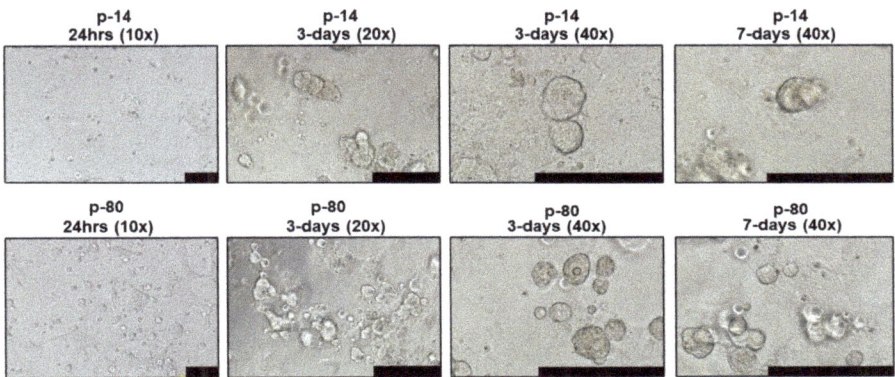

Figure 2. iSGEC-nSS2 early (p-14) and late (p-80) spheroid formation on matrigel. **Legend.** Cells were initially seeded at 4×10^4 per well. Cultures began to form spheroids at 24 h on matrigel (2 mg/mL). Early passages (e.g., p-14) formed larger, but overall fewer spheroids when assessed after 3 days. Spheroids appeared to reach their final size after 3–4 days. Scale bars represent 200 μm.

4.2. Characterization of iSGECs by qRT-PCR

mRNA expression of epithelial and acinar markers was determined by qRT-PCR in iSGECs, SGCLs, and Hela cells. Expression of epithelial and acinar cell markers showed slight deviation among all three iSGECs when grown as a monolayer culture (Figure 3A,B). Compared to SGCLs and Hela, A253 and HMC-3A showed the greatest similarity to iSGEC cultures. Mucoepidermoid carcinomas have been shown to exhibit increased expression of AQP5 and among all cell lines analyzed, HMC-3A expressed AQP5 highest (Figure 3A) [24].

The two consistently over-expressed pro-acinar genes by iSGEC-nSS2 were ANO1 and SLC12A2, compared to both iSGEC-pSS1 and -nSS1 (Figure 3A). We did not observe a difference in the pro-acinar expression of AMY1A, AQP5, STIM1, and STIM2 when comparing iSGEC-nSS2 to both iSGEC-pSS1 and -nSS1.

iSGEC-nSS1 exhibited the highest expression of both VIM and CST3, and the lowest expression of KRT19 (a ductal/epithelial cell maker of salivary glands) among iSGECs, indicating a heterologous mesenchymal phenotype (Figure 3B) [5,25]. KRT5 is a marker for progenitor and basal ductal cells of the salivary gland [26,27]. In agreement with the work by Jang et al. on primary SGECs, KRT5 was the gene with highest expression in iSGECs by qRT-PCR among the characterization markers, which did not differ significantly among all three iSGEC lines [5]. HSG, HSY, and HeLa cells expressed most transcripts consistently at the same level and exhibited a mesenchymal expression pattern reflected by iSGEC-nSS1 with low CDH1 and high VIM expression [25].

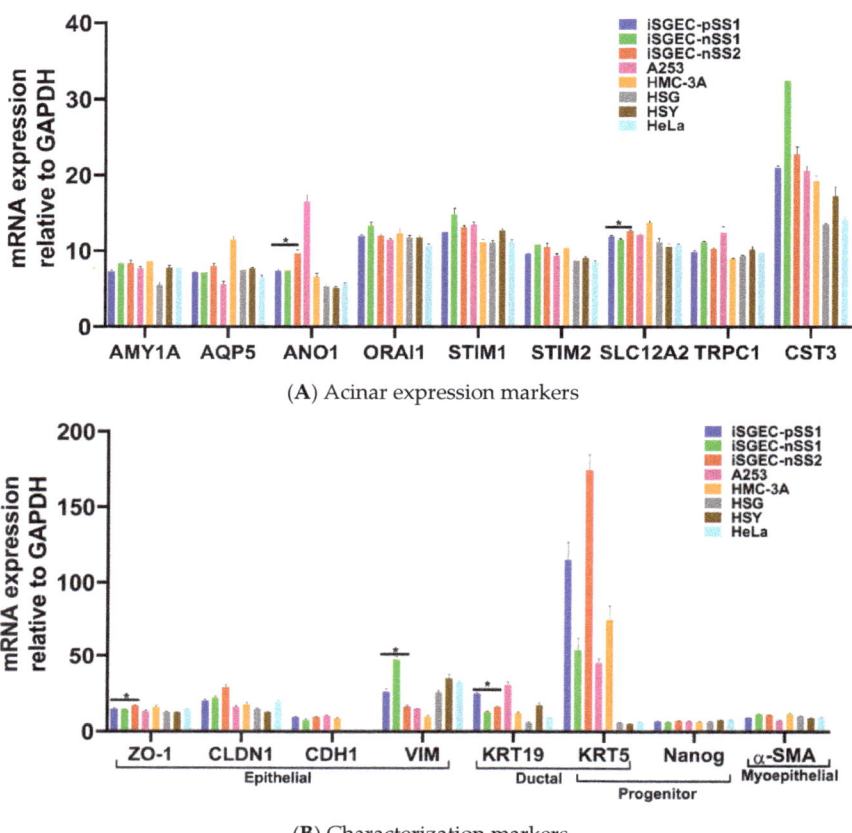

Figure 3. mRNA expression of acinar and characterization markers in monolayer cultured iSGECs, SGCLs, and HeLa cells by qRT-PCR. **Legend.** (**A**) Pro-acinar markers were highly expressed in all iSGECs. ANO1 and SLC12A2 were expressed highest in iSGEC-nSS2 compared to other iSGECs. (**B**) Characterization markers for epithelial, ductal, progenitor, and myoepithelial expression in all cell lines examined. The epithelial marker ZO-1 is an integral component of tight junctions and was overexpressed, whereas Vimentin (VIM) was under-expressed in iSGEC-nSS2. KRT-19, a ductal cell marker, was differentially expressed in iSGECs. * Indicates significant difference in expression determined by Student's t-test (alpha = 0.05) and corrected using the Holm–Šidák method. Error bars represent mean +/− SEM.

4.3. Changes in mRNA Expression among Early and Late Passage iSGECs by qRT-PCR

Expression of acinar and other characterization markers was assessed over early and late passages. iSGEC-pSS1 was the most stable cell line where only AMY1A and CST3 expression increased in later passages. Both iSGEC-nSS1 and -nSS2 exhibited pro-acinar changes in expression profiles at later passages where most markers increased (Figure 4A). In iSGEC-nSS1 p-45, pro-acinar markers (AMY1A, AQP5, ANO1, SLC12A2, CST3, and TRPC1) increased in expression compared to early (p-14) cultures (Figure 4A). iSGEC-nSS2 at p-80 expressed AMY1A, ORAI1, STIM1, SLC12A2, CST3, and TRPC1 higher, and only one marker lower (ANO1) compared to p-14. Both AQP5 and STIM2 were stably expressed during extended passaging in iSGEC-nSS2. Overall, AMY1A and CST3 increased during late passages of all three iSGECs lines, which could be important for maintaining pro-acinar characteristics.

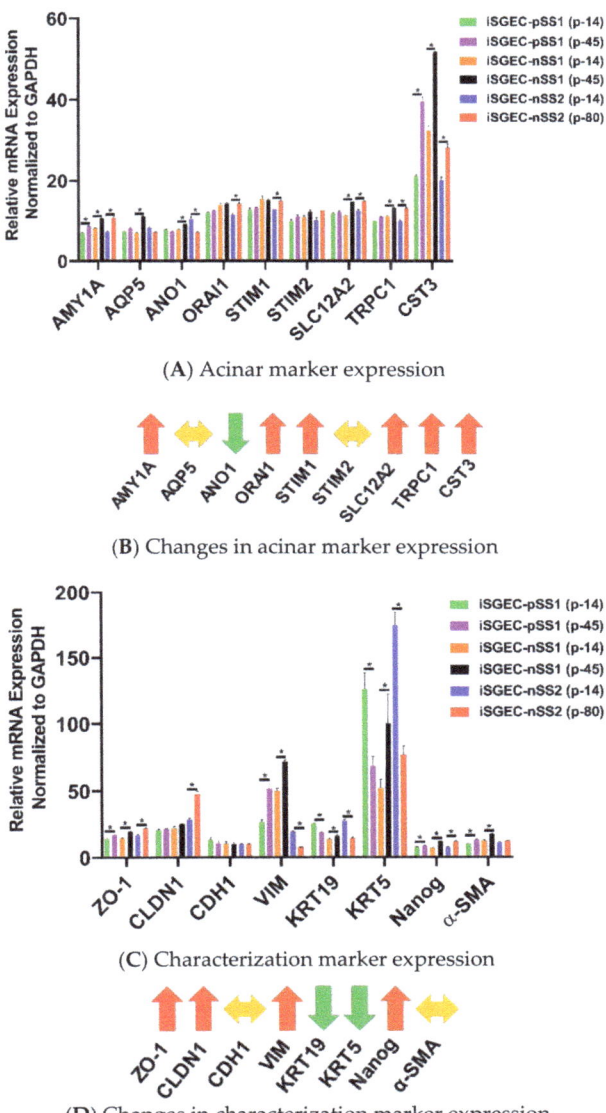

Figure 4. Changes in mRNA expression of early and late passaged iSGECs by qRT-PCR. **Legend.** mRNA expression of acinar (**A**) and characterization markers (**C**) in monolayer cultures of early and late passaged iSGECs by qRT-PCR (ΔCT). iSGECs increased in AMY1A (**A**), ZO-1 (**C**), and Nanog (**C**) in later passages. Changes in gene expression of iSGEC-nSS2 early (p-14) and late (p-80) are indicated with arrows: increased (**red**), decreased (**green**), and no change (**yellow**). (**B,D**) iSGEC-nSS2 differentially expressed several acinar and characterization markers in later passages. Significance of differences between the means was determined by Student's t-test and p-values corrected using the Holm–Šidák multiple comparisons post hoc test (alpha = 0.05). Error bars represent mean +/− SEM. * $p < 0.05$.

Characterization markers were the most differentially expressed and exhibited the greatest changes in late passaged iSGECs. Epithelial marker CDH1 was the only stably expressed gene among all characterization markers, whereas ZO-1 increased in late passages of all three iSGECs (Figure 4C,D). iSGEC-nSS2 maintained an epithelial expression pattern, including a decrease in the mesenchymal marker VIM and a significant increase in CLDN1 expression. Over passages, both KRT5 and KRT19 decreased in expression and the progenitor cell marker NANOG increased and could indicate a shift towards a less-differentiated cell population in iSGEC-nSS2.

4.4. Effects of Ca^{2+} on iSGECs mRNA Expression

Calcium concentrations in media affect SGEC expression of pro-acinar genes, including AQP5, ORAI1, STIM1 and STIM2 [5,28]. Jang et al. demonstrated an increase in the activity of the store-operated Ca^{2+} entry (SOCE) system that upregulates AQP5 expression through the nuclear factor of activated T-cells 1 (NFAT1) [28]. To evaluate changes produced by an increase in Ca^{2+}, we cultured iSGECs in 1.2 mM Ca^{2+} for three days and then assessed mRNA expression by qRT-PCR. Early iSGEC-nSS2 cultures (p-14) did not exhibit any alterations in expression of acinar markers when cultured in 1.2 mM Ca^{2+} (Figure 5A,B). Late iSGEC-nSS2 (p-80) cells supplemented with 1.2 mM Ca^{2+} demonstrated an increase in AQP5 and ANO1 mRNA expression and decreases in other acinar markers (AMY1A, ORAI1, STIM1, SLC12A2, TRPC1) (Figure 5A,B). Moreover, a change in ductal characterization marker KRT19 was decreased in p-14 iSGEC-nSS2 cells cultured in 1.2 mM Ca^{2+} (Figure 5C,D). Late (p-80) iSGEC-nSS2 responded differently via an increased expression of tight junction component ZO-1 and myoepithelial marker α-SMA. The lack of response to 1.2 mM Ca^{2+} in iSGC-nSS2 p14 cells reiterates the possibility of a de-differentiated cell population seen in Figure 4A,B, where p-80 demonstrated a response to increased Ca^{2+} that was more similar to other SGEC publications [5,28].

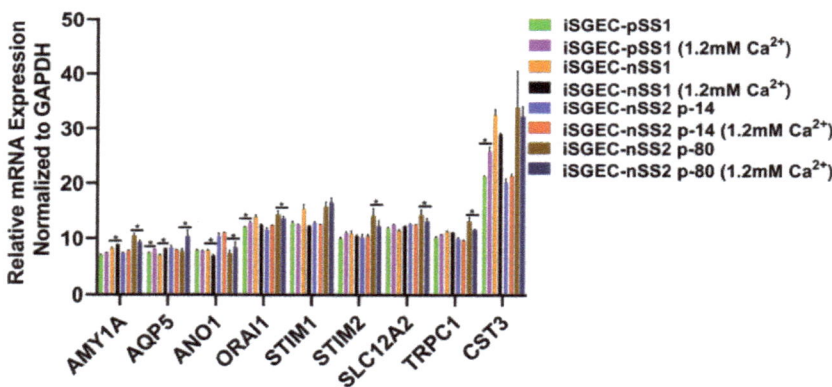

(**A**) Acinar marker expression

Figure 5. *Cont.*

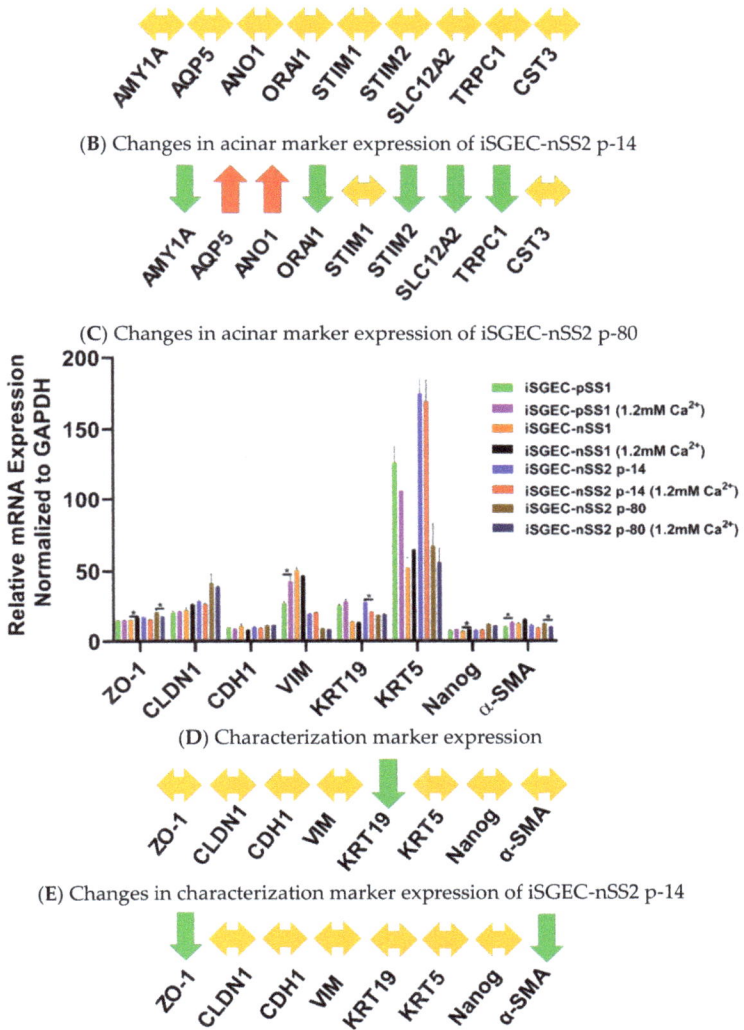

(B) Changes in acinar marker expression of iSGEC-nSS2 p-14

(C) Changes in acinar marker expression of iSGEC-nSS2 p-80

(D) Characterization marker expression

(E) Changes in characterization marker expression of iSGEC-nSS2 p-14

(F) Changes in characterization marker expression of iSGEC-nSS2 p-80

Figure 5. Changes in mRNA expression mediated by 1.2 mM Ca^{2+}. **Legend.** Changes in acinar (**A–C**) and characterization markers (**D–F**) gene expression in iSGECs when cultured in 1.2 mM Ca^{2+} for 72 h. Changes in gene expression of iSGEC-nSS2 are indicated with arrows: increased (**red**), decreased (**green**), and no change (**yellow**). (**B**) iSGEC-nSS2 p-14 did not display changes in expression whereas late passaged (p-80) exhibited increases in acinar markers AQP5 and ANO1. AMY1A, ORAI1, STIM2, SLC12A2, and TRPC1 expression decreased in 1.2 mM Ca^{2+} p-80 cells. (**C**) Overall, characterization markers exhibited little change in 1.2 mM Ca^{2+} supplemented medium. (**D**) Ductal cell marker (KRT19) decreased in early passage (p-14) iSGEC-nSS2 to levels similar in late (p-80) cells. Conversely, ZO-1 and α-SMA expression decreased in later passaged (p-80) iSGECs with 1.2 mM Ca^{2+} and did not change in early (p-14) cells. Results calculated by Student's *t*-test and *p*-values corrected by the Holm-Šídák multiple comparisons post hoc test (* $p < 0.05$). Error bars represent mean +/− SEM.

4.5. Characterization of iSGECs by ICC and Western Blot

4.5.1. ICC and Western Blot of iSGECs in Monolayer Culture

The cytokeratins KRT8, KRT18, and KRT19 are cytoplasmic proteins expressed in the salivary gland epithelium and are characterization markers for ductal and acinar cells [29,30]. We first characterized iSGECs by KRT8/18/19 protein expression and found iSGEC-nSS1 expressed all three epithelial markers more intensely and uniformly than iSGEC-pSS1 and -nSS2 (Table 2, Supplementary Figure S3). KRT19 protein localized within cells containing a larger cytoplasm and were dispersed throughout iSGEC-nSS2 cultures, whereas smaller cells demonstrated a low expression or a lack thereof (Supplementary Figure S3). KRT18 was the most uniform and ubiquitously expressed cytokeratin among iSGECs, whereas KRT8 exhibited focal protein expression in iSGEC-nSS2 (Supplementary Figure S3). Heterogenous expression of KRT19 and KRT8 could indicate multiple stages of differentiation among cells [26]. Overall, the expression of KRT8, KRT18, and KRT19 indicates these cell lines to be of ductal origin and reflects other long-term cultures of SGECs in both mice and humans [5,30,31].

Acinar cell markers, AQP5 and AMY1A, were expressed in all three iSGECs, and highest in both iSGEC-pSS1 and -nSS2. Within these cultures, cells in close contact expressed the highest levels of AQP5, unlike AMY1A where intercellular contact or proximity to other cells did not appear to have an influence. We observed an increase in AQP5 protein expression in both p-14 and p-80 iSGEC-nSS2 cultures when supplemented with 1.2 mM Ca^{2+}. Increased AQP5 protein was determined by ICC and replicated by Western blot using whole-cell lysates (Supplementary Figure S3, Figure 6A). ZO-1 expression was low in all iSGECs when accessed by ICC and confirmed by Western blot in whole-cell lysates. iSGEC-nSS1 exhibited the lowest expression of ZO-1 and CDH-1 and higher expression of VIM in monolayer culture, which reiterates the observed mesenchymal phenotype [25].

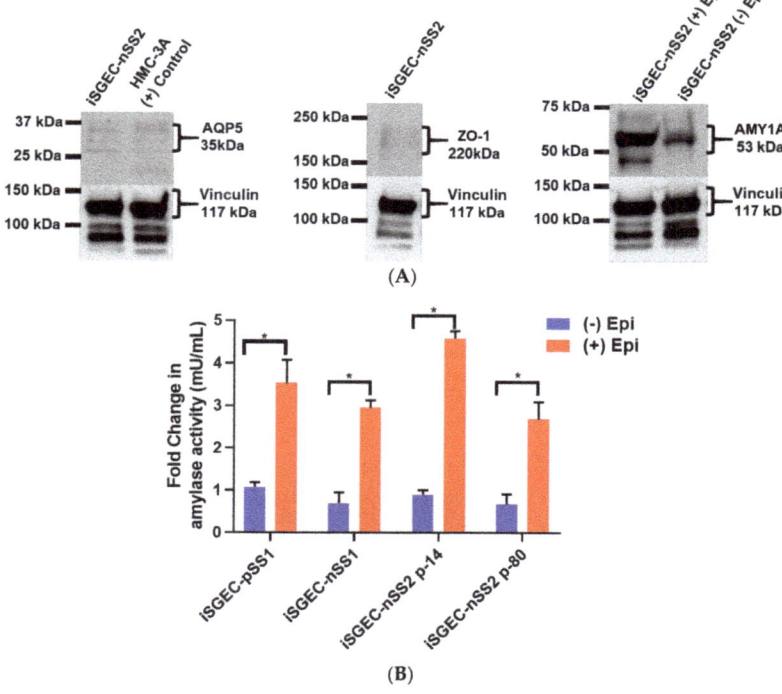

Figure 6. *Cont.*

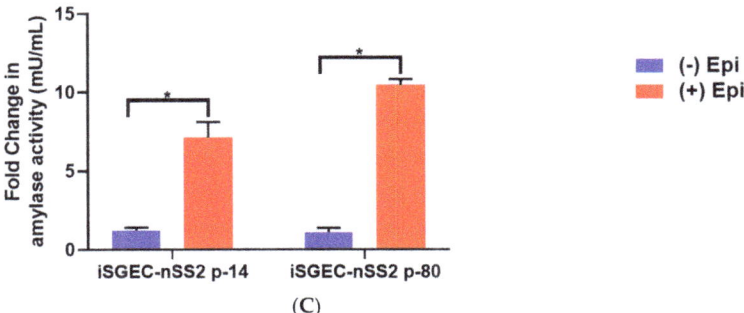

(C)

Figure 6. Protein expression of acinar and epithelial cell markers by Western blot in iSGEC-nSS2. **Legend.** (**A**) Protein expression of acinar (AQP5) (**left**) and epithelial (ZO-1) (**middle**) markers in whole-cell lysate of monolayer cultured iSGEC-nSS2. (**left**) Expression of AQP5 in iSGEC-nSS2 whole-cell lysate compared to HMC-3A, which was used as a (+) control for AQP5 in Western blots. (**right**) After stimulation with 10 µM epinephrine for 45 min ((+) Epi) cell culture supernatant was replaced, and cells were grown for 72 h before media were collected and concentrated. Cells without stimulation by media supplementation with 10µM epinephrine ((−) Epi) served as the control. Secreted α-amylase was detected in both stimulated ((+) Epi) and unstimulated ((−) Epi) cultures. 10µM epinephrine stimulated ((+) Epi) iSGEC-nSS2 cultures exhibited higher levels of α-amylase in cell culture supernatant than unstimulated cultures after 72 h. Western blots were normalized to vinculin expression in whole-cell lysate of their respective sample. (**B**,**C**) Media were harvested after stimulation with 10µM epinephrine for 45 min and amylase activity measured by colorimetric assay. (**B**) Supernatant of monolayer cultured iSGECs treated with 10µM ((+) Epi) had significantly higher α-amylase activity compared to untreated cells ((−) Epi). (**C**) Comparison of early (p-14) and late (p-80) passaged iSGEC-nSS2 secretion of α-amylase into media when cultured on matrigel. Results are listed as fold-change over the untreated control. Significance of differences between means was determined by Student's t-test and p-values corrected using the Holm–Šidák multiple comparisons test (alpha = 0.05). Error bars represent mean +/− SEM. * $p < 0.05$.

In the case of iSGEC-nSS2, α-SMA was not detected in either p-14 or p-80 monolayer cultures as compared to iSGEC-pSS1 and -nSS1, where it was expressed at very low levels (Supplementary Figure S3). Pringle et al. demonstrated low α-SMA expression in cultured salivary gland stem cells (SGSCs) likely originating from intercalated and striated ductal cells, which could explain these results [3]. Vimentin is a marker for mesenchymal cells within the salivary glands [32,33]. Vimentin was expressed sporadically in iSGEC-nSS2 monolayer culture and could indicate a small population of mesenchymal cells or epithelial cells reverting to a mesenchymal-like state within cultures (Supplementary Figure S3).

In all three iSGEC lines, α-amylase was secreted into the cell culture medium after β-adrenergic stimulation by epinephrine (Figure 6B). Additionally, iSGEC-nSS2 early (p-14) and late passages (p-80) secreted α-amylase into cell culture media with and without β-adrenergic stimulation (Figure 6B). iSGECs-nSS2 p-80 secrete α-amylase, demonstrating retention of pro-acinar cell characteristics after significant cellular expansion. Moreover, iSGEC-nSS2 cells cultured on matrigel formed spheroid structures and secreted α-amylase in response to 10 mM epinephrine stimulation (Figure 6C). An overall increase in α-amylase secretion when compared to unstimulated cells was observed in iSGEC-nSS2 and could indicate a stricter regulation of secretion within the differentiated cells.

4.5.2. 3D-Matrigel Spheroid Culture

Matrigel contains a mixture of basement membrane and extracellular matrix proteins, which have been shown to promote SGEC and salivary gland stem cell (SGSC) differentiation [3,11,34,35]. SGECs plated on matrigel form spheroids resembling a basic acinus structure, composed of differentiated acinar and ductal cells [3,34,35]. iSGECs began to form spheroids within 24 h of plating on matrigel (2 mg/mL) and were cultured for a total seven days. ICC–IF protein expression analysis of iSGEC-nSS2 spheroid cultures showed high localization of acinar and epithelial cell markers ZO-1, AQP5, and AMY1A within acinus-like spheroid structures (Figure 7). Cytokeratins KRT8, KRT18, and KRT19 were all expressed in iSGEC-nSS2 cultured on matrigel (Figure 7). We observed greater levels of KRT8 expression within interior cells of spheroids similar to previously described high expression in luminal cells [36]. At a matrigel concentration of 2 mg/mL, some cells formed monolayer sheets across the matrigel that expressed KRT18 and KRT19 at high levels (Figure 7). α-SMA protein expression was localized to myoepithelial-like cells located on the spheroid exteriors.

mRNA expression analysis by qRT-PCR of iSGEC-nSS2 matrigel cultures demonstrated an increase in pro-acinar cell expression of AQP5 compared to monolayer cultures (Figure 8A,C). Spheroids from late passaged iSGEC-nSS2 expressed AMY1A and AQP5 at levels higher than early (p-14) cultures while expressing ANO1 at significantly lower (Figure 8D). Most characterization markers in iSGEC-nSS2 (p-14 and p-80) cultured on matrigel were differentially expressed (Figure 8E–G). Two consistent differentially expressed genes were VIM and KRT19, where VIM increased in matrigel cultures and KRT19 decreased. Similar to monolayer cultures on plastic, p-80 expressed NANOG at higher and KRT19 at lower levels, indicating a potential dedifferentiation when cultured for extended periods. However, p-80 exhibited the same increase in AQP5 mRNA expression as p-14 iSGEC-nSS2 cells on matrigel, retaining their ability to differentiate.

5. Discussion

This is the first study to establish immortalized primary cultures of xerostomic female patients using LSG biopsy tissue. We generated three novel composite iSGEC lines, with one capable of growing over 100 passages and maintaining expression of characterization markers.

Characterization of iSGEC-nSS2 indicates these cells to be of an undifferentiated ductal cell origin due to their high mRNA expression of KRT5 and relatively spotty distribution of KRT19 protein by ICC during monolayer culture on plastic [37,38]. When grown on matrigel, expression of KRT19 protein appeared more uniform over cells spread across the dish as a monolayer and is a marker expressed in both acinar and ductal cells [29,39]. Although a low concentration of 2 mg/mL was used for the entirety of this study, we tested whether higher at concentrations of matrigel, those monolayer cells would remain. At a concentration of (4.5 mg/mL) those monolayer cells fully incorporated into spheroid structures.

Isolated acinar cells undergo dedifferentiation into ductal-like cells when explanted into cell culture plates [17]. Dedifferentiation of rat acinar cells can be halted by the inhibition of Src and p-38 pathways, allowing the cells to retain high cytoplasm complexity and size in culture [17]. Understanding the interactions between ductal and acinar cells within the salivary gland epithelium could provide more insight into acinar cell regeneration and population maintenance. Additionally, SGECs have demonstrated the ability to trans-differentiate into acinar-like cells in matrigel cultures [10,40]. Pathways regulating trans-differentiation would likely provide viable therapeutic targets, for example, with small-molecule inhibitors, bypassing the need for stem-cell implantation [41]. iSGEC-nSS2 spheroids resembled acinus-like structures with cells high in AQP5 expression and exterior surrounding myoepithelial-like cells expressing α-SMA (Figure 7). Changes in protein expression exemplified by a lack of α-SMA in iSGEC-nSS2 monolayer cultures and high expression in matrigel indicate cell differentiation during spheroid formation.

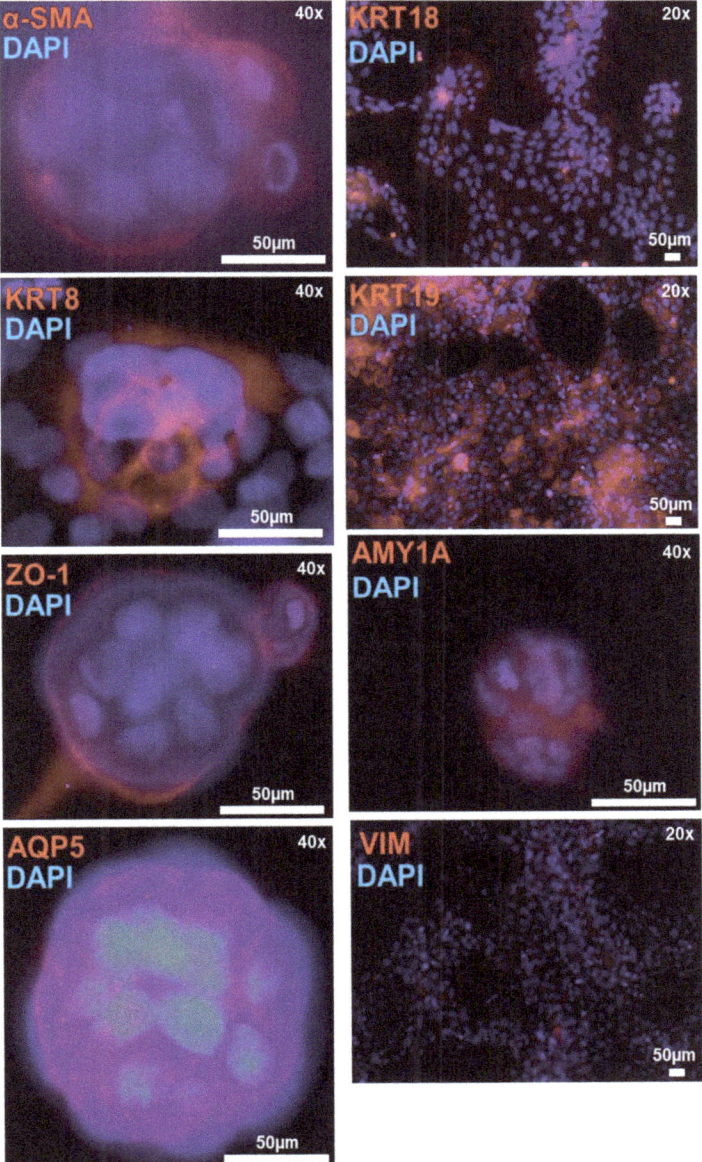

Figure 7. Immunofluorescence detection of salivary epithelium markers in matrigel cultured iSGEC-nSS2 cells. **Legend.** Detection of salivary epithelium markers (**red**) by immunofluorescence in matrigel cultures of iSGEC-nSS2 p-80 after 7 days. Spheroids expressed acinar cell markers (AQP5, AMY1A), tight-junction protein (ZO-1), and had clearly defined myoepithelial cells (α-SMA). Cells growing on the surface of the matrigel and spheroids expressed salivary epithelial markers KRT8, KRT18, and KRT19 proteins. Vimentin was expressed low and sparsely among cells and did not indicate regular staining patters. Scale bar represents 50 µm. DNA (**blue**) is highlighted with DAPI.

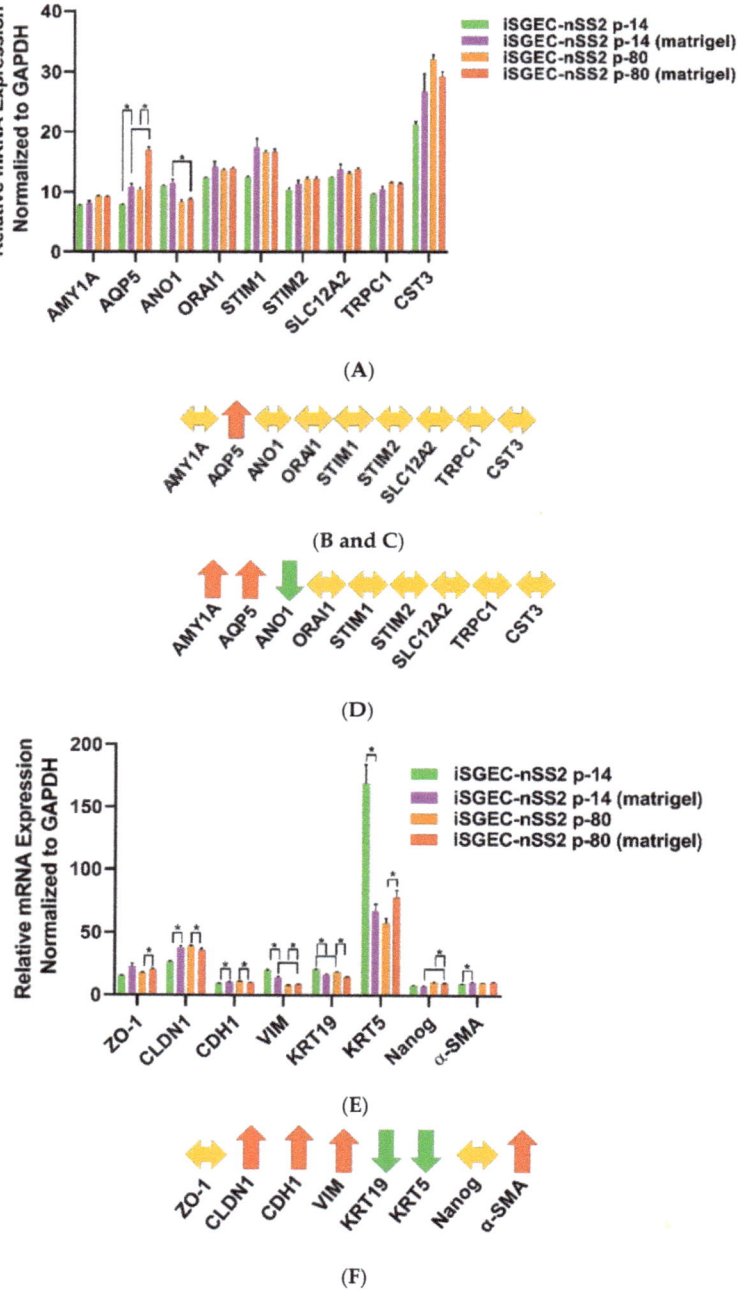

Figure 8. Cont.

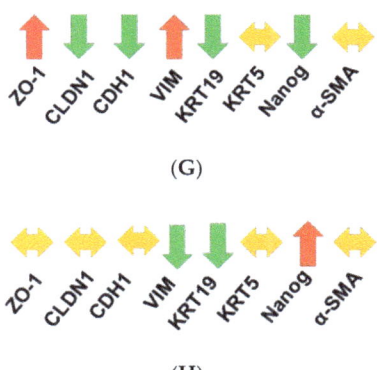

(G)

(H)

Figure 8. Changes in mRNA expression of early (p-14) and late (p-80) iSGEC-nSS2 cultures grown on matrigel. **Legend.** mRNA expression of early (p-14) and late (p-80) passaged iSGEC-nSS2 grown on either uncoated (monolayer) or matrigel coated plates by qRT-PCR (ΔCT). Changes in gene expression are indicated with arrows: increased (**red**), decreased (**green**), and no change (**yellow**). (**A–C**) AQP5 expression was the only acinar cell marker to increase in both p-14 (**B**) and p-80 (**C**) when cultured on matrigel (final: 2mg/mL) coated plates. In p-80 cells, matrigel had a greater effect on AQP5 expression compared to p-14. (**D**) Over extended passages, iSGEC-nSS2 expressed both AQP5 and AMY1A higher, whereas ANO1 decreased in expression over time. (**E–H**) The mRNAs of characterization markers CLDN1, CDH1, VIM, and KRT19 were differentially expressed in both p-14 and p-80 cultures, respectively, when grown as a monolayer or matrigel coated plates. (**F–G**) Only the ductal cell marker, KRT19, was consistently downregulated by matrigel. (**F–G**) Vimentin (VIM) can be an indicator of dedifferentiation in SGECs and was increased (**red**) in both p-14 and p-80 matrigel cultures. Results calculated by Student's *t*-test and *p*-values corrected by the Holm-Šídák multiple comparisons test (* $p < 0.05$). Error bars represent mean +/− SEM.

The KRT5 transcript was found highly expressed in our iSGEC cultures similar to non-transformed SGECs, which is in agreement with reported protein expression by progenitor and ductal basal cells within the salivary gland epithelium [5]. Under normal homeostatic conditions, KRT5-positive cells give rise to intercalated and striated ductal populations [42]. However, during radiation-induced salivary gland injury KRT5-expressing ductal cells are capable of differentiation into acinar cells [42]. KRT5-positive ductal cells demonstrate higher robustness than acinar cells to radiation induced salivary gland damage and represent a favorable target in restoring acinar cell populations within damaged salivary glands [38]. Importantly, SV40Lt immortalization has been shown to not affect the differentiation potential of immortalized progenitor cells [43]. iSGEC-nSS2 could be a suitable model for understanding the cellular factors associated with trans-differentiation potential due to their high KRT5 mRNA expression.

Early (p-14) and late (p-80) passaged iSGEC-nSS2 cells expressed AQP5 at higher levels in spheroid cultures (Figure 8B,C), possibly indicating a greater extent of differentiation and therefore displaying increased heterogeneity. However, the expression of characterization marker KRT19 decreased while VIM expression increased in iSGEC-nSS2 cells cultured on matrigel. Higher VIM expression may indicate an increase in stemness properties by dedifferentiation, along with reduced KRT19 expression (differentiated ductal cell marker), which could also indicate an increase in stemness [26,44]. Similarly, changes in VIM and KRT19 expression were observed in long term 2D cultured (p-80) cells (Figure 4D). Overall, dedifferentiation of iSGEC-nSS2 cells in both 2D and 3D cultures is likely associated with their high growth and differentiation potentials when cultured on matrigel. Last, iSGEC-nSS2 could offer an in vitro alternative for salivary gland developmental research due to its dedifferentiation properties.

Direct introduction of an AQP1 expressing AAV vector into salivary glands demonstrated favorable clinical trial results where participants experienced a subjective decrease in xerostomia symptoms [45]. Although the original rationale behind AQP1 AAV therapy was to increase water permeability in ductal cells, it was later found that acinar cells were responsible for the expression of AQP1 and saliva secretion [46]. As previously stated, KRT5 protein expressing ductal progenitor cells are more abundant and can differentiate into acinar cells after injury [38]. Spheroid cultures obtained via iSGEC-nSS2 differentiation could serve as a suitable model to investigate how KRT5-positive progenitor cells possibly contribute to the generation of AQP1-expressing acinar after salivary gland damage and AQP1 AAV therapy.

6. Limitations

SGECs express AQP5 mRNA and protein under established culturing conditions, although being commonly identified of ductal origin [5,12]. Moreover, a spontaneously immortalized mouse cell line expressing mixed ductal and myoepithelial protein markers when cultured as a monolayer showed mRNA expression of acinar markers in monolayer and 3D culture [40]. Markers of differentiated ductal cells include KRT8 and KRT19 among others [26]. The lack of uniform expression by either KRT8 and KRT19 in monolayer cultures of iSGEC-nSS2 indicates a potential progenitor cell population, which is capable of differentiation into acinar-like and ductal-like cells when cultured on matrigel. Following culture on matrigel, iSGEC-nSS2 cells could be replated onto plastic tissue culture plates and further grown, thereby potentially expanding the differentiated cell populations for further analysis. To determine the extent of differentiation among acinar-like cells, immunocytochemistry targeting the terminally differentiated acinar cell marker, MIST1, should be employed. Moreover, dual staining of acinar and differentiated ductal cell markers to better identify and characterize the iSGEC-nSS2 cell line could be required to determine the extent of heterogeneity within the monolayer cultured cells.

Further research is needed to analyze the presence of tight junctions and their location throughout the apical portion of the plasma membrane, an important feature for polarized secretion by acinar cells [47]. Previous studies have demonstrated trans-epithelial resistance and polarized secretion of α-amylase within monolayer SGEC cultures [5]. Among the several cell mechanisms dictating epithelial polarization and directional secretion, tight junction formation is a critical factor [47]. Techniques better visualizing the location of tight junctions within iSGEC-nSS2 spheroids should be employed to better determine the extent of polarization and direction secretion of the high AQP5-expressing acinar cells. Furthermore, ZO-1 was expressed at low levels in monolayer iSGEC cultures indicated by immunocytochemistry and its presence confirmed by Western blot. Spheroids were uncut during the immunocytochemistry procedure, which could have impacted the interior binding of the ZO-1 antibody or the visualization of the 3D architecture.

When salivary glands are damaged, acinar cells revert to a ductal-like state in mouse models [48]. Similar to the phenomenon observed in mice, rat acinar cells when extracted and cultured on plastic revert to a ductal like state, which can be reversed by inhibition of p-38 and/or Src pathways [16,17]. Due to the outlined characteristics of iSGEC-nSS2, populations of differentiated acinar–ductal cells and ductal–progenitor cells could be present. Overall expression of AQP5 protein within iSGEC-nSS2 monolayer cultures localized within the plasma membrane and cytoplasm. Confirmation of AQP5 protein was further demonstrated by Western blot and exhibited a level of protein expression comparable to HMC-3A, which expressed AQP5 mRNA highest among all cell lines tested. When transitioned to culture on matrigel, AQP5 protein expression appeared to increase substantially within spheroid formations by ICC–IF. The increase in AQP5 expression among cells in matrigel culture could be a result of either de-differentiated acinar cell populations or progenitor-like cell populations (KRT5-positive) further differentiating into acinar cells. Before iSGEC-nSS2 use in developing therapies for increasing AQP5 expressing cells within the salivary gland, further cell sorting would need to be employed to ensure a homogenous cell population to the extent possible for reproducibility in drug assays.

In addition, age, gender, and associated hormonal changes account for possible factors affecting expression profiles of iSGECs, impacting their biological properties. Moreover, acinar cells of lacrimal glands, acinar progenitor cells of salivary glands, and saliva DNA of pSS patients may have shortened telomeres, which could be more prominent with older age [3,49,50]. Extensive cell passaging due to age combined with chronically shortened telomeres could lead to chromosomal instability and changes in DNA expression. Short Tandem Repeat (STR) profiling would be useful in the future to determine the extent of chromosome stability when passaged for extended periods and to establish a unique identifier for iSGEC-nSS2.

Although spheroids were formed by iSGEC-nSS2 in both early and late cultured cells, lumen formation needs to be further visualized, which could be useful in determining the extent of differentiation and cell types present. Furthermore, a panel of cell lines derived from different types of xerostomic patients (i.e., nSS "sicca" or radiation-induced) may be needed to develop effective treatments.

7. Conclusions

The iSGECs generated in our study represent a preliminary model system for the development of therapies targeting salivary gland dysfunction. We have demonstrated that iSGEC-nSS2 cells derived from a sicca female patient retained the ability to form spheroids with differentiated cell types at late passages (p-80) and exhibited a significant proliferation capacity (>100 passages) when cultured as a monolayer. Overall, iSGECs could be used as an alternative to currently available cell culture models in salivary gland research.

Supplementary Materials: The following are available online at http://www.mdpi.com/2077-0383/9/12/3820/s1, Supplementary Table S1: RT-PCR primers; Supplementary Table S2: Antibodies and dilutions used in ICC and Western blots; Supplementary Figure S1: Semi-qRT-PCR analysis of SV40Lt expression in late-passaged iSGECs; Supplementary Figure S2A: Phase contrast images of iSGEC-nSS2 p-80 single-cell colonies; Supplementary Figure S2B–G: Phase contrast images of iSGEC-pSS1 and iSGEC-nSS1 spheroids; Supplementary Figure S3: expression of characterization markers in iSGEC-nSS2 cells by ICC.

Author Contributions: Experimentation, B.D.N., A.G.; conceptualization, B.D.N., J.-L.C.M., F.B.M., M.T.B.; manuscript preparation B.D.N., J.-L.C.M., F.B.M.; data analysis B.D.N., J.-L.C.M., F.B.M. All authors read and approved the final submitted version of this manuscript.

Funding: N/A. This work was supported by Atrium Health-Carolinas Healthcare Research Fund.

Acknowledgments: Salivary gland cell lines HSG and HSY were a generous gift from Bruce Baum (NIDCR, NIH). HMC-3A cells were a generous gift from Jacques E. Nör (University of Michigan School of Dentistry, Ann Arbor, MI, USA). We would like to thank our clinical research staff, Jenene Noll and Cathleen Peterson, for their help with patient recruitment, the collection of clinical data, and the collection and transport of LSG biopsy samples to the lab.

Conflicts of Interest: The authors declare no conflict of interest.

References

1. Guchelaar, H.J.; Vermes, A.; Meerwaldt, J.H. Radiation-induced xerostomia: Pathophysiology, clinical course and supportive treatment. *Support. Care Cancer Off. J. Multinatl. Assoc. Support. Care Cancer* **1997**, *5*, 281–288. [CrossRef] [PubMed]
2. Baum, B.J.; Ship, J.A.; Wu, A.J. Salivary gland function and aging: A model for studying the interaction of aging and systemic disease. *Crit. Rev. Oral Biol. Med. Off. Publ. Am. Assoc. Oral Biol.* **1992**, *4*, 53–64. [CrossRef] [PubMed]
3. Pringle, S.; Wang, X.; Verstappen, G.; Terpstra, J.H.; Zhang, C.K.; He, A.; Patel, V.; Jones, R.E.; Baird, D.M.; Spijkervet, F.K.L.; et al. Salivary Gland Stem Cells Age Prematurely in Primary Sjogren's Syndrome. *Arthritis Rheumatol.* **2019**, *71*, 133–142. [CrossRef] [PubMed]
4. Lin, L.C.; Elkashty, O.; Ramamoorthi, M.; Trinh, N.; Liu, Y.; Sunavala-Dossabhoy, G.; Pranzatelli, T.; Michael, D.G.; Chivasso, C.; Perret, J.; et al. Cross-contamination of the human salivary gland HSG cell line with HeLa cells: A STR analysis study. *Oral Dis.* **2018**, *24*, 1477–1483. [CrossRef]

5. Jang, S.I.; Ong, H.L.; Gallo, A.; Liu, X.; Illei, G.; Alevizos, I. Establishment of functional acinar-like cultures from human salivary glands. *J. Dent. Res.* **2015**, *94*, 304–311. [CrossRef]
6. Azuma, M.; Tamatani, T.; Kasai, Y.; Sato, M. Immortalization of normal human salivary gland cells with duct-, myoepithelial-, acinar-, or squamous phenotype by transfection with SV40 ori-mutant deoxyribonucleic acid. *Lab. Investig. J. Tech. Methods Pathol.* **1993**, *69*, 24–42.
7. Shirasuna, K.; Sato, M.; Miyazaki, T. A neoplastic epithelial duct cell line established from an irradiated human salivary gland. *Cancer* **1981**, *48*, 745–752. [CrossRef]
8. Giard, D.J.; Aaronson, S.A.; Todaro, G.J.; Arnstein, P.; Kersey, J.H.; Dosik, H.; Parks, W.P. In Vitro Cultivation of Human Tumors: Establishment of Cell Lines Derived From a Series of Solid Tumors2. *J. Natl. Cancer Inst.* **1973**, *51*, 1417–1423. [CrossRef]
9. Patel, R.; Shahane, A. The epidemiology of Sjögren's syndrome. *Clin. Epidemiol.* **2014**, *6*, 247–255. [CrossRef]
10. Nam, H.; Kim, J.-H.; Hwang, J.-Y.; Kim, G.-H.; Kim, J.-W.; Jang, M.; Lee, J.-H.; Park, K.; Lee, G. Characterization of Primary Epithelial Cells Derived from Human Salivary Gland Contributing to in vivo Formation of Acini-like Structures. *Mol. Cells* **2018**, *41*, 515–522. [CrossRef]
11. Dimitriou, I.D.; Kapsogeorgou, E.K.; Abu-Helu, R.F.; Moutsopoulos, H.M.; Manoussakis, M.N. Establishment of a convenient system for the long-term culture and study of non-neoplastic human salivary gland epithelial cells. *Eur. J. Oral Sci.* **2002**, *110*, 21–30. [CrossRef] [PubMed]
12. Kawanami, T.; Sawaki, T.; Sakai, T.; Miki, M.; Iwao, H.; Nakajima, A.; Nakamura, T.; Sato, T.; Fujita, Y.; Tanaka, M.; et al. Skewed production of IL-6 and TGFβ by cultured salivary gland epithelial cells from patients with Sjögren's syndrome. *PLoS ONE* **2012**, *7*, e45689. [CrossRef] [PubMed]
13. Ittah, M.; Miceli-Richard, C.; Gottenberg, J.E.; Lavie, F.; Lazure, T.; Ba, N.; Sellam, J.; Lepajolec, C.; Mariette, X. B cell-activating factor of the tumor necrosis factor family (BAFF) is expressed under stimulation by interferon in salivary gland epithelial cells in primary Sjögren's syndrome. *Arthritis Res.* **2006**, *8*, R51. [CrossRef] [PubMed]
14. Shiboski, C.H.; Shiboski, S.C.; Seror, R.; Criswell, L.A.; Labetoulle, M.; Lietman, T.M.; Rasmussen, A.; Scofield, H.; Vitali, C.; Bowman, S.J.; et al. 2016 American College of Rheumatology/European League Against Rheumatism Classification Criteria for Primary Sjogren's Syndrome: A Consensus and Data-Driven Methodology Involving Three International Patient Cohorts. *Arthritis Rheumatol.* **2017**, *69*, 35–45. [CrossRef]
15. Nguyen, V.T.; Dawson, P.; Zhang, Q.; Harris, Z.; Limesand, K.H. Administration of growth factors promotes salisphere formation from irradiated parotid salivary glands. *PLoS ONE* **2018**, *13*, e0193942. [CrossRef]
16. Fujita-Yoshigaki, J. Plasticity in Differentiation of Salivary Glands: The Signaling Pathway That Induces Dedifferentiation of Parotid Acinar Cells. *J. Oral Biosci.* **2010**, *52*, 65–71. [CrossRef]
17. Fujita-Yoshigaki, J.; Matsuki-Fukushima, M.; Sugiya, H. Inhibition of Src and p38 MAP kinases suppresses the change of claudin expression induced on dedifferentiation of primary cultured parotid acinar cells. *Am. J. Physiol. Cell Physiol.* **2008**, *294*, C774–C785. [CrossRef]
18. Ahuja, D.; Sáenz-Robles, M.T.; Pipas, J.M. SV40 large T antigen targets multiple cellular pathways to elicit cellular transformation. *Oncogene* **2005**, *24*, 7729–7745. [CrossRef]
19. Satyanarayana, A.; Greenberg, R.A.; Schaetzlein, S.; Buer, J.; Masutomi, K.; Hahn, W.C.; Zimmermann, S.; Martens, U.; Manns, M.P.; Rudolph, K.L. Mitogen stimulation cooperates with telomere shortening to activate DNA damage responses and senescence signaling. *Mol. Cell. Biol.* **2004**, *24*, 5459–5474. [CrossRef]
20. ATCC. A-253 (ATCC®HTB-41™). Available online: https://www.atcc.org/Global/Products/D/9/3/3/HTB-41.aspx (accessed on 24 November 2020).
21. Warner, K.A.; Adams, A.; Bernardi, L.; Nor, C.; Finkel, K.A.; Zhang, Z.; McLean, S.A.; Helman, J.; Wolf, G.T.; Divi, V.; et al. Characterization of tumorigenic cell lines from the recurrence and lymph node metastasis of a human salivary mucoepidermoid carcinoma. *Oral Oncol.* **2013**, *49*, 1059–1066. [CrossRef]
22. Bruno, S.; Darzynkiewicz, Z. Cell cycle dependent expression and stability of the nuclear protein detected by Ki-67 antibody in HL-60 cells. *Cell Prolif.* **1992**, *25*, 31–40. [CrossRef] [PubMed]
23. Schindelin, J.; Arganda-Carreras, I.; Frise, E.; Kaynig, V.; Longair, M.; Pietzsch, T.; Preibisch, S.; Rueden, C.; Saalfeld, S.; Schmid, B.; et al. Fiji: An open-source platform for biological-image analysis. *Nat. Methods* **2012**, *9*, 676–682. [CrossRef] [PubMed]
24. D'Agostino, C.; Elkashty, O.A.; Chivasso, C.; Perret, J.; Tran, S.D.; Delporte, C. Insight into Salivary Gland Aquaporins. *Cells* **2020**, *9*, 1547. [CrossRef] [PubMed]

25. Sisto, M.; Tamma, R.; Ribatti, D.; Lisi, S. IL-6 Contributes to the TGF-β1-Mediated Epithelial to Mesenchymal Transition in Human Salivary Gland Epithelial Cells. *Arch. Immunol. Ther. Exp.* **2020**, *68*, 27. [CrossRef]
26. May, A.J.; Cruz-Pacheco, N.; Emmerson, E.; Gaylord, E.A.; Seidel, K.; Nathan, S.; Muench, M.O.; Klein, O.D.; Knox, S.M. Diverse progenitor cells preserve salivary gland ductal architecture after radiation-induced damage. *Development* **2018**, *145*, dev166363. [CrossRef] [PubMed]
27. Kwak, M.; Ninche, N.; Klein, S.; Saur, D.; Ghazizadeh, S. c-Kit+ Cells in Adult Salivary Glands do not Function as Tissue Stem Cells. *Sci. Rep.* **2018**, *8*, 14193. [CrossRef] [PubMed]
28. Jang, S.I.; Ong, H.L.; Liu, X.; Alevizos, I.; Ambudkar, I.S. Up-regulation of Store-operated Ca^{2+} Entry and Nuclear Factor of Activated T Cells Promote the Acinar Phenotype of the Primary Human Salivary Gland Cells. *J. Biol. Chem.* **2016**, *291*, 8709–8720. [CrossRef]
29. Pringle, S.; Wang, X.; Bootsma, H.; Spijkervet, F.K.L.; Vissink, A.; Kroese, F.G.M. Small-molecule inhibitors and the salivary gland epithelium in Sjögren's syndrome. *Expert Opin. Investig. Drugs* **2019**, *28*, 605–616. [CrossRef]
30. Draeger, A.; Nathrath, W.B.; Lane, E.B.; Sundström, B.E.; Stigbrand, T.I. Cytokeratins, smooth muscle actin and vimentin in human normal salivary gland and pleomorphic adenomas. Immunohistochemical studies with particular reference to myoepithelial and basal cells. *Apmis Acta Pathol. Microbiol. Immunol. Scand.* **1991**, *99*, 405–415. [CrossRef]
31. Ikeura, K.; Kawakita, T.; Tsunoda, K.; Nakagawa, T.; Tsubota, K. Characterization of Long-Term Cultured Murine Submandibular Gland Epithelial Cells. *PLoS ONE* **2016**, *11*, e0147407. [CrossRef]
32. You, S.; Avidan, O.; Tariq, A.; Ahluwalia, I.; Stark, P.C.; Kublin, C.L.; Zoukhri, D. Role of Epithelial–Mesenchymal Transition in Repair of the Lacrimal Gland after Experimentally Induced Injury. *Investig. Ophthalmol. Vis. Sci.* **2012**, *53*, 126–135. [CrossRef] [PubMed]
33. Hosseini, Z.F.; Nelson, D.A.; Moskwa, N.; Sfakis, L.M.; Castracane, J.; Larsen, M. FGF2-dependent mesenchyme and laminin-111 are niche factors in salivary gland organoids. *J. Cell Sci.* **2018**, *131*, jcs208728. [CrossRef] [PubMed]
34. Shin, H.-S.; Hong, H.J.; Koh, W.-G.; Lim, J.-Y. Organotypic 3D Culture in Nanoscaffold Microwells Supports Salivary Gland Stem-Cell-Based Organization. *ACS Biomater. Sci. Eng.* **2018**, *4*, 4311–4320. [CrossRef]
35. Maria, O.M.; Zeitouni, A.; Gologan, O.; Tran, S.D. matrigel improves functional properties of primary human salivary gland cells. *Tissue Eng. Part A* **2011**, *17*, 1229–1238. [CrossRef] [PubMed]
36. Su, L.; Morgan, P.R.; Harrison, D.L.; Waseem, A.; Lane, E.B. Expression of keratin mRNAS and proteins in normal salivary epithelia and pleomorphic adenomas. *J. Pathol.* **1993**, *171*, 173–181. [CrossRef] [PubMed]
37. Knox, S.M.; Lombaert, I.M.A.; Reed, X.; Vitale-Cross, L.; Gutkind, J.S.; Hoffman, M.P. Parasympathetic Innervation Maintains Epithelial Progenitor Cells During Salivary Organogenesis. *Science* **2010**, *329*, 1645. [CrossRef] [PubMed]
38. Knox, S.M.; Lombaert, I.M.A.; Haddox, C.L.; Abrams, S.R.; Cotrim, A.; Wilson, A.J.; Hoffman, M.P. Parasympathetic stimulation improves epithelial organ regeneration. *Nat. Commun.* **2013**, *4*, 1494. [CrossRef]
39. Emmerson, E.; May, A.J.; Nathan, S.; Cruz-Pacheco, N.; Lizama, C.O.; Maliskova, L.; Zovein, A.C.; Shen, Y.; Muench, M.O.; Knox, S.M. SOX2 regulates acinar cell development in the salivary gland. *eLife* **2017**, *6*, e26620. [CrossRef]
40. Min, S.; Song, E.-A.C.; Oyelakin, A.; Gluck, C.; Smalley, K.; Romano, R.-A. Functional characterization and genomic studies of a novel murine submandibular gland epithelial cell line. *PLoS ONE* **2018**, *13*, e0192775. [CrossRef]
41. Lombaert, I.M.A.; Brunsting, J.F.; Wierenga, P.K.; Faber, H.; Stokman, M.A.; Kok, T.; Visser, W.H.; Kampinga, H.H.; de Haan, G.; Coppes, R.P. Rescue of Salivary Gland Function after Stem Cell Transplantation in Irradiated Glands. *PLoS ONE* **2008**, *3*, e2063. [CrossRef]
42. Weng, P.-L.; Aure, M.H.; Maruyama, T.; Ovitt, C.E. Limited Regeneration of Adult Salivary Glands after Severe Injury Involves Cellular Plasticity. *Cell Rep.* **2018**, *24*, 1464–1470.e3. [CrossRef] [PubMed]
43. Wang, Y.; Chen, S.; Yan, Z.; Pei, M. A prospect of cell immortalization combined with matrix microenvironmental optimization strategy for tissue engineering and regeneration. *Cell Biosci.* **2019**, *9*, 1–21. [CrossRef] [PubMed]
44. Costa, A.F.; Altemani, A.; Hermsen, M. Current Concepts on Dedifferentiation/High-Grade Transformation in Salivary Gland Tumors. *Pathol. Res. Int.* **2011**, *2011*, 325965. [CrossRef] [PubMed]

45. Baum, B.J.; Alevizos, I.; Zheng, C.; Cotrim, A.P.; Liu, S.; McCullagh, L.; Goldsmith, C.M.; Burbelo, P.D.; Citrin, D.E.; Mitchell, J.B.; et al. Early responses to adenoviral-mediated transfer of the aquaporin-1 cDNA for radiation-induced salivary hypofunction. *Proc. Natl. Acad. Sci. USA* **2012**, *109*, 19403–19407. [CrossRef]
46. Alevizos, I.; Zheng, C.; Cotrim, A.P.; Liu, S.; McCullagh, L.; Billings, M.E.; Goldsmith, C.M.; Tandon, M.; Helmerhorst, E.J.; Catalan, M.A.; et al. Late responses to adenoviral-mediated transfer of the aquaporin-1 gene for radiation-induced salivary hypofunction. *Gene* **2017**, *24*, 176–186. [CrossRef]
47. Baker, O.J. Tight junctions in salivary epithelium. *J. Biomed. Biotechnol.* **2010**, *2010*, 278948. [CrossRef]
48. Shubin, A.D.; Sharipol, A.; Felong, T.J.; Weng, P.-L.; Schutrum, B.E.; Joe, D.S.; Aure, M.H.; Benoit, D.S.W.; Ovitt, C.E. Stress or injury induces cellular plasticity in salivary gland acinar cells. *Cell Tissue Res.* **2020**, *380*, 487–497. [CrossRef]
49. Noll, B.; Mougeot, F.B.; Brennan, M.T.; Mougeot, J.C. Telomere erosion in Sjögren's syndrome: A multi-tissue comparative analysis. *J. Oral Pathol. Med. Off. Publ. Int. Assoc. Oral Pathol. Am. Acad. Oral Pathol.* **2020**, *49*, 63–71. [CrossRef]
50. Kawashima, M.; Kawakita, T.; Maida, Y.; Kamoi, M.; Ogawa, Y.; Shimmura, S.; Masutomi, K.; Tsubota, K. Comparison of telomere length and association with progenitor cell markers in lacrimal gland between Sjogren syndrome and non-Sjogren syndrome dry eye patients. *Mol. Vis.* **2011**, *17*, 1397–1404.

Publisher's Note: MDPI stays neutral with regard to jurisdictional claims in published maps and institutional affiliations.

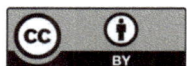

© 2020 by the authors. Licensee MDPI, Basel, Switzerland. This article is an open access article distributed under the terms and conditions of the Creative Commons Attribution (CC BY) license (http://creativecommons.org/licenses/by/4.0/).

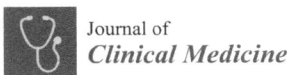

Article

First Report of Sublingual Gland Ducts: Visualization by Dynamic MR Sialography and Its Clinical Application

Tatsurou Tanaka [1], Masafumi Oda [1], Nao Wakasugi-Sato [1], Takaaki Joujima [1], Yuichi Miyamura [1], Manabu Habu [2], Masaaki Kodama [3], Osamu Takahashi [2], Teppei Sago [4], Shinobu Matsumoto-Takeda [1], Ikuko Nishida [5], Hiroki Tsurushima [6], Yasushi Otani [6], Daigo Yoshiga [6], Masaaki Sasaguri [2] and Yasuhiro Morimoto [1,*]

[1] Division of Oral and Maxillofacial Radiology, Kyushu Dental University, Kitakyushu 803-8580, Japan; t-tanaka@kyu-dent.ac.jp (T.T.); r07oda@fa.kyu-dent.ac.jp (M.O.); r16wakasugi@fa.kyu-dent.ac.jp (N.W.-S.); r16jojima@fa.kyu-dent.ac.jp (T.J.); r16miyamura@fa.kyu-dent.ac.jp (Y.M.); r17matsumoto@fa.kyu-dent.ac.jp (S.M.-T.)

[2] Division of Maxillofacial Surgery, Kyushu Dental University, Kitakyushu 803-8580, Japan; h-manabu@kyu-dent.ac.jp (M.H.); r07takahashi@fa.kyu-dent.ac.jp (O.T.); r13sasaguri@fa.kyu-dent.ac.jp (M.S.)

[3] Department of Oral and Maxillofacial Surgery, Japan Seafarers Relief Association Moji Ekisaikai Hospital, Kyushu 801-8550, Japan; kodama@ekisaikai-moji.jp

[4] Division of Dental Anesthesiology, Kyushu Dental University, Kitakyushu 803-8580, Japan; r07sagou@fa.kyu-dent.ac.jp

[5] Division of Developmental Stomatognathic Function Science, Kyushu Dental University, Kitakyushu 803-8580, Japan; nishida@kyu-dent.ac.jp

[6] Division of Oral Medicine, Kyushu Dental University, Kitakyushu 803-8580, Japan; r17tsurushima@fa.kyu-dent.ac.jp (H.T.); r17otani@fa.kyu-dent.ac.jp (Y.O.); r11yoshiga@fa.kyu-dent.ac.jp (D.Y.)

* Correspondence: rad-mori@kyu-dent.ac.jp; Tel./Fax: +81-93-285-3094

Received: 30 October 2020; Accepted: 11 November 2020; Published: 16 November 2020

Abstract: This study was done to determine whether the sublingual gland ducts could be visualized and/or their function assessed by MR sialography and dynamic MR sialography and to elucidate the clinical significance of the visualization and/or evaluation of the function of sublingual gland ducts by clinical application of these techniques. In 20 adult volunteers, 19 elderly volunteers, and 7 patients with sublingual gland disease, morphological and functional evaluations were done by MR sialography and dynamic MR sialography. Next, four parameters, including the time-dependent changes (change ratio) in the maximum area of the detectable sublingual gland ducts in dynamic MR sialographic images and data were analyzed. Sublingual gland ducts could be accurately visualized in 16 adult volunteers, 12 elderly volunteers, and 5 patients. No significant differences in the four parameters in detectable duct areas of sublingual glands were found among the three groups. In one patient with a ranula, the lesion could be correctly diagnosed as a ranula by MR sialography because the mass was clearly derived from sublingual gland ducts. This is the first report of successful visualization of sublingual gland ducts. In addition, the present study suggests that MR sialography can be more useful in the diagnosis of patients with lesions of sublingual gland ducts.

Keywords: MR sialography; dynamic; sublingual gland ducts

1. Introduction

There have been many studies of clinical applications of magnetic resonance imaging (MRI) for evaluation, in addition to the evaluation of morphology, due to the higher quality of MRI technology [1–8]. As for our study, the technique of "dynamic MR sialography" was named and introduced because of its clinical usefulness in visualizing the excretion of saliva from the parotid and submandibular glands, and in evaluating the diagnosis of morphology and functions for both glands and the outcomes of treatments for Sjögren's syndrome and xerostomia [1,9–12]. However, the visualization of the sublingual gland ducts is not considered even on MR imaging because it is difficult to visualize the very thin and short ducts, as seen in anatomy textbooks [13].

In our experience, the sublingual gland duct-like structures visualized and the possibility of visualizing the sublingual gland ducts by MR sialography needed to be elucidated.

In the present study, the sublingual gland ducts could be visualized. In addition, the clinical significance of the visualization and/or evaluation of the function of sublingual gland ducts was evaluated by clinical application of these techniques for some patients with sublingual gland diseases.

2. Materials and Methods

A total of 20 adult volunteers (9 males and 11 females, mean age 41.5 years, age range 18–56 years) and 19 elderly volunteers (8 males and 11 females, mean age 67.8 years, age range 60–80 years) over the age of 60 years, with no sublingual gland-related diseases, as confirmed by both a history and clinical examination, were recruited (Table 1). In addition, 7 consecutive patients (3 males and 4 females, mean age 43.4 years, age range 19–76 years) were also recruited, with 5 having inflammations of the oral floor, including the sublingual glands, and 2 with ranulas (Table 1). The image of a single side (randomly chosen) or a disease-related side of the sublingual gland ducts was used, since only single images could be acquired at one given time for functional evaluation. The total volume of the sublingual gland ducts was also analyzed using the images. Approval for the present study was obtained from the institutional review board of Kyushu Dental University (No. 20-27).

Table 1. Subjects.

	Male			Female		
	Number	Age (Mean ± SD)	Age Range	Number	Age (Mean ± SD)	Age Range
Adult volunteers	9	46.5 ± 8.7	29–55	11	40.3 ± 12.9	18–56
Elderly volunteers	8	68.1 ± 5.5	61–79	11	67.5 ± 6.5	60–80
Patients	3	37.3 ± 15.4	27–55	4	48.0 ± 24.3	19–76

As in our previous reports, all images were acquired using a 1.5T full-body MR system (EXCELART Vantage powered by Atlas PPP; Toshiba, Tokyo, Japan) with a head coil (Atlas Head SPEEDER) to visualize the sublingual gland ducts, such as the parotid and submandibular gland ducts, according to Oda et al. [14]. T1-weighted, short tau inversion recovery (STIR), three-dimensional (3D) fast asymmetric spin-echo, and 2D-FASE images were acquired for each subject. The MRI parameters that were used are shown in Table 2. The 2D-FASE images were acquired after a single excitation with specific encoding for each echo. Fat saturation suppressed signals from subcutaneous fat.

The 3D MR sialography for sublingual gland ducts was performed as described by Oda et al. [14]. Briefly, in the same session where conventional MR studies of the sublingual glands were obtained, MR sialography was performed using 3D-FASE sequencing. In the 3D-FASE imaging, after a single excitation, images were acquired with a specific encoding for each echo. Fat saturation suppressed the signals from the subcutaneous fat. The imaging volume was centered parasagittally for the midline of the sublingual gland. In all volunteers and patients, post-processing of the MR sialographic images was performed for maximum intensity projection (MIP) reconstructions. Since 3D acquisitions can be reformatted into any required orientation, the sublingual gland ducts were identified on an initial set of axial 3D-FASE images, and oblique sagittal acquisition was used to capture the image of the parotid gland and/or submandibular gland ducts. The imaging time required for MR sialographic 3D reconstruction images using 3D-FASE sequencing was less than 5 min.

Table 2. Imaging parameters of each sequence.

	Sequence			
	STIR	T1WI	2D-FASE	3D-FASE
TR (ms)	4700	820	6000	3.2
TE (ms)	75	15	250	1.6
Flip angle (°)	90	90	90	45
FOV (mm)	200 × 200	200 × 200	200 × 200	200 × 200
Section thickness (mm)	6	6	30–60	1.8
Matrix (pixels)	224 × 320	224 × 320	224 × 320	120 × 96
Acquisition time (min: s)	3:30	3:30	0:18 (12hase)	4:30–5:30

TR: Repetition time, TE: Echo time, FOV: Field of view, STIR: Short T1 inversion recovery, T1WI: T1-weighted image, 2D-FASE: 2-dimensional fast asymmetric spin-echo, 3D-FASE: 3-dimensional fast asymmetric spin-echo.

Dynamic MR sialographic images and data were acquired using the method described by Oda et al. [14]. First, 2D-FASE sequencing was repeated every 18 s of acquisition time and 12 s of interval time before and after the placement of several drops of 5% citric acid (1 mL) on the tongue, using a device similar to a syringe to acquire the dynamic MR sialography. Fat saturation was also applied for the suppression of signals from subcutaneous fat. The acquisition time of the dynamic MR sialography was about 7 min after stimulation. For the prevention of movement artifacts, head rests were used with a flat long cord with non-magnetic materials.

Each digitized image acquired by the dynamic MR sialography was linked to the Ziostation2 (Ziosoft, Tokyo, Japan). The detectable area in the parotid or submandibular gland ducts on the respective images and the time from post-stimulation to the return to the baseline state of the ducts pre-stimulation were measured using the scanner-computer analysis system. For each patient, the change in ratio of the detectable area in the sublingual gland ducts in respective images to the detectable area pre-citric acid stimulation was also analyzed. A graph demonstrated the connection between the time post-stimulation (x-axis) and the change ratio of the dynamic MR sialographic data (y-axis). We commonly used the graph to show the connection between the time, post-stimulation, and the change ratio for the standardization of volunteers and patients.

Using the graph of dynamic MR sialography, the diagnostic parameters were also analyzed as follows: (1) the maximum area of the sublingual gland ducts pre-citric acid stimulation; (2) the change ratio (change ratio = detectable area of sublingual gland ducts post-citric acid stimulation/detectable area pre-citric acid stimulation); (3) the time from the end of post-stimulation to the occurrence of the maximum area of the sublingual gland ducts; and (4) the time it took for the sublingual gland ducts to decrease from their maximum level to 50% of the pre-stimulation level.

The Mann–Whitney U test was used to examine the differences between the following: (1) the maximum area of the sublingual gland ducts between the adult and elderly volunteers; (2) the degree of difference between the maximum and minimum duct areas based on computer calculations between the adult and elderly volunteers; (3) the time from the end of citric acid stimulation to the occurrence of the maximum area of the sublingual gland ducts between the adult and elderly volunteers; and (4) the time required for the sublingual gland ducts to decrease from their maximum level to the 50% pre-citric acid stimulation level between the adult and elderly volunteers. p values less than 0.05 indicated a significant difference.

3. Results

3.1. Visualization of Sublingual Gland Ducts by MR Sialography

Extraglandular portions of the typical sublingual gland ducts on MR sialography could be identified as many bright, homogeneous, ascending linear structures in continuity with the sublingual glands (Figure 1). The MR sialographic 3D reconstruction images of the respective angles were more easily visualized when the angle was determined manually using the mouse accompanying the MRI system. Both sublingual glands and sublingual gland ducts could be accurately visualized in 16 of the 20 adult volunteers, 12 of the 19 elderly volunteers, and 4 of the 7 patients, but only the sublingual glands were visualized in 2 adult volunteers, 4 elderly volunteers, and 1 patient (Table 3).

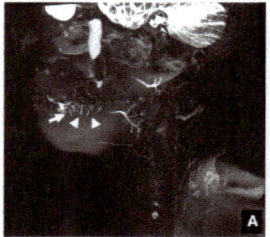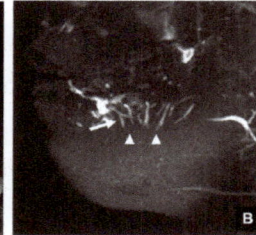

Figure 1. MR sialography of sublingual gland ducts. Extraglandular portions of the typical sublingual gland ducts in MR sialography ((**A**): overall image, (**B**): enlarged image of the sublingual gland area) can be identified as many bright, homogeneous, ascending linear structures (arrows) in continuity with the sublingual glands (arrowheads).

Table 3. Summary of visualization of sublingual gland ducts by MR sialography.

	Sublingual Glands and Ducts Visualized	Only Sublingual Glands Visualized
Adult volunteers ($n = 20$)	16	2
Elderly volunteers ($n = 19$)	12	4
Patients ($n = 7$)	5	1

3.2. Function of Sublingual Gland Ducts Evaluated by Dynamic MR Sialography

Normal dynamic MR sialography images obtained before and after citric acid stimulation are shown in Figure 2. The sublingual gland ducts were identified as many bright, homogeneous, ascending linear structures in continuity with the sublingual glands, as mentioned above (Figure 2A). The many ducts became slightly clearer in a time-dependent fashion gradually after citric acid stimulation and up to 30–60 s post-stimulation. Thereafter, the many ducts became slightly clearer in a time-dependent fashion. In the graph demonstrating the relationship between the time course post-citric acid stimulation and the change ratio of the detectable area in the sublingual gland ducts, the area was seen at first to only increase slightly to 30 s in a time-dependent fashion (Figure 2B).

The volunteers' data are summarized in Table 4. Before citric acid stimulation, the maximum area of the sublingual gland ducts was 10.0 mm^2 (mean ± SD = 10.0 ± 4.6 mm^2) in the 16 adult volunteers, 9.0 mm^2 (mean ± SD = 9.0 ± 3.4 mm^2) in the 3 elderly volunteers, and 10.2 mm^2 (mean ± SD = 10.2 ± 5.5 mm^2) in the 5 patients (adult vs. elderly: $p = 0.21$, adult vs. patients: $p = 0.46$, elderly vs. patients: $p = 0.92$; Mann–Whitney U test). After citric acid stimulation, the maximum area of the parotid gland duct was 13.2 mm^2 (mean ± SD = 13.2 ± 5.3 mm^2) in the 16 adult volunteers, 10.7 mm^2 (mean ± SD = 10.7 ± 4.4 mm^2) in the 12 elderly volunteers, and 11.0 mm^2 (mean ± SD = 11.0 ± 5.4 mm^2) in the 5 patients (adult vs. elderly: $p = 0.53$, adult vs. patients: $p = 0.94$, elderly vs. patients: $p = 0.67$; Mann–Whitney U test).

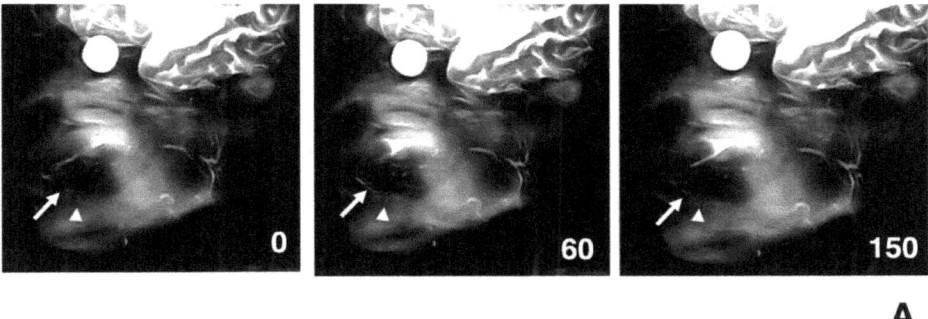

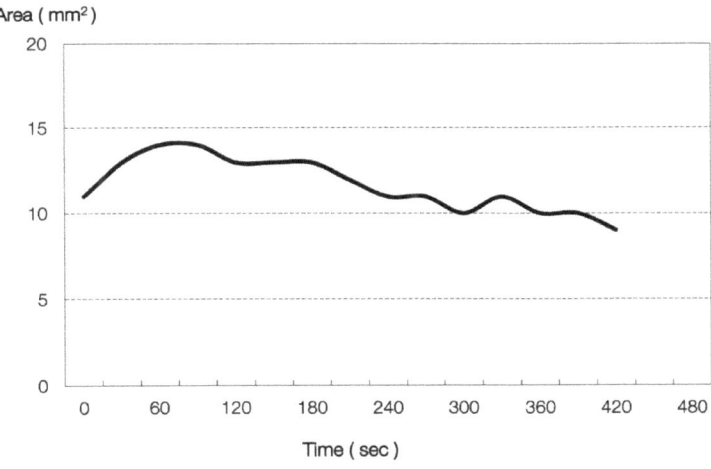

Figure 2. Dynamic MR sialographic images (**A**) and a graph (**B**) of sublingual gland ducts in a 26-year-old, healthy female volunteer. (**A**) The sublingual gland (arrowheads) and ducts (arrows) are gradually and slightly more clearly visualized after stimulation with citric acid for up to 60 s in a time-dependent manner. After 150 s, the many ducts became slightly clearer in a time-dependent fashion. (**B**) A graph of MR data of the sublingual gland ducts in Figure 2A demonstrates the connection between the time post-stimulation (x-axis) and the change ratio (y-axis). The area is seen at first to only increase slightly until 60 s in a time-dependent fashion. The maximum change ratio is about 1.2.

After stimulation, the time of occurrence of the maximum duct area varied from 30 s to 180 s in all subjects (mean ± SD = 62 ± 28 s in the 16 adult volunteers, mean ± SD = 63 ± 26 s in the 12 elderly volunteers, and mean ± SD = 54 ± 13 s in the 5 patients); (adult vs. elderly: $p = 0.92$, adult vs. patients: $p = 0.40$, elderly vs. patients: $p = 0.39$; Mann–Whitney U test). The time it took for the detectable duct area to return to almost 50% of its former area was about 115 s in all subjects (mean ± SD = 110 ± 39 s in the 12 adult volunteers, mean ± SD = 117 ± 57 s in the 12 elderly volunteers, and mean ± SD = 114 ± 25 s in the 5 patients); (adult vs. elderly: $p = 0.76$, adult vs. patients: $p = 0.82$, elderly vs. patients: $p = 0.89$; Mann–Whitney U test). No significant differences in the four parameters, including the change ratio (adult vs. elderly: $p = 0.24$, adult vs. patients: $p = 0.19$, elderly vs. patients: $p = 0.26$; Mann–Whitney U test) in the detectable duct area of the sublingual glands were found among the three groups (Table 4).

Table 4. Summary of physical and dynamic MR sialographic data.

	Area (mm^2)			Period to Occurrence of Maximum Area (s)	Period to Return to Its Pre-Citric Acid Stimulation 50% Level (s)
	Before Citric Acid Stimulation	After Citric Acid Stimulation	Change Ratio		
Adult volunteers ($n = 16$)	10.0 ± 4.6	13.2 ± 5.3	1.3 ± 1.1	62 ± 28	110 ± 39
Elderly volunteers ($n = 12$)	9.0 ± 3.4	10.7 ± 4.4	1.2 ± 1.3	63 ± 26	117 ± 57
Patients ($n = 5$)	10.2 ± 5.5	11.0 ± 5.4	1.1 ± 1.0	54 ± 13	114 ± 25

3.3. Clinical Application of MR Sialography for Patients with Sublingual Gland Diseases

In a 76-year-old man with inflammation of the right oral floor, many sublingual gland ducts continued with the sublingual glands in STIR, T1-weighted images, and MR sialography (Figure 3A–C).

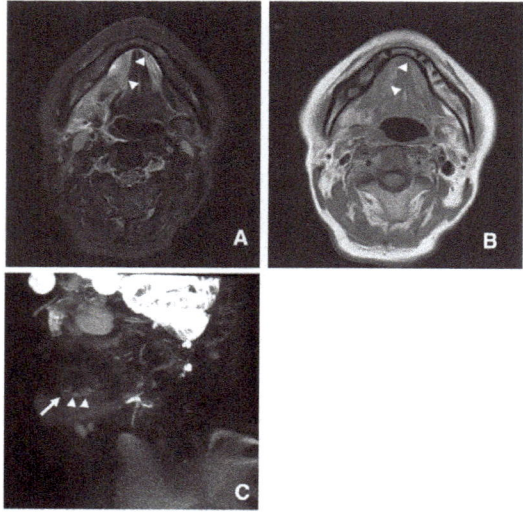

Figure 3. STIR (**A**), T1-weighted images (**B**), and MR sialography (**C**) of a 76-year-old man with inflammation of the right oral floor. The disappearance (arrows) of many sublingual gland ducts in continuity with the sublingual glands is visualized using MR sialography.

In a 30-year-old woman with a ranula on the left, the mass lesion was detected in continuity with the sublingual glands in STIR and T1-weighted images and was thus diagnosed as a ranula (Figure 4A,B). In addition, the mass was derived from one of the many sublingual gland ducts in images obtained using MR sialography (Figure 4C).

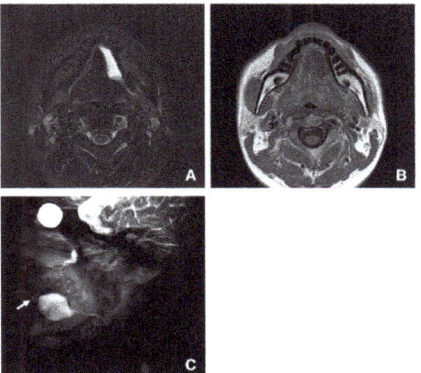

Figure 4. STIR (**A**), T1-weighted image (**B**), and MR sialography (**C**) of a 30-year-old woman with a ranula on the left. The mass lesion is seen in continuity with the sublingual glands in STIR (**A**) and T1-weighted images (**B**) and is diagnosed as a ranula. The mass is derived from one of many sublingual gland ducts (arrow) (**C**).

4. Discussion

The most interesting result of the present study is that it is the first to show the imaging characteristics of the sublingual gland ducts obtained by 3D MR sialography. It is otherwise difficult to visualize the very thin and very short ducts, with a diameter and length of only 1 mm, as shown in anatomy textbooks [13]. This is a very significant first success in salivary gland imaging. The extraglandular portions of the typical sublingual gland ducts appeared as many bright, homogeneous, ascending linear structures in continuity with the sublingual glands. The figures of the sublingual gland ducts obtained by MR sialography were the same as those in a textbook of oral anatomy [13]. Therefore, the images of the structures could be confirmed to be sublingual gland ducts using MR sialography. However, the sublingual gland duct could not be detected in all subjects as the detection rate was about 57.1%. One possible explanation is that the sublingual gland ducts are so thin and short that they cannot be visualized in all subjects using MR sialography.

So far, the reason the sublingual gland ducts, with their thin and short size, have not been visualized before, even in MR images, is that visualization has been considered technically impossible. In addition, it was thought that there was little clinical significance in the visualization of sublingual gland ducts. However, these very sublingual gland duct-like structures were visualized in the MR sialography of patients with submandibular and/or parotid gland-related diseases. Therefore, we planned the present study of the visualization of sublingual gland ducts using MR sialography.

One other interesting result of the present study is that the visualization of sublingual gland ducts indicates the clinical significance of sublingual gland-related diseases. The visualization of sublingual gland ducts concretely demonstrated a mass derived from one of many sublingual gland ducts. Based on the imaging, the mass should have been diagnosed as a ranula. At the same time, the disappearance of many sublingual gland ducts in continuity with sublingual glands was visualized using MR sialography in patients with inflammation on the right. We would like to elucidate the clinical significance of the MR sialography of sublingual gland ducts for many kinds of diseases in the oral floor, including sublingual gland-related diseases.

One reason for this first success in the visualization of sublingual gland ducts is that MR systems, 3D computer vision, and image processing techniques have been fast advancing due to the growing computational power of current computer systems. Rapid advances in 3D data acquisition and post-processing technologies are expanding the potential applications of 3D displays. In the 1.5T full-body MR system (EXCELART Vantage powered by Atlas PPP; Toshiba, Tokyo, Japan) with a head coil (Atlas Head SPEEDER), 3D-FASE was used for the sequencing of MR data sets through the acquisition of MR sialographic 3D reconstruction images, since this method was most likely to provide good resolution in a short period of time, as in our previous report [15]. That both types of images had good resolution using 3D-FASE sequencing may have been due to the section thickness being as little as 1 mm, despite the short acquisition time [16]. The section thickness was based on the advantage that 3D-FASE sequencing could excite a three-dimensional sample [17]. Thin slices produce images with good resolution while minimizing interference from partial volume effects and the formation of artifacts in the MR data and workstation. In addition, an adequate Fourier transform may be applied to 3D-FASE sequencing to produce high-resolution images [17]. Another advantage is that an image can be acquired using additional excitation, without conducting an additional imaging session, in cases when using a single excitation would not produce a satisfactory image. These unusual and useful characteristics of 3D-FASE sequencing allow for the avoidance of unnecessary exposure of patients to the RF pulse and an unnecessarily long acquisition time.

To our regret, little alteration of the dynamic curve was seen by dynamic MR sialography of sublingual gland ducts. This can be considered physiologically correct and reasonable [18,19]. Physiologically stimulated saliva production is the main role of the parotid glands [18,19]. The saliva flow rate of the parotid glands increases more quickly than that of the submandibular glands during citric acid stimulation [20–22]. Resting saliva is produced as the main role of the submandibular glands [18,19]. The salivary flow rate in the parotid gland during stimulation is twice as high as that in the rest phase, but less of an increase is found in the submandibular gland [23,24]. The main role of sublingual glands, however, is to keep the oral mucosa moist, but not to maintain resting and stimulated saliva flow. Therefore, little alteration of the dynamic curve via dynamic MR sialography of sublingual gland ducts was seen. We are now planning to elucidate the clinical significance of dynamic MR sialography of the sublingual gland ducts through its clinical application to many kinds of diseases in the oral floor, including sublingual gland-related diseases.

One possible limitation of the present data is the small sample size. The variables of race and sex could not be studied in this study sample. In addition, only a few clinical applications were examined. Therefore, further investigation is required. In the present study, there was little witness of movement artifacts by the volunteers, but we predicted that patients would move in MR examinations, despite our system preventing movement artifacts. Moreover, we paid attention to the possibility of visualizing sublingual gland ducts using dynamic MR sialography and its clinical application in the present study. Therefore, we could not elucidate the classification of the drainage of the sublingual glands in Bartholin's ducts and/or the duct of Rivinus. At the next stage, we should try to classify their drainage patterns. At the same time, we should try to elucidate how the presence of Bartholin's ducts may be related to ranula formation as the next stage. We added the sentence mentioned above in the revised manuscript.

5. Conclusions

MR sialography allows for the evaluation of function and morphology of the sublingual gland ducts. This technique appears to have many possible applications in the dental, medical, and biological fields.

Author Contributions: Analysis of this research data was performed by T.T. Statistical analysis was performed by T.T. and M.O. Data collection of this research was performed by T.T., M.O., N.W.-S., S.M.-T., T.J., Y.M. (Yuichi Miyamura), M.H., M.K., O.T., T.S., I.N., H.T., Y.O., D.Y. and M.S. Integration of this research was performed by Y.M. (Yasuhiro Morimoto). All authors have read and agreed to the published version of the manuscript.

Funding: This research received no external funding.

Acknowledgments: This study was supported in part by grants-in-aid for scientific research from the Ministry of Education, Science, Sports and Culture of Japan and from Kitakyushu City to Y.M.

Conflicts of Interest: The authors declare no conflict of interest.

References

1. Morimoto, Y.; Ono, K.; Tanaka, T.; Kito, S.; Inoue, H.; Seta, Y.; Yokota, M.; Inenaga, K.; Ohba, T. The functional evaluation of salivary glands using dynamic MR sialography following citric acid stimulation: A preliminary study. *Oral Surg. Oral Med. Oral Pathol. Oral Radiol. Endod.* **2005**, *100*, 357–364. [CrossRef] [PubMed]
2. Morimoto, Y.; Tanaka, T.; Kito, S.; Tominaga, K.; Yoshioka, I.; Yamashita, Y.; Shibuya, T.; Matsufuji, Y.; Kodama, M.; Takahashi, T.; et al. Utility of three dimension fast asymmetric spin-echo (3D-FASE) sequences in MR sialographic sequences: Model and volunteer studies. *Oral Dis.* **2005**, *11*, 35–43. [CrossRef] [PubMed]
3. Dirix, P.; De Keyzer, F.; Vandecaveye, V.; Stroobants, S.; Hermans, R.; Nuyts, S. Diffusion-weighted magnetic resonance imaging to evaluate major salivary gland function before and after radiotherapy. *Int. J. Radiat. Oncol. Biol. Phys.* **2008**, *71*, 1365–1371. [CrossRef]
4. Wada, A.; Uchida, N.; Yokokawa, M.; Yoshizako, T.; Kitagaki, H. Radiation-induced xerostomia: Objective evaluation of salivary gland injury using MR sialography. *AJNR Am. J. Neuroradiol.* **2009**, *30*, 53–58. [CrossRef] [PubMed]
5. Becker, M.; Marchal, F.; Becker, C.D.; Dulguerov, P.; Georgakopoulos, G.; Lehmann, W.; Terrier, F. Sialolithiasis and salivary ductal stenosis: Diagnostic accuracy of MR sialography with a three-dimensional extended-phase conjugate-symmetry rapid spin-echo sequence. *Radiology* **2000**, *217*, 347–358. [CrossRef]
6. Murakami, R.; Baba, Y.; Nishimura, R.; Baba, T.; Matsumoto, N.; Yamashita, Y.; Ishikawa, T.; Takahashi, M. MR sialography using half-Fourier acquisition single-shot turbo spin-echo (HASTE) sequences. *Am. J. Neuroradiol.* **1998**, *19*, 959–961.
7. Gadodia, A.; Seith, A.; Sharma, R.; Thakar, A.; Parshad, R. Magnetic resonance sialography using CISS and HASTE sequences in inflammatory salivary gland diseases: Comparison with digital sialography. *Acta Radiol.* **2010**, *51*, 156–163. [CrossRef]
8. Ohbayashi, N.; Yamada, I.; Yoshino, N.; Sasaki, T. Sjögren syndrome: Comparison of assessments with MR sialography and conventional sialography. *Radiology* **1998**, *209*, 683–688. [CrossRef]
9. Morimoto, Y.; Habu, M.; Tomoyose, T.; Ono, K.; Tanaka, T.; Yoshioka, I.; Tominaga, K.; Yamashita, Y.; Ansai, T.; Kito, S.; et al. Dynamic MR sialography as a new diagnostic technique for patients with Sjögren syndrome. *Oral Dis.* **2006**, *12*, 408–414. [CrossRef]
10. Tanaka, T.; Ono, K.; Ansai, T.; Yoshioka, I.; Habu, M.; Tomoyose, T.; Yamashita, Y.; Nishida, I.; Oda, M.; Kuroiwa, H.; et al. Dynamic magnetic resonance sialography for patients with xerostomia. *Oral Surg. Oral Med. Oral Pathol. Oral Radiol. Endod.* **2008**, *106*, 115–123. [CrossRef]
11. Habu, M.; Tanaka, T.; Tomoyose, T.; Ono, K.; Ansai, T.; Ozaki, Y.; Yoshioka, I.; Yamashita, Y.; Kodama, M.; Yamamoto, N.; et al. Significance of dynamic magnetic resonance sialography in prognostic evaluation of saline solution irrigation of the parotid gland for the treatment of xerostomia. *J. Oral Maxillofac. Surg.* **2010**, *68*, 768–776. [CrossRef]
12. Tanaka, T.; Ono, K.; Habu, M.; Inoue, H.; Tominaga, K.; Okabe, S.; Kito, S.; Yokota, M.; Fukuda, J.; Inenaga, K.; et al. Functional evaluations of the parotid and submandibular glands using dynamic magnetic resonance sialography. *Dentomaxillofac. Radiol.* **2007**, *36*, 218–223. [CrossRef] [PubMed]
13. Harold, E. *Clinical Anatomy*, 11th ed.; Blackwell Publishing: Hoboken, NJ, USA, 2018; pp. 272–274.
14. Oda, M.; Tanaka, T.; Habu, M.; Ono, K.; Kodama, M.; Kokuryo, S.; Yamamoto, N.; Kito, S.; Wakasugi-Sato, N.; Matsumoto-Takeda, S.; et al. Diagnosis and prognostic evaluation for xerostomia using dynamic MR sialography. *Curr. Med. Imaging Rev.* **2014**, *10*, 84–94. [CrossRef]
15. Morimoto, Y.; Tanaka, T.; Yoshioka, I.; Masumi, S.; Yamashita, M.; Ohba, T. Virtual endoscopic view of salivary gland ducts using MR sialography data from three dimension fast asymmetric spin-echo (3D-FASE) sequences: A preliminary study. *Oral Dis.* **2002**, *8*, 268–274. [CrossRef] [PubMed]
16. Morimoto, Y.; Tanaka, T.; Tominaga, K.; Yoshioka, I.; Kito, S.; Ohba, T. Clinical application of MR sialographic 3D-reconstruction imaging and MR virtual endoscopy for salivary gland duct analysis. *J. Oral Maxillofac. Surg.* **2004**, *62*, 1236–1244. [CrossRef]
17. Yang, D.; Kodama, T.; Tamura, S.; Watanabe, K. Evaluation of inner ear by 3D fast asymmetric spin echo (FASE) MR imaging: Phantom and volunteer studies. *Magn. Reson. Imaging* **1999**, *17*, 171–182. [CrossRef]
18. Markopoulos, A.K. *A Handbook of Oral Physiology and Oral Biology*; Bentham Science Publishers: Sharjah, UAE, 2010; pp. 44–50.

19. Moore, K.L. *Essential Clinical Anatomy*; Lippincott Williams and Wilkins Publishers: Philadelphia, PA, USA, 2010; pp. 560–570.
20. Carbognin, G.; Girardi, V.; Biasiutti, C.; Manfredi, R.; Frulloni, R.L.; Hermans, J.J.; Mucelli, R.P. Autoimmune pancreatitis: Imaging findings on contrast-enhanced MR, MRCP and dynamic secretin-enhanced MRCP. *Radiol. Med.* **2009**, *114*, 1214–1231. [CrossRef]
21. Park, H.S.; Lee, J.M.; Choi, H.K.; Hong, S.H.; Han, J.K.; Choi, B.I. Preoperative evaluation of pancreatic cancer: Comparison of gadolinium-enhanced dynamic MRI with MR cholangiopancreatography versus MDCT. *J. Magn. Reson. Imaging* **2009**, *30*, 586–595. [CrossRef]
22. Schlaudraff, E.; Wagner, H.J.; Klose, K.J.; Heverhagen, J.T. Prospective evaluation of the diagnostic accuracy of secretin-enhanced magnetic resonance cholangiopancreaticography in suspected chronic pancreatitis. *Magn. Reson. Imaging* **2008**, *26*, 1367–1373. [CrossRef]
23. Akisik, M.F.; Sandrasegaran, K.; Aisen, A.A.; Maglinte, D.D.; Sherman, S.; Lehman, G.A. Dynamic secretin-enhanced MR cholangiopancreatography. *Radiographics* **2006**, *26*, 665–677. [CrossRef]
24. Gillams, A.R.; Kurzawinski, T.; Lees, W.R. Diagnosis of duct disruption and assessment of pancreatic leak with dynamic secretin-stimulated MR cholangiopancreatography. *Am. J. Roentgenol.* **2006**, *186*, 499–506. [CrossRef] [PubMed]

Publisher's Note: MDPI stays neutral with regard to jurisdictional claims in published maps and institutional affiliations.

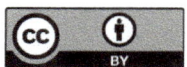 © 2020 by the authors. Licensee MDPI, Basel, Switzerland. This article is an open access article distributed under the terms and conditions of the Creative Commons Attribution (CC BY) license (http://creativecommons.org/licenses/by/4.0/).

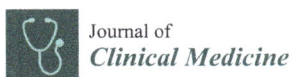 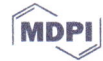

Article

Enhanced Salivary and General Oxidative Stress in Hashimoto's Thyroiditis Women in Euthyreosis

Katarzyna Morawska [1], Mateusz Maciejczyk [2,*], Łukasz Popławski [3], Anna Popławska-Kita [4], Adam Krętowski [4] and Anna Zalewska [5,*]

[1] Department of Restorative Dentistry, Medical University of Bialystok, 24A M. Sklodowskiej-Curie Street, 15-276 Bialystok, Poland; kmorawska1009@gmail.com
[2] Department of Hygiene, Epidemiology and Ergonomics, Medical University of Bialystok, 2c Mickiewicza Street, 15-022 Bialystok, Poland
[3] Department of Radiology, Medical University of Bialystok, 24A M. Sklodowskiej-Curie Street, 15-276 Bialystok, Poland; gajki91@o2.pl
[4] Department of Endocrinology, Diabetology and Internal Medicine, Medical University of Bialystok, 24A M. Sklodowskiej-Curie Street, 15-276 Bialystok, Poland; annapoplawskakita@op.pl (A.P.-K.); adamkretowski@wp.pl (A.K.)
[5] Laboratory of Experimental Dentistry, Medical University of Bialystok, 24A M. Sklodowskiej-Curie Street, 15-276 Bialystok, Poland
* Correspondence: mat.maciejczyk@gmail.com (M.M.); azalewska426@gmail.com (A.Z.);

Received: 5 June 2020; Accepted: 2 July 2020; Published: 3 July 2020

Abstract: Hashimoto's thyroiditis (HT) is one of the most common autoimmune diseases. Although HT is inextricably linked to oxidative stress, there have been no studies assessing salivary redox homeostasis or salivary gland function in patients with HT. This study is the first to compare antioxidant defense and oxidative stress biomarkers in non-stimulated (NWS) and stimulated (SWS) whole saliva and plasma/erythrocytes of HT patients compared to controls. The study included 45 women with HT in the euthyreosis period as well as an age- and gender-matched control group. We showed that NWS secretion was significantly lower in HT patients compared to healthy controls, similar to salivary amylase activity in NWS and SWS. Catalase and peroxidase activities were considerably higher in NWS and SWS of HT patients, while the concentrations of reduced glutathione and uric acid were significantly lower in comparison with healthy subjects. Total antioxidant potential was significantly lower, while total oxidant status and the level of oxidation products of proteins (advanced glycation end products, advanced oxidation protein products) and lipids (malondialdehyde, lipid hydroperoxides) were significantly higher in NWS, SWS and plasma of HT patients. In conclusion, in both salivary glands of women with HT in euthyreosis, the ability to maintain redox homeostasis was hindered. In HT patients we observed oxidative damage to salivary proteins and lipids; thus, some biomarkers of oxidative stress may present a potential diagnostic value.

Keywords: Hashimoto's disease; oxidative stress; saliva

1. Introduction

Hashimoto's disease (HT) is known as chronic lymphocytic thyroiditis. It is an autoimmune-mediated disease characterized by dense infiltrations of the thyroid gland by plasma cells, macrophages and, particularly, lymphocytes [1,2]. The T and B lymphocytes are stimulated against thyroglobulin and thyroid peroxidase, and induce a number of biochemical processes that lead to progressive destruction of thyrocytes, fibrosis, reduction of the thyroid gland size and its hypofunction [3]. Growing evidence indicates that HT is linked to lowered cellular antioxidant potential and enhanced oxidative stress (OS) [2–4].

OS is a situation in which balance between reactive oxygen species (ROS) and the body's ability to neutralize them is shifted in favor of oxidants [5]. This leads to a temporary or chronic elevation of ROS concentration as well as disturbed cell metabolism and degradation of cell components [5].

Evidence showed an altered antioxidant potential and enhanced OS in the plasma of HT patients. Lassoued et al. [6] demonstrated increased plasma malondialdehyde (MDA) concentration as well as the activities of superoxide dismutase (SOD) and catalase (CAT) compared to the controls. Rostami et al. [2] observed decreased reduced glutathione (GSH) concentration in the plasma of newly diagnosed hypothyroid HT patients. This study showed that GSH depletion initiates OS and development of immunological intolerance in the course of HT. Ates et al. [4] argued that higher OS levels in patients progressing to overt hypothyroidism may be evidence of redox balance shift towards oxidative reactions and could thus serve as a significant factor in the initiation and progression of this disease. Interestingly, in the study performed by Nanda et al. [7], OS levels were higher in the thyroid antibody-positive hypothyroid group than in the thyroid antibody-negative hypothyroid group. The authors concluded that the presence of autoimmune antibodies is a key factor for enhanced ROS production and increased concentrations of oxidative biomolecular modifications, while thyroid hormone levels are of secondary importance.

Systemic inflammation, elevated levels of thyroid antibodies, disturbed concentrations of thyroid hormones and chronically raised ROS levels in the course of HT lead to numerous systemic complications, including cardiological diseases, insulin resistance, mood disorders and salivary gland diseases [2,4,8].

Agha-Hosseini et al. [8] demonstrated significantly reduced unstimulated saliva flow rate and xerostomia among HT women in euthyreosis vs. healthy controls. The cause of salivary gland dysfunction in the course of HT has not been explained yet. It is noteworthy that they observed salivary gland dysfunction in patients in euthyreosis. Abnormalities in both the composition and the amount of the secreted saliva negatively affects oral health and the condition of the entire body. Therefore, it is important to understand the mechanisms leading to salivary gland dysfunction in the course of the described disease. Moreover, the oral cavity is exposed to numerous oxidizing agents capable of generating large amounts of ROS. Evidence showed that salivary and, to some extent, plasma antioxidants, constitute an important part of the antioxidant barrier in both oral cavity and the entire body. Salivary peroxidase (Px), together with catalase (CAT), neutralizes H_2O_2 formed in a dismutation reaction catalyzed by superoxide dismutase (SOD). Reduced glutathione (GSH) is the most important low molecular weight salivary antioxidant responsible for maintaining thiol groups of salivary proteins at a reduced level. Forty percent of the total salivary antioxidant barrier is provided by bloodborne uric acid (UA) [5]. Failure of these antioxidant systems may result in the development of oral cavity diseases, including periodontitis [9,10], precancerous lesions [11] and cancers [12]. Previous studies showed the alteration in the salivary antioxidants barrier and the contribution of OS in the development and progression of salivary gland dysfunction in the course of other autoimmune diseases: psoriasis vulgaris, systemic sclerosis, rheumatoid arthritis, diabetes type 1, multiple sclerosis, Sjögren's syndrome and systemic lupus erythematosus [13–21]. In general, reduced/elevated levels of endogenous, non-enzymatic antioxidants or enhanced/weakened activity of antioxidant enzymes and increased oxidative modification of salivary cell components are observed in the saliva of patients with autoimmune diseases. The salivary antioxidants in HT have not yet been determined, so in the light of the above, it appears necessary to assess the antioxidant potential of saliva and the role of OS in the development of salivary gland dysfunction in the course of HT.

The aim of this study was to evaluate antioxidative defense parameters and measurable oxidative stress effects in unstimulated and stimulated saliva and plasma/erythrocytes of patients with HT in euthyreosis and to compare the obtained results with those in the control group.

2. Materials and Methods

2.1. Patients

The study was approved by the Local Ethics Committee, permission number: R-I-002/386/2016. Each patient was informed of the purpose and the detailed procedure of the study and consented in writing to join the research project.

The study group consisted of 45 women diagnosed with HT. The disease was confirmed when anti-TG and/or anti-TPO levels in serum was above the normal range and occurred with the presence of parenchymal heterogeneity on thyroid ultrasonography (USG). Our experiment included patients with HT in euthyreosis (free thyroxine (fT4) and thyroid-stimulating hormones (TSH) within normal ranges), 24 treated with Eutyrox (doses from 50 to 150 mg; the last tablet taken 24 h before the hormone level test) and 21 untreated. Patients were reported for follow-up visits to the Department of Endocrinology, Diabetology and Internal Medicine of the Medical University of Bialystok. We decided to create only one group, because the results of particular redox balance assays did not differ between patients in the course of a hormone therapy and those not requiring it.

The reference group consisted of 45 generally healthy women, matched to the study group in terms of age and BMI, selected from those who reported for dental check-ups to the Department of Restorative Dentistry, MUB.

Exclusion and inclusion criteria:

Patients with HT and healthy controls did not suffer from any associated diseases, including other autoimmune diseases (type 1 diabetes, rheumatoid arthritis, scleroderma, psoriasis, lupus, Sjögren's syndrome, etc.) or depression. Participants from both the study and control group were qualified for further examinations only if they did not have periodontitis, gingivitis, or active foci of odontogenic infections. Participants had $18.5 \leq BMI \leq 25$. The subjects had not taken any drugs that could affect saliva secretion (mainly antidepressants or drugs for hypertension) or its redox status (vitamins, antioxidants) within 3 months prior to saliva collection, nor were they on any reducing diet. Patients and the controls who smoked tobacco or consumed any amount of alcohol or other stimulants were not included in the study. All the subjects in the control group had normal serum TSH, fT4, anti-TG and anti-TPO levels as well as thyroid imaging (homogenous parenchyma without nodules) on USG.

2.2. Blood Collection

A total of 10 mL of venous blood samples were collected in ethylenediaminetetraacetic acid (EDTA) tubes. The blood was then centrifuged 1500× g at 4 °C for 10 min. The acquired plasma was placed in Eppendorf tubes. The obtained erythrocyte mass was centrifuged three times in cold saline (0.9% NaCl) and then underwent osmotic lysis by adding a cold phosphate buffer (1:9, 50 mM, pH 7.4). In order to prevent sample oxidation and proteolysis, 10 µL 0.5 M BHT (butylated hydroxytoluene, BHT, Sigma-Aldrich, Germany) in acetonitrile was added per 1 mL of plasma and erythrocytes, and stored at −80 °C until assayed, but not for longer than 6 months.

Clinical details of patients and control subjects are presented in Table 1.

2.3. Saliva Collection

The assessment of the antioxidant barrier of saliva is complete when it includes analysis of both stimulated and unstimulated saliva. It has been shown that antioxidants produced by the parotid gland are aimed at combating deleterious foreign ROS that may penetrate oral cavity during eating, and antioxidants present in NWS for the rest of the time [22]. The studied material was non-stimulated (NWS) and stimulated (SWS) whole saliva collected via the spitting method. Participants were advised to refrain from consuming meals and drinks other than clean water, performing oral hygiene procedures for 2 h and taking any medications for 8 h before saliva collection. Saliva was collected between 8 a.m. and 10 a.m. to minimize the effect of daily changes on its secretion. The material was taken in a separate room so that patients did not feel uncomfortable or nervous. Participants had their saliva collected in a sitting position, with the head slightly inclined downwards, with minimized face and lip movements, upon a 5-min adaptation period. After that time, every patient rinsed their mouth three times with water at room temperature. The saliva collected during the first minute was discarded. Subsequent batches of saliva (the patient actively spat out the saliva accumulated in the bottom of the oral cavity) were collected into plastic centrifuge tubes placed in ice containers. The time of NWS collection was 15 min [15,16,22]. SWS was collected after a 5-min break, for 5 min. Its stimulation was triggered by dripping 100 µL 2% citric acid under the tongue every 20 s [23]. To avoid sample oxidation, 0.5 M BHT was added to the saliva (Sigma-Aldrich, Saint Louis, MO, USA; 10 µL/mL saliva) [24]. The volume of each sample was measured with a pipette calibrated to 0.1 mL. Saliva secretion was calculated by dividing the volume of the obtained saliva by the number of minutes of its collection. Then saliva was centrifuged (20 min, 4 °C, 10,000× g). Further tests were performed using the preserved supernatant fluid, which was frozen at −80 °C until assayed. Frozen samples were stored for no longer than 6 months.

Table 1. Clinical characteristics of the patients and control group.

Patients Variables	Control, $n = 45$ M (Min–Max)	HT, $n = 45$ M (Min–Max)	p
Age (years)	35 (29–43)	35 (29–43)	NS
BMI (kg/m^2)	19.25 (18.3–24.52)	23.15 (18.19–25.89)	NS
TSH (µU/mL)	1,99 (0.35–2.85)	2.85 (0.35–4.94)	NS
Free T4 (ng/mL)	1.2 (0.91–1.4)	1.1 (0.7–1.42)	NS
Free T3 (pg/mL)	2.56 (1.9–3.45)	2.4 (1.7–3.65)	NS
Anty TPO (IU/mL)	0.35 (0–2.1)	321.2 (108.25–652.1)	<0.0001
Anty TG (IU/mL)	0.32 (0–2.1)	153.8 (99.9–333.1)	<0.0001
PTH (pg/mL)	39.45 (10–62.2)	35.02 (15.51–63.56)	NS
Glucose (mg/dL)	86.37 (76.96–95.49)	84.11 (73.90–98.65)	NS
Euthyrox, n(%)	0	24 (53.3%)	

Abbreviations: HT—Hashimoto thyroiditis, C—control, BMI—body mass index, TSH—thyrotropic hormone, anty TPO—thyroid peroxidase antibody, anty TG—thyroid peroxidase antibody, PTH—parathyroid hormone.

2.4. Dental and Periodontal Examination

Dental examination was performed on the day of and immediately after saliva collection using a mirror, an explorer and a periodontal probe, in artificial light, by one calibrated dentist (K.M.). The study included dental evaluation, caries severity index (DMFT) as well as approximal plaque index (API), periodontal probing depth (PPD) and gingival index (GI). DMFT is an index that evaluates the condition of teeth, which consists in counting teeth with caries, removed due to caries or filled because of caries. GI is the assessment of the gingiva for possible inflammation. API is an index used to assess plaque located in interdental spaces. Finally, PPD is an index of the depth of probed gingival pockets. In 20 participants, the study was conducted by another experienced dentist (A. Z.) and the results were compared with those obtained by the head doctor (K. M.). The interrater reliability for DMFT was $r = 0.92$, for GI $r = 0.94$, for API $r = 0.98$ and for PPD $r = 100$.

2.5. Xerostomy Assessment and Schirmer Test

The women in both groups were asked to complete a questionnaire containing a list of symptoms associated with xerostomia and xerophthalmia listed in the American-European classification criteria for Sjögren's syndrome [15,24,25].

Tear secretion was assessed by the Schirmer I test from both eyes for over 5 min with no anesthesia used [26].

2.6. Selection of Patients and the Control Group Participants

Blood collection for the determination of hormones, antibodies and other clinical and oxidative stress parameters as well as ultrasound examination took place a day before saliva collection and dental examination, and included 70 patients and 70 control subjects. Based on the results of USG, thyroid hormone and TSH assays, the patients and the control group were qualified for further examinations (over 60 patients (10 patients had elevated TSH levels) and 59 control group participants (11 people from the control group had an abnormal ultrasound examination) were positively qualified for the experiment).

After the dental examination, 15 patients (PPD > 4 mm) and 5 control (gingival bleeding during probing) subjects were eliminated from the experiment due to the coexisting periodontal/gingival inflammation, and 9 additional participants were excluded from the control group as they did not match the other subjects in terms of BMI.

2.7. Biochemical Determinations: Salivary Amylase Activity and IL-1β Concentration

The salivary amylase activity (EC 3.2.1.1) was assessed spectrophotometrically using an alkaline solution of 3,5-dinitrosalicylic acid (DNS). The absorbance of samples was measured at 540 nm, accompanying the increased concentration of reducing sugars released during the hydrolysis of starch catalyzed by salivary amylase. Salivary amylase activity was determined in duplicate samples and expressed in μmol/mg protein [23].

Salivary interleukin 1β (IL-1β) concentration was determined by ELISA using a commercially available kit from EIAab Science Inc. Wuhan (Wuhan, China) in accordance with the manufacturer's instructions provided in the package.

2.8. Biochemical Determinations: Redox Assay

All analyses were performed in duplicate samples. Absorbance and fluorescence were measured with Infinite M200 PRO Multimode Tecan microplate reader. The results were standardized to 1 mg of total protein. The content of protein was evaluated by the bicinchoninic method (BCA) using a ready-made reagent kit (Thermo Scientific Pierce BCA Protein Assay Kit, Rockford, IL, USA) and a bovine serum albumin standard (BSA).

2.8.1. Enzymatic Antioxidants

The enzymatic antioxidant barrier was evaluated in saliva and erythrocyte samples by measuring the activity of SOD, CAT, Px and glutathione peroxidase (GPx).

Spectrophotometric evaluation of SOD activity (SOD, E.C. 1.15.1.1) was performed according to Misra and Fridovich [27], based on the adrenaline to adrenochrome oxidation rate. Absorbance measurements were taken at 480 nm wavelength.

Colorimetric measurement of CAT activity (CAT, E.C. 1.11.1.6) was based on the hydrogen peroxide degradation rate [28]. The unit of CAT activity (1 U) was determined as the amount of the enzyme decomposing 1 mmol H_2O_2 per minute. The measurements were performed at 240 nm wavelength.

The activity of Px (Px, E.C. 1.11.1.7) was determined colorimetrically according to the method by Mansson-Rahemtulla et al. [29] based on the reduction of 5,5'-dithiobis-(2-nitrobenzoic acid) (DTNB) to thionitrobenzoic acid at 412 nm wavelength.

The activity of GPx (GPx, E.C. 1.11.1.9) was measured spectrophotometrically using the Paglia and Valentine method [30], based on the reduction of organic peroxides in the presence of NADPH at 340 nm.

2.8.2. Non-Enzymatic Antioxidants

The non-enzymatic antioxidant barrier was assessed by measuring GSH and UA concentrations in NWS, SWS and plasma.

GSH concentration was determined colorimetrically based on the reaction with DTNB. Absorbance of the samples was measured at 412 nm wavelength [31].

UA concentration was determined spectrophotometrically at 490 nm using the ability of 2,4,6-Tris(2-pyridyl)-s-triazine to form a blue complex with iron ions in the presence of UA. We used a commercial set of reagents (QuantiChrom^{TM} Uric Acid Assay Kit DIUA-250; BioAssay Systems, Hayward, CA, USA).

Total antioxidant capacity (TAC) level in plasma was determined spectrophotometrically at 660 nm wavelength using 2,2′-azino-bis(3-ethylbenzothiazoline-6-sulphonic acid) (ATBS). The intensity of the color resulting from the reaction of ABTS radical cation was proportional to the content of antioxidants in the tested samples [32].

2.8.3. Total Oxidant Status (TOS) and Oxidative Stress Index (OSI)

TOS and OSI levels were determined in NWS, SWS and plasma.

TOS level was assayed bichromatically (560/800 nm) based on the oxidation of Fe_{2+} to Fe_{3+} in the sample. TOS level was calculated from the standard curve for H_2O^2 [33].

OSI was calculated based on the formula OSI = (TOS/TAC)/100 [34].

2.8.4. Oxidative Damage to Proteins and Lipids

Oxidative damage to proteins and lipids was assessed by measuring the concentration of advanced glycation end products (AGE) of proteins, advanced oxidation protein products (AOPP), lipid hydroperoxides (LOOH) and malondialdehyde (MDA) in saliva and plasma samples.

AGE content was assessed by measuring AGE-specific fluorescence at 350/440 nm wavelength, as described by Kalousová et al. [35].

The colorimetric measurement of AOPP content was determined fluorimetrically as described by Kalousová et al. [35] based on the oxidative capacity of iodine ions at 340 nm wavelength.

To measure AGE and AOPP concentrations, NWS, SWS and plasma samples were diluted with phosphate-buffered saline (PBS, pH 7.2) at a ratio of 1:5 (v/v).

The concentration of LOOH was evaluated spectrophotometrically from the reaction of iron ions (3+) with xylenol orange (XO). The absorbance of Fe-XO complex was measured at 560 nm wavelength [36].

MDA concentration was assessed colorimetrically based on the reaction with thiobarbituric acid (TBA) at 535 nm wavelength. 1,1,3,3-Tetraethoxypropane was used as a standard [24].

2.9. Statistical Analysis

Statistical analysis was performed using GraphPad Prism 8.3.0 for MacOS (GraphPad Software, Inc. La Jolla, CA, USA). The distribution of the obtained results was assessed using the Shapiro–Wilk test. Due to the lack of normal distribution, the Mann–Whitney U test was used for quantitative comparisons. Chi-square test with Yates's modification was used to analyze the differences in the prevalence of qualitative variables. Correlations of the results were assessed using the Spearman rank correlation coefficient. The statistical significance level was set at $p < 0.05$.

The number of subjects was determined based on our previous experiment, assuming that the power of the test would be equal to 0.9 (ClinCalc sample size calculator).

3. Results

3.1. Clinical Data

Saliva secretion in the group of HT patients was 32% lower than in the control group ($p = 0.02$). None of the patients had the rate of unstimulated saliva secretion below 0.1 mL/min. Moreover, stimulated saliva secretion did not differ between the groups. The concentration of total protein in unstimulated and stimulated saliva of HT patients was significantly higher than in the control group (↑46%, $p = 0.00002$ and ↑16%, $p = 0.0003$, respectively). Salivary amylase activity was considerably lower in NWS (↓50%, $p = 0.00001$) and SWS (↓114%, $p = 0.00001$) of HT patients compared to the controls (Table 2).

Table 2. Salivary gland function and dental indices of the patients and the control group.

Clinical Parameters	Control			HT			p
	Median	Minimum	Maximum	Median	Minimum	Maximum	
NWS mL/min	0.51	0.27	0.96	0.32	0.07	0.77	0.02
SWS mL/min	1.01	0.9	2	0.9	0.2	2	ns
TP NWS (mg/mL)	704.2	556.5	924.5	1293	979.4	1707	<0.0001
TP SWS (mg/mL)	1545	371.3	1672	1834	266.6	3861	<0.0001
Salivary amylase NWS (μmol/mg protein)	0.22	0.18	0.28	0.11	0.09	0.15	<0.0001
Salivary amylase SWS (μmol/mg protein)	0.3	0.19	0.38	0.14	0.1	0.16	<0.0001
Salivary IL-1β NWS (pg/mg protein)	0.91	0.27	2	2	0.4	3	<0.0001
Salivary IL-1β SWS (pg/mg)	5.1	2.7	6.8	7.8	4	12	<0.0001
Schirmer- I test (mm/5 min) Left eye Right eye	21 25	10 11	28 30	19 20	12 9	23 30	ns
Subjective dryness n (%) Xerostomiaxerophtalmia	1(2.22) 3(6.67)			26(57.7) 3(6.67)			0.003 ns
DMFT	15	0	25	16	3	28	ns
API	41.85	0	100	54.5	8.3	100	ns
GI	1	0	2	1	0	2	ns
PPD (mm)	1.898	1.14	2.55	1.99	1.33	3.64	ns

NWS—unstimulated saliva, SWS—stimulated saliva, TP—total protein, DMFT—decay, missing, filling teeth, API—approximal plaque index, GI—gingival index, PPD—periodontal pocket depth, ns—non-statistically important.

IL-1β concentration in NWS and SWS of patients with HT was significantly higher compared to the controls (↑119%, $p = 0.00001$ and, ↑52%, $p = 0.00002$, respectively).

Oral dryness was more prevalent in HT women than in healthy controls ($p = 0.003$). The prevalence of eye dryness was similar in both examined groups.

The median value of Schirmer I test for the left and right eye did not differ between the groups.

The analysis of dental data showed no differences in DMFT, API, GI and PPD between the study and the control group (Table 2).

3.2. Antioxidant Defense Parameters

3.2.1. NWS

SOD activity as well as the levels of GSH, UA and TAC (Figure 1) in NWS of HT patients were significantly lower than those in NWS of control patients (↓10%, $p = 0.03$; ↓28%, $p = 0.00003$; ↓38%, $p = 0.00003$; ↓34%, $p = 0.00005$, respectively). CAT and Px activities in NWS of HT patients were notably higher compared to those parameters found in NWS of the control group (↑66%, $p = 0.00002$; ↑66%, $p = 0.00003$, respectively) (Figure 1).

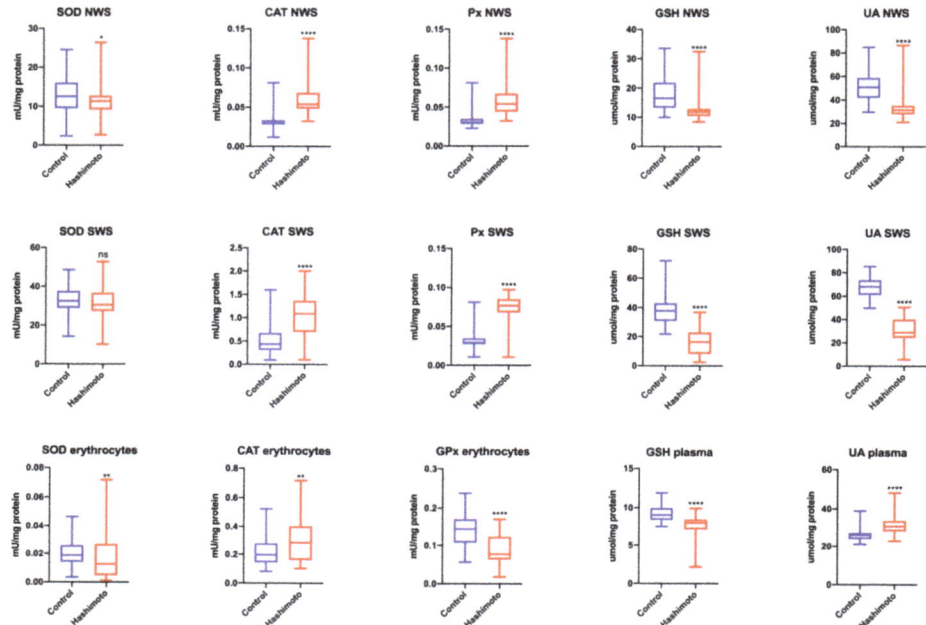

Figure 1. Enzymatic and nonenzymatic antioxidants in NWS, SWS and blood plasma/erythrocytes of the patients and control group. Data are shown as median (minimum–maximum). CAT—catalase; GPx—glutathione peroxidase; GSH—reduced glutathione; NWS—non-stimulated whole saliva; Px—salivary peroxidase; SOD—superoxide dismutase-1; SWS—stimulated whole saliva; UA—uric acid. * $p < 0.05$, ** $p < 0.01$, and **** $p < 0.0001$.

3.2.2. SWS

GSH, UA and TAC (Figure 2) concentrations in NWS of HT patients were significantly lower than in NWS of healthy controls (↓57%, $p = 0.000003$; ↓58%, $p = 0.00001$; ↓53%, $p = 0.00001$, respectively). CAT and Px activities in NWS of HT patients were considerably higher than in NWS of the control group (↑147%, $p = 0.00002$; ↑166%, $p = 0.00003$, respectively) (Figure 1).

3.2.3. Erythrocytes, Plasma

SOD and GPx activities in blood erythrocytes as well as GSH and TAC plasma concentrations (Figure 2) in HT patients were significantly lower than the discussed parameters in the erythrocytes and plasma of the control group (↓50%, $p = 0.009$; ↓45%, $p = 0.00001$; ↓13%, $p = 0.001$; ↓82%, $p = 0.00001$, respectively) (Figure 1).

3.2.4. TOS and OSI

We observed significantly increased values of TOS and OSI in NWS (↑81%, $p = 0.00001$; ↑191%, $p = 0.000001$, respectively), SWS (↑201%, $p = 0.00001$; ↑588%, $p = 0.000001$, respectively) and plasma (↑76%, $p = 0.00001$; ↑158%, $p = 0.000001$, respectively) of HT patients compared to the control group (Figure 2).

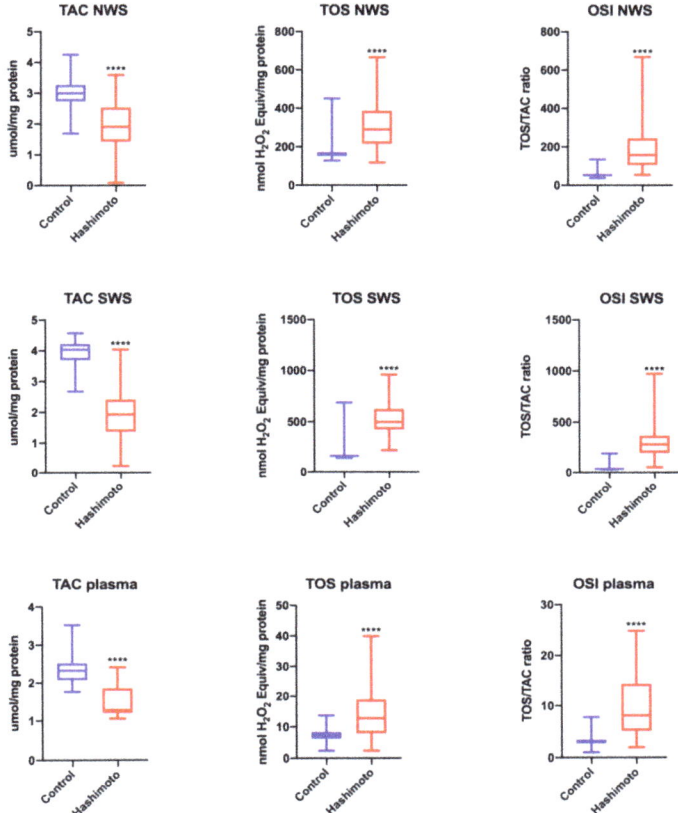

Figure 2. Redox status in NWS, SWS and plasma of the patients and control group. Data are shown as median (minimum–maximum). OSI—oxidative stress index; NWS—non-stimulated whole saliva; SWS—stimulated whole saliva; TAC—total antioxidant capacity; TOS— total oxidant status. **** $p < 0.0001$.

3.2.5. Products of Oxidative Modifications

The concentrations of all the evaluated products of oxidative modifications: AGE, AOPP, LOOH and MDA were considerably higher in NWS (↑80%, $p = 0.00001$; ↑232%, $p = 0.00002$; ↑91%, $p = 0.00001$; ↑194%, $p = 0.00001$, respectively), SWS (↑97%, $p = 0.00001$; ↑476%, $p = 0.00001$; ↑46%, $p = 0.00001$; ↑96%, $p = 0.00001$, respectively) and plasma (↑3%, $p = 0.0007$; ↑31%, $p = 0.0003$; ↑77%, $p = 0.00001$; ↑42%, $p = 0.00001$, respectively) of HT patients compared to the values of these parameters obtained in the control group (Figure 3).

3.2.6. Comparison of Antioxidants and Redox Balance Markers between NWS and SWS

Control

We observed significantly higher activity of SOD, CAT, Px ($p < 0.0001$, $p < 0.0001$, $p < 0.0001$, respectively) and GSH, UA, TAC, OSI, AOPP, LOOH and MDA ($p < 0.0001$, $p < 0.0001$, $p < 0.0001$, $p < 0.0001$, $p < 0.0001$, $p < 0.0001$, $p < 0.0001$, respectively) concentration in SWS vs. NWS of the control women.

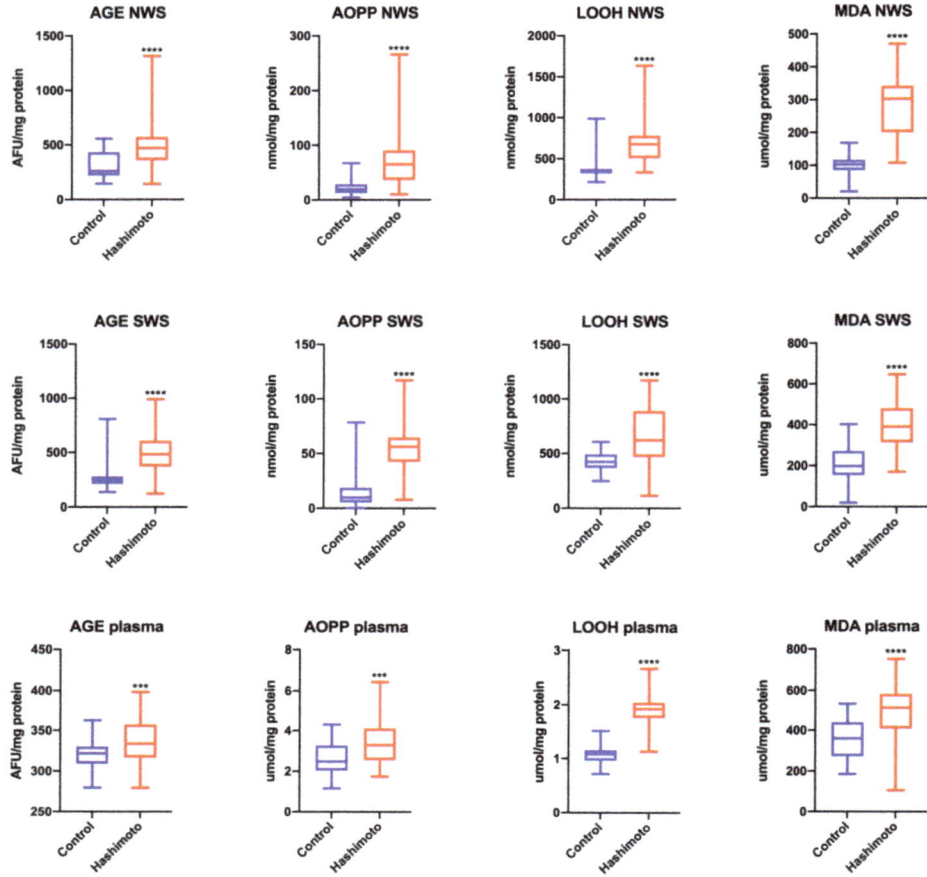

Figure 3. Oxidative damage in NWS, SWS and plasma of the patients and control group. Data are shown as median (minimum–maximum). AGE—advanced glycation end products; AOPP—advanced oxidation protein products; LOOH—lipid hydroperoxides; MDA—malondialdehyde; NWS—non-stimulated whole saliva; SWS—stimulated whole saliva. *** $p < 0.001$, and **** $p < 0.0001$.

HT Women

The activity of SOD, CAT, Px ($p < 0.0001$, $p < 0.0001$, $p < 0.0001$, respectively) and GSH, TOS, OSI and MDA ($p = 0.025$, $p < 0.0001$, $p < 0.0001$, $p < 0.0001$, respectively) concentrations were significantly higher in SWS compared to NWS of HT women (Table 3).

3.2.7. Saliva–Blood Ratio

NWS

CAT, Px, AGE AOPP, MDA ($p = 0.01$, $p < 0.0001$, $p < 0.0001$, $p < 0.0001$, $p < 0.0001$, respectively) salivary/blood ratio was significantly higher in NWS of HT women vs. control, while GSH and UA ($p = 0.0009$, $p < 0.0001$) salivary/blood ratio was significantly lower in NWS of HT women vs. control.

Table 3. Comparison of NWS to SWS.

Redox Parameters	Control							HT						
	NWS			SWS			p	NWS			SWS			p
	Median	Minimum	Maximum	Median	Minimum	Maximum		Median	Minimum	Maximum	Median	Minimum	Maximum	
SOD	12.63	2.439	24.6	32.67	14.42	48.69	<0.0001	11.38	2.746	26.41	30.61	10.28	52.8	<0.0001
CAT	0.0306	0.0121	0.0815	0.4379	0.1	1.603	<0.0001	0.0544	0.0326	0.1381	1.094	0.1058	2.006	<0.0001
Px	0.031	0.0234	0.0815	0.4379	0.1	1.603	<0.0001	0.0545	0.0326	0.1381	1.094	0.1058	2.006	<0.0001
GSH	16.61	10.09	33.62	37.94	21.98	72.11	<0.0001	11.94	8.543	32.52	16.52	2.634	36.96	0.0258
UA	51.12	29.86	85.09	68.21	50.05	85.52	<0.0001	31.53	21.19	86.65	28.98	5.787	50.67	ns
TAC	2.997	1.695	4.258	4.038	2.677	4.578	<0.0001	1.909	0.0935	3.594	1.934	0.2413	4.044	ns
TOS	160.3	129.1	451.2	165.4	147.2	689.9	ns	290.1	118.7	666.8	499.2	223.6	961.4	<0.0001
OSI	54.48	39.2	136.5	41.24	34.02	196.7	<0.0001	158.5	54.79	669.8	284	55.28	973.4	<0.0001
AGE	261.6	146.4	558.1	244.5	138.5	807.9	ns	471	143.2	1314	482.9	122	989.2	ns
AOPP	19.55	4.569	67.25	9.754	0.1632	78.37	<0.0001	65.01	10.37	265.8	56.21	7.779	117	ns
LOOH	352	218.1	989.5	424.5	249.6	607.5	<0.0001	675.2	334.4	1635	622.2	114.3	1172	ns
MDA	102.6	20.49	168.2	198.4	20.46	402.8	<0.0001	302.6	107.6	469.9	390.1	170.2	647.3	<0.0001

AGE—advanced glycation end products; AOPP—advanced oxidation protein products; AUC—area under the curve; CAT—catalase; GPx—glutathione peroxidase; GSH—reduced glutathione; LOOH—lipid hydroperoxides; MDA—malondialdehyde; NWS—non-stimulated whole saliva; OSI—oxidative stress index; Px—salivary peroxidase; ROS—reactive oxygen species; SOD—superoxide dismutase; SWS—stimulated whole saliva; TAC—total antioxidant capacity; TOS—total oxidant status; UA—uric acid.

SWS

CAT, Px, TOS, OSI, AGE, AOPP and MDA ($p = 0.005$, $p < 0.0001$, $p < 0.0001$, $p < 0.0001$, $p < 0.0001$, $p < 0.0001$, $p < 0.0001$, $p = 0.002$, respectively) salivary/blood ratio was significantly higher in SWS of HT women vs. control, while GSH, UA, TAC and LOOH ($p < 0.0001$, $p < 0.0001$, $p < 0.0001$, $p = 0.01$, respectively) salivary/blood ratio was significantly lower in SWS of HT women vs. control (Table 4).

Table 4. Saliva to blood ratio.

Salivary/Blood Ratio	Control			HT			p
	Median	Minimum	Maximum	Median	Minimum	Maximum	
SOD NWS	655.6	145.7	3580	816.4	113.1	10,113	ns
SOD SWS	1625	396.1	10,721	2312	414.4	29,459	ns
CAT NWS	0.1582	0.0411	0.8706	0.2144	0.0501	0.8531	0.0115
CAT SWS	1.988	0.3915	10.61	3.337	0.3794	14.38	0.0053
Px NWS	0.2378	0.1272	0.9917	0.6863	0.2076	4.777	<0.0001
Px SWS	3.186	0.6492	18.57	11.55	1.403	71.15	<0.0001
GSH NWS	1.819	0.9336	3.613	1.464	0.9591	8.705	0.0009
GSH SWS	4.051	2.369	9.534	2.216	0.5282	3.961	<0.0001
UA NWS	1.973	1.002	2.763	1.034	0.6256	2.508	<0.0001
UA SWS	2.525	1.851	3.556	0.9855	0.2191	1.775	<0.0001
TAC NWS	1.246	0.8213	2.401	1.356	0.0647	2.665	ns
TAC SWS	1.728	0.9485	2.466	1.268	0.1385	2.794	<0.0001
TOS NWS	22.5	11.08	54.29	23.78	6.919	161.5	ns
TOS SWS	23.61	11.63	100.9	38.81	9.852	155.5	<0.0001
OSI NWS	18.33	7.485	43.07	15.68	3.368	184	ns
OSI SWS	13.77	7.244	54	30.15	6.401	429.8	<0.0001
AGE NWS	0.8406	0.4666	1.786	1.366	0.4045	4.279	<0.0001
AGE SWS	0.761	0.4457	2.84	1.434	0.3307	3.133	<0.0001
AOPP NWS	7.951	1.338	31	18.88	2.203	69.16	<0.0001
AOPP SWS	3.725	0.0983	29.82	16.57	1.595	36.84	<0.0001
LOOH NWS	327.5	214.4	1255	334.5	177.6	805.8	ns
LOOH SWS	419.4	249.7	677	341.4	65.17	637	0.0135
MDA NWS	0.2532	0.0631	0.6355	0.5392	0.2124	3.402	<0.0001
MDA SWS	0.5698	0.0548	1.38	0.8321	0.2707	3.756	0.0024

AGE—advanced glycation end products; AOPP—advanced oxidation protein products; AUC—area under the curve; CAT—catalase; GPx—glutathione peroxidase; GSH—reduced glutathione; LOOH—lipid hydroperoxides; MDA—malondialdehyde; NWS—non-stimulated whole saliva; OSI—oxidative stress index; Px—salivary peroxidase; ROS—reactive oxygen species; SOD—superoxide dismutase; SWS—stimulated whole saliva; TAC—total antioxidant capacity; TOS—total oxidant status; UA—uric acid.

3.2.8. Correlations

In the study group we demonstrated a negative correlation between the plasma concentrations of anti-TPO antibodies and GSH ($r = -0.854$, $p < 0.0001$). We also observed a negative correlation between TAC in NWS ($r = -0.704$, $p < 0.0001$) and SWS ($r = -0.759$, $p < 0.0001$) and serum concentration of anti-TPO.

We also found a positive correlation between MDA in NWS and thyroglobulin antibodies (r = 0.851, $p < 0.0001$) as well as between LOOH in SWS and anti-TG (r = 0.839, $p < 0.0001$).

We showed a negative correlation between SOD activity in SWS and plasma glucose concentration ($r = -0.851$, $p < 0.0001$) in the HT group.

In the study group we found a negative correlation between GSH and AOPP concentrations in SWS ($r = -0.730$, $p < 0.0001$). Moreover, IL-1β correlated positively with LOOH concentrations (r = 0.886, $p < 0.0001$) and negatively with GSH levels in SWS ($r = -0.849$, $p < 0.0001$).

The minute flow of unstimulated saliva correlated negatively with IL-1β concentration in NWS ($r = -0.891$, $p < 0.0001$). We also observed a negative correlation between salivary α-amylase activity and TOS in NWS ($r = -0.8$, $p < 0.0001$). The remaining correlations were included in the supplementary materials.

4. Discussion

In the presented experiment we employed a wide range of biochemical assays to search for a link between OS expressed as antioxidant activity/concentration and oxidative damage products and salivary gland function in patients with HT in euthyreosis. To the best of our knowledge, this study is the first to assess the function of salivary glands and their redox balance in patients with HT in euthyreosis.

OS is the result of an imbalance between ROS production and neutralization, which leads to oxidative damage to tissues. In the case of autoimmune thyroiditis, OS is considered to be the result of a deficiency of thyroid hormones as well as autoimmunity and the associated inflammation. During the synthesis of thyroid hormones, iodine is oxidized by nicotinamide adenine dinucleotide phosphate oxidase (NOX). Hydrogen peroxide (H_2O_2) formed in this reaction is used for the production of thyroid hormones [37]. Excess of H_2O_2, e.g., due to excessive iodine substitution or deficiency of glutathione peroxidase (GPx, an enzyme involved in the neutralization of hydrogen peroxide and protecting thyroid tissue from oxidative damage), leads to apoptosis and necrosis of thyrocytes. Interestingly, in the presented study we demonstrated a 45% decrease of GPx activity in blood erythrocytes of HT patients, which, in our opinion, largely contributes to the observed increase in the generation of oxygen free radicals (↑76% TOS in serum). In the situation of increased concentration of ROS, particularly H_2O_2, increased immunogenicity of thyroid specific antigens (thyroglobulin and thyroid peroxidase) and intensified intercellular adhesion molecule-1 (ICAM-1) expression are observed, which results in increased generation of antibodies and autoimmune response as well as raises in inflammation [38]. The latter, in turn, directly increases H_2O_2 in thyroid epithelial cells and activates NOX in T and B lymphocytes, which further boosts ROS production [3].

The existence and extent of OS can be assessed based on the behavior of numerous biomarkers, including the measurement of the concentration/activity of antioxidants as well as the evaluation of the concentrations of oxidative modification products [39]. In our research, we used a wide panel of biomarkers of oxidative stress, because there is a belief that a single parameter does not reflect the size and severity of the OS phenomenon [40]. The parameters helpful in the assessment of OS are also total antioxidant capacity (TAC), total oxidative status (TOS) and oxidative stress index (OSI) [41]. It has been evidenced that TAC expresses the efficiency of both enzymatic and non-enzymatic antioxidant defense mechanisms, whereas TOS is the sum of all oxidants present in the sample. OSI illustrates the relationship between antioxidant mechanisms and oxidative molecules [42].

Our results showed a decrease in antioxidant potential (82%↓TAC) and increased production of free radicals as well as all products of oxidative modifications in the serum of patients with HT in euthyreosis compared to the controls, which confirms a shift in the redox balance towards oxidation and the existence of general OS. Decreased concentration of GSH deserves special attention as the reduction of GSH concentration is considered a causative factor in the development of autoimmune diseases by inhibition of IL-1 and T-cell receptor-mediated transduction signaling [1]. Increased concentration of GSH has been evidenced to be the result of GSH use through oxidation, conjugation or extrusion from the cell, and indicates highly raised OS [40]. Interestingly, we demonstrated a negative correlation between anti-TPO antibody and GSH concentrations, which is consistent with the results of Rostami et al. [2]. According to these authors, their findings prove that the presence of antibodies is a causative factor for excessive ROS production and that GSH is capable of inhibiting complement-mediated damage in HT. They also presume that GSH deficiency may indicate the occurrence of processes leading to oxidative stress activation and the development of immune intolerance.

Interestingly, changes in the salivary redox balance seem to reflect those observed in the blood, but it should be noted that the changes in saliva are more intense. Only for UA we see different directionality. Its reduced salivary concentration in patients with HT vs. control suggests that in the oral cavity UA behaves as an antioxidant. It has been shown, that the increased concentration of UA, that we observe in the serum of patients with HT, shifts the redox balance towards the oxidation reaction and OS and may be a factor predisposing to cardiovascular diseases [43]. Moreover, the performed analyses did not reveal any correlation between the redox balance parameters in blood and saliva. The lack of correlation and saliva/blood ratio analysis may suggest that oxidative stress in the salivary glands is independent of general oxidative stress in the course of HT. What's more, the higher saliva/blood ratio with respect to some of the parameters studied, in the HT women group compared to the control, indicates that the observed changes are the result of processes occurring in the salivary glands, and are not the result of their passive blood transitions.

The large salivary glands together produce about 90% of the total saliva volume. The largest of them—the parotid gland—produces saliva mainly in response to the applied stimulation, hence any changes in stimulated saliva composition and amount are considered to reflect the function of the parotid gland. At rest, 2/3 of the total saliva amount is produced by the submandibular glands. Therefore, any variations in the composition and amount of NWS reflect the functioning of the latter glands [44,45].

Our study demonstrated a reduction in the antioxidant potential of parotid and submandibular salivary glands, confirmed by a 34% decrease in TAC in NWS and a 53% decrease in TAC in SWS, which manifests the inefficiency of antioxidant systems of these glands to eradicate ROS. Although we observed significantly increased CAT and Px activities in NWS and SWS, which may—to some extent—prove an adaptive mechanism of the salivary glands in response to excessive ROS production and be of great importance to oral health. Px and CAT maintain concentration salivary H_2O_2 at a level 8 to 14 µM [46], which is non-toxic to oral fibroblasts [47] and epithelial cells [48].

In the euthyreosis status in the course of HT, the causes of reduced antioxidant response should be seen as a result of depletion of the resources in the process of ROS neutralization or of the oxidative modification of polypeptide chains rather than as a result of decreased synthesis caused by reduced production of thyroid hormones. The impaired antioxidant defense may also be caused by non-enzymatic glycation of these enzymes, which explains the negative correlation between SOD activity in SWS and plasma glucose concentration in HT group [49], despite the fact that diabetes as well as insulin resistance were excluded in HT patients. Moreover, the negative correlation between TAC in NWS and SWS and the serum concentration of anti-TPO as well as between GSH and IL-1β concentrations in SWS confirm that the exhaustion of antioxidant sources in salivary glands is related to an elevated oxidative stress level due to autoimmunity-related inflammation and that increased concentration of autoimmune antibodies is a key factor for the enhancement of ROS production.

As our results show, the impaired saliva antioxidant barrier results in an increase in oxidative modifications of salivary proteins and lipids. So it is advisable to use exogenous antioxidants supporting endogenous antioxidant mechanisms. The results of our study revealed a significantly greater percentage increase in the concentration of TOS and OSI in SWS (↑201% and ↑588%, respectively) compared to NWS (↑81% and ↑191%, respectively) in HT female patients. A significant reduction of GSH concentration in SWS (↓57%) vs. NWS (↓23%) in HT women as well as a negative correlation between AOPP and GSH levels in SWS may be helpful in understanding the intensification of oxidative modifications to proteins in the parotid vs. submandibular salivary glands. It has been evidenced that the main role of GSH is in maintaining thiol groups of proteins at a reduced level, i.e., protecting proteins against oxidation [50,51]. We also found a positive correlation between MDA in NWS and anti-TG, LOOH in SWS as well as between anti-TG and LOOH in SWS and IL-1β concentration in SWS, which proves that oxidative damage to the lipids contained in salivary glands is boosted with an increase in autoimmunity-related inflammation in the course of HT.

The main physiological difference between the parotid and submandibular saliva is the fact that the former type of saliva is secreted mainly during eating, whereas the latter type is produced continuously and is responsible for maintaining the integrity of oral structures [22]. Maintaining the appropriate rate of both types of secretion is therefore equally important for the functioning of the body. Despite a higher intensity of OS and a more pronounced decrease in antioxidant defense in the parotid glands, the rate of stimulated saliva secretion did not differ significantly between the groups. However, our study demonstrated that HT patients lose the unstimulated salivary gland function. The median values of NWS and SWS secretion were within the standard limits assumed for proper saliva secretion. It is noteworthy that in 15 patients, NWS secretion was lower than 0.2 mL/min (but higher than 0.1 mL/min) and 5 HT group patients secreted stimulated saliva at a level lower than 0.7 mL/min, which proves the developed salivary gland failure in these patients, referred to as hyposalivation, and explains the significant intensification of subjective symptoms of reduced saliva secretion reported when completing the survey on a dry mouth. The performed analyses excluded Sjögren's syndrome, but, to be 100% certain, a biopsy of the salivary glands would be advisable. However, we were not granted permission for its performance from the Bioethics Committee. Evidence showed that proinflammatory cytokines, including the evaluated IL-1β, induce the activity of metalloproteinases, which leads to changes in the basement membrane of the salivary glands and the structure of receptors for neurotransmitters associated with saliva secretion [52]. A higher increase in IL-1β concentration in NWS (↑119%) vs. SWS (↑52%) as well as in the observed relationship between NWS and IL-1β concentration may confirm the destruction of acinar cell-basement membrane interaction by excessive production of MMPs followed by a decreased number of secretory units (acini and ducts) [53,54]. It has also been demonstrated that the presence of IL-β in the inflamed environment may inhibit the release of acetylcholine from the residual nerves, resulting in reduced saliva secretion [13,14,55]. The described phenomenon of extracellular matrix remodeling has been demonstrated as a cause of reduced saliva secretion in Sjögren's syndrome patients [56] and reduced activity of muscarinic neurotransmitters/receptors in the submandibular glands of diabetic patients [55].

Changes in salivary amylase activity are considered a determinant of sympathetic nervous system (SNS) activity. The stimulation of β-adrenergic receptor activity results in increased production/secretion and activity of salivary α-amylase and other salivary proteins [57]. In our study, we observed decreased salivary α-amylase activity with a simultaneous increase in protein concentration in both SWS and NWS, which could suggest a higher activity of this branch of autonomic nervous system. The negative correlation between salivary α-amylase activity and TOS in NWS may suggest that lowered activity of salivary α-amylase results from the use of this enzyme in the elimination of excessive amounts of ROS (↑TOS) or, more likely, from the oxidative modification of its polypeptide chain, leading to a loss of/significant reduction in enzymatic activity.

One of the limitations of this paper is the fact of determining only some parameters characterizing the redox balance. Perhaps the use of other biomarkers would change the results and conclusions, which of course can be considered a weak point of this experiment.

5. Conclusions

(1) Parotid as well as submandibular salivary glands of HT female patients in euthyreosis had an impaired ability to maintain the redox status at the level observed in the salivary glands of the control women.
(2) The saliva of patients with HT in euthyreosis demonstrated a reduced antioxidant potential. Moreover, a significant increase in oxidatively modified molecules in NWS and SWS suggests the failure of the salivary gland antioxidant barrier to combat excess ROS production.
(3) OS in NWS and SWS of HT women appears to be closely connected with autoimmunity-related inflammation, and not with the level of thyroid hormones or TSH.
(4) The secretory function of the submandibular glands of HT female patients in euthyreosis is decreased, which is manifested as a significant reduction of unstimulated saliva secretion.

Supplementary Materials: The following are available online at http://www.mdpi.com/2077-0383/9/7/2102/s1, Table S1: Spearman r coeficient of variables, Table S2: p value of correlations.

Author Contributions: Conceptualization, A.Z., M.M. and K.M.; Data curation, A.Z., M.M. and K.M.; Formal analysis, A.Z., M.M. and K.M.; Funding acquisition, A.Z. and M.M.; Investigation, K.M., A.Z. and M.M.; Methodology, A.Z., M.M. and K.M.; Material collection, K.M., Ł.P. and A.P.-K.; Supervision, A.Z., A.P.-K. and A.K.; Validation, A.Z. and M.M.; Visualization, A.Z. and M.M.; Writing—original draft, K.M., A.Z. and M.M.; Writing—review and editing, K.M., A.Z. and M.M. All authors have read and agreed to the published version of the manuscript.

Funding: This work was supported by the Medical University of Bialystok, Poland (grant number: SUB/1/DN/20/002/1209). Mateusz Maciejczyk, was supported by the Foundation for Polish Science (FNP).

Conflicts of Interest: The authors declare no conflict of interest.

References

1. Rose, N.R.; Bonita, R.; Burek, C.L. Iodine: An environmental trigger of thyroiditis. *Autoimmun Rev.* **2002**, *1*, 97–103. [CrossRef]
2. Rostami, R.; Aghasi, M.R.; Mohammadi, A.; Nourooz-Zadeh, J. Enhanced oxidative stress in Hashimoto's thyroiditis: Inter-relationships to biomarkers of thyroid function. *Clin. Biochem.* **2013**, *46*, 308–312. [CrossRef] [PubMed]
3. Ates, I.; Yilmaz, F.M.; Altay, M.; Yilmaz, N.; Berker, D.; Guler, S. The relationship between oxidative stress and autoimmunity in Hashimoto's thyroiditis. *Eur. J. Endocrinol* **2015**, *173*, 791–799. [CrossRef]
4. Ates, I.; Arikan, M.F.; Altay, M.; Yilmaz, F.M.; Yilmaz, N.; Berker, D.; Guler, S. The effect of oxidative stress on the progression of Hashimoto's thyroiditis. *Arch. Physiol. Biochem.* **2018**, *124*, 351–356. [CrossRef]
5. Knaś, M.; Maciejczyk, M.; Waszkiel, D.; Zalewska, A. Oxidative stress and salivary antioxidants. *Dent. Med. Probl.* **2013**, *50*, 461–466.
6. Lassoued, S.; Mseddi, M.; Mnif, F.; Abid, M.; Guermazi, F.; Masmoudi, H.; El Feki, A.; Attia, H. A comparative study of the oxidative profile in Graves' disease, Hashimoto's thyroiditis, and papillary thyroid cancer. *Biol. Trace Elem. Res.* **2010**, *138*, 107–115. [CrossRef]
7. Nanda, N.; Bobby, Z.; Hamide, A. Oxidative stress in anti thyroperoxidase antibody positive hypothyroid patients. *Asian J. Biochem.* **2012**, *7*, 54–58.
8. Agha-Hosseini, F.; Shirzad, N.; Moosavi, M.S. Evaluation of Xerostomia and salivary flow rate in Hashimoto's Thyroiditis. *Med. Oral Patol. Oral Cir. Bucal* **2016**, *21*, e1–e5. [CrossRef] [PubMed]
9. Toczewska, J.; Konopka, T.; Zalewska, A.; Maciejczyk, M. Nitrosative stress biomarkers in the non-stimulated and stimulated saliva, as well as gingival crevicular fluid of patients with periodontitis: Review and clinical study. *Antioxidants* **2020**, *9*, 259. [CrossRef]
10. Toczewska, J.; Konopka, T. Activity of enzymatic antioxidants in periodontitis: A systematic overview of the literature. *Dent. Med. Probl.* **2019**, *56*, 419–426. [CrossRef]
11. Darczuk, D.; Krzyściak, W.; Bystrowska, B.; Kęsek, B.; Kościelniak, D.; Chomyszyn-Gajewska, M.; Kaczmarzyk, T. The relationship between the concentration of salivary tyrosine and antioxidants in patients with oral lichen planus. *Oxid. Med. Cell Longev.* **2019**, *2019*, 5801570. [CrossRef] [PubMed]
12. Babiuch, K.; Bednarczyk, A.; Gawlik, K.; Pawlica-Gosiewska, D.; Kęsek, B.; Darczuk, D.; Stępień, P.; Chomyszyn-Gajewska, M.; Kaczmarzyk, T. Evaluation of enzymatic and non-enzymatic antioxidant status and biomarkers of oxidative stress in saliva of patients with oral squamous cell carcinoma and oral leukoplakia: A pilot study. *Acta Odont. Scand.* **2019**, *77*, 408–418. [CrossRef] [PubMed]
13. Skutnik-Radziszewska, A.; Maciejczyk, M.; Flisiak, I.; Kolodziej, J.K.U.; Kotowska-Rodziewicz, A.; Klimiuk, A.; Zalewska, A. Enhanced inflammation and nitrosative stress in the saliva and plasma of patients with plaque psoriasis. *J. Clin. Med.* **2020**, *9*, 745. [CrossRef]
14. Skutnik-Radziszewska, A.; Maciejczyk, M.; Fejfer, K.; Krahel, J.; Flisiak, I.; Kołodziej, U.; Zalewska, A. Salivary antioxidants and oxidative stress in psoriatic patients: Can salivary total oxidant status and oxidative stress index be a plaque psoriasis biomarker? *Oxid. Med. Cell Longev.* **2020**, *2020*, 9086024. [CrossRef] [PubMed]
15. Zalewska, A.; Knaś, M.; Waszkiewicz, N.; Waszkiel, D.; Sierakowski, S.; Zwierz, K. Rheumatoid arthritis patients with xerostomia have reduced production of key salivary constituents. *Oral Surg. Oral Med. Oral Pathol.* **2013**, *115*, 483–490. [CrossRef] [PubMed]

16. Zalewska, A.; Knaś, M.; Waszkiewicz, N.; Klimiuk, A.; Litwin, K.; Sierakowski, S.; Waszkiel, D. Salivary antioxidants in patients with systemic sclerosis. *J. Oral Pathol. Med.* **2014**, *43*, 61–68. [CrossRef]
17. Zalewska, A.; Knaś, M.; Kuźmiuk, A.; Waszkiewicz, N.; Niczyporuk, M.; Waszkiel, D.; Zwierz, K. Salivary innate defense system in type 1 diabetes mellitus in children with mixed and permanent dentition. *Acta Odont. Scand.* **2013**, *71*, 1493–1500. [CrossRef]
18. Norheim, K.B.; Jonsson, G.; Harboe, E.; Hanasand, M.; Gøransson, L.; Omdal, R. Oxidative stress, as measured by protein oxidation, is increased in primary Sjøgren's syndrome. *Free Radic. Res.* **2012**, *46*, 141–146. [CrossRef]
19. Karlík, M.; Valkovič, P.; Hančinová, V.; Krížová, L.; Tóthová, L'.; Celec, P. Markers of oxidative stress in plasma and saliva in patients with multiple sclerosis. *Clin. Biochem.* **2015**, *48*, 24–28. [CrossRef]
20. Su, H.; Baron, M.; Benarroch, M.; Velly, A.M.; Gravel, S.; Schipper, H.M.; Gornitsky, M. Altered salivary redox homeostasis in patients with systemic sclerosis. *J. Rheumatol.* **2010**, *37*, 1858–1863. [CrossRef]
21. Zaieni, S.H.; Derakhshan, Z.; Sariri, R. Alternations of salivary antioxidant enzymes in systemic lupus erythematosus. *Lupus* **2015**, *24*, 1400–1405. [CrossRef] [PubMed]
22. Nagler, R.M.; Klein, I.; Zarzhevsky, N.; Drigues, N.; Reznick, A.Z. Characterization of the differentiated antioxidant profile of human saliva. *Free Radic. Biol. Med.* **2002**, *32*, 268–277. [CrossRef]
23. Klimiuk, A.; Zalewska, A.; Sawicki, R.; Knapp, M.; Maciejczyk, M. Salivary oxidative stress increases with the progression of chronic heart failure. *J. Clin. Med.* **2020**, *9*, 769. [CrossRef] [PubMed]
24. Buege, J.A.; Aust, S.D. Microsomal lipid peroxidation. *Methods Enzymol.* **1978**, *52*, 302–310.
25. Vitali, C.; Bombardieri, S.; Jonsson, R.; Moutsopoulos, H.M.; Alexander, E.L.; Carsons, S.E.; Daniels, T.E.; Fox, R.I.; Kasson, S.S.; Pillemer, S.R.; et al. Classification criteria for Sjogren's syndrome: A revised version of the European criteria proposed by American-European Consensus Group. *Ann. Rheum. Dis.* **2002**, *61*, 554–558. [CrossRef]
26. Schirmer, O. Studien zur physiologie der tranenabsonderung und tranenabfuhr. *Arch. Opthalmol.* **1903**, *56*, 197–221. [CrossRef]
27. Misra, H.P.; Fridovich, I. The role of superoxide anion in the autoxidation of epinephrine and a simple assay for superoxide dismutase. *J. Biol. Chem.* **1972**, *247*, 3170–3175. [PubMed]
28. Aebi, H. Catalase in vitro. *Methods Enzymol.* **1984**, *105*, 121–126. [PubMed]
29. Mansson-Rahemtulla, B.; Baldone, D.C.; Pruitt, K.M.; Rahemtulla, F. Specific assays for peroxidases in human saliva. *Arch. Oral Biol.* **1986**, *31*, 661–668. [CrossRef]
30. Paglia, D.E.; Valentine, W.N. Studies on the quantitative and qualitative characterization of erythrocyte glutathione peroxidase. *J. Lab. Clin. Med.* **1967**, *70*, 158–169.
31. Griffith, O.W. Determination of glutathione and glutathione disulfide using glutathione reductase and 2-vinylpyridine. *Anal. Biochem.* **1980**, *106*, 207–212. [CrossRef]
32. Erel, O. A novel automated direct measurement method for total antioxidant capacity using a new generation, more stable ABTS radical cation. *Clin. Biochem.* **2004**, *37*, 227–285. [CrossRef] [PubMed]
33. Erel, O. A new automated colorimetric method for measuring total oxidant status. *Clin. Biochem.* **2005**, *38*, 1103–1111. [CrossRef]
34. Kołodziej, U.; Maciejczyk, M.; Niklińska, W.; Waszkiel, D.; Żendzian-Piotrowska, M.; Żukowski, P.; Zalewska, A. Chronic high-protein diet induces oxidative stress and alters the salivary gland function in rats. *Arch. Oral Biol.* **2017**, *84*, 6–12. [CrossRef] [PubMed]
35. Kalousová, M.; Skrha, J.; Zima, T. Advanced glycation end-products and advanced oxidation protein products in patients with diabetes mellitus. *Physiol. Res.* **2002**, *51*, 597–604. [PubMed]
36. Grintzalis, K.; Zisimopoulos, D.; Grune, T.; Weber, D.; Georgiou, C.D. Method for the simultaneous determination of free/protein malondialdehyde and lipid/protein hydroperoxides. *Free Radic. Biol. Med.* **2013**, *59*, 27–35. [CrossRef] [PubMed]
37. Duthoit, C.; Estienne, V.; Giraud, A.; Durand-Gorde, J.M.; Rasmussen, A.K.; Feldt-Rasmussen, U.; Carayon, P.; Ruf, J. Hydrogen peroxide-induced production of a 40 kDa immunoreactive thyroglobulin fragment in human thyroid cells: The onset of thyroid autoimmunity? *Biochem. J.* **2001**, *360*, 557–562. [CrossRef]
38. Burek, C.L.; Rose, N.R. Autoimmune thyroiditis and ROS. *Autoimmun. Rev.* **2008**, *7*, 530–537. [CrossRef]
39. Lushchak, V.L. Free radicals, reactive oxygen species, oxidative stress and its classification. *Chem. Biol. Interact.* **2014**, *224*, 164–175. [CrossRef]
40. Lushchak, V.L. Classification of oxidative stress based on its intensity. *Exp. Clin. Sci.* **2014**, *13*, 922–937.

41. Knaś, M.; Maciejczyk, M.; Sawicka, K.; Hady Razak, H.; Niczyporuk, M.; Ładny, J.R.; Matczuk, J.; Waszkiel, D.; Żendzian-Piotrowska, M.; Zalewska, A. Impact of morbid obesity and bariatric surgery on antioxidant/oxidant balance of the unstimulated and stimulated saliva. *J. Oral Pathol. Med.* **2016**, *45*, 455–464. [CrossRef]
42. Knaś, M.; Maciejczyk, M.; Daniszewska, I.; Klimiuk, A.; Matczuk, J.; Kołodziej, U.; Waszkiel, D.; Ładny, J.R.; Żendzian-Piotrowska, M.; Zalewska, A. Oxidative damage to the salivary glands of rats with streptozotocin-induced diabetes-temporal study: Oxidative stress and diabetic salivary glands. *J. Diabetes Res.* **2016**, *2016*, 4583742. [CrossRef]
43. Viazzi, F.; Garneri, D.; Leoncini, G.; Gonnella, A.; Muiesan, M.L.; Ambrosioni, E.; Costa, F.V.; Leonetti, G.; Pessina, A.C.; Trimarco, B.; et al. Serum uric acid and its relationship with metabolic syndrome and cardiovascular risk profile in patients with hypertension: Insights from the I-DEMAND study. *Nutr. Metab. Cardiovasc. Dis.* **2014**, *24*, 921–927. [CrossRef] [PubMed]
44. Matczuk, J.; Zendzian-Piotrowska, M.; Maciejczyk, M.; Kurek, K. Salivary lipids: A review. *Adv. Clin. Exp. Med.* **2017**, *26*, 1021–1029. [CrossRef] [PubMed]
45. Zalewska, A.; Waszkiel, D.; Łuczaj-Cepowicz, D.; Szajda, S.D.; Waszkiewicz, N. Salivary gland involvement in rheumatoid arthritis: Salivary peroxidase and the flow rate. *Pol. J. Environ. Stud.* **2010**, *19*, 321–325.
46. Pruitt, K.M.; Tenovuo, J.; Mansson-Rahemtulla, B.; Harrington, P.; Baldone, D.C. Is thiocyanate peroxidation at equilibrium in vivo? *Biochim. Biophys. Acta* **1986**, *870*, 385–391. [CrossRef]
47. Tenovuo, J.; Larjava, H. The protective effect of peroxidase and thiocyanate against hydrogen peroxide toxicity assessed by the uptake of [3H]-thymidine by human gingival fibroblasts cultured in vitro. *Arch. Oral Biol.* **1984**, *29*, 445–451. [CrossRef]
48. Hanstrom, L.; Johansson, A.; Carlsson, J. Lactoperoxidase and thiocyanate protect cultured mammalian cells against hydrogen peroxide toxicity. *Med. Biol.* **1983**, *61*, 268–274.
49. Erejuwa, O.O.; Gurtu, S.; Sulaiman, S.A.; Wahab, M.S.A.; Sirajudeen, K.N.; Salleh, M.S. Hypoglycemic and antioxidant effects of honey supplementation in streptozotocin-induced diabetic rats. *Int. J. Vitam. Nutr. Res.* **2010**, *80*, 74–82.
50. Cooper, A.J.; Pinto, J.T.; Callery, P.S. Reversible and irreversible protein glutathionylation: Biological and clinical aspects. *Expert Opin. Drug Metab. Toxicol.* **2011**, *7*, 891–910. [CrossRef]
51. Lushchak, V.I. Glutathione homeostasis and functions: Potential targets for medical interventions. *J. Amino Acids* **2012**, *2012*, 736837. [CrossRef] [PubMed]
52. Azuma, M.; Aota, K.; Tamatani, T.; Motegi, K.; Yamashita, T.; Ashida, Y.; Hayashi, Y.; Sato, M. Suppression of tumor necrosis factor alpha-induced matrix metalloproteinase 9 production in human salivary gland acinar cells by cepharanthine occurs via down-regulation of nuclear factor kappaB: A possible therapeutic agent for preventing the destruction of the acinar structure in the salivary glands of Sjogren's syndrome patients. *Arthr. Rheum.* **2002**, *46*, 1585–1594. [CrossRef]
53. Bozzato, A.; Burger, P.; Zenk, J.; Ulter, W.; Iro, H. Salivary gland biometry in female patients with eating disorders. *Eur. Arch. Otorhinolaryngol.* **2008**, *265*, 1095–1102. [CrossRef] [PubMed]
54. Heo, M.S.; Lee, S.C.; Lee, S.S.; Choi, H.M.; Choi, S.C.; Park, T.W. Quantitative analysis of normal major salivary glands using computed tomography. *Oral Surg. Oral Med. Oral Pathol. Oral Radiol. Endod.* **2001**, *92*, 240–244. [CrossRef]
55. Watanabe, M.; Yamagishi-Wang, H.; Kawaguchi, M. Lowered susceptibility of muscarinic receptor involved in salivary secretion of streptozotocin-induced diabetic rats. *Jpn. J. Pharmacol.* **2001**, *87*, 117–124. [CrossRef] [PubMed]
56. Hanemaaijer, R.; Visser, H.; Konttinen, Y.T.; Koolwijk, P.; Verheijen, J.H. A novel and simple immunocapture assay for determination of gelatinase-B (MMP-9) activities in biological fluids: Saliva from patients with Sjogren's syndrome contain increased latent and active gelatinase-B levels. *Matrix Biol.* **1998**, *17*, 657–665. [CrossRef]
57. Skov Olsen, P.; Kirkegaard, P.; Rasmussen, T.; Magid, E.; Poulsen, S.S.; Nexø, E. Adrenergic effects on secretion of amylase from the rat salivary glands. *Digestion* **1988**, *41*, 34–38. [CrossRef]

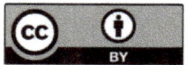

© 2020 by the authors. Licensee MDPI, Basel, Switzerland. This article is an open access article distributed under the terms and conditions of the Creative Commons Attribution (CC BY) license (http://creativecommons.org/licenses/by/4.0/).

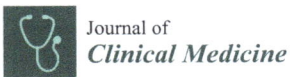

Article

Salivary Gland Dysfunction, Protein Glycooxidation and Nitrosative Stress in Children with Chronic Kidney Disease

Mateusz Maciejczyk [1,*], Julita Szulimowska [2], Katarzyna Taranta-Janusz [3], Anna Wasilewska [3] and Anna Zalewska [4]

1. Department of Hygiene, Epidemiology and Ergonomics, Medical University of Bialystok, 2c Mickiewicza Street, 15-233 Bialystok, Poland
2. Department of Pedodontics, Medical University of Bialystok, 24a M. Sklodowskiej-Curie Street, 15-274 Bialystok, Poland; szulimowska.julita@gmail.com
3. Department of Pediatrics and Nephrology, Medical University of Bialystok, 24a M. Sklodowskiej-Curie Street, 15-274 Bialystok, Poland; katarzyna.taranta@wp.pl (K.T.-J.); annwasil@interia.pl (A.W.)
4. Experimental Dentistry Laboratory, Medical University of Bialystok, 24a M. Sklodowskiej-Curie Street, 15-274 Bialystok, Poland; anna.zalewska1@umb.edu.pl or azalewska426@gmail.com
* Correspondence: mat.maciejczyk@gmail.com or mateusz.maciejczyk@umb.edu.pl

Received: 31 March 2020; Accepted: 27 April 2020; Published: 29 April 2020

Abstract: This study is the first to evaluate protein glycooxidation products, lipid oxidative damage and nitrosative stress in non-stimulated (NWS) and stimulated whole saliva (SWS) of children with chronic kidney disease (CKD) divided into two subgroups: normal salivary secretion ($n = 18$) and hyposalivation (NWS flow < 0.2 mL min^{-1}; $n = 12$). Hyposalivation was observed in all patients with severe renal failure (4–5 stage CKD), while saliva secretion > 0.2 mL/min in children with mild-moderate CKD (1–3 stage) and controls. Salivary amylase activity and total protein content were significantly lower in CKD children with hyposalivation compared to CKD patients with normal saliva secretion and control group. The fluorescence of protein glycooxidation products (kynurenine, N-formylkynurenine, advanced glycation end products), the content of oxidative damage to lipids (4-hydroxynonneal, 8-isoprostanes) and nitrosative stress (peroxynitrite, nitrotyrosine) were significantly higher in NWS, SWS, and plasma of CKD children with hyposalivation compared to patients with normal salivary secretion and healthy controls. In CKD group, salivary oxidation products correlated negatively with salivary flow rate, α-amylase activity and total protein content; however, salivary oxidation products do not reflect their plasma level. In conclusion, children with CKD suffer from salivary gland dysfunction. Oxidation of salivary proteins and lipids increases with CKD progression and deterioration of salivary gland function.

Keywords: chronic kidney disease; salivary gland dysfunction; salivary biomarkers; oxidative stress; nitrosative stress

1. Introduction

Chronic kidney disease (CKD) is a multi-symptomatic syndrome resulting from a reduction in the number of active nephrons. The diagnosis of CKD is based on anatomical and/or functional renal abnormalities as well as glomerular filtration rate (GFR) below 60 mL/min/1.73 m^2 [1]. Although the prevalence of CKD in children is much lower than in adults, the disease is a significant clinical problem in the child population. Indeed, mortality in CKD children remains high and is about 30 times higher than the expected mortality at any given age [2]. The most common causes of CKD in children are urological defects, glomerulopathies, congenital nephropathies, and kidney dysplasia [2,3]. Their effect is the reduction of active nephrons, leading to intraglomerular hypertension in the remaining nephrons and their hypertrophy. This also leads to proteinuria, progressive hardening of the glomeruli as well as fibrosis of the renal interstitial tissue [1,4]. However, CKD complications can affect just about every organ [1]. These include cardiovascular disease (hypertrophy of the left ventricle, coronary heart disease), respiratory system (pulmonary edema, "uremic lung"), endocrine disorders (glucose intolerance, dyslipidemia), hematological (normochromic anemia, hemorrhagic diathesis) or mineral and bone disorders (vitamin D deficiency, hypoparathyroidism) [1,4]. In the CKD pathogenesis, the key role of oxidative stress has recently been stressed [5–7].

The increased production of free radicals in CKD leads to oxidative stress which initiates oxidative damage to proteins and lipids. This increases the accumulation of oxidized proteins in the kidney parenchyma and leads to a progressive impairment of its function [5–7]. It has been proven that the advanced oxidation protein products (AOPP) and advanced glycation end products (AGE) intensify the RAAS (renin–angiotensin–aldosterone system) activation, increase the expression of NF-κB (nuclear factor-κB) pathway and impair nitric oxide (NO) production [8,9]. The oxidation protein products increase synthesis of collagen and fibronectin in the mesangial cells, activate the NADPH oxidase (NOX) through the protein kinase C dependent pathway, enhance the activity of caspase-3, the expression of the p58 protein and Bax. Therefore, the protein oxidation products play a critical role in proteinuria and thickening of the renal glomeruli progression, decreasing the number of podocytes through apoptosis [10–13]. Moreover, as a result of peroxidation of kidney lipids, the activity of membrane enzymes and transporting proteins is inhibited, which disturbs the integrity of cell membranes [5–7]. Nevertheless, it is suggested that the accumulation of oxidized proteins and lipids may also disrupt other organs [5–7].

A number of systemic diseases affect the function of salivary glands. Reduced saliva production, disturbances of protein secretion into saliva as well as xerostomia (subjective dryness of oral mucosa) were observed in patients with diabetes, obesity, hypertension, psoriasis, and rheumatoid arthritis [14–18]. It is suggested that oxidative stress may play a key role in the pathogenesis of salivary hypofunction. In fact, the oral cavity is the only place in the body exposed to so many environmental factors such as food, stimulants (alcohol, tobacco smoke), air pollution, medicines, or dental materials [19]. Although all of them can generate oxygen free radicals, patients with systemic diseases are particularly predisposed to salivary oxidative stress [14–17]. Indeed, in a situation of reduced antioxidant capacity, systemic oxidative stress can affect the oxidative-reductive balance of the oral cavity. Products of protein/lipid oxidation can aggregate and accumulate in the salivary glands leading to damage of secretory cells. Protein oxidation products can also increase reactive oxygen species (ROS) formation (by activating NOX and NF-κB signaling), which, on a positive feedback, enhances local oxidative stress [20,21].

In our earlier studies we have shown that oxidative stress in CKD children affects not only the kidneys but also the oral cavity [3,22,23]. Indeed, we have shown disturbances of the enzymatic and non-enzymatic antioxidant barrier and increased oxidative damage to salivary proteins [3]. Moreover, salivary FRAP (ferric ion reducing antioxidant power) with high sensitivity (100%) and specificity (100%) differentiates children with mildly to moderately decreased kidney function from those with severe renal impairment [22]. Additionally, CKD patients are much more likely to develop oral diseases such as dental caries, candidiasis or tooth erosion [24]. However, still little is known about salivary gland function in children with CKD. We suppose that as in other oxidative stress-related diseases, CKD causes a decrease in saliva production and disturbances of protein secretion into saliva [20,25–27]. This may be due to the accumulation of protein oxidation products in the salivary glands, which damage their parenchyma and lead to hyposalivation. As in obesity, insulin resistance or psoriasis, salivary gland hypofunction may also result from the impairment of NO bioavailability and the damaging effect of nitrosative stress mediators (especially peroxynitrite) [20,25,26]. Therefore, our study is the first to evaluate salivary glycooxidation products, oxidative damage to lipids and nitrosative stress biomarkers in CKD children with normal and decreased saliva secretion. In addition to the non-stimulated and stimulated salivary flow, we also assessed other indicators of salivary gland function, such as salivary amylase activity and total protein content. An important part of our study is also the assessment of salivary-blood correlation of the analyzed redox biomarkers.

2. Material and Methods

2.1. Ethical Issues

The study was approved by the Local Bioethics Committee at the Medical University of Bialystok (permission number R-I-002/43/2018). All patients and/or their legal guardians have been acquainted with the research project and gave written consent to participate in the experiment.

2.2. Patients

The study included 30 children with CKD treated in the Department of Pediatrics and Nephrology of the Medical University of Bialystok, Poland. Patients were divided into two subgroups based on the rate of non-stimulated salivary flow (NWS): normal salivary secretion (normal salivation, CKD NS) and reduced salivary secretion (hyposalivation; CKD HS). Hyposalivation was defined as NWS flow below 0.2 mL/min [16,26,28].

CKD was defined according to the Kidney Disease Improving Global Outcomes (KDIGO) criteria based on different eGFR distribution: Stage 1: >90 mL/min/1.73 m^2; Stage 2: 60–89 mL/min/1.73 m^2; Stage 3: 30–59 mL/min/1.73 m^2; Stage 4: 15–29 mL/min/1.73 m^2; and Stage 5: <15 mL/min/1.73 m^2 [1]. The estimated glomerular filtration rate (eGFR) was calculated using the updated Schwartz formula-eGFR (mL/min/1.73 m^2) = 0.413 × (height in cm/serum creatinine (Cr)) [29]. Upon the diagnosis of CKD, all patients were on a renal diet that was low in sodium and/or phosphorous and/or protein depending on patients' condition and CKD stage [30]. Office blood pressure (BP) was measured by means of either the manual auscultatory technique or an automated oscillometric device after the subject had rested for 5 min in a sitting position. The average values of the second and third measurements of systolic and diastolic BP were used. Hypertension was defined when the average value of the systolic and/or diastolic BP were ≥95th percentile for age, gender, and height [31].

The causes of CKD were urological defects (33.3%), glomerulopathies (33.3%), congenital nephropathies (13.3%), kidney dysplasia (13.3%), and undetermined etiology (6.8%).

The control group consisted of 30 healthy children attending the Specialist Dental Clinic of the Medical University of Bialystok, Poland for regular check-ups. The control was matched by age and gender to the study group. All patients in the control group had an NWS flow > 0.2 mL/min.

The exclusion criterion in the study and control groups was the occurrence of general diseases: metabolic (insulin resistance, type 1 and 2 diabetes), autoimmune (thyroiditis, systemic sclerosis, arthritis, lupus erythematosus, Crohn's disease, ulcerative colitis), infectious, gastrointestinal and pulmonary diseases. Patients taking antibiotics, non-steroidal anti-inflammatory drugs (NSAIDs), glucocorticosteroids, vitamins and dietary supplements for at least 1 months before saliva collection were excluded from the study, similarly to children with acute inflammatory states. Subjects with poor oral hygiene (Approximal Plaque Index, API > 20) and gingivitis (Sulcus Bleeding Index, SBI > 0.5; Gingival Index, GI > 0.5) were also excluded from the experiment (see: dental examination).

Since pharmacotherapy significantly affects saliva secretion [16,27], patients with CKD taking 5 and more drugs were eliminated from the study.

Detailed characteristics of the patients and the control group are presented in Table 1.

2.3. Saliva Collection

The research material was non-stimulated (NWS) and stimulated (SWS) whole saliva collected by the spitting method. In order to eliminate the influence of physical exercise and daily rhythm on saliva secretion, samples were taken from subjects who were not physically active for the last 24 h, after an all-night rest, always between 7 a.m. and 9 a.m. Subjects did not consume any meals or drinks (other than water), and refrained from performing any oral hygiene procedures at least 2 h before saliva collection. Additionally, children did not take any medications for at least 8 h prior to saliva collection [16,28].

The subjects were instructed to rinse their mouth two times with distilled water and to spit saliva into a sterile Falcon tube placed in an ice container. Saliva collection was done by the patient when sitting with the head down (with minimized facial and lip movements), after at least a 5-min adaptation, always in the same child-friendly room. The time of NWS collection was 15 min. Then, saliva was stimulated by dropping 10 µl of citric acid (2%, w/v) solution on the tip of the tongue every 30 s [16,17,26,28]. The time of SWS collection was 5 min [16,28].

Immediately after collection, the volume of saliva was measured with a pipette set to 100 µL. The salivary flow rate was calculated by dividing the volume of saliva by the time necessary for its secretion (mL min^{-1}). The pH of saliva was also analyzed using Seven Multi pH meter (Mettler Toledo, Greifensee, Switzerland).

After measuring the salivary pH, the samples were immediately centrifuged (3000× g, 4 °C, 20 min) and the supernatant was preserved for further analysis [32]. To protect against sample oxidation, butylated hydroxytoluene (BHT, Sigma-Aldrich, Nümbrecht, Germany) was added (10 µL 0.5 M BHT in acetonitrile (ACN)/1 mL NWS/SWS) [32]. The samples were portioned into 200 µL aliquots and frozen at −80 °C. Frozen samples were stored for no more than six months.

In order to identify samples contaminated with blood, the concentration of transferrin in saliva was assessed (Human Transferrin ELISA Kit; Abcam; Cambridge, UK). However, no blood contamination was confirmed in any of the samples.

The activity of salivary amylase (EC 3.2.1.1) was assessed for the evaluation of salivary gland function [33,34]. A spectrophotometric method with 3,5-dinitrosalicylic acid (DNS) was used and absorbance was measured at 540 nm.

2.4. Dental Examination

A clinical examination in artificial lighting (10,000 lux) was also performed. According to the World Health Organization criteria [35], a mirror, an explorer and a periodontal probe were used. The incidence of caries was assessed using DMFT index (decay, missing, filled teeth). DMFT is the sum of teeth with caries (D), teeth extracted because of caries (M), and teeth filled because of caries (F). DMFT for deciduous teeth (dmft) was also evaluated. API (approximal plaque index) was used to assess the status of oral hygiene and determines the percentage of tooth surface with plaque. GI (Gingival Index) and SBI (Sulcus Bleeding Index) were used to assess the condition of gums. GI described qualitative changes in the gingiva, while SBI showed the intensity of bleeding from the gingival sulcus after probing [35].

Clinical dental examinations were performed by the same experienced pedodontist (J. S.). In 10 children, the inter-rater agreements between the examiner and another experienced pedodontist (A. Z.) were assessed. The reliability for all dental indices was >0.97.

2.5. Blood Collection

Whole blood was collected after an all-night rest, always between 6 and 8 a.m. We used S-Monovette® K3 EDTA blood collection system (Sarstedt, Nümbrecht, Germany). Samples were immediately centrifuged (1500× g; 4 °C, 10 min) [32] and the top layer (plasma) was preserved for further analyses. Similarly to NWS and SWS, BHT (10 µL 0.5 M BHT/1 mL plasma) was added to samples that were then frozen at −80 °C [32].

2.6. Total Protein Assay

The total protein content was determined colorimetrically using the bicinchoninic acid (BCA) method (Thermo Scientific PIERCE BCA Protein Assay (Rockford, IL, USA)). Bovine serum albumin (BSA) was used as a standard.

2.7. Redox Assays

All reagents were purchased from Sigma-Aldrich (Nümbrecht, Germany and/or Saint Louis, MO, USA). The absorbance/fluorescence was measured using Infinite M200 PRO Multimode Microplate Reader Tecan. The results were standardized to 1 mg of total protein. All determinations were performed in duplicate samples.

2.8. Protein Glycooxidation Products

The content of dityrosine, kynurenine, N-formylkynurenine and tryptophan was assessed fluorimetrically. The characteristic fluorescence at 330/415, 365/480, 325/434, and 295/340 nm, respectively, was measured [36,37]. Immediately before determination, saliva and plasma samples were diluted in 0.1 M H_2SO_4 (1:5, v/v) [32]. The results were normalized to fluorescence of 0.1 mg/mL quinine sulfate in 0.1 M H_2SO_4 and expressed in arbitrary fluorescence units (AFU)/mg protein.

The content of advanced glycation end products (AGE) was assessed fluorimetrically. The characteristic fluorescence of pentosidine, pyraline, carboxymethyl lysine (CML), and furyl-furanyl-imidazole (FFI) was measured at 350/440 nm [38]. Immediately before determination, saliva and plasma samples were diluted in 0.1 M H_2SO_4 (1:5, v/v) [32]. The results were expressed in arbitrary fluorescence units (AFU)/mg protein.

2.9. Oxidative Stress Products

The total thiols concentration was measured colorimetrically using the Ellman's reagent (5,5-dithio-bis-(2-nitrobenzoic acid)) [39]. The absorbance was measured at 412 nm and total thiols concentration was expressed in µmol/mg protein.

4-hydroxynonneal protein adducts (4-HNE) and 8-isoprostanes (8-isop) concentration was measured using ELISA kits (Cell Biolabs, Inc. San Diego, CA, USA; Cayman Chemicals, Ann Arbor, MI, USA, respectively), following the manufacturer's instructions. The results were expressed in nmol/mg protein and pmol/mg protein, respectively.

2.10. Nitrosative Stress Products

Nitric oxide (NO) concentration was measured colorimetrically using sulfanilamide and NEDA·2 HCl (N-(1-naphthyl)-ethylenediamine dihydrochloride). Nitrate was converted to nitrite using nitrate reductase and total NO was measured [40,41]. The absorbance was measured at 490 nm and NO concentration was expressed in µmol/mg protein.

S-nitrosothiols concentration was measured colorimetrically based on the reaction of the Griess reagent with Cu^{2+} ions [41,42]. The absorbance was measured at 490 nm and S-nitrosothiols concentration was expressed in nmol/mg protein.

Peroxynitrite concentration was measured colorimetrically based on peroxynitrite-mediated nitration resulting in the formation of nitrophenol [43]. The absorbance was measured at 320 nm and peroxynitrite concentration was expressed in nmol/mg protein.

Nitrotyrosine concentration was measured colorimetrically by the ELISA method, using a commercial diagnostic kit (Immundiagnostik AG; Bensheim, Germany). Nitrotyrosine concentration was expressed in pmol/mg protein.

2.11. Statistical Analysis

Statistical analysis was performed using GraphPad Prism 8 for Mac (GraphPad Software, La Jolla, USA). The Shapiro–Wilk test was used to determine the normality of distribution while one-way ANOVA and Tukey's multiple comparisons test were used to compare the tested groups. The value of $p < 0.05$ was considered statistically significant. Multiplicity adjusted p value vas also calculated. The results were presented as mean ± SD. The correlation of the obtained results was measured using the Pearson correlation coefficient. The number of patients was set a priori based on the previous clinical study. Online sample size calculator (ClinCalc) was used and 0.9 was assumed as the test power.

3. Results

3.1. Clinical Characteristics

Clinical characteristics of the subjects are presented in Table 1.

Interestingly, hyposalivation was observed in all patients with severe renal failure (4–5 stage CKD), while saliva secretion >0.2 mL/min in children with mild-moderate CKD (1–3 stage) and controls.

Table 1. Clinical characteristics of children with chronic kidney disease (CKD) and healthy controls.

		C (n = 30)	CKD NS (n = 18)	CKD HS (n = 12)	ANOVA p
NWS flow (mL min^{-1})	mean ± SD	0.495 ± 0.1	0.338 ± 0.09	0.138 ± 0.04	<0.0001
	min	0.292	0.219	0.0730	
	max	0.682	0.494	0.199	
Men n		15	7	8	NA
Age (years)		13 ± 3.5	14 ± 3.2	12 ± 3.7	NS
CKD n	stage 1	-	6	0	NA
	stage 2	-	5	0	NA
	stage 3	-	7	0	NA
	stage 4	-	0	6	NA
	stage 5	-	0	6	NA
eGFR (mL/min/1.73 m^2)		136 ± 6.9	84 ± 43	18 ± 7.4	< 0.0001
Serum creatinine (mg/dL)		0.41 ± 0.09	1.2 ± 0.54	4.6 ± 0.58	<0.0001
Serum urea (mg/dL)		18 ± 2.6	44 ± 4.7	124 ± 13	<0.0001
Albuminuria (mg/24 h)		8 ± 0.9	51 ± 23	815 ± 236	<0.0001
Proteinuria (mg/24 h)		58.4 ± 3.5	403 ± 165	845 ± 248	<0.0001
Hgb (g/dL)		14.5 ± 0.3	13 ± 0.49	11 ± 0.51	<0.0001
Hct (%)		39.7 ± 1.1	38 ± 1.2	33 ± 1.3	<0.0001
Serum iron (μg/dL)		82 ± 2.1	68 ± 6.7	91 ± 8.6	<0.0001
Hypertension n		-	1	11	NA
Dialysis n		-	0	6	NA
Drugs per day n	0	-	2	0	NA
	1–2	-	10	4	NA
	3–4	-	6	8	NA
Drugs n	iron	-	9	10	NA
	loop diuretics	-	10	9	NA
	ACEI	-	10	9	NA
	β-blockers	-	3	5	NA
	CCB	-	3	3	NA

ACEI—Angiotensin-converting enzyme inhibitors; C—Healthy controls; CCB—Calcium channel blockers; CKD NS—CKD patients with normal salivary secretion; CKD HS—CKD patients with reduced salivary secretion; NA—not applicable; NWS—Non-stimulated whole saliva; eGFR—estimated glomerular filtration rate; Hct—Hematocrit; Hgb—Hemoglobin.

3.2. Salivary Gland Function and Salivary pH

The non-stimulated and stimulated salivary secretion was significantly lower in CKD children with hyposalivation compared to patients with normal salivary secretion and control group. Similarly, total protein content and salivary amylase activity were significantly lower in NWS and SWS of CKD children with hyposalivation as compared to other groups. The pH of non-stimulated saliva was significantly higher in CKD children with decreased salivary secretion compared to controls (Figure 1).

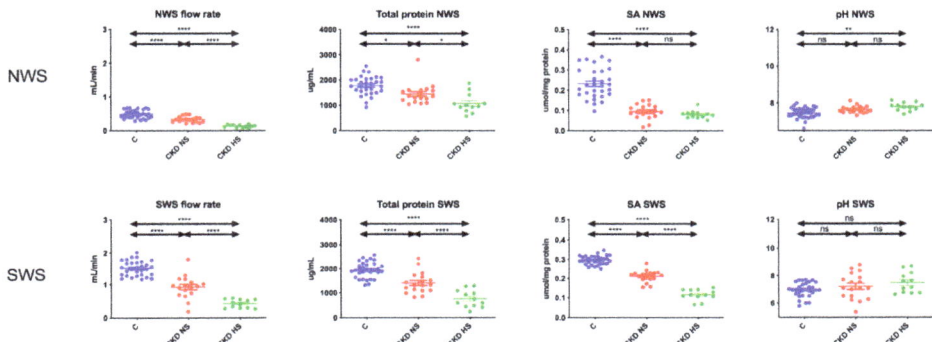

Figure 1. Salivary gland function and salivary pH of children with chronic kidney disease (CKD) and healthy controls. C—Healthy controls; CKD NS—CKD patients with normal salivary secretion; CKD HS—CKD patients with reduced salivary secretion; NWS—Non-stimulated whole saliva; SA—Salivary amylase; SWS—Stimulated whole saliva. Differences statistically significant at: * $p < 0.05$, ** $p < 0.005$, **** $p < 0.0001$.

3.3. Dental Examination

Oral hygiene (DMFT, dmft, API) and periodontal condition (GI, SBI) did not differ significantly between groups (Table 2). The children had all permanent teeth completely erupted (up to the seventh tooth). There was no active eruption of eighth teeth in any child.

Table 2. Dental examination of children with chronic kidney disease (CKD) and healthy controls.

	C ($n = 30$)	CKD NS ($n = 18$)	CKD HS ($n = 12$)	ANOVA p
DMFT	2.5 ± 0.5	2.7 ± 0.7	2.8 ± 0.6	NS
dmft	9.8 ± 0.5	10.1 ± 0.5	10.3 ± 0.7	NS
GI	0 ± 0.1	0 ± 0.2	0 ± 0.2	NS
SBI	0 ± 0.1	0 ± 0.1	0 ± 0.1	NS

C—healthy controls; CKD NS—CKD patients with normal salivary secretion; CKD HS—CKD patients with hyposalivation; DMFT—decay, missing, filled teeth (for permanent teeth); dmft—decay, missing, filled teeth (for milk teeth); NS—not significant; SBI—Sulcus Bleeding Index; GI—Gingival Index.

3.4. Glycooxidation Products

Generally, the fluorescence of glycooxidation products (dityrosine, kynurenine, N-formylkynurenine and AGE) was significantly higher in NWS, SWS and plasma of CKD children with hyposalivation compared to patients with normal salivary secretion and control group. Tryptophan fluorescence was significantly lower in stimulated saliva and plasma of patients with CKD (both groups) as compared to controls (Figure 2).

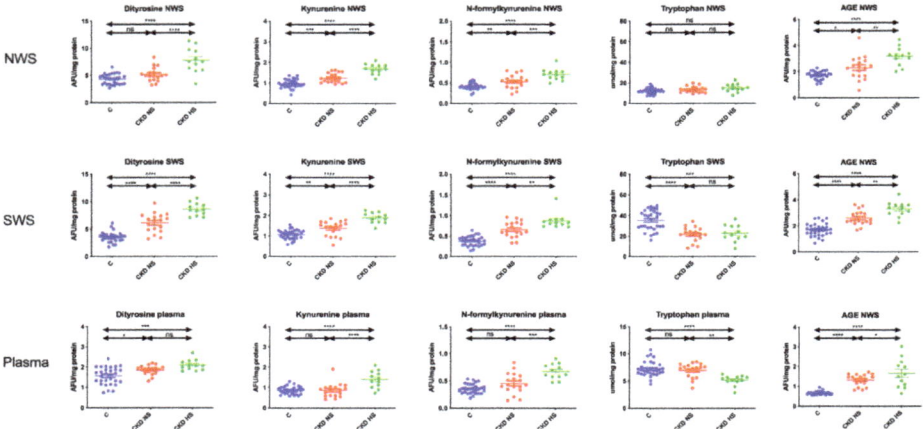

Figure 2. Glycooxidation products in children with chronic kidney disease (CKD) and healthy controls. AGE—Advanced glycation end products; C—Healthy controls; CKD NS—CKD patients with normal salivary secretion; CKD HS—CKD patients with reduced salivary secretion; NWS—Non-stimulated whole saliva; SWS—Stimulated whole saliva. Differences statistically significant at: * $p < 0.05$, ** $p < 0.005$, *** $p < 0.0005$, **** $p < 0.0001$.

3.5. Oxidative Stress Products

Oxidative damage to proteins (total thiols) and lipids (4-HNE and 8-isop) was significantly higher in NWS, SWS and plasma of children with chronic kidney disease and hyposalivation compared to patients with normal salivary secretion and control group (Figure 3).

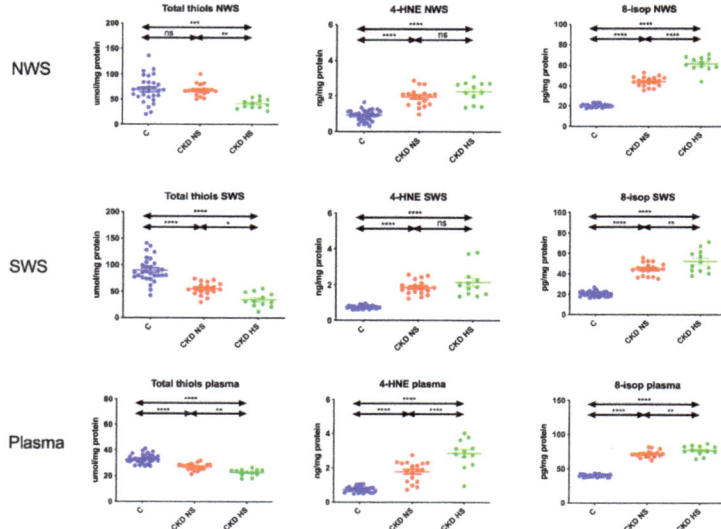

Figure 3. Oxidative damage to proteins and lipids in children with chronic kidney disease (CKD) and healthy controls. 4-HNE—4-hydroxynoneal protein adducts; 8-isop—8-isoprostanes; C—Healthy controls; CKD NS—CKD patients with normal salivary secretion; CKD HS—CKD patients with reduced salivary secretion; NWS—Non-stimulated whole saliva; SWS—Stimulated whole saliva. Differences statistically significant at: * $p < 0.05$, ** $p < 0.005$, *** $p < 0.0005$, **** $p < 0.0001$.

3.6. Nitrosative Stress Products

NO concentration was significantly lower in NWS, SWS, and plasma in CKD children with hyposalivation compared to other groups. The concentration of S-nitrosothiols was significantly higher in NWS and SWS of children with chronic kidney disease and hyposalivation compared to CKD patients with normal salivary secretion and healthy controls. However, it did not differ significantly in plasma. The content of peroxynitrite and nitrotyrosine was significantly higher in NWS, SWS and plasma of CKD children with hyposalivation in comparison with the other groups (Figure 4).

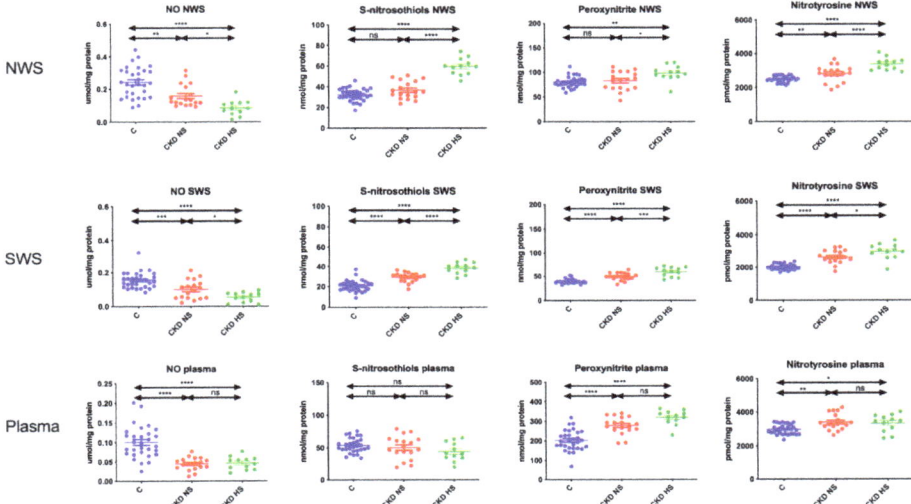

Figure 4. Nitrosative stress in children with chronic kidney disease (CKD) and healthy controls. CKD NS—CKD patients with normal salivary secretion; CKD HS—CKD patients with reduced salivary secretion; NO—nitric oxide; NWS—non-stimulated whole saliva; SWS—stimulated whole saliva. Differences statistically significant at: * $p < 0.05$, ** $p < 0.005$, **** $p < 0.0001$.

3.7. Correlations

In CKD children the concentration of redox biomarkers in NWS and SWS correlated negatively with eGFR and positively with serum creatinine and urea (except for total thiols and tryptophan). However, no correlation with renal function parameters was generally observed in healthy subjects (Table 3).

In children with CKD, the concentration of protein and lipid oxidation products correlates negatively with salivary flow rate, salivary amylase activity and total protein content. Only salivary tryptophan and thiol groups correlated positively with salivary glands activity (Table 4). In NWS, glycooxidation products (except tryptophan), 4-HNE, 8-isop and peroxynitrite correlated positively with salivary pH. However, there was no relationship between the assessed biomarkers in saliva and plasma (except for kynurenine) (Table 5).

In the control group, dityrosine, kynurenine, tryptophan, AGE, and 4-HNE in non-stimulated saliva correlates positively with their plasma levels (Table 5). However, no relationships between cellular oxidation products and salivary gland function were demonstrated (except for AGE in SWS) (Table 4).

Table 3. Correlations between analyzed redox biomarkers and renal function of children with chronic kidney disease (CKD) and healthy controls.

	C (n = 30)			CKD (n = 30)		
	eGFR	serum Cr	serum urea	eGFR	serum Cr	serum urea
Dityrosine NWS	0.086	0.163	0.22	*−0.579*	*0.72*	*0.713*
Kynurenine NWS	0.17	0.246	0.057	*−0.562*	*0.71*	*0.691*
N-formylkynurenine NWS	0.225	0.322	0.118	*−0.527*	*0.641*	*0.585*
Tryptophan NWS	0.095	0.218	0.216	0.203	−0.102	−0.097
AGE NWS	0.228	0.041	−0.015	*−0.531*	*0.555*	*0.568*
Total thiols NWS	0.13	−0.164	−0.144	*0.431*	*−0.675*	*−0.649*
4-HNE NWS	0.135	0.154	0.163	*−0.512*	*0.533*	*0.476*
8-isop NWS	−0.017	0.096	−0.032	*−0.592*	*0.819*	*0.76*
NO NWS	−0.072	−0.089	−0.132	*0.609*	*−0.594*	*−0.531*
S-nitrosothiols NWS	−0.014	0.268	*0.543*	*−0.675*	*0.551*	*0.525*
Peroxynitrite NWS	0.039	−0.073	−0.236	*−0.537*	*0.631*	*0.579*
Nitrotyrosine NWS	0.194	0.018	−0.034	*−0.565*	*0.625*	*0.593*
Dityrosine SWS	0.037	0.076	−0.349	*−0.632*	*0.721*	*0.601*
Kynurenine SWS	0.217	−0.249	−0.146	*−0.48*	*0.586*	*0.626*
N-formylkynurenine SWS	0.219	*−0.456*	−0.028	*−0.457*	*0.509*	*0.49*
Tryptophan SWS	0.041	0.247	0.049	0.255	−0.296	−0.193
AGE SWS	−0.138	−0.134	−0.123	*−0.413*	*0.372*	*0.39*
Total thiols SWS	0.106	0.379	0.007	*0.674*	*−0.736*	*−0.657*
4-HNE SWS	−0.057	−0.251	−0.081	*−0.286*	*0.306*	*0.227*
8-isop SWS	−0.136	−0.306	0.203	*−0.417*	*0.464*	*0.55*
NO SWS	−0.123	0.176	*0.353*	*0.661*	*−0.52*	*−0.452*
S-nitrosothiols SWS	−0.484	0.106	0.257	*−0.357*	*0.448*	*0.417*
Peroxynitrite SWS	0.198	*−0.459*	−0.031	−0.29	*0.341*	*0.243*
Nitrotyrosine SWS	−0.068	−0.015	−0.156	*−0.41*	0.367	0.2

4-HNE – 4-hydroxynoeal protein adducts; 8-isop—8-isoprostanes; AGE—Advanced glycation end products; C—Healthy controls; Cr—Creatinine; CKD—patients with chronic kidney disease; eGFR—estimated glomerular filtration rate; NWS—Non-stimulated whole saliva; SWS—Stimulated whole saliva. Statistically significant correlations ($p < 0.05$) are highlighted as bold and italics.

Table 4. Correlations between analyzed redox biomarkers and salivary gland function and salivary pH of children with chronic kidney disease (CKD) and healthy controls.

	C (n = 30)					CKD (n = 30)			
	NWS Flow	Total Protein NWS	SA NWS	pH NWS		NWS Flow	Total Protein NWS	SA NWS	pH NWS
Dityrosine NWS	−0.092	−0.128	0.061	0.002		**−0.754**	**−0.633**	**−0.522**	**0.561**
Kynurenine NWS	−0.042	0.051	0.123	−0.152		**−0.722**	**−0.521**	**−0.362**	**0.388**
N-formylkynurenine NWS	−0.166	0.255	0.154	−0.133		**−0.663**	**−0.52**	−0.24	**0.545**
Tryptophan NWS	−0.009	−0.107	−0.073	−0.217		0.242	0.363	0.348	−0.14
AGE NWS	−0.111	−0.236	−0.063	−0.141		**−0.618**	**−0.358**	**−0.367**	**0.403**
Total thiols NWS	−0.013	0.265	0.063	−0.18		**0.6**	**0.395**	0.09	−0.34
4-HNE NWS	0.161	0.156	−0.12	−0.191		**−0.628**	**−0.632**	**−0.403**	**0.619**
8-isop NWS	0.163	0.335	0.043	−0.254		**−0.711**	**−0.385**	**−0.316**	**0.422**
NO NWS	−0.24	0.149	0.183	−0.093		**0.577**	**0.343**	**0.439**	0.032
S-nitrosothiols NWS	0.214	0.259	0.058	−0.332		**−0.725**	**−0.397**	−0.255	0.285
Peroxynitrite NWS	−0.069	−0.021	0.297	0.101		**−0.666**	**−0.872**	**−0.486**	**0.508**
Nitrotyrosine NWS	0.063	0.094	−0.282	0.538		**−0.594**	**−0.402**	**−0.354**	0.268
	SWS Flow	Total Protein SWS	SA SWS	pH SWS		SWS Flow	Total Protein SWS	SA SWS	pH SWS
Dityrosine SWS	−0.041	0.082	−0.118	0.152		**−0.534**	**−0.513**	**−0.584**	0.088
Kynurenine SWS	0.16	−0.168	0.155	0.039		**−0.466**	**−0.394**	**−0.473**	0.099
N-formylkynurenine SWS	0.24	0.06	−0.129	0.143		**−0.442**	**−0.482**	**−0.478**	−0.016
Tryptophan SWS	0.277	−0.301	−0.055	−0.192		0.026	0.083	−0.026	0.035
AGE SWS	**−0.488**	0.078	−0.051	−0.123		**−0.553**	**−0.401**	**−0.513**	−0.008
Total thiols SWS	0.037	0.177	−0.271	−0.202		**0.566**	**0.509**	**0.538**	−0.192
4-HNE SWS	−0.127	0.126	0.11	0.22		−0.119	0.02	−0.151	0.014
8-isop SWS	0.045	−0.114	−0.027	0.116		−0.216	−0.318	**−0.369**	**−0.346**
NO SWS	0.245	−0.267	−0.091	−0.066		**0.589**	**0.448**	**0.612**	−0.187
S-nitrosothiols SWS	0.152	0.302	−0.294	−0.051		**−0.466**	**−0.329**	**−0.47**	0.052
Peroxynitrite SWS	**0.349**	−0.001	0.036	0.239		−0.242	−0.297	**−0.516**	−0.095
Nitrotyrosine SWS	0.084	0.025	−0.003	0.074		−0.266	**−0.521**	−0.232	0.067

4-HNE—4-hydroxynonenal protein adducts; 8-isop—8-isoprostanes; AGE—Advanced glycation end products; C—Healthy controls; CKD—patients with chronic kidney disease; NWS—Non-stimulated whole saliva; SA—Salivary amylase; SWS—Stimulated whole saliva. Statistically significant correlations ($p < 0.05$) are highlighted as bold and italics.

Table 5. Correlations between salivary and plasma redox biomarkers in children with chronic kidney disease (CKD) and healthy controls.

	C ($n = 30$)		CKD ($n = 30$)	
	NWS & plasma	SWS & plasma	NWS & plasma	SWS & plasma
Dityrosine	*0.825*	−0.106	0.173	0.106
Kynurenine	*0.698*	0.140	*0.504*	*0.629*
N-formylkynurenine	0.327	−0.019	0.268	0.060
Tryptophan	*0.507*	0.208	*−0.374*	0.043
AGE	*0.781*	*0.461*	−0.268	0.314
Total thiols	−0.042	0.084	*0.387*	0.335
4-HNE	*0.473*	0.210	0.257	0.262
8-isop	0.041	−0.208	0.349	0.350
NO	0.030	−0.209	0.016	−0.078
S-nitrosothiols	−0.045	0.174	−0.059	0.025
Peroxynitrite	0.121	−0.340	0.224	0.334
Nitrotyrosine	0.096	−0.054	0.165	0.140

4-HNE—4-hydroxynoneal protein adducts; 8-isop—8-isoprostanes; AGE—Advanced glycation end products; C—Healthy controls; CKD—Patients with chronic kidney disease; NWS—Non-stimulated whole saliva; SA—Salivary amylase; SWS—Stimulated whole saliva. Statistically significant correlations ($p < 0.05$) are highlighted as bold and italics.

4. Discussion

This study is the first to evaluate protein glycooxidation products, lipid oxidative damage and nitrosative stress in non-stimulated and stimulated saliva and plasma in children with chronic kidney disease. We have shown that in CKD there is a dysfunction of salivary glands, which intensifies with the oxidation of salivary proteins/lipids and nitrosative damage. Interestingly, in children with CKD, salivary oxidation products did not correlate with their plasma content. Therefore, disturbances in salivary redox homeostasis may occur independently of alterations at the central level (plasma).

In the course of CKD, pathological changes of oral mucosa, susceptibility to fungal infections and olfactory and taste disorders were observed [44]. Therefore, it is not surprising that non-stimulated and stimulated saliva secretion was significantly lower in all children with CKD in comparison to controls. However, hyposalivation (NWS flow < 0.2 mL/min) was observed only in patients with severe renal failure (4–5 stage CKD). This indicates the progression of salivary hypofunction according to the CKD severity. This may also explain the increased incidence of dental caries and periodontal disease in children with advanced stages of CKD [44]. However, total protein content and salivary amylase activity were also significantly lower in CKD children with hyposalivation compared to other subjects (CKD children with normal salivary secretion and healthy controls). Indeed, it should be recalled that α-amylase is not only involved in the degradation of food polysaccharides [33]. This enzyme is synthesized in acinar cells (i.e., major secretory cells) of the salivary glands, where it is stored in granules before secretion. Secretory granules are transported to the apical membrane, fuse with the membrane and secrete their contents into the secretory ducts by exocytosis. Therefore, α-amylase can be an indicator of protein secretion through exocytosis [33,45]. Many studies have also shown a relationship between the decrease in α-amylase activity and impairment of secretory function of salivary glands [17,33]. Consequently, CKD is not only associated with reduced saliva secretion, but also with impaired protein secretion into saliva (Figure 1).

Salivary oxidative/nitrosative stress was significantly higher in children with CKD and hyposalivation (4–5 stage CKD) compared to patients with normal salivary secretion (1–3 stage CKD).

Therefore, both salivary glycooxidation and lipoperoxidation intensify with the progression of CKD. Interestingly, salivary oxidation products correlate negatively with salivary flow rate, α-amylase activity and total protein content.

As a result of protein oxidation, many structural and functional changes occur. Indeed, the amino acids are modified, the protein chain is fragmented and cross-linkages between the amino acids are formed. Interestingly, thiol groups (-SH) are the first to be oxidized [46]. Thus, it is no surprising that the salivary thiol levels in CKD have decreased. However, ROS also react with side chains of amino acids (e.g., tyrosine, lysine, arginine, or threonine). In our study we observed a quenching of tryptophan fluorescence (probably due to enhanced oxidation of salivary albumin [47]) as well as an increase in the fluorescence of protein glycooxidation products. Interestingly, the fluorescence of glycooxidation products was significantly higher in both NWS and SWS of CKD children with hyposalivation (↑dityrosine, ↑kynurenine, ↑N-formylkynurenine, and ↑AGE) compared to patients with normal salivary secretion. Under inflammatory conditions, there is an increased production of reactive chlorates that combine with tyrosine or kynurenine. The resulting aggregates tend to accumulate in the tissues [46]. AGE, products of non-enzymatic glycation of proteins, can react with a specific receptor (RAGE, receptor for advanced glycation end products) to activate multiple signalling pathways (e.g., NF-κB, NJK, p21RAS) [48]. Another important source of free radicals in CKD is activation of RAAS and increased expression of xanthine oxidase (XO), which also increases uric acid production [6]. Furthermore, by stimulating various reductases (e.g., aldose reductase), carbonyl stress is increased (↑AGE). However, carbonylation of proteins is an irreversible process. Although oxidized proteins can be degraded, the ability of proteasomes to remove them is limited and depends on the degree of protein oxidation [46]. Therefore, oxidized proteins can disrupt the function of different organs, including impairing saliva secretion [20,21,49]. The prolonged accumulation of glycooxidation products (especially AGE) may also enhance the infiltration of macrophages and neutrophils in the parenchyma of the salivary glands, increasing, on a positive feedback, the production of free radicals [48]. In our study, the potential relationship between protein glycooxidation and salivary gland dysfunction in CKD children may be indicated by negative correlations between NWS/SWS flow and the fluorescence of oxidative modification products. Importantly, no such dependence was observed in the control group.

However, it is not proteins but lipids that are particularly susceptible to oxidation. In our study we assessed the concentration of 4-HNE protein adducts and 8-isop, which was significantly higher in NWS and SWS of CKD children with reduced saliva secretion. It was shown that lipid peroxidation products modify the physical properties of cell membranes. This increases the cell membrane permeability and reduces the difference in electrical potentials on both sides of the lipid bi-layer. Lipid oxidation may also affect the secretory function of the salivary glands, particularly since oxidized lipids induce further oxidative damage to proteins and DNA [20,21,49]. In our study, salivary 8-isop and 4-HNE correlated negatively with salivary flow, protein content and α-amylase activity. Increased levels of malondialdehyde (MDA) were observed in salivary glands of rats with experimental chronic kidney disease [50] as well as in saliva of children with CKD [3]. 4-HNE protein adducts may also increase the expression of matrix metalloproteinases, which not only damage the parenchyma of the salivary glands but also the nerves involved in salivary secretion [21,51]. However, this issue requires further research, especially in the context of CKD.

Binding of various neurotransmitters to salivary gland duct/secretory acini receptors initiates the excretion of primary saliva. At the parasympathetic nerve endings, NO is secreted, which by increasing the level of calcium ions is responsible for opening water channels (aquaporins) [52]. It is therefore not surprising that the concentration of total NO was significantly lower in CKD children with hyposalivation. Indeed, in children with CKD there is a reduced NO synthesis and increased endothelial production of the endogenous NO synthase inhibitor (asymmetric dimethylarginine, ADMA) [53]. However, the decrease in NO bioavailability can be explained not only by the impairment of endothelial cells but also by increased production of peroxynitrite. It is formed in the reaction of nitric oxide with superoxide radical anion. The resulting peroxynitrite is a weaker vasodilatant (than NO), but also a much stronger and more stable oxidant. It has been shown that peroxynitrite oxidizes thiol groups of proteins, initiates lipid peroxidation and inhibits mitochondrial respiratory chain (also in the salivary glands [14,20,21]). In our study, peroxynitrite levels were significantly higher in NWS, SWS, and plasma of CKD children with hyposalivation compared to those with normal salivary secretion. Although our methodology is routinely used to assess nitrosative stress in frozen saliva samples [54,55], it should be remembered that NO and peroxynitrite have a very short half-life and this may understate the results obtained.

An important part of the study was also the evaluation of the saliva-blood correlation coefficients. In children with CKD, salivary glycooxidation products, lipid oxidation damage and nitrosative stress products did not correlate with their plasma content. Thus, salivary biomarkers do not reflect the central redox homeostasis of CKD children. It is well known that the products of protein and lipid oxidation are not only produced in the salivary glands. By passive and active transport, these compounds can be transported from plasma to the oral cavity. Nevertheless, our study indicates that oxidative/nitrosative stress are different at the local (NWS, SWS) and central (plasma) levels. The influence of several environmental factors on salivary redox homeostasis is not without significance [19]. The oxidative-reductive balance of the oral cavity may also be varied by a distinctive microbiota composition of CKD patients [56].

However, correlations between salivary and plasma oxidation products were observed in the control group. Indeed, in healthy children, adults and the elderly, the concentration of oxidative stress products in NWS generally reflects their plasma content [28]. However, also in some systemic diseases, salivary oxidation products correlates with their blood level [32,55]. Salivary redox biomarkers can therefore be used in the diagnosis of systemic diseases, but only when salivary hypofunction is not present [57].

Hyposalivation was also observed in adults with CKD [23,58,59]. Although the cause of disturbed salivary gland function in CKD is still unknown, it is assumed that apart from changes in NO bioavailability, pharmacotherapy may also affect salivary secretion. Indeed, numerous drugs, including those used in CKD therapy, may influence the quantitative and qualitative composition of saliva. Some of them affect the water-electrolyte balance of salivary glands, while others block muscarinic/adrenergic receptors involved in the initiation of saliva secretion. Since pharmacotherapy is one of the major causes of hyposalivation [16,27], in this study we excluded children taking 5 and more medications. What is important, we did not observe any significant differences in salivary flow/redox biomarkers depending on the number of drugs.

Finally, please note the limitations of our manuscript. Firstly, the method of saliva collection using citric acid may affect the pH of the stimulated saliva. For analysis of components in SWS, mastication of no-taste gum could be a better method. Secondly, we only assessed the selected biomarkers of oxidative/nitrosative damage. Therefore, we cannot fully characterize salivary redox homeostasis in CKD children. Since oxidative stress promotes inflammation, the assessment of pro-inflammatory mediators in saliva is also indicated. Moreover, we cannot eliminate the impact of pharmacotherapy on saliva secretion and composition. Nevertheless, the study was carried out on children from whom non-stimulated and stimulated saliva as well as plasma were taken. The study and control groups are also carefully selected for accompanying diseases and periodontal status.

5. Conclusions

Chronic kidney disease is associated with salivary gland dysfunction and increased oxidative and nitrosative damage. Oxidation of salivary proteins and lipids increases with the progression of the disease and the degree of salivary gland damage. The assessment of salivary gland function should be an integral part of a dental examination in patients with CKD. Antioxidant supplementation may be considered in CKD children; nevertheless, further research is necessary, especially in a larger population of patients.

Author Contributions: Conceptualization, M.M. and A.Z.; Data curation, M.M.; Formal analysis, M.M.; Funding acquisition, M.M. and A.Z.; Investigation, M.M., K.T.-J., and A.Z.; Methodology, M.M. and A.Z.; Project administration, M.M. and A.Z.; Resources, M.M., J.S., K.T.-J., A.W., and A.Z.; Software, M.M.; Supervision, A.W. and A.Z.; Validation, M.M.; Visualization, M.M.; Writing—original draft, M.M.; Writing—review and editing M.M., K.T.-J., and A.Z. All authors have read and agreed to the published version of the manuscript.

Funding: This work was supported by grants from the Medical University of Bialystok, Poland (grant numbers: SUB/1/DN/20/002/1209; SUB/1/DN/20/002/3330).

Acknowledgments: The authors would like to thank Anna Skutnik and Izabela Zieniewska for their help in collecting material for research.

Conflicts of Interest: The authors declare no conflict of interest.

References

1. Levey, A.S.; De Jong, P.E.; Coresh, J.; Nahas, M.E.; Astor, B.C.; Matsushita, K.; Gansevoort, R.T.; Kasiske, B.L.; Eckardt, K.U. The definition, classification, and prognosis of chronic kidney disease: A KDIGO Controversies Conference report. *Kidney Int.* **2011**. [CrossRef] [PubMed]
2. Becherucci, F.; Roperto, R.M.; Materassi, M.; Romagnani, P. Chronic kidney disease in children. *Clin. Kidney J.* **2016**. [CrossRef] [PubMed]
3. Maciejczyk, M.; Szulimowska, J.; Skutnik, A.; Taranta-Janusz, K.; Wasilewska, A.; Wiśniewska, N.; Zalewska, A. Salivary Biomarkers of Oxidative Stress in Children with Chronic Kidney Disease. *J. Clin. Med.* **2018**, *7*, 209. [CrossRef] [PubMed]
4. Tomino, Y. Pathogenesis and treatment of chronic kidney disease: A review of our recent basic and clinical data. *Kidney Blood Press. Res.* **2014**. [CrossRef] [PubMed]
5. Modaresi, A.; Nafar, M.; Sahraei, Z. Oxidative stress in chronic kidney disease. *Iran. J. Kidney Dis.* **2015**, *9*, 165–179. [PubMed]
6. Putri, A.Y.; Thaha, M. Role Of Oxidative Stress On Chronic Kidney Disease Progression. *Acta Med. Indones.* **2014**, *46*, 244–252.
7. Sureshbabu, A.; Ryter, S.W.; Choi, M.E. Oxidative stress and autophagy: Crucial modulators of kidney injury. *Redox Biol.* **2015**, *4*, 208–214. [CrossRef]
8. Beetham, K.S.; Howden, E.J.; Small, D.M.; Briskey, D.R.; Rossi, M.; Isbel, N.; Coombes, J.S. Oxidative stress contributes to muscle atrophy in chronic kidney disease patients. *Redox Rep.* **2015**, *20*, 126–132. [CrossRef]
9. Li, H.Y.; Hou, F.F.; Zhang, X.; Chen, P.Y.; Liu, S.X.; Feng, J.X.; Liu, Z.Q.; Shan, Y.X.; Wang, G.B.; Zhou, Z.M.; et al. Advanced Oxidation Protein Products Accelerate Renal Fibrosis in a Remnant Kidney Model. *J. Am. Soc. Nephrol.* **2007**, *18*, 528–538. [CrossRef]
10. Fogo, A.B. Mechanisms of progression of chronic kidney disease. *Pediatr. Nephrol.* **2007**. [CrossRef]
11. Zhou, L.L.; Cao, W.; Xie, C.; Tian, J.; Zhou, Z.; Zhou, Q.; Zhu, P.; Li, A.; Liu, Y.; Miyata, T.; et al. The receptor of advanced glycation end products plays a central role in advanced oxidation protein products-induced podocyte apoptosis. *Kidney Int.* **2012**, *82*, 759–770. [CrossRef]
12. Zhou, L.; Hou, F.F.; Wang, G.B.; Yang, F.; Xie, D.; Wang, Y.P.; Tian, J.W. Accumulation of advanced oxidation protein products induces podocyte apoptosis and deletion through NADPH-dependent mechanisms. *Kidney Int.* **2009**, *76*, 1148–1160. [CrossRef] [PubMed]
13. Nakanishi, T.; Kuragano, T.; Nanami, M.; Nagasawa, Y.; Hasuike, Y. Misdistribution of Iron and Oxidative Stress in Chronic Kidney Disease. *Free Radic. Biol. Med.* **2018**. [CrossRef] [PubMed]
14. Zalewska, A.; Ziembicka, D.; Żendzian-Piotrowska, M.; Maciejczyk, M. The Impact of High-Fat Diet on Mitochondrial Function, Free Radical Production, and Nitrosative Stress in the Salivary Glands of Wistar Rats. *Oxid. Med. Cell. Longev.* **2019**, *2019*, 2606120. [CrossRef] [PubMed]
15. Fejfer, K.; Buczko, P.; Niczyporuk, M.; Ładny, J.R.; Hady, H.R.; Knaś, M.; Waszkiel, D.; Klimiuk, A.; Zalewska, A.; Maciejczyk, M. Oxidative Modification of Biomolecules in the Nonstimulated and Stimulated Saliva of Patients with Morbid Obesity Treated with Bariatric Surgery. *Biomed Res. Int.* **2017**, *2017*. [CrossRef] [PubMed]
16. Maciejczyk, M.; Taranta-Janusz, K.; Wasilewska, A.; Kossakowska, A.; Zalewska, A. A Case-Control Study of Salivary Redox Homeostasis in Hypertensive Children. Can Salivary Uric Acid be a Marker of Hypertension? *J. Clin. Med.* **2020**, *9*, 837. [CrossRef]

17. Skutnik-Radziszewska, A.; Maciejczyk, M.; Fejfer, K.; Krahel, J.; Flisiak, I.; Kołodziej, U.; Zalewska, A. Salivary Antioxidants and Oxidative Stress in Psoriatic Patients: Can Salivary Total Oxidant Status and Oxidative Status Index Be a Plaque Psoriasis Biomarker? *Oxid. Med. Cell. Longev.* **2020**, *2020*, 9086024. [CrossRef]
18. Silvestre-Rangil, J.; Bagán, L.; Silvestre, F.J.; Bagán, J.V. Oral manifestations of rheumatoid arthritis. A cross-sectional study of 73 patients. *Clin. Oral Investig.* **2016**. [CrossRef]
19. Żukowski, P.; Maciejczyk, M.; Waszkiel, D. Sources of free radicals and oxidative stress in the oral cavity. *Arch. Oral Biol.* **2018**, *92*, 8–17. [CrossRef]
20. Zalewska, A.; Maciejczyk, M.; Szulimowska, J.; Imierska, M.; Błachnio-Zabielska, A. High-Fat Diet Affects Ceramide Content, Disturbs Mitochondrial Redox Balance, and Induces Apoptosis in the Submandibular Glands of Mice. *Biomolecules* **2019**, *9*, 877. [CrossRef]
21. Maciejczyk, M.; Matczuk, J.; Żendzian-Piotrowska, M.; Niklińska, W.; Fejfer, K.; Szarmach, I.; Ładny, J.R.; Zieniewska, I.; Zalewska, A. Eight-Week Consumption of High-Sucrose Diet Has a Pro-Oxidant Effect and Alters the Function of the Salivary Glands of Rats. *Nutrients* **2018**, *10*, 1530. [CrossRef] [PubMed]
22. Maciejczyk, M.; Szulimowska, J.; Taranta-Janusz, K.; Werbel, K.; Wasilewska, A.; Zalewska, A. Salivary FRAP as A Marker of Chronic Kidney Disease Progression in Children. *Antioxidants* **2019**, *8*, 409. [CrossRef] [PubMed]
23. Maciejczyk, M.; Żukowski, P.; Zalewska, A. Salivary Biomarkers in Kidney Diseases. In *Saliva in Health and Disease*; Tvarijonaviciute, A., Martínez-Subiela, S., López-Jornet, P., Lamy, E., Eds.; Springer International Publishing: Cham, Switzerland, 2020; pp. 193–219. ISBN 978-3-030-37681-9.
24. Klassen, J.T.; Krasko, B.M. The dental health status of dialysis patients. *J. Can. Dent. Assoc.* **2002**.
25. Zalewska, A.; Kossakowska, A.; Taranta-Janusz, K.; Zięba, S.; Fejfer, K.; Salamonowicz, M.; Kostecka-Sochoń, P.; Wasilewska, A.; Maciejczyk, M. Dysfunction of Salivary Glands, Disturbances in Salivary Antioxidants and Increased Oxidative Damage in Saliva of Overweight and Obese Adolescents. *J. Clin. Med.* **2020**, *9*, 548. [CrossRef] [PubMed]
26. Skutnik-Radziszewska, A.; Maciejczyk, M.; Flisiak, I.; Kołodziej, J.K.U.; Kotowska-Rodziewicz, A.; Klimiuk, A.; Zalewska, A. Enhanced Inflammation and Nitrosative Stress in the Saliva and Plasma of Patients with Plaque Psoriasis. *J. Clin. Med.* **2020**, *9*, 745. [CrossRef]
27. Saleh, J.; Figueiredo, M.A.Z.; Cherubini, K.; Salum, F.G. Salivary hypofunction: An update on aetiology, diagnosis and therapeutics. *Arch. Oral Biol.* **2015**, *60*, 242–255. [CrossRef]
28. Maciejczyk, M.; Zalewska, A.; Ładny, J.R. Salivary Antioxidant Barrier, Redox Status, and Oxidative Damage to Proteins and Lipids in Healthy Children, Adults, and the Elderly. *Oxid. Med. Cell. Longev.* **2019**, *2019*, 1–12. [CrossRef]
29. Schwartz, G.J.; Muñoz, A.; Schneider, M.F.; Mak, R.H.; Kaskel, F.; Warady, B.A.; Furth, S.L. New Equations to Estimate GFR in Children with CKD. *J. Am. Soc. Nephrol.* **2009**, *20*, 629–637. [CrossRef]
30. National Kidney Foundation K/DOQI clinical practice guidelines for chronic kidney disease: Evaluation, classification, and stratification. *Am. J. Kidney Dis.* **2002**, *39*, S1–S266.
31. NIH The Fourth Report on the Diagnosis, Evaluation, and Treatment of High Blood Pressure in Children and Adolescents. *Natl. Inst. Health* **2005**, *05–5267*, 1–60. [CrossRef]
32. Klimiuk, A.; Maciejczyk, M.; Choromańska, M.; Fejfer, K.; Waszkiewicz, N.; Zalewska, A. Salivary Redox Biomarkers in Different Stages of Dementia Severity. *J. Clin. Med.* **2019**, *8*, 840. [CrossRef] [PubMed]
33. Maciejczyk, M.; Kossakowska, A.; Szulimowska, J.; Klimiuk, A.; Knaś, M.; Car, H.; Niklińska, W.; Ładny, J.R.; Chabowski, A.; Zalewska, A. Lysosomal Exoglycosidase Profile and Secretory Function in the Salivary Glands of Rats with Streptozotocin-Induced Diabetes. *J. Diabetes Res.* **2017**, *2017*, 1–13. [CrossRef] [PubMed]
34. Bernfeld, P. Amylases, alpha and beta. *Methods Enzymol. I* **1955**. [CrossRef]
35. World Health Organization. *Oral Health Surveys: Basic Methods*; WHO Publications Center USA: Albany, NY, USA, 2013. ISBN 9789241548649.
36. Borys, J.; Maciejczyk, M.; Krętowski, A.J.; Antonowicz, B.; Ratajczak-Wrona, W.; Jablonska, E.; Zaleski, P.; Waszkiel, D.; Ladny, J.R.; Zukowski, P.; et al. The redox balance in erythrocytes, plasma, and periosteum of patients with titanium fixation of the jaw. *Front. Physiol.* **2017**, *8*. [CrossRef]

37. Rice-Evans, C.A.; Diplock, A.T.; Symons, M.C.R. Assay of antioxidant nutrients and antioxidant enzymes. *Lab. Tech. Biochem. Mol. Biol.* **1991**, *22*, 185–206. [CrossRef]
38. Kalousová, M.; Zima, T.; Tesař, V.; Dusilová-Sulková, S.; Škrha, J. Advanced glycoxidation end products in chronic diseases - Clinical chemistry and genetic background. *Mutat. Res.-Fundam. Mol. Mech. Mutagen.* **2005**.
39. Ellman, G.L. Tissue sulfhydryl groups. *Arch. Biochem. Biophys.* **1959**, *82*, 70–77. [CrossRef]
40. Grisham, M.B.; Johnson, G.G.; Lancaster, J.R. Quantitation of nitrate and nitrite in extracellular fluids. *Methods Enzymol.* **1996**, *268*, 237–246. [CrossRef]
41. Borys, J.; Maciejczyk, M.; Antonowicz, B.; Krętowski, A.; Sidun, J.; Domel, E.; Dąbrowski, J.R.; Ładny, J.R.; Morawska, K.; Zalewska, A. Glutathione Metabolism, Mitochondria Activity, and Nitrosative Stress in Patients Treated for Mandible Fractures. *J. Clin. Med.* **2019**, *8*, 127. [CrossRef]
42. Wink, D.A.; Kim, S.; Coffin, D.; Cook, J.C.; Vodovotz, Y.; Chistodoulou, D.; Jourd'heuil, D.; Grisham, M.B. Detection of S-nitrosothiols by fluorometric and colorimetric methods. *Methods Enzymol.* **1999**, *301*, 201–211. [CrossRef]
43. Beckman, J.S.; Ischiropoulos, H.; Zhu, L.; van der Woerd, M.; Smith, C.; Chen, J.; Harrison, J.; Martin, J.C.; Tsai, M. Kinetics of superoxide dismutase- and iron-catalyzed nitration of phenolics by peroxynitrite. *Arch. Biochem. Biophys.* **1992**, *298*, 438–445. [CrossRef]
44. Davidovich, E.; Schwarz, Z.; Davidovitch, M.; Eidelman, E.; Bimstein, E. Oral findings and periodontal status in children, adolescents and young adults suffering from renal failure. *J. Clin. Periodontol.* **2005**. [CrossRef]
45. Bosch, J.A.; Veerman, E.C.I.; de Geus, E.J.; Proctor, G.B. α-Amylase as a reliable and convenient measure of sympathetic activity: Don't start salivating just yet! *Psychoneuroendocrinology* **2011**, *36*, 449–453. [CrossRef] [PubMed]
46. Beal, M.F. Oxidatively modified proteins in aging and disease. *Free Radic. Biol. Med.* **2002**. [CrossRef]
47. Ghisaidoobe, A.B.T.; Chung, S.J. Intrinsic tryptophan fluorescence in the detection and analysis of proteins: A focus on Förster resonance energy transfer techniques. *Int. J. Mol. Sci.* **2014**, *15*, 22518–22538. [CrossRef]
48. Ott, C.; Jacobs, K.; Haucke, E.; Navarrete Santos, A.; Grune, T.; Simm, A. Role of advanced glycation end products in cellular signaling. *Redox Biol.* **2014**, *2*, 411–429. [CrossRef]
49. Knaś, M.; Maciejczyk, M.; Daniszewska, I.; Klimiuk, A.; Matczuk, J.; Kołodziej, U.; Waszkiel, D.; Ładny, J.R.; Żendzian-Piotrowska, M.; Zalewska, A. Oxidative Damage to the Salivary Glands of Rats with Streptozotocin-Induced Diabetes-Temporal Study: Oxidative Stress and Diabetic Salivary Glands. *J. Diabetes Res.* **2016**, *2016*, 1–13. [CrossRef]
50. Nogueira, F.N.; Romero, A.C.; da Silva Pedrosa, M.; Ibuki, F.K.; Bergamaschi, C.T. Oxidative stress and the antioxidant system in salivary glands of rats with experimental chronic kidney disease. *Arch. Oral Biol.* **2020**, *113*, 104709. [CrossRef]
51. Pérez, P.; Kwon, Y.J.; Alliende, C.; Leyton, L.; Aguilera, S.; Molina, C.; Labra, C.; Julio, M.; Leyton, C.; González, M.J. Increased acinar damage of salivary glands of patients with Sjögren's syndrome is paralleled by simultaneous imbalance of matrix metalloproteinase 3/tissue inhibitor of metalloproteinases 1 and matrix metalloproteinase 9/tissue inhibitor of metalloprotein. *Arthritis Rheum.* **2005**. [CrossRef]
52. Proctor, G.B.; Carpenter, G.H. Regulation of salivary gland function by autonomic nerves. *Auton. Neurosci.* **2007**, *133*, 3–18. [CrossRef]
53. Chaudhary, K.; Malhotra, K.; Sowers, J.; Aroor, A. Uric acid-key ingredient in the recipe for cardiorenal metabolic syndrome. *CardioRenal Med.* **2013**. [CrossRef] [PubMed]
54. Clodfelter, W.H.; Basu, S.; Bolden, C.; Dos Santos, P.C.; King, S.B.; Kim-Shapiro, D.B. The relationship between plasma and salivary NOx. *Nitric oxide Biol. Chem.* **2015**, *47*, 85–90. [CrossRef]
55. Klimiuk, A.; Zalewska, A.; Sawicki, R.; Knapp, M.; Maciejczyk, M. Salivary Oxidative Stress Increases With the Progression of Chronic Heart Failure. *J. Clin. Med.* **2020**, *9*, 769. [CrossRef] [PubMed]
56. Hu, J.; Iragavarapu, S.; Nadkarni, G.N.; Huang, R.; Erazo, M.; Bao, X.; Verghese, D.; Coca, S.; Ahmed, M.K.; Peter, I. Location-Specific Oral Microbiome Possesses Features Associated With CKD. *Kidney Int. Rep.* **2018**. [CrossRef] [PubMed]
57. Maciejczyk, M.; Zalewska, A.; Gerreth, K. Salivary Redox Biomarkers in Selected Neurodegenerative Diseases. *J. Clin. Med.* **2020**, *9*, 497. [CrossRef]

58. López-Pintor, R.-M.; López-Pintor, L.; Casañas, E.; de Arriba, L.; Hernández, G. Risk factors associated with xerostomia in haemodialysis patients. *Med. Oral Patol. Oral Cir. Bucal* **2017**, *22*, e185–e192. [CrossRef] [PubMed]
59. de Azambuja Berti-Couto, S.; Couto-Souza, P.H.; Jacobs, R.; Nackaerts, O.; Rubira-Bullen, I.R.F.; Westphalen, F.H.; Moysés, S.J.; Ignácio, S.A.; da Costa, M.B.; Tolazzi, A.L. Clinical diagnosis of hyposalivation in hospitalized patients. *J. Appl. Oral Sci.* **2012**. [CrossRef]

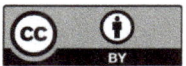

© 2020 by the authors. Licensee MDPI, Basel, Switzerland. This article is an open access article distributed under the terms and conditions of the Creative Commons Attribution (CC BY) license (http://creativecommons.org/licenses/by/4.0/).

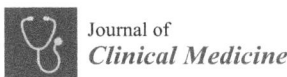 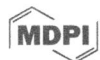

Article

Intra-Cystic (In Situ) Mucoepidermoid Carcinoma: A Clinico-Pathological Study of 14 Cases

Saverio Capodiferro [1,†], Giuseppe Ingravallo [2,*,†], Luisa Limongelli [1], Mauro Giuseppe Mastropasqua [2], Angela Tempesta [1], Gianfranco Favia [1] and Eugenio Maiorano [2]

1   Department of Interdisciplinary Medicine – Section of Odontostomatology, University of Bari Aldo Moro, Italy, Piazza G. Cesare, 11, 70124 Bari, Italy; capodiferro.saverio@gmail.com (S.C.); lululimongelli@gmail.com (L.L.); angelatempesta1989@gmail.com (A.T.); gianfranco.favia@uniba.it (G.F.)
2   Department of Emergency and Organ Transplantation – Section of Pathological Anatomy, University of Bari Aldo Moro, Italy, Piazza G. Cesare, 11, 70124 Bari, Italy; mauro.mastropasqua@uniba.it (M.G.M.); eugenio.maiorano@uniba.it (E.M.)
*   Correspondence: giuseppe.ingravallo@uniba.it
†   These authors contributed equally to this work.

Received: 1 April 2020; Accepted: 14 April 2020; Published: 18 April 2020

Abstract: Aims: To report on the clinico-pathological features of a series of 14 intra-oral mucoepidermoid carcinomas showing exclusive intra-cystic growth. Materials and methods: All mucoepidermoid carcinomas diagnosed in the period 1990–2012 were retrieved; the original histological preparations were reviewed to confirm the diagnosis and from selected cases, showing exclusive intra-cystic neoplastic components, additional sections were cut at three subsequent 200 m intervals and stained with Hematoxylin–Eosin, PAS, Mucicarmine and Alcian Blue, to possibly identify tumor invasion of the adjacent tissues, which could have been overlooked in the original histological preparations. Additionally, pertinent findings collected from the clinical charts and follow-up data were analyzed. Results: We identified 14 intraoral mucoepidermoid carcinomas treated by conservative surgery and with a minimum follow up of five years. The neoplasms were located in the hard palate (nine cases), the soft palate (two), the cheek (two) and the retromolar trigone (one). In all instances, histological examination revealed the presence of a single cystic space, containing clusters of columnar, intermediate, epidermoid, clear and mucous-producing cells, the latter exhibiting distinct intra-cytoplasmic mucin production, as confirmed by PAS, Mucicarmine and Alcian Blue stains. The cysts were entirely circumscribed by fibrous connective tissue, and no solid areas or infiltrating tumor cell clusters were detected. Conservative surgical resection was performed in all cases, and no recurrences or nodal metastases were observed during follow up. Conclusions: Mucoepidermoid carcinomas showing prominent (>20%) intra-cystic proliferation currently are considered low-grade tumors. In addition, we also unveil the possibility that mucoepidermoid carcinomas, at least in their early growth phase, may display an exclusive intra-cystic component and might be considered as in situ carcinomas, unable to infiltrate adjacent tissues and metastasize.

Keywords: salivary glands; minor salivary glands; salivary gland carcinoma; mucoepidermoid carcinoma; in situ carcinoma; intra-cystic carcinoma

1. Introduction

Mucoepidermoid carcinoma (MEC) was firstly described by Volkmann in 1895; subsequently, Stewart et al. (1945) defined such lesion as a "mucoepidermoid tumor", and identified tumors with "relatively favorable" and "highly unfavorable" clinical outcomes. Later on, Jakobsson et al. and many other authors [1–4] proposed to separate MECs into low, intermediate and high grades, based on the relative proportion of cell types, a distinction that still persisted in the WHO classification of tumors of 2017 [5]. MEC is one of the most common salivary gland malignancies, showing distinctive morphological features, such as mucous, intermediate and epidermoid cells in variable proportions [5–7]. Less than half of the cases arise in minor salivary glands, the palate being the most common intra-oral localization of MEC [8–12]. The architectural configuration of MEC may vary, but a cystic component is commonly present and may sometimes predominate [5,6,13–15]. Nevertheless, most MECs also show a solid growth pattern and infiltration of adjacent structures [16,17].

Though considered a tumor with low malignant potential in most instances, about 10% of the patients affected by MEC experience tumor-related death [10,11,18,19]. In this regard, MECs located in the submandibular gland and those showing a high histopathologic grade are considered more aggressive [8–10,20,21]. It should be noticed that the greater extension of the intra-cystic component correlates with lower grade of MEC, and therefore, this tumor characteristic per se may influence the clinical outcome [5–8,18,19,22].

Based on these premises, while retrospectively re-evaluating all MECs examined in the period 1990–2012, we focused our attention on those cases showing prevalent/exclusive intra-cystic components to further characterize their relevance in the clinic-pathological presentations and clinical outcomes of the affected patients.

2. Materials and Methods

All cases diagnosed as MEC at our institution during the years 1990–2012 were retrieved from the files of the Section of Pathological Anatomy of the University of Bari Aldo Moro, along with the pertinent clinical charts and follow-up data updated as of January 2019. All cases were fixed in 10% neutral buffered formalin, embedded in paraffin and routinely stained with Hematoxylin–Eosin; Periodic Acid–Shiff (PAS), with and without diastase pre-treatment; Mucicarmine; and Alcian Blue. The original histological preparations were reviewed to confirm the diagnoses, based on the occurrence of the distinct cell types (squamoid, mucous-producing and intermediate cells) that characterize MEC [5]. Additional sections at 3 subsequent 200 µm intervals were cut of selected cases showing exclusive tumoral intra-cystic components and stained with the above procedures, to possibly identify tumor invasion of the adjacent tissues that could have been overlooked in the original histological preparations.

3. Results

During the observational period, 128 MECs were identified, 82 involving the major and 46 the minor salivary glands; among these, 14 showed an exclusive intra-cystic tumoral component in the absence of infiltration of the adjacent tissues, as confirmed by the evaluation of additional cutting levels, the salient clinico-pathological features of which are reported in Table 1. Among such patients there were three males and 11 females, with a median age of 36.8 years; nine MECs involved the hard palate, two cases the soft palate, two the cheek mucosa and one case the retromolar trigone. In all instances, the neoplasms appeared as intra-oral nodules (Figure 1), sometimes with slight erosion/ulceration of the surface epithelium; and showed painless, slow growth and hard consistency, without evident infiltration of the adjacent soft and hard tissues, as confirmed by MR (conventional acronym for Magnetic Resonance) and CT scans. The tumor dimensions were relatively small, with a minimum clinical diameter of 0.5 cm up to a maximum of 1.8 cm. No loco-regional node involvement was detectable by clinical inspection or imaging techniques in any instance. All patients underwent conservative surgical excision with a rim of normal tissue. It should be emphasized that all the tumors of this cohort were localized in minor salivary glands and we were unable to identify "pure" intra-cystic (in situ) MEC in major glands.

Table 1. Clinico-pathological features of the patients with intra-cystic mucoepidemoid carcinoma (all alive without evidence of disease after the specified follow-up interval).

Case #	Age	Sex	Site	Size (cm)	Follow-up (months)
1	51	F	Hard palate	0.6	66
2	26	F	Hard palate	1.8	62
3	20	M	Soft palate	1.3	88
4	25	F	Hard palate	0.7	74
5	36	F	Hard palate	0.5	84
6	35	F	Cheek	0.9	68
7	34	F	Hard Palate	1.0	74
8	41	F	Cheek	1.2	62
9	28	M	Soft palate	0.8	68
10	46	F	Hard palate	1.1	62
11	50	M	Hard palate	1.8	120
12	39	F	Hard palate	1.2	95
13	45	F	Retromolar trigone	1.6	66
14	40	F	Hard palate	1.2	68

= conventional symbol for "number".

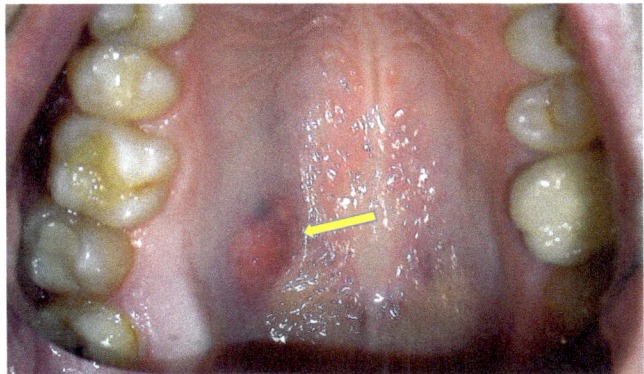

Figure 1. Clinical presentation MEC of the hard palate as a rather well-demarcated nodule with slight erosion of the covering mucosa.

Gross examination disclosed well defined cystic lesions, and microscopically, at scanning magnification, a single cystic space was detectable in all samples, showing parietal proliferation of clusters of epithelial cells with a focal cribriform growth pattern (Figure 2). The central part of the cyst was filled with proteinaceous material and cholesterol crystals, while a distinct and complete rim of collagenous stroma separated the cyst from the surface epithelium and from adjacent lobules of mucous salivary glands. The clusters of epithelial proliferation (Figure 3) were composed by small columnar and intermediate cells, cells with prominent cytoplasmic clearing and marginated nuclei, scattered flat to polygonal cells showing epidermoid differentiation and a reduced number of large mucous-producing cells with multivacuolated cytoplasm. The latter were better highlighted with Alcian Blue (Figure 4) and Mucicarmine stains and also showed PAS-positivity, which was partly abolished after diastase treatment. Occasionally, smaller cystic spaces with cribriform appearance were evident within the neoplastic epithelial clusters, which were lined by cuboidal to columnar cells. Nuclear pleomorphism was minimal, as was mitotic activity (<1/10 high power fields), while inflammatory infiltration, necrosis and perineural invasion were undetectable; additionally, tumor-free margins (> 1 mm) were assessed in all cases. Patients had been followed-up for a minimum of five years (range: 62–120 mo.; median: 68 mo.) and had remained without evidence of disease up to January 2019.

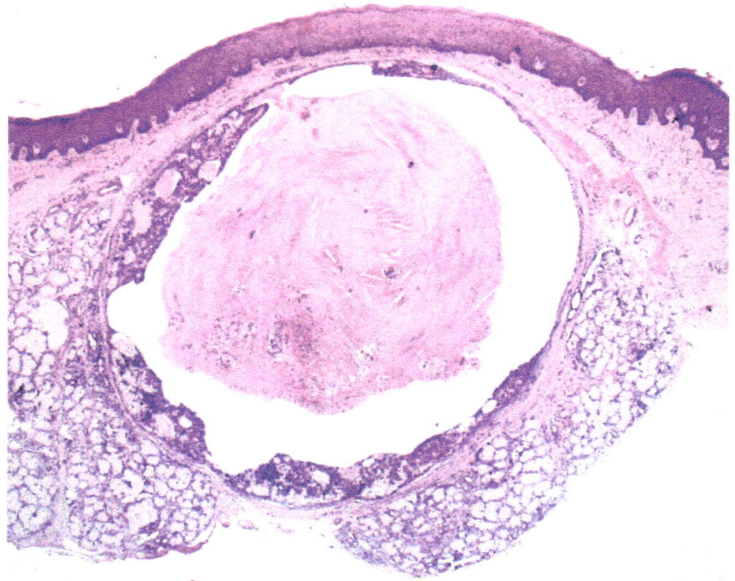

Figure 2. Under scanning magnification, the tumor was composed of a single cystic space, partly filled with proteinaceous material and cholesterol crystals, and showed parietal growth of epithelial cells and complete peripheral demarcation by fibrous connective tissue. (H&E, x1).

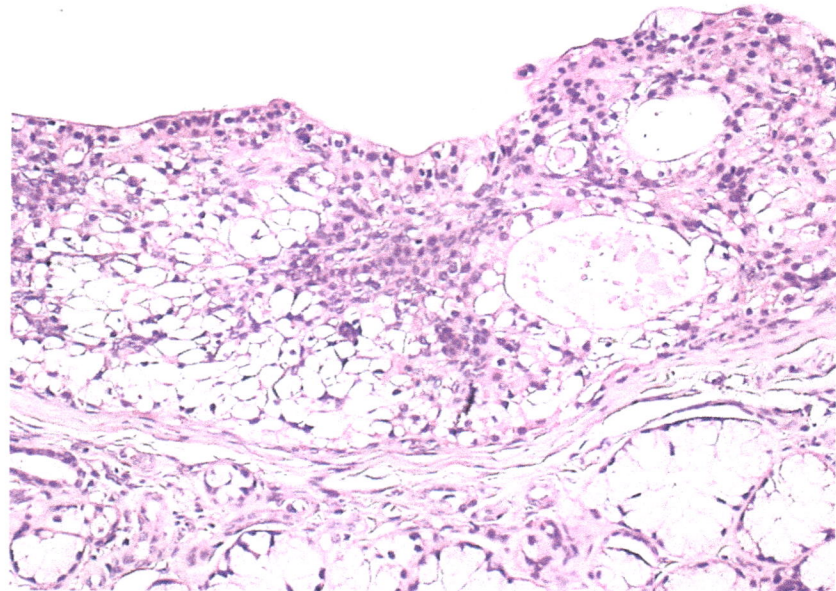

Figure 3. The epithelial component consisted of small columnar and intermediate cells, cells with prominent cytoplasmic clearing, rare flat to polygonal cells showing epidermoid differentiation and a reduced number of large mucous-producing cells with multivacuolated cytoplasm. (H&E, x10).

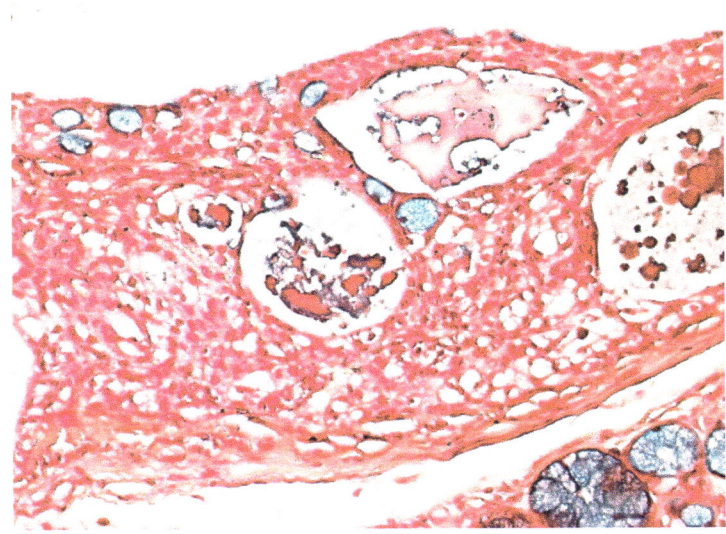

Figure 4. Epithelial cells with multi-vacuolated cytoplasms and marginated nuclei demonstrate consistent Alcian Blue positivity, indicating mucous production. (Alcian Blue, x20).

4. Discussion

Salivary gland carcinomas represent about 5% of all head and neck carcinomas and 0.5% of all malignancies [5,8–10,23–25], with an incidence of 1.1/100000 per year in the Caucasian population [9,25–27], and have been classified into 20 different types by the World Health Organization in 2017 [5].

MEC is the most common malignant tumor of the salivary glands (12%–29%) in children and young adults [9,25,28,29], and according to some authors, the most common malignancy in minor salivary glands [8–13,20]; its peak incidence is between the third and sixth decade, with predilection for females [25,28,29]. As confirmed by the results of the present study, the palate remains the most common site for MECs occurring in minor salivary glands, while they less frequently occur in the retromolar area, the floor of the mouth, the buccal mucosa, the lips and the tongue [3,5,18,23].

The cases reported herein showed the distinctive morphological features of "classical" MEC [5,30,31]; i.e., an epithelial tumor composed of intermediate, epidermoid, mucous-producing and clear cells, arranged in irregular clusters of variable size, but at variance with conventional MEC, no foci of stromal invasion were detected and the neoplastic proliferation manifested an exclusive intra-cystic growth. It is our opinion that the presence of a continuous rim of collagen around the neoplastic proliferation better testifies its in situ nature, and the presence of minimal stromal invasion or isolated tumor cell clusters should be accurately excluded, by examining the sample at multiple cutting levels. Immunohistochemical stains for myoepithelial (e.g., smooth muscle actin, calponin, smooth muscle myosin heavy chain) or basal cell markers (e.g., cytokeratin 14, p63) could possibly help to clarify this issue. Nevertheless, as for breast in situ carcinomas, residual ductal myoepithelial cells are not usually present as a continuous layer; therefore, it is somewhat misleading to assess the true in situ nature of the tumor. Additionally, anti-cytokeratin 14 and p63 antibodies do not stain residual ductal cells only; variable proportions of neoplastic MEC cells are positive for these markers as well.

Traditionally, MEC is considered a tumor with low malignant potential, though cases showing local recurrence, nodal and distant metastases and tumor-related death have been repeatedly reported [8,9,14,17,19,27]. Tumor aggressiveness is strictly related to histological grade, and although there is not complete agreement on the grading systems proposed so far, a three-tiered scale considering low, intermediate and high grade MECs has been more commonly adopted and proven useful for prognostic purposes [5,6,13,25,31]. Such systems take into account the extension of the intra-cystic component, the presence of neural invasion and necrosis, the mitotic index and cellular anaplasia [12,14,15,24,31]. At this regard, the cases of the present series, while fitting into the morphological diagnosis of "conventional" MEC as to their cell components, did not show but minimal nuclear pleomorphism, and occasional, if any, mitotic figures, in the absence of perineural/bone invasion and necrosis, thereby qualifying as low grade tumors, with indolent clinical behavior. Herewith, we provide morphological evidence to postulate that a less aggressive form of MEC may be identified, as for epithelial tumors occurring in other organs (e.g., breast and prostate), which could be considered an in situ carcinoma. This novel tumor subtype, characterized by exclusive intra-cystic growth, should be, by definition, incapable of infiltrating adjacent tissues and giving raise to nodal or distant metastases, thereby being easily curable with conservative surgery. Such clinico-pathological features parallel those of in situ (lobular/ductal/papillary) carcinomas of the breast and support the concept that early identification of such neoplasms may allow less aggressive treatments.

Furthermore, based on the classical morphological features of MEC, intraductal papilloma, cystadenoma, adenosquamous carcinoma, salivary duct carcinoma and salivary gland clear cell carcinomas could be considered in the differential diagnosis [21,22,30–32]. The lack of any papillary growth pattern and the presence of distinct and frequently prevalent clusters of intermediate cells help to rule out intraductal papilloma and cystadenoma, respectively. Adenosquamous carcinoma and salivary duct carcinoma may closely mimic MECs, but such tumor types are devoid of intermediate cells and usually show higher degrees of cellular pleomorphism and mitotic activity. In addition, evident mucin production within the neoplastic cells contributes to excluding other types of salivary gland carcinomas with clear cells (e.g., acinic cell carcinoma, hyalinizing carcinoma), which also lack an intermediate cell population [14,22,32].

It is well known that MECs may harbor MAML2 gene fusion, but in view of the typical morphologic features of all case of the present series, we considered the assessment of the status of MAML2 would have not added much to this study. In fact, it is generally accepted that up to 75%–80% of MECs, especially low and intermediate grades, harbor gene fusions involving MAML2 [33–36]. Despite its high specificity, MAML2 testing is no longer considered a useful prognostic indicator for already diagnosed MECs, and may be avoided when the diagnosis of MEC is reached straightforwardly, based on typical morphologic features [34,35,37]. Consequently, MAML2 testing as an ancillary diagnostic tool should be reserved for MECs showing unusual histological appearances [38,39], such as the oncocytic variant of MEC, to rule out oncocytoma and oncocytic carcinoma; and the Whartin-like variant and the recently described ciliated MEC variant, to rule out benign developmental cysts and ciliated, HPV-related squamous cell carcinomas [40,41].

In addition, we would also like to emphasize that we were unable to identify MECs with exclusive intra-cystic (in situ) growth in major salivary glands, but this may be related to the higher chances of detecting such tumors at earlier growth phases when located in intra-oral sites, in view of easier accessibility to inspection and palpation. In other words, we cannot exclude that intra-cystic (in situ) MECs may be present in major salivary glands, but they possibly remain undetected for longer times and are disclosed when infiltration of adjacent tissues has already occurred.

The pathogenesis of malignant salivary gland neoplasms, as well as the occurrence of genetic and epigenetic alterations still remain unclear. However, it would be interesting to explore whether the typical chromosomal translocation t (11;19) (MECT1-MAML2), which is detected in >50% of "conventional" MEC, is already present in tumors at early stages of tumorigenesis, such as those of the present series, and whether additional genetic alterations might be responsible for further progression to frankly invasive MEC.

In conclusion, we provide evidence that MECs with exclusive intra-cystic (in situ) components showed indolent clinical behavior, with no evidence of recurrence or metastases even after prolonged follow up, and may be more conservatively treated. Therefore, we strongly suggest adopting the designation intra-cystic (in situ) MEC in diagnostic reports to properly manage patients and avoid unnecessary over-treatments.

Author Contributions: Clinical data curation, S.C., L.L., A.T.; histological data curation, G.I., M.G.M., E.M.; investigation, G.I., E.M.; methodology, S.C., G.F.; supervision, G.F. and E.M.; validation, M.G.M.; writing–original draft, S.C.; writing – review and editing, G.I., E.M. All authors have read and agreed to the published version of the manuscript.

Funding: This research received no external funding.

Acknowledgments: No acknowledgments due.

Conflicts of Interest: The authors declare no conflict of interest.

References

1. Eversole, L.R.; Rovin, S.; Sabes, W.R. Mucoepidermoid carcinoma of minor salivary glands: Report of 17 cases with follow-up. *J. Oral Surg.* **1972**, *30*, 107–112. [PubMed]
2. Eversole, L.R. Mucoepidermoid carcinoma: Review of 815 reported cases. *J. Oral Surg.* **1970**, *28*, 490–499. [PubMed]
3. Evans, H.L. Mucoepidermoid Carcinoma of Salivary Glands: A Study of 69 Cases with Special Attention to Histologic Grading. *Am. J. Clin. Pathol.* **1984**, *81*, 696–701. [CrossRef] [PubMed]
4. Auclair, P.L.; Goode, R.K.; Ellis, G.L. Mucoepidermoid carcinoma of intraoral salivary glands evaluation and application of grading criteria in 143 cases. *Cancer* **1992**, *69*, 2021–2030. [CrossRef]
5. El-Naggar, A.K.; Grandis, J.R.; Takata, T.; Grandis, J.; Slootweg, P. (Eds.) *WHO Classification of Head and Neck Tumours*, 4th ed.; IARC: Lyon, France, 2017.
6. Saluja, K.; Butler, R.T.; Pytynia, K.B.; Zhao, B.; Karni, R.J.; Weber, R.S.; El-Naggar, A.K. Mucoepidermoid carcinoma post−radioactive iodine treatment of papillary thyroid carcinoma: Unique presentation and putative etiologic association. *Hum. Pathol.* **2017**, *68*, 189–192. [CrossRef]
7. Goode, R.K.; Auclair, P.L.; Ellis, G.L. Mucoepidermoid carcinoma of the major salivary glands: Clinical and histopathologic analysis of 234 cases with evaluation of grading criteria. *Cancer* **1998**, *82*, 1217–1224. [CrossRef]
8. Galdirs, T.M.; Kappler, M.; Reich, W.; Eckert, A.W. Current aspects of salivary gland tumors—A systematic review of the literature. *GMS Interdiscip. Plast. Reconstr. Surg. DGPW* **2019**, *8*. [CrossRef]
9. Lawal, A.O.; Adisa, A.O.; Kolude, B.; Adeyemi, B.F. Malignant salivary gland tumours of the head and neck region: A single institutions review. *Pan Afr. Med. J.* **2015**, *20*, 121. [CrossRef] [PubMed]
10. Da Silva, L.P.; Serpa, M.S.; Viveiros, S.K.; Sena, D.A.C.; Pinho, R.F.D.C.; Guimarães, L.D.D.A.; Andrade, E.S.D.S.; Pereira, J.R.D.; Da Silveira, M.M.F.; Sobral, A.P.V.; et al. Salivary gland tumors in a Brazilian population: A 20-year retrospective and multicentric study of 2292 cases. *J. Cranio-Maxillofac. Surg.* **2018**, *46*, 2227–2233. [CrossRef] [PubMed]
11. González, A.C.; Skinner, H.R.; Díaz, A.V.; Ramírez, A.L.; Espildora, I.G.; González, A.S. Perfil epidemiológico de neoplasias epiteliales de glándulas salivales. *Rev. Med. Chil.* **2018**, *146*, 1159–1166. [CrossRef] [PubMed]
12. Abrahao, A.; Dos Santos, T.C.R.B.; Netto, J.D.N.S.; Pires, F.R.; Cabral, M.G. Clinicopathological characteristics of tumours of the intraoral minor salivary glands in 170 Brazilian patients. *Br. J. Oral Maxillofac. Surg.* **2016**, *54*, 30–34. [CrossRef] [PubMed]
13. Fu, J.-Y.; Wu, C.; Shen, S.-K.; Zheng, Y.; Zhang, C.-P.; Zhang, Z.-Y. Salivary gland carcinoma in Shanghai (2003–2012): An epidemiological study of incidence, site and pathology. *BMC Cancer* **2019**, *19*, 350. [CrossRef]
14. Cipriani, N.A.; Lusardi, J.J.; McElherne, J.; Pearson, A.T.; Olivas, A.D.; Fitzpatrick, C.; Lingen, M.W.; Blair, E.A. Mucoepidermoid Carcinoma. *Am. J. Surg. Pathol.* **2019**, *43*, 885–897. [CrossRef] [PubMed]
15. Seethala, R.R. An Update on Grading of Salivary Gland Carcinomas. *Head Neck Pathol.* **2009**, *3*, 69–77. [CrossRef] [PubMed]
16. Mücke, T.; Robitzky, L.K.; Kesting, M.R.; Wagenpfeil, S.; Holhweg-Majert, B.; Wolff, K.-D.; Hölzle, F. Advanced malignant minor salivary glands tumors of the oral cavity. *Oral Surg. Oral Med. Oral Pathol. Oral Radiol. Endodontol.* **2009**, *108*, 81–89. [CrossRef] [PubMed]

17. Kolokythas, A.; Connor, S.; Kimgsoo, D.; Fernandes, R.P.; Ord, R.A. Low-Grade Mucoepidermoid Carcinoma of the Intraoral Minor Salivary Glands With Cervical Metastasis: Report of 2 Cases and Review of the Literature. *J. Oral Maxillofac. Surg.* **2010**, *68*, 1396–1399. [CrossRef]
18. Ord, R.A.; Salama, A. Is it necessary to resect bone for low-grade mucoepidermoid carcinoma of the palate? *Br. J. Oral Maxillofac. Surg.* **2012**, *50*, 712–714. [CrossRef]
19. Lee, S.-Y.; Shin, H.A.; Rho, K.J.; Chung, H.J.; Kim, S.-H.; Choi, E. Characteristics, management of the neck, and oncological outcomes of malignant minor salivary gland tumours in the oral and sinonasal regions. *Br. J. Oral Maxillofac. Surg.* **2013**, *51*, e142–e147. [CrossRef]
20. Guzzo, M.; Andreola, S.; Sirizzotti, G.; Cantù, G. Mucoepidermoid carcinoma of the salivary glands: Clinicopathologic review of 108 patients treated at the National Cancer Institute of Milan. *Ann. Surg. Oncol.* **2002**, *9*, 688–695. [CrossRef]
21. Brandwein, M.S.; Ivanov, K.; Wallace, D.I.; Hille, J.J.; Wang, B.; Fahmy, A.; Bodian, C.; Urken, M.; Gnepp, D.R.; Huvos, A.; et al. Mucoepidermoid Carcinoma. *Am. J. Surg. Pathol.* **2001**, *25*, 835–845. [CrossRef]
22. Maiorano, E.; Altini, M.; Favia, G. Clear cell tumours of the salivary glands, jaws and oral mucosa. *Semin. Diagn. Pathol.* **1997**, *14*, 203–212. [PubMed]
23. Sultan, I.; Rodriguez-Galindo, C.; Al-Sharabati, S.; Guzzo, M.; Casanova, M.; Ferrari, A. Salivary gland carcinomas in children and adolescents: A population-based study, with comparison to adult cases. *Head Neck* **2010**, *33*, 1476–1481. [CrossRef] [PubMed]
24. Speight, P.M.; Barrett, A. Salivary gland tumours. *Oral Dis.* **2002**, *8*, 229–240. [CrossRef] [PubMed]
25. Bradley, P.J.; Eisele, D.W. Salivary Gland Neoplasms in Children and Adolescents. *Adv. Otorhinolaryngol.* **2016**, *78*, 175–181. [CrossRef] [PubMed]
26. Ettl, T.; Schwarz-Furlan, S.; Gosau, M.; Reichert, T.E. Salivary gland carcinomas. *Oral Maxillofac. Surg.* **2012**, *16*, 267–283. [CrossRef]
27. Bradley, P.J. Primary malignant parotid epithelial neoplasm. *Curr. Opin. Otolaryngol. Head Neck Surg.* **2015**, *23*, 91–98. [CrossRef]
28. Ba, N.D.D.; Wolter, N.E.; Irace, A.L.; Cunningham, M.J.; Mack, J.W.; Marcus, K.J.; Vargas, S.O.; Perez-Atayde, A.R.; Robson, C.D.; Rahbar, R. Mucoepidermoid carcinoma of the head and neck in children. *Int. J. Pediatr. Otorhinolaryngol.* **2019**, *120*, 93–99. [CrossRef]
29. Chiaravalli, S.; Guzzo, M.; Bisogno, G.; De De Pasquale, M.D.; Migliorati, R.; De Leonardis, F.; Collini, P.; Casanova, M.; Cecchetto, G.; Ferrari, A. Salivary gland carcinomas in children and adolescents: The Italian TREP project experience. *Pediatr. Blood Cancer* **2014**, *61*, 1961–1968. [CrossRef]
30. Schwarz, S.; Stiegler, C.; Müller, M.; Ettl, T.; Brockhoff, G.; Zenk, J.; Agaimy, A. Salivary gland mucoepidermoid carcinoma is a clinically, morphologically and genetically heterogeneous entity: A clinicopathological study of 40 cases with emphasis on grading, histological variants and presence of the t(11;19) translocation. *Histopathology* **2011**, *58*, 557–570. [CrossRef]
31. Pinheiro, J.; Fernandes, M.S.; Pereira, A.R.; Lopes, J.M. Histological Subtypes and Clinical Behavior Evaluation of Salivary Gland Tumors. *Acta Med. Port.* **2018**, *31*, 641–647. [CrossRef]
32. Rooper, L.M. Challenges in Minor Salivary Gland Biopsies: A Practical Approach to Problematic Histologic Patterns. *Head Neck Pathol.* **2019**, *13*, 476–484. [CrossRef] [PubMed]
33. Behboudi, A.; Enlund, F.; Winnes, M.; Andrén, Y.; Nordkvist, A.; Leivo, I.; Flaberg, E.; Szekely, L.; Mäkitie, A.; Grenman, R.; et al. Molecular classification of mucoepidermoid carcinomas—Prognostic significance of theMECT1–MAML2 fusion oncogene. *Genes Chromosom. Cancer* **2006**, *45*, 470–481. [CrossRef] [PubMed]
34. Chiosea, S.I.; Dacic, S.; Nikiforova, M.N.; Seethala, R.R. Prospective testing of mucoepidermoid carcinoma for the MAML2 translocation: Clinical Implications. *Laryngoscope* **2012**, *122*, 1690–1694. [CrossRef] [PubMed]
35. Seethala, R.R.; Dacic, S.; Cieply, K.; Kelly, L.M.; Nikiforova, M.N. A reappraisal of the MECT1/MAML2 translocation in salivary mucoepidermoid carcinomas. *Am. J. Surg. Pathol.* **2010**, *34*, 1106–1121. [CrossRef] [PubMed]
36. Okabe, M.; Miyabe, S.; Nagatsuka, H.; Terada, A.; Hanai, N.; Yokoi, M.; Shimozato, K.; Eimoto, T.; Nakamura, S.; Nagai, N.; et al. MECT1-MAML2 Fusion Transcript Defines a Favorable Subset of Mucoepidermoid Carcinoma. *Clin. Cancer Res.* **2006**, *12*, 3902–3907. [CrossRef]
37. Seethala, R.R.; Chiosea, S.I. MAML2 Status in Mucoepidermoid Carcinoma Can No Longer Be Considered a Prognostic Marker. *Am. J. Surg. Pathol.* **2016**, *40*, 1151–1153. [CrossRef]

38. Saade, R.E.; Bell, D.; Garcia, J.; Roberts, D.; Weber, R. Role of CRTC1/MAML2 Translocation in the Prognosis and Clinical Outcomes of Mucoepidermoid Carcinoma. *JAMA Otolaryngol. Head Neck Surg.* **2016**, *142*, 234–240. [CrossRef]
39. Ishibashi, K.; Ito, Y.; Masaki, A.; Fujii, K.; Beppu, S.; Sakakibara, T.; Takino, H.; Takase, H.; Ijichi, K.; Shimozato, K.; et al. Warthin-like Mucoepidermoid Carcinoma. *Am. J. Surg. Pathol.* **2015**, *39*, 1479–1487. [CrossRef]
40. Bishop, J.A.; Westra, W.H. Ciliated HPV-related Carcinoma. *Am. J. Surg. Pathol.* **2015**, *39*, 1591–1595. [CrossRef]
41. Radkay-Gonzalez, L.; Faquin, W.; McHugh, J.B.; Lewis, J.S.; Tuluc, M.; Seethala, R.R. Ciliated Adenosquamous Carcinoma: Expanding the Phenotypic Diversity of Human Papillomavirus-Associated Tumors. *Head Neck Pathol.* **2015**, *10*, 167–175. [CrossRef]

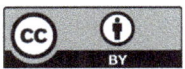

© 2020 by the authors. Licensee MDPI, Basel, Switzerland. This article is an open access article distributed under the terms and conditions of the Creative Commons Attribution (CC BY) license (http://creativecommons.org/licenses/by/4.0/).

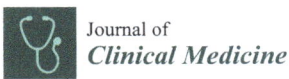
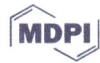

Review

Role of Viral Infections in the Pathogenesis of Sjögren's Syndrome: Different Characteristics of Epstein-Barr Virus and HTLV-1

Hideki Nakamura *, Toshimasa Shimizu and Atsushi Kawakami

Department of Immunology and Rheumatology, Unit of Advanced Preventive Medical Sciences, Division of Advanced Preventive Medical Sciences, Nagasaki University Graduate School of Biomedical Sciences, Nagasaki 852-8501, Japan; toshimasashimizu2000@yahoo.co.jp (T.S.); atsushik@nagasaki-u.ac.jp (A.K.)
* Correspondence: nhideki@nagasaki-u.ac.jp; Tel.: +81-95-819-7262

Received: 15 April 2020; Accepted: 6 May 2020; Published: 13 May 2020

Abstract: Viruses are possible pathogenic agents in several autoimmune diseases. Sjögren's syndrome (SS), which involves exocrine dysfunction and the appearance of autoantibodies, shows salivary gland- and lacrimal gland-oriented clinical features. Epstein-Barr virus (EBV) is the most investigated pathogen as a candidate that directly induces the phenotype found in SS. The reactivation of the virus with various stimuli induced a dysregulated form of EBV that has the potential to infect SS-specific B cells and plasma cells that are closely associated with the function of an ectopic lymphoid structure that contains a germinal center (GC) in the salivary glands of individuals with SS. The involvement of human T-cell leukemia virus type 1 (HTLV-1) in SS has been epidemiologically established, but the disease concept of HTLV-1-associated SS remains unexplained due to limited evidence from basic research. Unlike the cell-to-cell contact between lymphocytes, biofilm-like structures are candidates as the mode of HTLV-1 infection of salivary gland epithelial cells (SGECs). HTLV-1 can infect SGECs with enhanced levels of inflammatory cytokines and chemokines that are secreted from SGECs. Regardless of the different targets that viruses have with respect to affinitive lymphocytes, viruses are involved in the formation of pathological alterations with immunological modifications in SS.

Keywords: viral infection; Epstein-Barr virus; HTLV-1; salivary gland epithelial cell

1. Introduction

The pathogenesis of Sjögren's syndrome (SS), which affects salivary glands (SGs) as well as lacrimal glands (LGs), involves multiple factors including genetic elements [1–3] and subsequent environmental factors [4]. The clinical characteristics of individuals with SS are exocrine dysfunction (e.g., xerostomia and xerophthalmia) with the appearance of autoantibodies (including anti-Ro/SS-A and La/SS-B antibodies) [5]. With respect to genetic elements of SS, human leukocyte antigen (HLA) alleles have shown the strongest association with SS, and significant variations in HLA alleles by ethnicity have been revealed. Environmental factors that affect gender differences or the production of various autoantibodies may exert estrogen deficiency-mediated immunological effects [6] or alterations of the oral microbiome [7].

In addition, viral infections are profoundly associated with the activation of innate immunity, followed by an acquired immune response. Recognition of single-stranded ribonucleic acid (RNA) by toll-like captor 7/9 was a representative sensor of innate immunity in SS [8,9]. With the activation of an innate immunity signal with an interferon-gamma (IFN-γ) signature in viruses, the subsequent function of antigen presentation through the induction of major histocompatibility complex (MHC) is followed by an expansion of antigen-specific autoreactive T cells. In contrast, some viruses have a unique characteristic, i.e., a so-called in vivo 'reactivation' by various stimuli up to years after the initial infection [10]. In this review, we provide a comprehensive explanation of the roles of viruses that cause a breakdown of immune tolerance or modulation of the immune system in the pathogenesis of SS, and we describe the various detection analyses that have been used for these viruses. We focus on the actions of Epstein-Barr virus (EBV) and retroviruses by comparing the effects of these viruses in salivary glands of individuals with Sjögren's syndrome, as well as on the epidemiological and immunological findings.

2. Viral Infection and Autoimmune Diseases (AIDs)

2.1. Possible Mechanism Triggered by Viral Infection in AIDs

An acute or chronic viral infection is thought to play a crucial role as a triggering phase of the immunological instability that is required for the formulation of the chronic inflammatory condition in AIDs. As an initial step of innate immunity that involves several functions of cytotoxic T lymphocytes or natural killer T cells, the recognition of mobilized pathogens by receptors of innate immunity is required. Pathogen-associated molecular patterns (PAMPs) are common structures detected in pathogenic microbes that contribute to the initiation of innate immunity [11]. In concert with the detection of PAMPs, the concept of pattern recognition receptors (PRRs) was defined; PRRs have several molecules including toll-like receptors (TLRs), C-type lectin receptors, nucleotide-binding oligomerization domain (NOD)-like receptors (NLRs), and retinoic acid inducible gene-I (RIG-I)-like receptors (RLRs) [12–14]. Toll-like receptor 7 (TLR7) in particular is known to recognize single-stranded RNA viruses in exosomes of plasmatoid dendritic cells (pDCs) followed by a MyD88-dependent activation of the nuclear factor kappa B pathway after the assembly of tumor necrosis factor (TNF)-receptor associated factor-6 or interferon (IFN)-regulatory factor-7 (IRF-7) [15], which are associated with the induction of type I IFNs.

In our previous study, the expression of downstream signal transduction after stimulation with the TLR7 ligand was confirmed in the salivary glands of patients with SS and in an in vitro investigation using cultured epithelial cells obtained from SS patients [8], and pDCs appeared to be a source of type I IFN (including IFN-α and IFN-β). Regarding the close association between retinoic acid-inducible gene I (RIG-I)-like family signaling and SS, Maria et al. [16] demonstrated that RIG-I and melanoma differentiation associated gene-5 (MDA-5) were strongly expressed in mononuclear cells (MNCs) of salivary glands from SS patients. They also demonstrated that TLR7 stimulation had the potential to activate the signaling pathway of RIG-I-like family members in vitro. These observations suggested that TLRs and RLRs that were stimulated in salivary gland pDCs or monocytes are closely associated with RNA-sensing receptor-mediated innate immunity with the presentation of the type I IFN signature.

2.2. The Relationship between Autoimmune Conditions and Viral Infection

A relationship between typical AIDs and viral infection has been clarified over the past three decades. With respect to outbreaks of type 1 diabetes mellitus, the involvement of coxsackie B virus (an enterovirus) has been suggested, but the epidemiological evidence remains controversial regardless of a systematic review of 26 case-control studies [17]. In contrast, in a clinical study [18] using autopsied specimen RIG-I and MDA-5, type I IFNs were also strongly expressed in cells of enterovirus-infected pancreas in patients with fulminant type 1 diabetes mellitus.

Regarding the relationship between pathogens and the axonal form of Guillain-Barré Syndrome (GBS) with the appearance of antibodies against GM1 or GD1b, the involvement of Campylobacter infection as an exposure to bacteria has been discussed [19], and the involvement of Campylobacter toward GBS from a molecular biological perspective has been clarified. In addition, Zika virus infections in Columbia [20] were reported to be associated with GBS accompanied by a high degree of cranial nerve involvement or autonomic dysfunction.

Concerning connective tissue diseases, there are debates with respect to the relationship between systemic lupus erythematosus (SLE) and some viruses [21], and the involvement of parvovirus and EBV was discussed in serological research. It was reported that 3.9% of sera from SLE patients had a viral genome toward parvovirus, and among these patients, those with secondary anti-phospholipid syndrome (APS) had antibodies against parvovirus [22], suggesting a close association between APS-related antibody production and parvovirus. Regarding the relevance of the association between EBV and pathogenesis in SLE, the impairment of EBV-specific CD8+ T cells was reported to be associated with the activation of B cells in SLE patients who had high EBV viral loads [23]. The involvement of viral infection in rheumatoid arthritis (RA) has also been suspected for many years, but there is no definitive evidence regarding this matter. In a Norwegian study [24], there were no differences between patients with RA and healthy controls with respect to IgG antibodies against EBV and parvovirus B19 in sera.

Human T-cell leukemia virus type 1 (HTLV-1) has been vigorously investigated because HTLV-1 transgenic mice showed chronic erosive arthritis that resembled the synovitis observed in RA [25,26]. However, evidence that HTLV-1 infection directly induces typical RA has not yet been obtained in human studies, although the expression of HTLV-1-related antigen was demonstrated in synovial tissue obtained from RA patients [27]. Rather, there is concern regarding responsiveness to molecular targeted drugs including biologics (such as TNF inhibitors) among HTLV-1-seropositive patients with RA when therapeutic strategies are being considered [28,29]. No change of viral load or clonality was observed in HTLV-1-seropositive RA patients who were treated with a TNF inhibitor [28], and the efficacy of a TNF inhibitor was attenuated in HTLV-1-seropositive RA patients, especially in those who were anti-citrullinated protein antibody-positive [29]. For the treatment of HTLV-1-seropositive RA patients in endemic areas, the molecular targeted drugs' response rates and tumorigenesis remain serious concerns.

3. EBV Infection and Sjögren's Syndrome

3.1. Characteristics of the Infection Mechanism in EBV

EBV is a member of the family of herpes viruses. It is a double-stranded DNA virus, and the nomenclature of EBV is human herpes virus 4 (HHV-4). EBV was originally isolated from culture medium of Burkitt tumor cells [30], and EBV was an etiological agent for infectious mononucleosis or nasopharyngeal carcinoma in China [31]. Clinical issues of concern are the activation of EBV in specific conditions; for example, the reactivation of EBV was observed in the early infection phase of human immunodeficiency virus (HIV), and EBV reactivation within six months was observed before HIV seroconversion [32]. The reactivation of EBV has also been frequently detected under immunosuppressive conditions. The management of EBV reactivation in cases of stem cell transplantation under intensive immunosuppression is a serious issue [33].

In the field of rheumatology, the involvement of EBV in methotrexate (MTX)-associated lymphoproliferative disorder (MTX-LPD) is a considerable problem in the era of molecular-targeted therapy for RA [34]. In addition, chronic active EBV (CAEBV) infection [35] was classified as a new entity in the revised version of World Health Organization (WHO) criteria, in which EBV can infect not only B cells but also T cells and natural killer cells, resulting in a poor prognosis. There is a specific mode of infection in EBV that includes a latent and lytic infection phase during the EBV life cycle [36]. The latent infection of EBV was usually observed in peripheral blood B cells with the expression of latent membrane protein (LMP), which is associated with B-cell transformation [37]. In addition, the latency of EBV was categorized into four patterns (from 0 to III) based on the host cells' condition [38] with various expression patterns of EB nuclear antigen (EBNA)1 or EB-encoding regions (EBERs). In the latent phase, viral particles are not produced with the expression of non-structural protein in B cells. In contrast, the latent phase was switched to the lytic phase by LMP1 that was induced by BRLF1 [39], and once EBV had entered the lytic cycle, emitted EBV virions infected mucosal epithelial cells of the pharynx or ductal epithelial cells of salivary glands.

3.2. Chronological Changes in the Interpretations of EBV Infection in SS

With respect to the relationship between SS and EBV infection, our PubMed search identified 149 reports, with many conflicting results and opinions regarding SS per se and EBV-associated hematological tumors. Representative studies about the detection of EBV in SS are listed in Table 1.

Table 1. Representative publications suggesting involvement of Epstein-Barr virus (EBV) infection in patients with Sjögren's syndrome.

Authors [Ref.]	Origin	Year	Detection	Key Points
Venables [40]	UK	1985	Indirect IF	IgG antibody against EBVCA was detected in sicca syndrome patients, RA patients, and healthy subjects.
Fox [41]	USA	1986	Immunostaining, IB, slot hybridization	EA-D was detected in 8 of 14 SGs and EBVDNA was detected in 8 of 20 saliva samples from SS patients.
Yamaoka [42]	Japan	1988	Indirect IF	IgG and IgM antibodies against EBV capsid antigen and EBV excretion from the oropharynx were observed in SS patients.
Saito [43]	USA	1989	PCR	The usefulness of PCR was shown, revealing viral DNA in SG epithelial cells from SS patients.
Venables [44]	UK	1989	ISH, IF, immunostaining	EBVDNA was detected in SGs from 60% of healthy subjects and 17% of SS patients.
Mariette [45]	France	1991	ISH, PCR	A combination of ISH and PCR was introduced, showing a high positive rate in patients with SS.
Inoue [46]	Japan	1991	ELISA, IB	Elevated IgG antibody against EBNA antigens was detected in sera from SS patients.
Fox [45]	USA	1989	RFLP	Two SS patients with B-cell lymphoma showed an unusual RFLP pattern.
Tateishi [47]	Japan	1993	FCM, PCR	Massive EBV production was confirmed in an SS PBMC-derived B-cell line.
Newkirk [48]	Canada	1996	ELISA	Antibodies against early EBV peptides such as BHRF1 were detected in SS patients.
Merne [49]	Finland	1996	ISH, PCR	ISH detected EBVDNA in SGs from 19% of SS patients and 3% of controls.
Inoue [50]	Japan	2001	IF, RT-PCR, IB	ZEBRA mRNA in SGs from SS patients was observed, and EBV-activated lymphocyte mediated the production of 120-kDa alpha-fodrin.
Inoue [51]	Japan	2012	Luciferase assay	With the use of saliva from SS patients, dioxin augmented the transcription of BZLF1 that stimulated conversion to the lytic phase in EBV.
Pasoto [52]	Brazil	2013	ELISA	Frequent anti-EA-D antibodies were observed in SS patients.
Croia [53]	UK	2014	RT-PCR, ISH, immunostaining	Affinity of lytic phase EBV toward PCs in ELS was shown. Perifollicular PCs showed reactivity toward Ro52.

EA-D: EBV-encoded early antigen, ELS: ectopic lymphoid structure, FCM: flow cytometry, IF: immunofluorescence, IB: immunoblot, ISH: in situ hybridization, PBMC: peripheral blood mononuclear cell, PCR: polymerase chain reaction, PC: plasma cell, RA: rheumatoid arthritis, RFLP: restriction fragment length polymorphism, RT: reverse transcription, SG: salivary gland.

A first definitive study [40] regarding EBV in Sjögren's syndrome was conducted in 41 patients with RA; IgG antibody against EBV capsid antigen (EBVCA) was detected in all 41 RA patients, 26 patients with sicca syndrome, and 26 healthy subjects. Subsequently, Fox et al. [41] reported that EBV DNA revealed by slot hybridization was detected in 8 of 20 parotid saliva samples from SS patients, whereas EBV DNA was not detected in saliva from control subjects. Fox et al. also reported positive cytoplasmic staining of EBV-encoded early antigen (EA-D) in 8 of 14 salivary gland samples from SS patients. Whittingham et al. [54] hypothesized that EBV is an etiological agent of SS (especially for early-stage SS) in light of their observation of the binding of anti-La/SS-B antibody to viral RNAs or molecules encoded by EBV.

It was reported that, compared to control subjects, the titer of anti-ENBA antibodies but not that of anti-cytomegalovirus (CMV) antibodies was higher in sera from SS patients, and anti-EBNA antibodies were dominantly detected in anti-La/SS-B antibody-positive patients with SS [55]. Venables et al. subsequently reported that EBV DNA was present in the salivary gland biopsy specimen of 6 of 10 control subjects (60%) compared to 17% in the salivary gland biopsy specimens of SS patients [44]. They also detected EBV DNA in the salivary glands of five control subjects without HLA-class II antigen, suggesting that EBV infection was not specific for SS. With respect to the tumorigenicity of EBV, Fox et al. used a restriction fragment length polymorphism technique and reported that EBV or HHV-6 was associated with the onset of lymphomas [56]. In a study applying probes for both EBV and HHV-6 in cultured salivary gland epithelial cells (SGECs), only HHV-6 was detected, but HHV-6 was not related to SS [46].

Because benign lymphoepithelial lesions (BLELs) are unique pathological features in SS, Di Giuseppe et al. examined the involvement of EBV in BLELs [57]: they detected no EBER1 expression in salivary glands from SS patients and suggested that there is no involvement of latent EBV infection in SS. Regarding the relationship between CMV and EBV, their DNA in labial salivary glands (LSGs) from SS patients and subjects with non-specific sialadenitis was examined by polymerase chain reaction (PCR), which revealed no significant difference between the two patient groups [58]. Di Giuseppe et al. also contended that the persistence of these two viruses after the initial infection in LSGs was reasonable, but a direct involvement of EBV in the pathogenesis of SS was not suggested by their findings. Other investigators detected EBV DNA by in situ hybridization (ISH) and PCR in 19% of their SS patients versus 3% of the control subjects [49]. In contrast, EBV LMP was identified in 17% of their SS patients and 22% of the control subjects, indicating that the involvement of EBV can be influenced by the presence of undetermined factors.

Regarding the involvement of EBV in the pathogenesis of lymphomas, Royer et al. examined the occurrence of non-Hodgkin's lymphoma (NHL) and they identified cases with low-grade marginal zone lymphoma (MZL) and mucosa-associated lymphoid tissue (MALT) lymphoma; however, no obvious association between these SS and EBV infection was observed based on the presence of LMP proteins and EBER RNA [59]. In addition, the clinical implications of EBV in relation to the frequency of the detection of EBV DNA and related proteins have not been established. Regarding the association between the disease activity of SS and EBV infection, it was first demonstrated that significant levels of anti-EA-D antibodies were present in SS patients with articular manifestations described by items of the EULAR Sjögren's Syndrome Disease Activity Index (ESSDAI) [52]. Croia et al. took ectopic lymphoid structures (ELSs) into account, considering the selectivity of active EBV infection in SS as described below in the Pathogenesis section (Section 3.4) [53]. Regarding lymphoma observed in SS, it was demonstrated that among 382 patients with SS, 2.6% ($n = 10$) were diagnosed with EBV-associated follicular lymphoma, and 8 of these 10 patients showed a positive expression of LMP1 [60].

3.3. The Reactivation and Detection of EBV in SS

The word 'reactivation' in SS was first used in the 1980s by researchers examining the reactivity of monoclonal antibodies against EBV in salivary glands of individuals with SS [61,62]. Since then, the interpretation of the concept of reactivation has changed, as have the techniques for detecting EBV DNA and proteins. Saito et al. [55] demonstrated the usefulness of a PCR method to detect and monitor EBV DNA in salivary gland epithelial cells and peripheral blood. They also highlighted the importance of the rapid detection of EBV reactivation under immunosuppressive conditions and in lymphoproliferative disorders. Mariette et al. [56] introduced a combination of ISH using BamH1-W fragment and PCR reaction to detect EBV DNA in salivary glands from SS patients and control subjects. They observed positivity predominantly in the specimens from the SS patients, but they reported that there was no evidence to show that EBV infection was directly involved in the destruction of the glandular structure.

ISH was later used to detect EBV-specific DNA in patients with secondary SS in which epithelial cells positive for EBV DNA were observed around areas with salivary gland destruction or lymphoepithelial lesions [63]. By using an enzyme-linked immunosorbent assay (ELISA) and a western blot analysis, Inoue et al. then observed high IgG antibody titers against EBNA antigens in sera from SS patients compared to sera from normal subjects [46]. With respect to the reactivation of EBV, Saito et al. used reverse transcriptase PCR coupled with PCR and immunohistochemistry (IHC), which revealed a strong expression of thioredoxin (TRX) in infiltrating B cells and epithelial cells in salivary glands from most of their SS patients [64]. In addition, an anatomical association between TRX and EBV as well as the co-expression of TRX message and EBV DNA were confirmed. In an in vitro experiment by those authors, B-cell lines that were infected with EBV frequently expressed TRX. These findings were the first to suggest the usefulness of detecting factors of EBV reactivation.

Regarding a link between tumorigenesis and EBV reactivation, increased reactivity was demonstrated toward EBV EA proteins such as BHRF1 (which is a viral homologue of Bcl-2 in rheumatic diseases including SS) [48]. A clear and frequent expression of interleukin (IL)-12 in infiltrating B cells and salivary gland tissue of SS patients was shown to correspond to EBV DNA [65], suggesting a relationship between EBV reactivation and Th1 cytokine. The involvement of the aryl hydrocarbon receptor (AhR, which binds to 2, 3, 7, 8-tetrachlorodibenzo-p-dioxin, or TCDD) in the reactivation of EBV was also reported [51]; that research group demonstrated an enhancement of BZLF1 transcription that mediated the switch to the lytic form, as well as a BZLF1 message and EBV DNA due to TCDD. These findings suggest that the ligation of AhR had the potential to induce the reactivation of EBV in both B cells and salivary epithelial cells.

3.4. EBV-Mediated Pathogenesis Observed in SS

Immunological and virological considerations have shaped the perspective on the involvement of EBV in the pathogenesis of Sjögren's syndrome. Yamaoka et al. reported an increase in the proportion of polyclonal B cells in accord with the elevation of antiviral capsid antigen in SS [54]. Different findings were obtained by using a fusion protein (C28k) and synthetic peptides in an ELISA: there was no significant difference in the level of IgG antibodies in SS patients and healthy controls [66]. A counter-argument regarding these findings could be offered based on the differences in antigenic epitopes or the isolation of EBV from SS patients with additional in vitro observations.

Regarding the hypothesis of the direct involvement of EBV in SS, positive reactivity to EBV-related nucleo-cytoplasmic antigen was reported in 24 patients with SS, although the reactivity data differed between immunofluorescence and immunoblot analyses [67]. Correlations between aqueous tear deficiency and an elevated titer of EBV antigens as well as between SS and human leukocyte antigen (HLA)-DR+ CD8 lymphocytes were observed in lacrimal glands (LGs) [68], suggesting the presence of acquired immunological dysfunction in SS. With respect to the direct involvement of EBV in B-cell immunity, the production of EBV from a B-cell line that was newly established from peripheral blood mononuclear cells of patients with SS was demonstrated [47,69].

Alpha-fodrin was indicated as a possible autoantigen for SS [70], and Inoue et al. revealed that lymphoid cells that were reactivated by EBV had the potential to cleave alpha-fodrin as a 120-kDa fragment [50]. ZEBRA mRNA was shown to be a marker of the activation of the lytic cycle [71]. These findings showed novel functions that involved an apoptotic protease capability of reactivated EBV as an integrated concept in the pathogenesis of SS. Notably, the production of alpha-fodrin cleaved by EBV might be associated with antigen presentation, because 120-kDa alpha-fodrin was detected in sera from SS patients [70]; it may thus be involved in the pathogenesis of SS. A study regarding saliva as a soluble factor for EBV reactivation demonstrated that BZLF1 promotor was also activated in saliva under the presence of transforming growth factor-beta 1 (TGF-β1) induced by mitogen-activated protein kinase [72].

In the most recent development regarding the pathogenesis of SS, Croia et al. demonstrated SS-specific B-cell reactivation by EBV in their examination of ectopic lymphoid structures (ELSs) [53]. Although ELSs, which are an ectopic germinal center (GC) are known as a locus for B-cell activation and subsequent autoantibody production (as well as posing a risk for the development of lymphoma) [73,74], the affinity of EBV toward ELSs is a unique and crucial point. Croia et al. [53] described the following six important observations: (1) Lytic EBV infection was exclusively present in ELSs of salivary glands from patients with SS. (2) $CD20^+$ B cells and $CD138^+$ plasma cells around ELSs expressed EBER. (3) The expression of epithelial LMP was observed in both SS and nonspecific sialadenitis. (4) An antigen expressed during the lytic cycle, BFRF-positive CD138+ plasma cells that EBV lytically infected around ELSs, displayed Ro52. (5) SCID mice that received transplants of SS salivary gland tissue containing ELSs exhibited the ability to produce anti-Ro52/SS-A and anti-La/SS-B antibodies. (6) EBV that had increased affinity to ELSs in SS salivary glands was closely associated with impaired $CD8^+$ T-cell cytotoxicity. These observations clearly demonstrated that the lytic phase of EBV has affinity to both ELSs and plasma cells with the capability to produce SS-specific autoantibodies.

4. HTLV-1 Infection and SS

4.1. Retrovirus Infection (Other Than HTLV-1 Infection) and SS

Representative studies on the involvement of retroviruses in SS are listed in Table 2.

Table 2. Representative publications suggesting involvement of retroviruses (other than HTLV-1) with Sjögren's syndrome.

Author [Ref. No]	Origin	Year	Findings
Schiødt [75]	USA	1989	9 patients with HIV-SGD showed parotid gland enlargement and 11 patients with xerostomia. CD8 T cells showed in LSGs. No EBV and CMV was detected.
Garry [76]	USA	1990	Particles of human intracisternal A-type retrovirus that were similar to HIV were observed in LSGs of SS patients.
Talal [77,78]	USA	1990	Antibodies against HIV-1 were detected in 30% of SS patients and 1 among 120 normal subjects. Seropositive SS patients reacted p24 (gag) only.
Itescu [79]	USA	1990	Among 17 HIV patients showed, 14 patients had xerostomia and 11 patients had abnormal Gallium uptake. CD8 cells in LSGs and HLA-DR5 were associated with these patients.
Itescu [80]	USA	1991	Concept of diffuse infiltrative lymphocytosis syndrome (DILS) in patients with HIV was released. CD8 T cell infiltration and involvement of exocrine glands and other tissues were shown.
Dwyer [81]	USA	1993	Sharing of the sequences of 59 beta-chains in 5 DILS patients was shown. Additionally, appearance of certain common V beta and J beta gene segments was found. Usage of TCR beta chains was different from primary SS patients.
Kordossis [82]	Greece	1998	The prevalence of SLS in HIV-1-positive patients was 7.79%, in which 6 out of 14 patients showed sialadenitis with CD8 T cell dominancy. These patients had no anti-Ro/SS-A and La/SS-B antibodies but had hypergammaglobulinemia.
Williams [83]	USA	1998	Among 523 patients with HIV, 15 patients (3%) showed DILS with racial differences. DILS patients had high CD8 counts and clinical stage of DILS patients was less than non-DILS patients.
Yamano S [84]	Japan	1997	Sera from 33% SS patients reacted against p24 (gag) and LSGs from 47% SS patients reacted against anti-p24 monoclonal antibody. Additionally, A-type-like retroviral particles were detected by electron microscopy in LSGs from SS patients.

Table 2. Cont.

Author [Ref. No]	Origin	Year	Findings
Rigby [85]	UK	1997	By nested PCR, 1 non-SS patient and 1 secondary SS patient showed positive for human retrovirus-5 (HRV-5) among 92 samples. Three different sequences of HRV-5 were 98% identical to originally detected sequence.
Panayiotakopoulos [86]	Greece	2001	Reduced prevalence of SLS after introduction of the highly active anti-retroviral therapy (HAART) was detected with only 2 positive findings among 17 SGs biopsy. Prevalence of 7.8% in pre-HAART period disappeared after execution of HAART.

CMV: cytomegalovirus, ELS; ectopic lymphoid structures, HIV: human immunodeficiency, HRV: human retrovirus, PCR; polymerase chain reaction, SGD: salivary gland disease, SGs; salivary glands, SLS: Sjögren's-like syndrome, TCR: T cell receptor.

The possibility of retrovirus infections other than HTLV-1 infection in individuals with SS was a research focus in the early 1990s. In 1989 it was reported that patients with HIV-associated salivary gland disease (HIV-SGD) showed a high frequency of parotid enlargement, sicca symptoms, and a low CD4/8 ratio in LSG biopsy specimens [75]. Interestingly, no anti-Ro/SS-A or La/SS-B antibodies were detected in the enrolled patients. Garry and colleagues described a human intracisternal A-type retroviral particle that was closely associated with HIV which they detected in lymphoid cells that were exposed to homogenates of salivary gland tissue from SS patients [76]. In investigations of the presence of serum antibodies of retrovirus, sera from 30% of healthy subjects had positive reactivity toward p24 (gag) but not gp41 or gp120 (env), with low reactivity to Ro/SS-A and La/SS-B [77,78]. Itescu et al. reported cases of HIV-positive patients demonstrating parotid enlargement, sicca symptoms, and CD8 T-lymphocyte dominance with HLA-DR5 [79], and the term 'diffuse infiltrative lymphocytosis syndrome (DILS)' was proposed [80].

The diagnostic criteria of DILS are as follows: (1) HIV infection with positive serology, (2) bilateral salivary gland enlargement or xerostomia, (3) persistence of signs or symptoms for ≥6 months, and (4) histologic confirmation of salivary or lacrimal gland lymphocytic infiltration without granulomatosis or neoplastic involvement. All four of these criteria must be met for the diagnosis of DILS. A difference in the T-cell receptor (TCR) beta-chains was also revealed between SS patients and subjects with DILS [81]. In a cohort study in Greece, SS-like syndrome (SLS) was confirmed in 7.79% of HIV-positive subjects, in whom $CD8^+$ T cell-dominant infiltration was observed in salivary gland biopsy specimens without anti-Ro/SS-A, La/SS-B antibody [82]. An assessment of the prevalence of DILS at an HIV outpatient clinic in the U.S. revealed that 3% of the HIV-seropositive patients (15/523) had DILS with enlargement of the parotid gland and sicca symptoms [83]. In their study of HIV-associated antigen, Yamano et al. observed that 33% of the sera and 47% of the salivary gland specimens from SS patients reacted with p24 (gag) of HIV, although target genes for HIV were not detected in either type of samples from SS patients [84]. Their findings suggest the involvement not of HIV but of an unknown retrovirus in SS.

The presence of human retrovirus-5 (HRV-5) in salivary glands was examined by nested PCR in 55 SS patients and 37 non-SS subjects, and no association of HRV-5 with SS was observed [85]. The estimated prevalence of SLS among 131 HIV patients under an intensive anti-retroviral strategy, i.e., highly active anti-retroviral therapy (HAART), was 7.8% [86]. As of 2020, the number of publications concerning a relationship between SS and HIV has decreased, probably because of the development of HAART and the 2002 description of HIV infection as well as hepatitis C infection in the exclusion criteria in the classification of SS provided by the American-European Consensus Group (AECG) [87].

4.2. Clinical and Epidemiological Findings of HTLV-1 Infection in SS

In parallel with investigations of involvement of the HIV in Sjögren's syndrome, the engagement of HTLV-1 in SS has been researched. In this section, we summarize the clinical and epidemiological studies of the association between HTLV-1 infection and SS. HTLV-1, a member of the type C delta-retrovirus family [88], is a causative agent of adult T-cell leukemia (ATL), which is a hematological neoplastic disorder first described by Takatsuki et al. in 1977 [89]. After HTLV-1 was recognized as causative virus for ATL, the whole base sequence [90] and the function of Tax protein [91] were determined. HTLV-1 is also a causative agent for the tropical spastic paraparesis/HTLV-1-associated myelopathy (HAM) identified in the Caribbean basin and the southeast area of Japan; patients with HAM exhibit slowly progressive neurological symptoms such as spastic gait and bladder and rectal disturbance [92,93]. HTLV-1-associated uveitis [94] is also observed in HTLV-1 carriers, and the frequent complication of Grave's disease is reported [95]. Broncho-alveolitis is an example of organ involvement in HTLV-1 infection as a pulmonary complication [96]. As transmission pathways of HTLV-1, maternal infection with various levels of HTLV-1 proviral DNA during pregnancy was reported [97]. Representative publications about the detection of genes and proteins in HTLV-1-associated SS are listed in Table 3.

Table 3. Detection of HTLV-1-related genes and proteins in sera or SGs from patients with Sjögren's syndrome.

Authors [Ref.]	Origin	Year	Detection	Key Points
Green [98]	USA	1989	IB, IHC	Tax protein expression was detected in SGs and muscle of *tax* transgenic mice as a first mouse model of SS.
Shattles [99]	UK	1992	Indirect IF	HTLV-1 p19 was detected in 31% of epithelial cytoplasm of SS patients by using a monoclonal antibody specific for retrovirus.
Mariette [100]	France	1993	ISH, PCR	*tax* gene only was detected in 2/9 LSGs from SS patients, although these patients did not react to anti-HTLV-1 antibodies.
Sumida [101]	Japan	1994	RT-PCR	*tax* gene only was detected in 4 of 14 LSGs from Japanese SS patients. The *pXIV* region sequence had homology to MT-2 cells.
Terada [102]	Japan	1994	IB, PCR	Salivary IgA antibodies to SS patients with anti-HTLV-1 antibody and high prevalence of HTLV-1 in SS patients were observed.
Yamazaki [103]	Japan	1997	RT-PCR	Transgenic rats with env-pX gene showed chronic sialadenitis as well as arthritis, vasculitis, and polymyositis.
Ohyama [104]	Japan	1998	PCR, in situ PCR hybridization	Extracted DNA from HTLV-1 seropositive SS contained full proviral DNA. Infiltrating T cells had proviral DNA in the nucleus.
Tangy [105]	France	1999	PCR, ISH	Expression of tax was observed in SGs of HTLV-1-seropositive SS and HTLV-1-seronegative SS patients and sicca subjects.
Sasaki [106]	Japan	2000	PCR, SSCP, sequencing of cDNA	Use of TCR Vβ5.2, 6, and 7 in LSGs from HTLV-1-seropositive SS patients. Vβ7 with conserved AA motif was observed in these patients.
Mariette [107]	France	2000	PCR	*tax* gene was detected in LSGs from 30% of SS patients, 28% of patients with inflammatory diseases, and 4% of healthy subjects.
Lee [108]	Korea	2012	PCR, nested PCR, IHC	*tax* gene but not *pX*, *p19* or *pol* was observed in PBMCs from 3.8% of SS patients. p19 and Tax were expressed in LSGs.
Nakamura [109]	Japan	2015	In situ PCR, IF	Expressions of proviral DNA, Gag, and chemokines were observed on SGECs co-cultured with a HTLV-1-positive cell line.
Nakamura [110]	Japan	2018	Real-time PCR, ISH, IHC	In LSGs of HAM-SS, dominant *tax* and *HBZ* was observed with the expression of Foxp3 in LSGs from HAM-SS and ATL patients.
Nakamura [111]	Japan	2019	IF, EM	A biofilm-like structure but not virus synapses was involved in the transmission of HTLV-1 virions from HTLV-1-positive cells to SGECs.

AA: amino acid, EM: electron microscopy, HAM: HTLV-1-associated myelopathy, IF: immunofluorescence, IB: immunoblot, IHC: immunohistochemistry, ISH: in situ hybridization, LSG: labial salivary gland, PBMC: peripheral blood mononuclear cell, PCR: polymerase chain reaction, RA: rheumatoid arthritis, RT: reverse transcription, SG: salivary gland, SGEC: salivary gland epithelial cell, SSCP: single-strand confirmation polymorphism, TCR: T-cell receptor.

Although several case reports regarding SS associated with HTLV-1 infection are available, it was initially reported that HTLV-1 carriers with SS showed high frequencies of extra-glandular manifestations including uveitis and myopathy [112]. It was subsequently demonstrated that in Nagasaki, Japan (an endemic area for HTLV-1), the prevalence of HTLV-1 in SS patients was significantly higher than that of 27,284 blood donors [113]. In addition, a serum antibody toward HTLV-1 in HTLV-1-seropositive SS patients was similar to that from patients with HTLV-1-associated myelopathy (HAM). In a study conducted in Chile, among 48 patients with HAM, 29.1% of the patients who lacked autoantibodies including anti-Ro/SS-A antibody or rheumatoid factor (RF) showed chronic dacryosialadenitis without being classified as having SS [110]. We observed that 60% of a series of HAM patients fulfilled the preliminary European Community criteria for SS with positive mononuclear cell infiltration in LSGs [114], and these HAM patients with SS showed low frequencies of anti-Ro/SS-A antibody, anti-nuclear antibody, and RF compared to those observed in typical SS.

The high prevalence of SS in HAM patients was also observed in a later investigation in which chronic sialadenitis and exocrine dysfunction were detected by Saxon test and Schirmer's test, respectively [115]. Magnetic resonance imaging (MRI) revealed that 92% of HAM patients with SS lacked typical characteristics usually found in SS, although the salivary flow rate of these patients was similar to that of SS patients without HAM [99]. We subsequently documented a low frequency of abnormal findings in HTLV-1-seropositive patients with SS compared to those of HTLV-1-seronegative patients with SS [100], although the aforementioned MRI findings showed much clearer imaging differences than those in sialography. The relationship between abnormality in such images and the pathogenesis of SS is discussed later in this review. With reference to our previous study [88] that showed a high frequency of myopathy in HTLV-1-seropositive SS, Cruz et al. [101] noted that their study conducted in Brazil revealed that 38% of HTLV-1-seropositve subjects had fibromyalgia, and their HTLV-1-seropositive subjects had a high prevalence of rheumatic diseases. We found that among atomic-bomb survivors in Japan, the prevalence of HTLV-1 infection in SS patients was higher than that in non-SS subjects [102].

We also re-evaluated the complications of SS experienced by patients with HAM 18 years after we reported the association [116], because the classification criteria were revised as AECG criteria [87] and the aging of HTLV-1-seropositive subjects with the changes in the composition of the population in Japan was established [117,118]. As a result, 38.5% of our patients with HAM were classified as having SS based on the AECG criteria, and the prevalence of anti-Ro/SS-A antibody was significantly lower than that in HTLV-1 carriers complicated with SS. A cross-sectional study performed in Brazil demonstrated that in a group of 272 HTLV-1-seropositive participants at an HTLV-1 clinic, 59 (21.7%) patients (none of whom had HAM) showed sicca symptoms without anti-Ro/SS-A, La/SS-B antibodies [119]. That study also revealed that proinflammatory cytokines were elevated in HTLV-1-seropositive subjects with sicca symptoms regardless of the presence/absence of SS, suggesting that HTLV-1 itself has the potential to induce nonspecific inflammation in salivary glands regardless of the presence of autoimmune disease.

Vale et al. [104] examined the association between HTLV-1 infection and the presence of SS in 129 HTLV-1-seropositive subjects in Brazil; they observed xerostomia and xerophthalmia in 35.7% and 13.95% of the subjects, respectively. In contrast, these HTLV-1-seropositive subjects showed only 0.77% anti-La/SS-B antibody. Regarding pulmonary involvement in SS, we detected an increased frequency of airway diseases in HTLV-1-seropositive SS patients [120], indicating an influence of HTLV-1 infection as a systemic manifestation.

4.3. The Detection of HTLV-1 Genes and Proteins in SGs in SS

Similar to the involvement of EBV in SS, the infection of salivary glands by HTLV-1 has also been debated. In 1992, it was reported that the expression of HTLV-1 p19 (a member of the family of gag antigens) was observed in SGECs from 31% of SS patients, 24% of RA patients with SS, and 21% of patients with sicca [105], suggesting the possibility of the presence of an endogenous retrovirus other than the human endogenous retroviral sequence (HRES-1). Mariette et al. [106] reported that *tax* gene (but not *gag*, *pol*, *env*) was detected by both ISH and PCR in labial salivary glands of two of nine patients with SS. They also observed the localization of *tax* in the nuclei of both SGECs and lymphocytes. Sumida et al. [107] later described similar findings with the positive expression of *tax* gene in labial salivary glands from Japanese patients with SS, and they reported that the nucleotide sequence of the *pX* region in labial salivary glands was completely identical to that of the MT-2 cell line, suggesting that the findings of these two studies [106,107] support the concept that at least *tax* gene might be involved in the pathogenesis of SS.

In an aforementioned study conducted in Nagasaki [113], the serum titers of anti-HTLV-1 antibody in patients with HTLV-1-seropositive SS was as high as that in HAM patients, and IgM-class antibodies were frequently detected in the former group. Interestingly, salivary IgA antibodies to HTLV-1 were observed in HTLV-1-seropositive SS patients although a low frequency of these antibodies was observed in the HAM patients and healthy carriers. Four responses to that study [113] arose from France and Austria [108], in which there were similar observations regarding the detection of these antibodies with additional observations in HTLV-1-seropositive SS patients. In these responses, the involvement of *tax* gene and the local synthesis of IgA class anti-HTLV-1 antibody in saliva was discussed. In contrast, a study of salivary glands from 49 patients with SS in Great Britain demonstrated no *tax* expression unlike that of ERV-3, an endogenous human retrovirus [110], suggesting differences in regional characteristics between endemic and non-endemic areas as well as the possibility of PCR contamination.

With respect to HTLV-1-seropositive patients with SS, an investigation using an in situ PCR technique detected HTLV-1 proviral DNA in infiltrating MNCs but not salivary gland epithelial cells of these patients [121]. In contrast, we detected *tax* gene in 18% of the salivary glands of HTLV-1-seronegative SS patients by nested PCR [122], suggesting that the involvement of HTLV-1 in HTLV-1-seronegative patients might be limited because the viral load in salivary glands from HTLV-1-seronegative SS patients was much lower than that from HTLV-1-seropositive patients. A study conducted in France and using ISH detected HTLV-1 RNA in both salivary gland epithelial cells and lymphoid cells of HTLV-1-seronegative SS patients, although *tax* gene was expressed in LSGs from these patients [123]. Sasaki et al. later described the presence of TCR Vbeta gene in infiltrating lymphocytes of salivary glands from HTLV-1-seropositive SS patients, in which specific T cells with Vbeta5.2, 6, and 7 were used, indicating the involvement of an HTLV-1-driven T-cell activation in SS [124].

As for other inflammatory conditions, Mariette et al. examined the expression of *tax* gene in LSGs from SS patients and patients with chronic inflammatory diseases [125]. They detected *tax* gene in 30% of the SS patients and 28% of the non-SS patients. These results suggested that HTLV-1 may contribute to the development of chronic inflammation regardless of the presence/absence of SS. Although the number of publications concerning HTLV-1-related genes in the salivary glands of individuals with SS has decreased since 2000, a 2012 report from Korea noted that *tax* gene was detected in 3.8% of a series of SS patients, and HTLV-1 p19 or Tax protein was revealed by IHC in LSGs from >40% of the SS patients [126]. With regard to HTLV-1 genes other than the previously reported genes, we examined the expressions of HTLV-1 bZIP factor (*HBZ*) and *tax* gene by ISH, which showed that both genes expressed in infiltrating MNCs and SGECs from HAM-SS patients and a patient with adult T-cell leukemia (ATL), although the expression of *tax* gene was dominant in MNCs of the HAM-SS patients [127] (Figure 1A,B).

HBZ gene, which is encoded by a minus strand of the HTLV-1 provirus, is known to induce chronic inflammation in ATL through the expression of Foxp3, and it was suggested that the expression of *HBZ* has the potential to induce Foxp3 gene transcription in CD4$^+$ T cells from *HBZ* transgenic mice [111,128]. In accord with these experimental observations, we also observed a high expression of Foxp3 in salivary gland tissue from a patient with ATL and patients with HAM-SS. The involvement of *HBZ* gene in HTLV-1-seropositive SS patients was newly considered after the observed outbreak of chronic inflammation in this population.

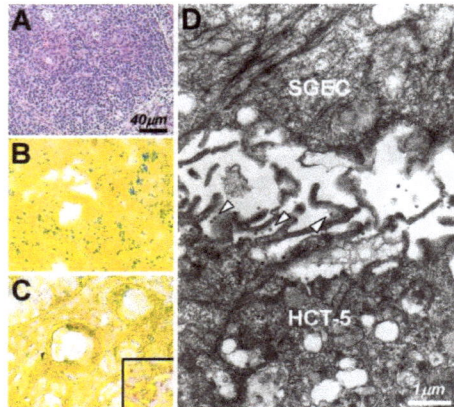

Figure 1. The expression of *tax/HBZ* and HTLV-1 virions in salivary glands (SGs) of patients with Sjögren's syndrome (SS). (**A**) Massive lymphocytic infiltration was by hematoxylin-eosin staining in a labial salivary gland from a patient with sicca symptoms and adult T-cell leukemia (ATL). The expression of *tax*/HTLV-1 bZIP factor (*HBZ*) in SGs from a patient with ATL (**B**) and patients with HTLV-1-associated myelopathy complicated with SS (**C**), examined by in situ hybridization. A dominant expression of *HBZ* (*green*) was observed in the ATL SGs in both infiltrating mononuclear cells (MNCs) and ducts (**B**). In contrast, a dominant expression of *tax* (*red*) was observed in MNCs of salivary glands from patients with HAM-SS (**C**). Electron microscopy (**D**) revealed the existence of HTLV-1 virions (*arrowheads*) at the contact face between HCT-5 cells (an HTLV-1-infected cell line) and salivary gland epithelial cells (SGECs).

4.4. The Mode of HTLV-1 Infection in SS Salivary Glands

As a potential mechanism of HTLV-1 transmission to salivary glands, a brief discussion of the concept of HTLV-1 transmission between lymphocytes is presented next. Generally, an efficient HTLV-1 infection requires cell-to-cell contact [98]; cell-free viral transmission is insufficient. HTLV-1 preferentially infects CD4$^+$ T cells but has shown a low frequency of infection of CD8$^+$ T cells. Two theories and an additional proposal have been published with regard to the cell-to-cell transmission of HTLV-1 virions. Igakura et al. proposed a concept that they named the 'viral synapse' which consists of an assembly of HTLV-1 gag protein complex and viral genomes at the microtube-organizing center, with a polarized contact surface between HTLV-1-infected and uninfected cells [103]. Another theory was proposed by Pais-Correia and colleagues, who demonstrated that extracellular matrix and linker structures including collagen, agrin, tetherin, and galectin-3 are involved in the delivery of the HTLV-1 viral particles at the contact surface [129,130]. In this system, a biofilm-like viral assembly with extracellular components on the HTLV-1-infected CD4$^+$ T cell contacts an uninfected CD4$^+$ T cell, resulting in the transmission of virions by cell-to-cell contact.

As an additional system to convey HTLV-1 virions from infected to uninfected CD4$^+$ T cells, the concept of a cellular conduit was described by Van Prooyen et al. [131]. They showed that cellular conduits that expressed HTLV-1 p8 protein with an accumulation of lymphocyte function-associated antigen (LFA-1) acted as an intermediary with respect to the transmission of HTLV-1 virions. This novel concept was introduced as a third pathway for the transmission of HTLV-1 virions in concert with the function of p8 accessory protein [132]. In coming to detection of the initial dynamic state of HTLV-1 infection of salivary glands, we investigated the involvement of these three pathways in an in vitro study as a single publication [133] by using an HTLV-1-infected cell line, HCT-5. Although agrin, tetherin, and galectin-3 were expressed on the surface of HCT-5 cells, agrin and tetherin were observed with HTLV-1 Gag-positive particles on cultured SGECs after a co-culture with HCT-5 cells

(Figure 1C). We observed no formation of virological synapses between HCT-5 cells and SGECS, although an immunofluorescence analysis suggested the possibility of the involvement of a cellular conduit (Figure 2).

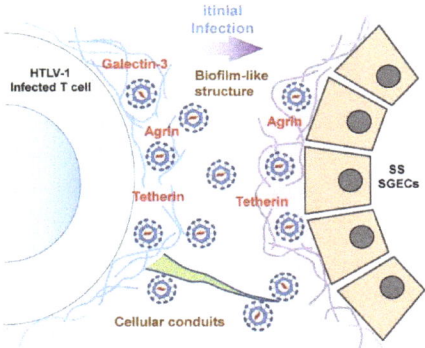

Figure 2. A hypothetical scheme of the initial transmission of HTLV-1 virions. HTLV-1 virions exist with extracellular matrix proteins or linker proteins including galectin-3, agrin, and tetherin. After the initial contact of HCT-5 cells with SGECs, HTLV-1 virions are Table 1. virions by the extension of a long structure that is stretched from the surface of HCT-5 cells.

The handing over of HTLV-1 virions between HTLV-1-infected cells and SGECs was confirmed by electron microscopy, although we found no endogenous virions on SGECs after a co-culture with an uninfected T-cell line.

4.5. Immunological Modulation of HTLV-1 Infection in SS

The association between the pathogenesis of SS and HTLV-1 infection has been addressed with experimental approaches including in vitro studies, animal studies, and studies with human tissue samples including salivary gland tissue. As a catalyst of experimental studies, Green et al. developed HTLV-1 *tax* gene transgenic (Tg) mice [134]. Interestingly, the *tax* Tg mice showed human SS-like pathology including cellular infiltration as well as a proliferation of ductal epithelial cells. It was also demonstrated that the introduction of *env-pX* gene to Wistar-King-Aptekman-Hokudai (WKAH) rats induced human SS-like characteristics such as chronic sialadenitis and dacryoadenitis as well as arthritis, necrotizing arteritis, polymyositis, myocarditis and dermatitis with elevated RF [135]. These characteristics in *env-pX* rats showed a direct involvement of HTLV-1 infection in the induction of autoimmunity.

Concerning the involvement of HTLV-1 infection in WKAH rats, Yoshiki et al. showed that one of their WKAH rats that possessed the RT1k haplotype presented neurological symptoms resembling HAM [136], suggesting that differences in the HTLV-1 haplotype might influence the clinical phenotypes. With respect to the involvement of HTLV-1 in apoptosis, we examined the frequency of terminal deoxynucleotidyl transferase-mediated dUTP nick-end labeling (TUNEL) staining [137] and Fas/Fas ligand (FasL) [138,139] staining of HTLV-1-seropositive and -seronegative SS patients because Fas/FasL system-mediated apoptosis has been shown to play a role in the pathogenesis of many autoimmune diseases [140]. Although we observed a low frequency of TUNEL-positive apoptosis in both SGECs and infiltrating MNCs, there was no significant between-cell type difference regardless of the presence/absence of anti-HTLV-1 antibody.

In our study of the involvement of anti-apoptotic molecules in HTLV-1-seropositive SS patients, we investigated the expression of Bcl-2 family proteins in PBMCs and LSGs from SS patients [141], because HTLV-1-mediated bcl-2 family proteins inhibited the apoptosis of T-cell lines including JPX-9 cells (a subline of Jurkat human T cells) and a mouse T-cell line (CTLL-2) through the activation of nuclear factor kappa B [142,143]. We observed, that compared to the Bax expression in the LSGs and PBMCs, there was a dominant expression of Bcl-2 as well as CD40/CD40 ligand in the LSGs regardless of HTLV-1 infection.

We subsequently detected members of the mitogen-activated protein kinase (MAPK) superfamily [144] including c-Jun N-terminal kinase and p38 that were accompanied by CD40 or X-chromosome-linked inhibitor of apoptosis protein (XIAP) [145] in salivary gland tissue from SS patients, but the differences in expression of XIAP were not determined by HTLV-1 infection. We then focused on the characteristics of the imaging of glands from HTLV-1-seropositive SS patients [100,101] and germinal centers (GCs) because it is known that GCs are a specific site for B-cell activation and selection [146,147]. Notably, Amft et al. showed that lymphoid tissue-homing chemokine B cell-attracting chemokine (BCA-1, also known as C-X-C motif chemokine ligand 13, or CXCL13) was specifically expressed in the GC structure and endothelial cells in salivary glands from SS patients. CXCL13 had the effect of specifically attracting human B cells that expressed BLR1, which was later named CXCR5 [109]. We observed a low number of GCs as well as a low expression of CXCL13 in HTLV-1-seropositive SS cases, and the HAM-SS cases in particular lacked GC formation, suggesting that HTLV-1 infection might inhibit the formation of GCs and the subsequent selection of high-affinity B cells that develop into plasma cells.

Concerning chronic lymphocytic infiltration in salivary glands without specific autoantibodies in SS, the DILS observed in salivary glands of individuals affected by HIV with the infiltration of $CD8^+$ T cells [148] is a reminder that the dominant infiltration of $CD4^+$ T cells in the salivary glands of HAM-SS patients with hypergammaglobulinemia resembles that observed in DILS. In addition, we treated an ATL patient with bilateral parotid gland enlargement, xerostomia, and xerophthalmia [149], and although this patient showed a massive infiltration of $CD4^+$ T cell-dominant lymphocytes, antibodies against Ro/SS-A, La/SS-B were negative. There are differences in the phenotypes of infiltrating T cells, but the existence of DILS in HIV-positive patients and a patient with ATL suggests the possibility that a massive infiltration of T cells with sicca symptoms would fulfill the classification criteria of SS [87,150].

Lastly, we discuss the immunological alterations observed in that area after the integration of HTLV-1 into host non-lymphoid cells including SGECs. HTLV-1 infection confirmed by semiquantitative PCR or ELISA was observed in 2.6% of retinal glial cells along with the production of inflammatory cytokines including IL-6 and TNF-α [151]. A similar in vitro study using synovial cells showed that a co-culture of synovial cells with HTLV-1-infected T-cell lines led to the expression of HTLV-1 core antigen and HTLV-1 proviral DNA on the synovial cells along with the production of granulocyte/macrophage colony-stimulating factor [152]. Interestingly, Carvalho Barros et al. demonstrated that HTLV-1 infected thymic epithelial cells (TECs), and the TECs had the potential to convey HTLV-1 virions to $CD4^+$ T cells [153].

Regarding the HTLV-1 infection of SGECs from SS patients, we confirmed HTLV-1 proviral DNA and proteins by in situ PCR and immunofluorescence, respectively after co-culture with an HTLV-1-infected T-cell line [154]; in addition, the concentrations of soluble intracellular adhesion molecule (ICAM)-1 and RANTES (regulated on activation, normal T cell expressed and secreted) and IFN-γ-inducible 10-kD protein (IP)-10 increased after the co-culture of SGECs from SS patients with HCT-5 cells. It was striking that the cytoplasmic expression of ICAM-1, CXCL1, RANTES, IL-8, and IP-10 on SGECs was also augmented after co-culture. Our findings indicated that HTLV-1 had the capability to infect SGECs, and these SGECs also expressed inflammatory cytokines or chemokines. However, these phenomena are currently limited to in vitro findings.

5. Overview of the Involvement of Viruses in SS

We have outlined the involvement of viruses (centering on EBV and HTLV-1 as environmental factors) in the pathogenesis of SS (Figure 3). These two viruses have distinct directionalities in the phenotypes of lymphocytes with respect to the formation of clinical characteristics (including exocrine dysfunction) in SS. The existence of conflicting findings with regard to the involvement of viruses in the development of SS must be considered, but it is anticipated that these viruses also have some unique actions in the formation of ELSs, i.e., ectopic GCs and the autoantibody production system.

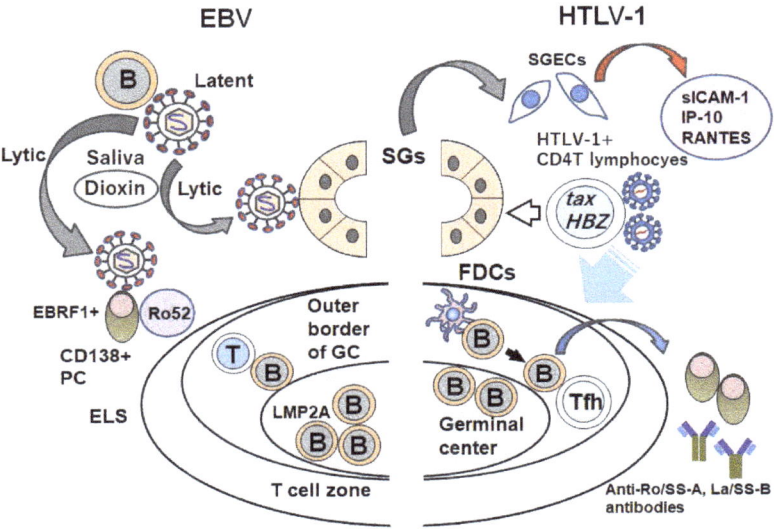

Figure 3. The different roles of EBV and HTLV-1 in the pathogenesis of SS. EBV exists in B cells and/or B cells that expresses LMP2A in ectopic lymphoid structures (ELSs) as a latent phase. Once the reactivation of EBV is induced by environmental factors (including dioxin), EBV changes to the lytic phase. Lytic EBV can infect SGECs and perifollicular EBRF$^+$ plasma cells (PCs) that can react with Ro52. In contrast, HTLV-1 that bears *tax* and HTLV-1 bZIP factor (*HBZ*) infects salivary glands of patients with SS. An in vitro study showed that after the HTLV-1 infection of salivary glands, SGECs express inflammatory cytokines or chemokines including soluble ICAM-1, IP-10, and RANTES. Inhibitory effects of HTLV-1 toward ELS components (including B cells), PCs that produce anti-Ro/SS-A, La/SS-B antibodies, follicular dendritic cells (FDCs), and follicular helper T cells (Tfh) have been considered.

EBV showed robust affinity to the ELS, whereas HTLV-1 infection might inhibit the formation of the ELS in accord with its proviral load (PVL). In addition, EBV has high affinity to B cells or plasma cells (PCs) in accord with the alteration of its phase from the latent mode to the lytic mode, which is suggested to be stimulated by environmental substances. However, SS patients with HAM who show higher PVLs than HTLV-1 carriers have a low frequency of the autoantibodies that are found in typical SS patients. Regarding the HTLV-1-mediated induction of SS, various theories have attempted to explain the pathogenesis of SS. A definite epidemiological relationship between HTLV-1 infection and SS has been established by the findings obtained in *tax* or *env-pX* Tg animal models and in vitro studies. However, unlike EBV infection, in HTLV-1-infected subjects there is no direct evidence indicating molecular biological effects on the production of autoantibodies in SS patients.

To address this scarcity of evidence, it is necessary to determine whether HTLV-1 infection has immunological influences on specific autoantibody production systems. In other words, it should be clarified whether or not HTLV-1 simply modulates the pathogenesis of existing typical SS. For example, HTLV-1 might influence immune cells including B cells, PCs, and/or T follicular helper cells in the ELS to reduce autoantibody production. It is also possible that CD4$^+$ T cells mobilized by HTLV-1 infection simply form an aggregation of DILS-like lymphocytes as observed in HIV infection or the sialadenitis observed in ATL. Unlike HIV infection with sialadenitis, a great mass of HTLV-1 infection occurs by maternal infection; in contrast, SS usually develops in middle age. Clinicians should thus be concerned about the effects and or the immunological modulation of HTLV-1 infection during the 40–50 years before the development of SS.

In cases of EBV infection, it is suspected that reactivation in the lytic phase promotes immunological dysfunction. However, when HTLV-1 infection occurs by maternal infection, HTLV-1 that shows no change of infective form continues to infect $CD4^+$ T cells for several decades. Investigations that may determine the triggers of the formation of SS-like sialadenitis in salivary glands over a prolonged period are further research tasks that will also elucidate the differences in engagement between EBV and HTLV-1.

6. Conclusions

Molecular biological approaches have enhanced our understanding of the contribution of Epstein-Barr virus to the pathogenesis of Sjögren's syndrome. The involvement of HTLV-1 has been thought to vary among endemic areas, whereas EBV infection is ubiquitously observed regardless of regional characteristics. In addition, the aging of HTLV-1-infected populations might influence the prevalence of HTLV-1-seropositive SS. To determine the direct contribution of both EBV and HTLV-1 in the pathogenesis of SS, the integration of epidemiological and experimental studies including virological and molecular immunological approaches is strongly desired.

Author Contributions: All authors were involved in drafting the article or revising it critically for important intellectual content, and all authors approved the final version for publication. H.N. has full access to all of the data in the study and takes responsibility for the integrity of the data and the accuracy of the data analysis. Study conception and design: H.N. Interpretation and critical reading of this review: H.N., T.S., A.K. All authors have read and agreed to the published version of the manuscript.

Funding: No external funding was involved in this review.

Acknowledgments: This review was supported in part by the JSPS KAKENHI (grant no. JP19K08884).

Conflicts of Interest: The authors declare no conflict of interest.

Abbreviations

AhR	aryl hydrocarbon receptor
AID	autoimmune disease
APS	anti-phospholipid syndrome
ATL	adult T-cell leukemia
BCA	B cell-attracting
BLEL	benign lymphoepithelial lesion
CAEBV	chronic active EBV
CMV	cytomegalovirus
CXCL	C-X-C motif chemokine ligand
DILS	diffuse infiltrative lymphocytosis syndrome
EA	early antigen
EBER	EB encoding region
EBNA	EB nuclear antigen
EBV	Epstein-Barr virus
EBVCA	EBV capsid antigen
ELISA	enzyme-linked immunosorbent assay
ELS	ectopic lymphoid structures
ESSDAI	EULAR Sjögren's Syndrome Disease Activity Index
FasL	Fas ligand
GC	germinal center
GBS	Guillain-Barré Syndrome
HAART	highly active anti-retroviral therapy

HHV	human herpes virus
HIV	human immunodeficiency virus
HLA	human leukocyte antigen
HRV	human retrovirus
HTLV-1	human T-cell leukemia virus type 1
HRES	human endogenous retroviral sequence
ICAM	intracellular adhesion molecule
IFN	interferon
IHC	immunohistochemistry
IL	interleukin
IP	interferon-γ-inducible 10-kD protein
IRF	IFN-regulatory factor
ISH	in situ hybridization
LFA	lymphocyte function-associated antigen
LG	lacrimal gland
LSG	labial salivary gland
LMP	latent membrane protein
LPD	lymphoproliferative disorder
MALT	mucosa-associated lymphoid tissues
MAPK	mitogen activated protein kinase
MDA	melanoma differentiation associated gene
MHC	major histocompatibility complex
MNC	mononuclear cell
MTX	methotrexate
MZL	marginal zone lymphoma
NHL	non-Hodgkin's lymphoma
NOD	nucleotide-binding oligomerization domain
NLR	(NOD)-like receptor
PAMP	pathogen-associated molecular pattern
pDC	plasmatoid dendritic cell
PCR	polymerase chain reaction
PCs	plasma cells
PVL	proviral load
RA	rheumatoid arthritis
RANTES	regulated on activation, normal T cell expressed and secreted
RF	rheumatoid factor
RIG-I	retinoic acid inducible gene-I
RLR	RIG-I-like receptor
RNA	ribonucleic acid
SG	salivary gland
SGEC	SG epithelial cell
SLE	systemic lupus erythematosus
SLS	SS-like syndrome
SS	Sjögren's syndrome
TCDD	tetrachlorodibenzo-p-dioxin
TCR	T-cell receptor
TEC	thymic epithelial cell
Tg	transgenic
TLR	toll-like receptor
TNF	tumor necrosis factor
TRX	thioredoxin
TUNEL	terminal deoxynucleotidyl transferase-mediated dUTP nick-end labeling
XIAP	X-chromosome-linked inhibitor of apoptosis protein
WKAH	Wistar-King-Aptekman-Hokudai

References

1. Karameris, A.; Gorgoulis, V.; Iliopoulos, A.; Frangia, C.; Kontomerkos, T.; Ioakeimidis, D.; Kalogeropoulos, N.; Sfikakis, P.; Kanavaros, P. Detection of the Epstein Barr viral genome by an in situ hybridization method in salivary gland biopsies from patients with secondary Sjögren's syndrome. *Clin. Exp. Rheumatol.* **1992**, *10*, 327–332. [PubMed]
2. Nakamura, H.; Takahashi, Y.; Yamamoto-Fukuda, T.; Horai, Y.; Nakashima, Y.; Arima, K.; Nakamura, T.; Koji, T.; Kawakami, A. Direct infection of primary salivary gland epithelial cells by human T lymphotropic virus type I in patients with Sjögren's syndrome. *Arthritis Rheumatol.* **2015**, *67*, 1096–1106. [CrossRef]
3. Ice, J.A.; Li, H.; Adrianto, I.; Lin, P.C.; Kelly, J.A.; Montgomery, C.G.; Lessard, C.J.; Moser, K.L. Genetics of Sjögren's syndrome in the genome-wide association era. *J. Autoimmun.* **2012**, *39*, 57–63. [CrossRef] [PubMed]
4. Li, Y.; Zhang, K.; Chen, H.; Sun, F.; Xu, J.; Wu, Z.; Li, P.; Zhang, L.; Du, Y.; Luan, H.; et al. A genome-wide association study in Han Chinese identifies a susceptibility locus for primary Sjögren's syndrome at 7q11.23. *Nat. Genet.* **2013**, *45*, 1361–1365. [CrossRef] [PubMed]
5. Mariette, X.; Criswell, L.A. Primary Sjögren's Syndrome. *N. Engl. J. Med.* **2018**, *379*, 97. [CrossRef] [PubMed]
6. Nakamura, H.; Kawakami, A.; Eguchi, K. Mechanisms of autoantibody production and the relationship between autoantibodies and the clinical manifestations in Sjögren's syndrome. *Transl. Res.* **2006**, *148*, 281–288. [CrossRef]
7. Ishimaru, N.; Arakaki, R.; Watanabe, M.; Kobayashi, M.; Miyazaki, K.; Hayashi, Y. Development of autoimmune exocrinopathy resembling Sjögren's syndrome in estrogen-deficient mice of healthy background. *Am. J. Pathol.* **2003**, *163*, 1481–1490. [CrossRef]
8. Moon, J.; Choi, S.H.; Yoon, C.H.; Kim, M.K. Gut dysbiosis is prevailing in Sjögren's syndrome and is related to dry eye severity. *PLoS ONE* **2020**, *15*, e0229029. [CrossRef]
9. Shimizu, T.; Nakamura, H.; Takatani, A.; Umeda, M.; Horai, Y.; Kurushima, S.; Michitsuji, T.; Nakashima, Y.; Kawakami, A. Activation of Toll-like receptor 7 signaling in labial salivary glands of primary Sjögren's syndrome patients. *Clin. Exp. Immunol.* **2019**, *196*, 39–51. [CrossRef]
10. Brauner, S.; Folkersen, L.; Kvarnström, M.; Meisgen, S.; Petersen, S.; Franzén-Malmros, M.; Mofors, J.; Brokstad, K.A.; Klareskog, L.; Jonsson, R.; et al. H1N1 vaccination in Sjögren's syndrome triggers polyclonal B cell activation and promotes autoantibody production. *Ann. Rheum. Dis.* **2017**, *76*, 1755–1763. [CrossRef]
11. Kerr, J.R. Epstein-Barr virus (EBV) reactivation and therapeutic inhibitors. *J. Clin. Pathol.* **2019**, *7*, 651–658. [CrossRef] [PubMed]
12. Hayashi, F.; Smith, K.D.; Ozinsky, A.; Hawn, T.R.; Yi, E.C.; Goodlett, D.R.; Eng, J.K.; Akira, S.; Underhill, D.M.; Aderem, A. The innate immune response to bacterial flagellin is mediated by Toll-like receptor 5. *Nature* **2001**, *410*, 1099–1103. [CrossRef] [PubMed]
13. Akira, S.; Takeda, K.; Kaisho, T. Toll-like receptors: Critical proteins linking innate and acquired immunity. *Nat. Immunol.* **2001**, *2*, 675–680. [CrossRef] [PubMed]
14. Bochud, P.Y.; Bochud, M.; Telenti, A.; Calandra, T. Innate immunogenetics: A tool for exploring new frontiers of host defence. *Lancet Infect. Dis.* **2007**, *7*, 531–542. [CrossRef]
15. Melchjorsen, J.; Jensen, S.B.; Malmgaard, L.; Rasmussen, S.B.; Weber, F.; Bowie, A.G.; Matikainen, S.; Paludan, S.R. Activation of innate defense against a paramyxovirus is mediated by RIG-I and TLR7 and TLR8 in a cell-type-specific manner. *J. Virol.* **2005**, *79*, 12944–12951. [CrossRef]
16. Lund, J.M.; Alexopoulou, L.; Sato, A.; Karow, M.; Adams, N.C.; Gale, N.W.; Iwasaki, A.; Flavell, R.A. Recognition of single-stranded RNA viruses by Toll-like receptor 7. *Proc. Natl. Acad. Sci. USA* **2004**, *101*, 5598–5603. [CrossRef] [PubMed]
17. Maria, N.I.; Steenwijk, E.C.; IJpma, A.S.; van Helden-Meeuwsen, C.G.; Vogelsang, P.; Beumer, W.; Brkic, Z.; van Daele, P.L.; van Hagen, P.M.; van der Spek, P.J.; et al. Contrasting expression pattern of RNA-sensing receptors TLR7, RIG-I and MDA5 in interferon-positive and interferon-negative patients with primary Sjögren's syndrome. *Ann. Rheum. Dis.* **2017**, *76*, 721–730. [CrossRef] [PubMed]
18. Green, J.; Casabonne, D.; Newton, R. Coxsackie B virus serology and Type 1 diabetes mellitus: A systematic review of published case-control studies. *Diabet. Med.* **2004**, *21*, 507–514. [CrossRef]
19. Aida, K.; Nishida, Y.; Tanaka, S.; Maruyama, T.; Shimada, A.; Awata, T.; Suzuki, M.; Shimura, H.; Takizawa, S.; Ichijo, M.; et al. RIG-I- and MDA5-initiated innate immunity linked with adaptive immunity accelerates beta-cell death in fulminant type 1 diabetes. *Diabetes* **2011**, *60*, 884–889. [CrossRef]

20. Ogawara, K.; Kuwabara, S.; Koga, M.; Mori, M.; Yuki, N.; Hattori, T. Anti-GM1b IgG antibody is associated with acute motor axonal neuropathy and Campylobacter jejuni infection. *J. Neurol. Sci.* **2003**, *210*, 41–45. [CrossRef]
21. Uncini, A.; González-Bravo, D.C.; Acosta-Ampudia, Y.Y.; Ojeda, E.C.; Rodríguez, Y.; Monsalve, D.M.; Ramírez-Santana, C.; Vega, D.A.; Paipilla, D.; Torres, L.; et al. Clinical and nerve conduction features in Guillain-Barré syndrome associated with Zika virus infection in Cúcuta, Colombia. *Eur. J. Neurol.* **2018**, *25*, 644–650. [CrossRef] [PubMed]
22. Illescas-Montes, R.; Corona-Castro, C.C.; Melguizo-Rodríguez, L.; Ruiz, C.; Costela-Ruiz, V.J. Infectious processes and systemic lupus erythematosus. *Immunology* **2019**, *158*, 153–160. [CrossRef]
23. Hod, T.; Zandman-Goddard, G.; Langevitz, P.; Rudnic, H.; Grossman, Z.; Rotman-Pikielny, P.; Levy, Y. Does parvovirus infection have a role in systemic lupus erythematosus? *Immunol. Res.* **2017**, *65*, 447–453. [CrossRef]
24. Larsen, M.; Sauce, D.; Deback, C.; Arnaud, L.; Mathian, A.; Miyara, M.; Boutolleau, D.; Parizot, C.; Dorgham, K.; Papagno, L.; et al. Exhausted cytotoxic control of Epstein-Barr virus in human lupus. *PLoS Pathog.* **2011**, *7*, e1002328. [CrossRef] [PubMed]
25. Jørgensen, K.T.; Wiik, A.; Pedersen, M.; Hedegaard, C.J.; Vestergaard, B.F.; Gislefoss, R.E.; Kvien, T.K.; Wohlfahrt, J.; Bendtzen, K.; Frisch, M. Cytokines, autoantibodies and viral antibodies in premorbid and postdiagnostic sera from patients with rheumatoid arthritis: Case-control study nested in a cohort of Norwegian blood donors. *Ann. Rheum. Dis.* **2008**, *67*, 860–866. [CrossRef] [PubMed]
26. Iwakura, Y.; Tosu, M.; Yoshida, E.; Takiguchi, M.; Sato, K.; Kitajima, I.; Nishioka, K.; Yamamoto, K.; Takeda, T.; Hatanaka, M. Induction of inflammatory arthropathy resembling rheumatoid arthritis in mice transgenic for HTLV-I. *Science* **1991**, *253*, 1026–1028. [CrossRef]
27. Yamamoto, H.; Sekiguchi, T.; Itagaki, K.; Saijo, S.; Iwakura, Y. Inflammatory polyarthritis in mice transgenic for human T cell leukemia virus type I. *Arthritis Rheum.* **1993**, *36*, 1612–1620. [CrossRef] [PubMed]
28. Ziegler, B.; Gay, R.E.; Huang, G.Q.; Fassbender, H.G.; Gay, S. Immunohistochemical localization of HTLV-I p19- and p24-related antigens in synovial joints of patients with rheumatoid arthritis. *Am. J. Pathol.* **1989**, *35*, 1–5.
29. Umekita, K.; Umeki, K.; Miyauchi, S.; Ueno, S.; Kubo, K.; Kusumoto, N.; Takajo, I.; Nagatomo, Y.; Okayama, A. Use of anti-tumor necrosis factor biologics in the treatment of rheumatoid arthritis does not change human T-lymphotropic virus type 1 markers: A case series. *Mod. Rheumatol.* **2015**, *25*, 794–797. [CrossRef]
30. Suzuki, T.; Fukui, S.; Umekita, K.; Miyamoto, J.; Umeda, M.; Nishino, A.; Okada, A.; Koga, T.; Kawashiri, S.Y.; Iwamoto, N.; et al. Brief report: Attenuated effectiveness of tumor necrosis factor inhibitors for anti-human T lymphotropic virus type I antibody-positive rheumatoid arthritis. *Arthritis Rheumatol.* **2018**, *70*, 1014–1021. [CrossRef]
31. Klein, G.; Pearson, G.; Nadkarni, J.S.; Nadkarni, J.J.; Klein, E.; Henle, G.; Henle, W.; Clifford, P. Relation between Epstein-Barr viral and cell membrane immunofluorescence of Burkitt tumor cells. I. Dependence of cell membrane immunofluorescence on presence of EB virus. *J. Exp. Med.* **1968**, *128*, 1011–1020. [CrossRef] [PubMed]
32. Lam, W.K.J.; Jiang, P.; Chan, K.C.A.; Cheng, S.H.; Zhang, H.; Peng, W.; Tse, O.Y.O.; Tong, Y.K.; Gai, W.; Zee, B.C.Y.; et al. Sequencing-based counting and size profiling of plasma Epstein-Barr virus DNA enhance population screening of nasopharyngeal carcinoma. *Proc. Natl. Acad. Sci. USA* **2018**, *115*, E5124. [CrossRef] [PubMed]
33. Rahman, M.A.; Kingsley, L.A.; Atchison, R.W.; Belle, S.; Breinig, M.C.; Ho, M.; Rinaldo, C.R., Jr. Reactivation of Epstein-Barr virus during early infection with human immunodeficiency virus. *J. Clin. Microbiol.* **1991**, *29*, 1215–1220. [CrossRef] [PubMed]
34. Meijer, E.; Slaper-Cortenbach, I.C.; Thijsen, S.F.; Dekker, A.W.; Verdonck, L.F. Increased incidence of EBV-associated lymphoproliferative disorders after allogeneic stem cell transplantation from matched unrelated donors due to a change of T cell depletion technique. *Bone Marrow Transplant.* **2002**, *29*, 335–339. [CrossRef]
35. Katsuyama, T.; Sada, K.E.; Yan, M.; Zeggar, S.; Hiramatsu, S.; Miyawaki, Y.; Ohashi, K.; Morishita, M.; Watanabe, H.; Katsuyama, E.; et al. Prognostic factors of methotrexate-associated lymphoproliferative disorders associated with rheumatoid arthritis and plausible application of biological agents. *Mod. Rheumatol.* **2017**, *27*, 773–777. [CrossRef]

36. Dojcinov, S.D.; Fend, F.; Quintanilla-Martinez, L. EBV-positive lymphoproliferations of B- T- and NK-cell derivation in non-immunocompromised hosts. *Pathogens* **2018**, *7*, 28. [CrossRef]
37. Anderson, A.G.; Gaffy, C.B.; Weseli, J.R.; Gorres, K.L. Inhibition of Epstein-Barr virus lytic reactivation by the atypical antipsychotic drug clozapine. *Viruses* **2019**, *11*, 450. [CrossRef]
38. Wang, F.; Gregory, C.; Sample, C.; Rowe, M.; Liebowitz, D.; Murray, R.; Rickinson, A.; Kieff, E. Epstein-Barr virus latent membrane protein (LMP1) and nuclear proteins 2 and 3C are effectors of phenotypic changes in B lymphocytes: EBNA-2 and LMP1 cooperatively induce CD23. *J. Virol.* **1990**, *64*, 2309–2318. [CrossRef]
39. Murata, T.; Sato, Y.; Kimura, H. Modes of infection and oncogenesis by the Epstein-Barr virus. *Rev. Med. Virol.* **2014**, *24*, 242–253. [CrossRef]
40. Nawandar, D.M.; Ohashi, M.; Djavadian, R.; Barlow, E.; Makielski, K.; Ali, A.; Lee, D.; Lambert, P.F.; Johannsen, E.; Kenney, S.C. Differentiation-dependent LMP1 expression is required for efficient lytic Epstein-Barr virus reactivation in epithelial cells. *J. Virol.* **2017**, *91*, e02438-16. [CrossRef]
41. Venables, P.J.; Ross, M.G.; Charles, P.J.; Melsom, R.D.; Griffiths, P.D.; Maini, R.N. A seroepidemiological study of cytomegalovirus and Epstein-Barr virus in rheumatoid arthritis and sicca syndrome. *Ann. Rheum. Dis.* **1985**, *44*, 742–746. [CrossRef] [PubMed]
42. Fox, R.I.; Pearson, G.; Vaughan, J.H. Detection of Epstein-Barr virus-associated antigens and DNA in salivary gland biopsies from patients with Sjögren's syndrome. *J. Immunol.* **1986**, *137*, 3162–3168.
43. Yamaoka, K.; Miyasaka, N.; Yamamoto, K. Possible involvement of Epstein-Barr virus in polyclonal B cell activation in Sjögren's syndrome. *Arthritis Rheum.* **1988**, *31*, 1014–1021. [CrossRef] [PubMed]
44. Saito, I.; Servenius, B.; Compton, T.; Fox, R.I. Detection of Epstein-Barr virus DNA by polymerase chain reaction in blood and tissue biopsies from patients with Sjogren's syndrome. *J. Exp. Med.* **1989**, *169*, 2191–2198. [CrossRef] [PubMed]
45. Venables, P.J.; Teo, C.G.; Baboonian, C.; Griffin, B.E.; Hughes, R.A. Persistence of Epstein-Barr virus in salivary gland biopsies from healthy individuals and patients with Sjögren's syndrome. *Clin. Exp. Immunol.* **1989**, *75*, 359–364. [PubMed]
46. Mariette, X.; Gozlan, J.; Clerc, D.; Bisson, M.; Morinet, F. Detection of Epstein-Barr virus DNA by in situ hybridization and polymerase chain reaction in salivary gland biopsy specimens from patients with Sjögren's syndrome. *Am. J. Med.* **1991**, *90*, 286–294. [CrossRef]
47. Pflugfelder, S.C.; Tseng, S.C.; Pepose, J.S.; Fletcher, M.A.; Klimas, N.; Feuer, W. Epstein-Barr virus infection and immunologic dysfunction in patients with aqueous tear deficiency. *Ophthalmology* **1990**, *97*, 313–323. [CrossRef]
48. Saito, I.; Shimuta, M.; Terauchi, K.; Tsubota, K.; Yodoi, J.; Miyasaka, N. Increased expression of human thioredoxin/adult T cell leukemia-derived factor in Sjögren's syndrome. *Arthritis Rheum.* **1996**, *39*, 773–782. [CrossRef]
49. Maitland, N.; Flint, S.; Scully, C.; Crean, S.J. Detection of cytomegalovirus and Epstein-Barr virus in labial salivary glands in Sjögren's syndrome and non-specific sialadenitis. *J. Oral Pathol. Med.* **1995**, *24*, 293–298. [CrossRef]
50. Haneji, N.; Nakamura, T.; Takio, K.; Yanagi, K.; Higashiyama, H.; Saito, I.; Noji, S.; Sugino, H.; Hayashi, Y. Identification of alpha-fodrin as a candidate autoantigen in primary Sjögren's syndrome. *Science* **1997**, *276*, 604–607. [CrossRef]
51. Horiuchi, M.; Yamano, S.; Inoue, H.; Ishii, J.; Nagata, Y.; Adachi, H.; Ono, M.; Renard, J.N.; Mizuno, F.; Hayashi, Y.; et al. Possible involvement of IL-12 expression by Epstein-Barr virus in Sjögren syndrome. *J. Clin. Pathol.* **1999**, *52*, 833–837. [CrossRef] [PubMed]
52. Royer, B.; Cazals-Hatem, D.; Sibilia, J.; Agbalika, F.; Cayuela, J.M.; Soussi, T.; Maloisel, F.; Clauvel, J.P.; Brouet, J.C.; Mariette, X. Lymphomas in patients with Sjogren's syndrome are marginal zone B-cell neoplasms, arise in diverse extranodal and nodal sites, and are not associated with viruses. *Blood* **1997**, *90*, 766–775. [CrossRef]
53. Pasoto, S.G.; Natalino, R.R.; Chakkour, H.P.; Viana Vdos, S.; Bueno, C.; Leon, E.P.; Vendramini, M.B.; Neto, M.L.; Bonfa, E. EBV reactivation serological profile in primary Sjögren's syndrome: An underlying trigger of active articular involvement? *Rheumatol. Int.* **2013**, *33*, 1149–1157. [CrossRef] [PubMed]
54. Inoue, H.; Mishima, K.; Yamamoto-Yoshida, S.; Ushikoshi-Nakayama, R.; Nakagawa, Y.; Yamamoto, K.; Ryo, K.; Ide, F.; Saito, I. Aryl hydrocarbon receptor-mediated induction of EBV reactivation as a risk factor for Sjögren's syndrome. *J. Immunol.* **2012**, *188*, 4654–4662. [CrossRef]

55. Fox, R.I.; Chilton, T.; Scott, S.; Benton, L.; Howell, F.V.; Vaughan, J.H. Potential role of Epstein-Barr virus in Sjögren's syndrome. *Rheum. Dis. Clin. N. Am.* **1987**, *13*, 275–292.
56. Origgi, L.; Hu, C.; Bertetti, E.; Asero, R.; D'Agostino, P.; Radelli, L.; Riboldi, P. Antibodies to Epstein-Barr virus and cytomegalovirus in primary Sjogren's syndrome. *Boll. Ist. Sieroter. Milan.* **1988**, *67*, 265–274.
57. Inoue, N.; Harada, S.; Miyasaka, N.; Oya, A.; Yanagi, K. Analysis of antibody titers to Epstein-Barr virus nuclear antigens in sera of patients with Sjögren's syndrome and with rheumatoid arthritis. *J. Infect. Dis.* **1991**, *164*, 22–28. [CrossRef]
58. DiGiuseppe, J.A.; Wu, T.C.; Corio, R.L. Analysis of Epstein-Barr virus-encoded small RNA 1 expression in benign lymphoepithelial salivary gland lesions. *Mod. Pathol.* **1994**, *7*, 555–559.
59. Merne, M.E.; Syrjänen, S.M. Detection of Epstein-Barr virus in salivary gland specimens from Sjögren's syndrome patients. *Laryngoscope* **1996**, *106*, 1534–1539. [CrossRef]
60. Croia, C.; Astorri, E.; Murray-Brown, W.; Willis, A.; Brokstad, K.A.; Sutcliffe, N.; Piper, K.; Jonsson, R.; Tappuni, A.R.; Pitzalis, C.; et al. Implication of Epstein-Barr virus infection in disease-specific autoreactive B cell activation in ectopic lymphoid structures of Sjögren's syndrome. *Arthritis Rheumatol.* **2014**, *66*, 2545–2557. [CrossRef]
61. Mackrides, N.; Campuzano-Zuluaga, G.; Maque-Acosta, Y.; Moul, A.; Hijazi, N.; Ikpatt, F.O.; Levy, R.; Verdun, R.E.; Kunkalla, K.; Natkunam, Y.; et al. Epstein-Barr virus-positive follicular lymphoma. *Mod. Pathol.* **2017**, *30*, 519–529. [CrossRef]
62. Fox, R.I.; Howell, F.V. Reactivation of Epstein-Barr virus in Sjögren's syndrome. *Ric. Clin. Lab.* **1987**, *17*, 273–277. [PubMed]
63. Fox, R.I.; Saito, I.; Chan, E.K.; Josephs, S.; Salahuddin, S.Z.; Ahlashi, D.V.; Staal, F.W.; Gallo, R.; Pei-Ping, H.; Le, C.S. Viral genomes in lymphomas of patients with Sjögren's syndrome. *J. Autoimmun.* **1989**, *2*, 449–455. [CrossRef]
64. Clark, D.A.; Lamey, P.J.; Jarrett, R.F.; Onions, D.E. A model to study viral and cytokine involvement in Sjögren's syndrome. *Autoimmunity* **1994**, *18*, 7–14. [CrossRef] [PubMed]
65. Newkirk, M.M.; Shiroky, J.B.; Johnson, N.; Danoff, D.; Isenberg, D.A.; Shustik, C.; Pearson, G.R. Rheumatic disease patients, prone to Sjögren's syndrome and/or lymphoma, mount an antibody response to BHRF1, the Epstein-Barr viral homologue of BCL-2. *Br. J. Rheumatol.* **1996**, *35*, 1075–1081. [CrossRef] [PubMed]
66. Whittingham, S.; McNeilage, L.J.; Mackay, I.R. Epstein-Barr virus as an etiological agent in primary Sjögren's syndrome. *Med. Hypotheses.* **1987**, *22*, 373–386. [CrossRef]
67. Venables, P.J.; Baboonian, C.; Maini, R.N. Normal serologic response to Epstein-Barr virus in patients with Sjögren's syndrome. *Arthritis Rheum.* **1989**, *32*, 811–812. [CrossRef] [PubMed]
68. Nagasaki, M.; Morikawa, S.; Harada, T.; Miyasaka, N. A novel EBV-related nucleo-cytoplasmic antigen in a null cell-line (HLN-STL-C) reactive to antibodies in the sera from patients with Sjögren's syndrome. *J. Autoimmun.* **1989**, *2*, 457–462. [CrossRef]
69. Tateishi, M.; Saito, I.; Yamamoto, K.; Miyasaka, N. Spontaneous production of Epstein-Barr virus by B lymphoblastoid cell lines obtained from patients with Sjögren's syndrome. Possible involvement of a novel strain of Epstein-Barr virus in disease pathogenesis. *Arthritis Rheum.* **1993**, *36*, 827–835. [CrossRef]
70. Miyasaka, N.; Saito, I.; Haruta, J. Possible involvement of Epstein-Barr virus in the pathogenesis of Sjogren's syndrome. *Clin. Immunol. Immunopathol.* **1994**, *72*, 166–170. [CrossRef]
71. Inoue, H.; Tsubota, K.; Ono, M.; Kizu, Y.; Mizuno, F.; Takada, K.; Yamada, K.; Yanagi, K.; Hayashi, Y.; Saito, I. Possible involvement of EBV-mediated alpha-fodrin cleavage for organ-specific autoantigen in Sjogren's syndrome. *J. Immunol.* **2001**, *166*, 5801–5809. [CrossRef] [PubMed]
72. Wang'ondu, R.; Teal, S.; Park, R.; Heston, L.; Deleceluse, H.; Miller, G. DNA damage signaling is induced in the absence of Epstein-Barr virus (EBV) lytic DNA replication and in response to expression of ZEBRA. *PLoS ONE* **2015**, *10*, e0126088. [CrossRef] [PubMed]
73. Nagata, Y.; Inoue, H.; Yamada, K.; Higashiyama, H.; Mishima, K.; Kizu, Y.; Takeda, I.; Mizuno, F.; Hayashi, Y.; Saito, I. Activation of Epstein-Barr virus by saliva from Sjogren's syndrome patients. *Immunology* **2004**, *111*, 223–229. [CrossRef] [PubMed]
74. Salomonsson, S.; Jonsson, M.V.; Skarstein, K.; Brokstad, K.A.; Hjelmström, P.; Wahren-Herlenius, M.; Jonsson, R. Cellular basis of ectopic germinal center formation and autoantibody production in the target organ of patients with Sjögren's syndrome. *Arthritis Rheum.* **2003**, *48*, 3187–3201. [CrossRef]

75. Sène, D.; Ismael, S.; Forien, M.; Charlotte, F.; Kaci, R.; Cacoub, P.; Diallo, A.; Dieudé, P.; Lioté, F. Ectopic germinal center-like structures in minor salivary gland biopsy tissue predict lymphoma occurrence in patients with primary Sjögren's Syndrome. *Arthritis Rheumatol.* **2018**, *70*, 1481–1488. [CrossRef] [PubMed]
76. Schiødt, M.; Greenspan, D.; Daniels, T.E.; Nelson, J.; Leggott, P.J.; Wara, D.W.; Greenspan, J.S. Parotid gland enlargement and xerostomia associated with labial sialadenitis in HIV-infected patients. *J. Autoimmun.* **1989**, *2*, 415–425. [CrossRef]
77. Garry, R.F.; Fermin, C.D.; Hart, D.J.; Alexander, S.S.; Donehower, L.A.; Luo-Zhang, H. Detection of a human intracisternal A-type retroviral particle antigenically related to HIV. *Science* **1990**, *250*, 1127–1129. [CrossRef]
78. Talal, N.; Dauphinée, M.J.; Dang, H.; Alexander, S.S.; Hart, D.J.; Garry, R.F. Detection of serum antibodies to retroviral proteins in patients with primary Sjögren's syndrome (autoimmune exocrinopathy). *Arthritis Rheum.* **1990**, *33*, 774–781. [CrossRef] [PubMed]
79. Talal, N. Immunologic and viral factors in Sjögren's syndrome. *Clin. Exp. Rheumatol.* **1990**, *8*, 23–26. [PubMed]
80. Itescu, S.; Brancato, L.J.; Buxbaum, J.; Gregersen, P.K.; Rizk, C.C.; Croxson, T.S.; Solomon, G.E.; Winchester, R. A diffuse infiltrative CD8 lymphocytosis syndrome in human immunodeficiency virus (HIV) infection: A host immune response associated with HLA-DR5. *Ann. Intern. Med.* **1990**, *112*, 3–10. [CrossRef] [PubMed]
81. Itescu, S. Diffuse infiltrative lymphocytosis syndrome in human immunodeficiency virus infection—A Sjögren's-like disease. *Rheum. Dis. Clin. N. Am.* **1991**, *17*, 99–115.
82. Dwyer, E.; Itescu, S.; Winchester, R. Characterization of the primary structure of T cell receptor beta chains in cells infiltrating the salivary gland in the sicca syndrome of HIV-1 infection. Evidence of antigen-driven clonal selection suggested by restricted combinations of V beta J beta gene segment usage and shared somatically encoded amino acid residues. *J. Clin. Investig.* **1993**, *92*, 495–502. [PubMed]
83. Kordossis, T.; Paikos, S.; Aroni, K.; Kitsanta, P.; Dimitrakopoulos, A.; Kavouklis, E.; Alevizou, V.; Kyriaki, P.; Skopouli, F.N.; Moutsopoulos, H.M. Prevalence of Sjögren's-like syndrome in a cohort of HIV-1-positive patients: Descriptive pathology and immunopathology. *Br. J. Rheumatol.* **1998**, *37*, 691–695. [CrossRef] [PubMed]
84. Williams, F.M.; Cohen, P.R.; Jumshyd, J.; Reveille, J.D.; Williams, F.M.; Cohen, P.R.; Jumshyd, J.; Reveille, J.D. Prevalence of the diffuse infiltrative lymphocytosis syndrome among human immunodeficiency virus type 1-positive outpatients. *Arthritis Rheum.* **1998**, *41*, 863–868. [CrossRef]
85. Yamano, S.; Renard, J.N.; Mizuno, F.; Narita, Y.; Uchida, Y.; Higashiyama, H.; Sakurai, H.; Saito, I. Retrovirus in salivary glands from patients with Sjögren's syndrome. *J. Clin. Pathol.* **1997**, *50*, 223–230. [CrossRef]
86. Rigby, S.P.; Griffiths, D.J.; Weiss, R.A.; Venables, P.J. Human retrovirus-5 proviral DNA is rarely detected in salivary gland biopsy tissues from patients with Sjögren's syndrome. *Arthritis Rheum.* **1997**, *40*, 2016–2021. [CrossRef]
87. Panayiotakopoulos, G.D.; Aroni, K.; Kyriaki, D.; Paikos, S.; Vouyioukas, N.; Vlachos, A.; Kontos, A.N.; Kordossis, T. Paucity of Sjogren-like syndrome in a cohort of HIV-1-positive patients in the HAART era. Part II. *Rheumatology (Oxford)* **2003**, *42*, 1164–1167. [CrossRef]
88. Vitali, C.; Bombardieri, S.; Jonsson, R.; Moutsopoulos, H.M.; Alexander, E.L.; Carsons, S.E.; Daniels, T.E.; Fox, P.C.; Fox, R.I.; Kassan, S.S.; et al. Classification criteria for Sjögren's syndrome: A revised version of the European criteria proposed by the American-European Consensus Group. *Ann. Rheum. Dis.* **2002**, *61*, 554–558. [CrossRef]
89. Yoshida, M.; Inoue, J.; Fujisawa, J.; Seiki, M. Molecular mechanisms of regulation of HTLV-1 gene expression and its association with leukemogenesis. *Genome* **1989**, *31*, 662–667. [CrossRef]
90. Takatsuki, K. Discovery of adult T-cell leukemia. *Retrovirology* **2005**, *2*, 16. [CrossRef]
91. Yoshida, M.; Miyoshi, I.; Hinuma, Y. Isolation and characterization of retrovirus from cell lines of human adult T-cell leukemia and its implication in the disease. *Proc. Natl. Acad. Sci. USA* **1982**, *79*, 2031–2035. [CrossRef] [PubMed]
92. Jeang, K.T.; Widen, S.G.; Semmes, O.J., 4th; Wilson, S.H. HTLV-I trans-activator protein, tax, is a trans-repressor of the human beta-polymerase gene. *Science* **1990**, *247*, 1082–1084. [CrossRef] [PubMed]
93. Osame, M.; Matsumoto, M.; Usuku, K.; Izumo, S.; Ijichi, N.; Amitani, H.; Tara, M.; Igata, A. Chronic progressive myelopathy associated with elevated antibodies to human T-lymphotropic virus type I and adult T-cell leukemialike cells. *Ann. Neurol.* **1987**, *21*, 117–122. [CrossRef] [PubMed]
94. Izumo, S.; Umehara, F.; Osame, M. HTLV-I-associated myelopathy. *Neuropathology* **2000**, *20*, S65–S68. [CrossRef]

95. Kamoi, K.; Mochizuki, M. HTLV infection and the eye. *Curr. Opin. Ophthalmol.* **2012**, *23*, 557–561. [CrossRef]
96. Ono, A.; Ikeda, E.; Mochizuki, M.; Matsuoka, M.; Yamaguchi, K.; Sawada, T.; Yamane, S.; Tokudome, S.; Watanabe, T. Provirus load in patients with human T-cell leukemia virus type 1 uveitis correlates with precedent Graves' disease and disease activities. *Jpn. J. Cancer Res.* **1998**, *89*, 608–614. [CrossRef]
97. Sugimoto, M.; Kitaichi, M.; Ikeda, A.; Nagai, S.; Izumi, T. Chronic bronchioloalveolitis associated with human T-cell lymphotrophic virus type I infection. *Curr. Opin. Pulm. Med.* **1998**, *4*, 98–102. [CrossRef]
98. Yamamoto-Taguchi, N.; Satou, Y.; Miyazato, P.; Ohshima, K.; Nakagawa, M.; Katagiri, K.; Kinashi, T.; Matsuoka, M. HTLV-1 bZIP factor induces inflammation through labile Foxp3 expression. *PLoS Pathog.* **2013**, *9*, e1003630. [CrossRef]
99. Nakamura, H.; Kawakami, A.; Tominaga, M.; Hida, A.; Yamasaki, S.; Migita, K.; Kawabe, Y.; Nakamura, T.; Eguchi, K. Relationship between Sjögren's syndrome and human T-lymphotropic virus type I infection: Follow-up study of 83 patients. *J. Lab. Clin. Med.* **2000**, *135*, 139–144. [CrossRef]
100. Izumi, M.; Nakamura, H.; Nakamura, T.; Eguchi, K.; Nakamura, T. Sjögren's syndrome (SS) in patients with human T cell leukemia virus I associated myelopathy: Paradoxical features of the major salivary glands compared to classical SS. *J. Rheumatol.* **1999**, *26*, 2609–2614.
101. Nakamura, H.; Takagi, Y.; Kawakami, A.; Ida, H.; Nakamura, T.; Nakamura, T.; Eguchi, K. HTLV-I infection results in resistance toward salivary gland destruction of Sjögren's syndrome. *Clin. Exp. Rheumatol.* **2008**, *26*, 653–655. [PubMed]
102. Cruz, B.A.; Catalan-Soares, B.; Proietti, F. Higher prevalence of fibromyalgia in patients infected with human T cell lymphotropic virus type, I.J. *Rheumatol.* **2006**, *33*, 2300–2303.
103. Gross, C.; Thoma-Kress, A.K. Molecular Mechanisms of HTLV-1 Cell-to-Cell Transmission. *Viruses* **2016**, *8*, 74. [CrossRef]
104. Lima, C.M.; Santos, S.; Dourado, A.; Carvalho, N.B.; Bittencourt, V.; Lessa, M.M.; Siqueira, I.; Carvalho, E.M. Association of sicca syndrome with proviral load and proinflammatory cytokines in HTLV-1 infection. *J. Immunol. Res.* **2016**, *2016*, 8402059. [CrossRef]
105. Kakugawa, T.; Sakamoto, N.; Ishimoto, H.; Shimizu, T.; Nakamura, H.; Nawata, A.; Ito, C.; Sato, S.; Hanaka, T.; Oda, K.; et al. Lymphocytic focus score is positively related to airway and interstitial lung diseases in primary Sjögren's syndrome. *Respir. Med.* **2018**, *137*, 95–102. [CrossRef] [PubMed]
106. Shattles, W.G.; Brookes, S.M.; Venables, P.J.; Clark, D.A.; Maini, R.N. Expression of antigen reactive with a monoclonal antibody to HTLV-1 P19 in salivary glands in Sjögren's syndrome. *Clin. Exp. Immunol.* **1992**, *89*, 46–51. [CrossRef] [PubMed]
107. Mariette, X.; Agbalika, F.; Daniel, M.T.; Bisson, M.; Lagrange, P.; Brouet, J.C.; Morinet, F. Detection of human T lymphotropic virus type I tax gene in salivary gland epithelium from two patients with Sjögren's syndrome. *Arthritis Rheum.* **1993**, *36*, 1423–1428. [CrossRef]
108. Sumida, T.; Yonaha, F.; Maeda, T.; Kita, Y.; Iwamoto, I.; Koike, T.; Yoshida, S. Expression of sequences homologous to HTLV-I tax gene in the labial salivary glands of Japanese patients with Sjögren's syndrome. *Arthritis Rheum.* **1994**, *37*, 545–550. [CrossRef]
109. Amft, N.; Bowman, S.J. Chemokines and cell trafficking in Sjögren's syndrome. *Scand. J. Immunol.* **2001**, *54*, 62–69. [CrossRef] [PubMed]
110. Terada, K.; Katamine, S.; Eguchi, K.; Moriuchi, R.; Kita, M.; Shimada, H.; Yamashita, I.; Iwata, K.; Tsuji, Y.; Nagataki, S. Antibodies to HTLV-I in Sjögren's syndrome. *Lancet* **1994**, *344*, 1116–1119. [CrossRef]
111. Satou, Y.; Yasunaga, J.; Zhao, T.; Yoshida, M.; Miyazato, P.; Takai, K.; Shimizu, K.; Ohshima, K.; Green, P.L.; Ohkura, N.; et al. HTLV-1 bZIP factor induces T-cell lymphoma and systemic inflammation in vivo. *PLoS Pathog.* **2011**, *7*, e1001274. [CrossRef] [PubMed]
112. Fuchi, N.; Miura, K.; Tsukiyama, T.; Sasaki, D.; Ishihara, K.; Tsuruda, K.; Hasegawa, H.; Miura, S.; Yanagihara, K.; Masuzaki, H. Natural course of human T-cell leukemia virus type 1 proviral DNA levels in carriers during pregnancy. *J. Infect. Dis.* **2018**, *217*, 1383–1389. [CrossRef] [PubMed]
113. Eguchi, K.; Matsuoka, N.; Ida, H.; Nakashima, M.; Sakai, M.; Sakito, S.; Kawakami, A.; Terada, K.; Shimada, H.; Kawabe, Y.; et al. Primary Sjögren's syndrome with antibodies to HTLV-I: Clinical and laboratory features. *Ann. Rheum. Dis.* **1992**, *51*, 769–776. [CrossRef]
114. Cartier, L.; Castillo, J.L.; Cea, J.G.; Villagra, R. Chronic dacryosialadenitis in HTLV I associated myelopathy. *J. Neurol. Neurosurg. Psychiatry* **1995**, *58*, 244–246. [CrossRef] [PubMed]

115. Nakamura, H.; Eguchi, K.; Nakamura, T.; Mizokami, A.; Shirabe, S.; Kawakami, A.; Matsuoka, N.; Migita, K.; Kawabe, Y.; Nagataki, S. High prevalence of Sjögren's syndrome in patients with HTLV-I associated myelopathy. *Ann. Rheum. Dis.* **1997**, *56*, 167–172. [CrossRef] [PubMed]
116. Hida, A.; Imaizumi, M.; Sera, N.; Akahoshi, M.; Soda, M.; Maeda, R.; Nakashima, E.; Nakamura, H.; Ida, H.; Kawakami, A.; et al. Association of human T lymphotropic virus type I with Sjogren syndrome. *Ann. Rheum. Dis.* **2010**, *69*, 2056–2057. [CrossRef] [PubMed]
117. Nakamura, H.; Shimizu, T.; Takagi, Y.; Takahashi, Y.; Horai, Y.; Nakashima, Y.; Sato, S.; Shiraishi, H.; Nakamura, T.; Fukuoka, J.; et al. Reevaluation for clinical manifestations of HTLV-I-seropositive patients with Sjögren's syndrome. *BMC Musculoskelet. Disord.* **2015**, *16*, 335. [CrossRef]
118. Satake, M.; Yamaguchi, K.; Tadokoro, K. Current prevalence of HTLV-1 in Japan as determined by screening of blood donors. *J. Med. Virol.* **2012**, *84*, 327–335. [CrossRef]
119. Satake, M.; Iwanaga, M.; Sagara, Y.; Watanabe, T.; Okuma, K.; Hamaguchi, I. Incidence of human T-lymphotropic virus 1 infection in adolescent and adult blood donors in Japan: A nationwide retrospective cohort analysis. *Lancet Infect. Dis.* **2016**, *16*, 1246–1254. [CrossRef]
120. Vale, D.A.D.; Casseb, J.; de Oliveira, A.C.P.; Bussoloti Filho, I.; de Sousa, S.C.O.M.; Ortega, K.L. Prevalence of Sjögren's syndrome in Brazilian patients infected with human T-cell lymphotropic virus. *J. Oral Pathol. Med.* **2017**, *46*, 543–548. [CrossRef]
121. Rigby, S.P.; Cooke, S.P.; Weerasinghe, D.; Venables, P.J. Absence of HTLV-1 tax in Sjögren's syndrome. *Arthritis Rheum.* **1996**, *39*, 1609–1611. [CrossRef] [PubMed]
122. Ohyama, Y.; Nakamura, S.; Hara, H.; Shinohara, M.; Sasaki, M.; Ikebe-Hiroki, A.; Mouri, T.; Tsunawaki, S.; Abe, K.; Shirasuna, K.; et al. Accumulation of human T lymphotropic virus type I-infected T cells in the salivary glands of patients with human T lymphotropic virus type I-associated Sjögren's syndrome. *Arthritis Rheum.* **1998**, *41*, 1972–1978. [CrossRef]
123. Mizokami, A.; Eguchi, K.; Moriuchi, R.; Futsuki, Y.; Terada, K.; Nakamura, H.; Miyamoto, T.; Katamine, S. Low copy numbers of human T-cell lymphotropic virus type I (HTLV-I) tax-like DNA detected in the salivary gland of seronegative patients with Sjögren's syndrome in an HTLV-I endemic area. *Scand. J. Rheumatol.* **1998**, *27*, 435–440. [CrossRef] [PubMed]
124. Tangy, F.; Ossondo, M.; Vernant, J.C.; Smadja, D.; Blétry, O.; Baglin, A.C.; Ozden, S. Human T cell leukemia virus type I expression in salivary glands of infected patients. *J. Infect. Dis.* **1999**, *179*, 497–502. [CrossRef]
125. Sasaki, M.; Nakamura, S.; Ohyama, Y.; Shinohara, M.; Ezaki, I.; Hara, H.; Kadena, T.; Kishihara, K.; Yamamoto, K.; Nomoto, K.; et al. Accumulation of common T cell clonotypes in the salivary glands of patients with human T lymphotropic virus type I-associated and idiopathic Sjögren's syndrome. *J. Immunol.* **2000**, *164*, 2823–2831. [CrossRef]
126. Mariette, X.; Agbalika, F.; Zucker-Franklin, D.; Clerc, D.; Janin, A.; Cherot, P.; Brouet, J.C. Detection of the tax gene of HTLV-I in labial salivary glands from patients with Sjögren's syndrome and other diseases of the oral cavity. *Clin. Exp. Rheumatol.* **2000**, *18*, 341–347.
127. Lee, S.J.; Lee, J.S.; Shin, M.G.; Tanaka, Y.; Park, D.J.; Kim, T.J.; Park, Y.W.; Lee, S.S. Detection of HTLV-1 in the labial salivary glands of patients with Sjögren's syndrome: A distinct clinical subgroup? *J. Rheumatol.* **2012**, *39*, 809–815. [CrossRef]
128. Nakamura, H.; Hasegawa, H.; Sasaki, D.; Takatani, A.; Shimizu, T.; Kurushima, S.; Horai, Y.; Nakashima, Y.; Nakamura, T.; Fukuoka, J.; et al. Detection of human T lymphotropic virus type-I bZIP factor and tax in the salivary glands of Sjögren's syndrome patients. *Clin. Exp. Rheumatol.* **2018**, *36* (Suppl. 112), 51–60.
129. Igakura, T.; Stinchcombe, J.C.; Goon, P.K.; Taylor, G.P.; Weber, J.N.; Griffiths, G.M.; Tanaka, Y.; Osame, M.; Bangham, C.R. Spread of HTLV-I between lymphocytes by virus-induced polarization of the cytoskeleton. *Science* **2003**, *299*, 1713–1716. [CrossRef]
130. Pais-Correia, A.M.; Sachse, M.; Guadagnini, S.; Robbiati, V.; Lasserre, R.; Gessain, A.; Gout, O.; Alcover, A.; Thoulouze, M.I. Biofilm-like extracellular viral assemblies mediate HTLV-1 cell-to-cell transmission at virological synapses. *Nat. Med.* **2010**, *16*, 83–89. [CrossRef]
131. Thoulouze, M.I.; Alcover, A. Can viruses form biofilms? *Trends Microbiol.* **2011**, *19*, 257–262. [CrossRef] [PubMed]
132. Van Prooyen, N.; Gold, H.; Andresen, V.; Schwartz, O.; Jones, K.; Ruscetti, F.; Lockett, S.; Gudla, P.; Venzon, D.; Franchini, G. Human T-cell leukemia virus type 1 p8 protein increases cellular conduits and virus transmission. *Proc. Natl. Acad. Sci. USA* **2010**, *107*, 20738–20743. [CrossRef] [PubMed]

133. Malbec, M.; Roesch, F.; Schwartz, O. A new role for the HTLV-1 p8 protein: Increasing intercellular conduits and viral cell-to-cell transmission. *Viruses* **2011**, *3*, 254–259. [CrossRef] [PubMed]
134. Nakamura, H.; Shimizu, T.; Takatani, A.; Suematsu, T.; Nakamura, T.; Kawakami, A. Initial human T-cell leukemia virus type 1 infection of the salivary gland epithelial cells requires a biofilm-like structure. *Virus Res.* **2019**, *269*, 197643. [CrossRef]
135. Green, J.E.; Hinrichs, S.H.; Vogel, J.; Jay, G. Exocrinopathy resembling Sjögren's syndrome in HTLV-1 tax transgenic mice. *Nature* **1989**, *341*, 72–74. [CrossRef]
136. Yamazaki, H.; Ikeda, H.; Ishizu, A.; Nakamaru, Y.; Sugaya, T.; Kikuchi, K.; Yamada, S.; Wakisaka, A.; Kasai, N.; Koike, T.; et al. A wide spectrum of collagen vascular and autoimmune diseases in transgenic rats carrying the env-pX gene of human T lymphocyte virus type, I. *Int. Immunol.* **1997**, *9*, 339–346. [CrossRef]
137. Yoshiki, T.; Ikeda, H.; Tomaru, U.; Ohya, O.; Kasai, T.; Yamashita, I.; Morita, K.; Yamazaki, H.; Ishizu, A.; Nakamaru, Y.; et al. Models of HTLV-I-induced diseases. Infectious transmission of HTLV-I in inbred rats and HTVL-I env-pX transgenic rats. *Leukemia* **1997**, *11* (Suppl. 3), 245–246.
138. Gavrieli, Y.; Sherman, Y.; Ben-Sasson, S.A. Identification of programmed cell death in situ via specific labeling of nuclear DNA fragmentation. *J. Cell Biol.* **1992**, *119*, 493–501. [CrossRef]
139. Itoh, N.; Yonehara, S.; Ishii, A.; Yonehara, M.; Mizushima, S.; Sameshima, M.; Hase, A.; Seto, Y.; Nagata, S. The polypeptide encoded by the cDNA for human cell surface antigen Fas can mediate apoptosis. *Cell* **1991**, *66*, 233–243. [CrossRef]
140. Suda, T.; Nagata, S. Purification and characterization of the Fas-ligand that induces apoptosis. *J. Exp. Med.* **1994**, *179*, 873–879. [CrossRef]
141. Nakamura, H.; Horai, Y.; Shimizu, T.; Kawakami, A. Modulation of apoptosis by cytotoxic mediators and cell-survival molecules in Sjögren's syndrome. *Int. J. Mol. Sci.* **2018**, *19*, 2369. [CrossRef] [PubMed]
142. Nakamura, H.; Kawakami, A.; Tominaga, M.; Migita, K.; Kawabe, Y.; Nakamura, T.; Eguchi, K. Expression of CD40/CD40 ligand and Bcl-2 family proteins in labial salivary glands of patients with Sjögren's syndrome. *Lab. Investig.* **1999**, *79*, 261–269.
143. Tsukahara, T.; Kannagi, M.; Ohashi, T.; Kato, H.; Arai, M.; Nunez, G.; Iwanaga, Y.; Yamamoto, N.; Ohtani, K.; Nakamura, M.; et al. Induction of Bcl-x(L) expression by human T-cell leukemia virus type 1 Tax through NF-kappaB in apoptosis-resistant T-cell transfectants with Tax. *J. Virol.* **1999**, *73*, 7981–7987. [CrossRef] [PubMed]
144. Kawakami, A.; Nakashima, T.; Sakai, H.; Urayama, S.; Yamasaki, S.; Hida, A.; Tsuboi, M.; Nakamura, H.; Ida, H.; Migita, K.; et al. Inhibition of caspase cascade by HTLV-I tax through induction of NF-kappaB nuclear translocation. *Blood* **1999**, *94*, 3847–3854. [CrossRef] [PubMed]
145. Nakamura, H.; Kawakami, A.; Yamasaki, S.; Kawabe, Y.; Nakamura, T.; Eguchi, K. Expression of mitogen activated protein kinases in labial salivary glands of patients with Sjögren's syndrome. *Ann. Rheum. Dis.* **1999**, *58*, 382–385. [CrossRef]
146. Nakamura, H.; Kawakami, A.; Yamasaki, S.; Nakashima, T.; Kamachi, M.; Migita, K.; Kawabe, Y.; Nakamura, T.; Koji, T.; Hayashi, Y.; et al. Expression and function of X chromosome-linked inhibitor of apoptosis protein in Sjögren's syndrome. *Lab. Investig.* **2000**, *80*, 1421–1427. [CrossRef]
147. Bohnhorst, J.Ø.; Bjørgan, M.B.; Thoen, J.E.; Natvig, J.B.; Thompson, K.M. Bm1-Bm5 classification of peripheral blood B cells reveals circulating germinal center founder cells in healthy individuals and disturbance in the B cell subpopulations in patients with primary Sjögren's syndrome. *J. Immunol.* **2001**, *167*, 3610–3618. [CrossRef]
148. Legler, D.F.; Loetscher, M.; Roos, R.S.; Clark-Lewis, I.; Baggiolini, M.; Moser, B. B cell-attracting chemokine 1, a human CXC chemokine expressed in lymphoid tissues, selectively attracts B lymphocytes via BLR1/CXCR5. *J. Exp. Med.* **1998**, *187*, 655–660. [CrossRef]
149. Ghrenassia, E.; Martis, N.; Boyer, J.; Burel-Vandenbos, F.; Mekinian, A.; Coppo, P. The diffuse infiltrative lymphocytosis syndrome (DILS). A comprehensive review. *J. Autoimmun.* **2015**, *59*, 19–25. [CrossRef]
150. Nakamura, H.; Iwamoto, N.; Horai, Y.; Takagi, Y.; Ichinose, K.; Kawashiri, S.Y.; Taguchi, J.; Hayashi, T.; Nakamura, T.; Kawakami, A. A case of adult T-cell leukemia presenting primary Sjögren's syndrome-like symptoms. *Int. J. Rheum. Dis.* **2013**, *16*, 489–492. [CrossRef]

151. Shiboski, C.H.; Shiboski, S.C.; Seror, R.; Criswell, L.A.; Labetoulle, M.; Lietman, T.M.; Rasmussen, A.; Scofield, H.; Vitali, C.; Bowman, S.J.; et al. 2016 American College of Rheumatology/European League against Rheumatism Classification Criteria for Primary Sjögren's Syndrome: A consensus and data-driven methodology involving three international patient cohorts. *Arthritis Rheumatol.* **2017**, *69*, 35–45. [CrossRef] [PubMed]
152. Sato, Y.; Ito, K.; Moritoyo, T.; Fujino, Y.; Masuda, K.; Yamaguchi, K.; Mochizuki, M.; Izumo, S.; Osame, M.; Watanabe, T. Human T-cell lymphotropic virus type 1 can infect primary rat retinal glial cells and induce gene expression of inflammatory cytokines. *Curr. Eye Res* **1997**, *16*, 782–791. [CrossRef] [PubMed]
153. Sakai, M.; Eguchi, K.; Terada, K.; Nakashima, M.; Yamashita, I.; Ida, H.; Kawabe, Y.; Aoyagi, T.; Takino, H.; Nakamura, T. Infection of human synovial cells by human T cell lymphotropic virus type I. Proliferation and granulocyte/macrophage colony-stimulating factor production by synovial cells. *J. Clin. Investig.* **1993**, *92*, 1957–1966. [CrossRef] [PubMed]
154. Carvalho Barros, L.R.; Linhares-Lacerda, L.; Moreira-Ramos, K.; Ribeiro-Alves, M.; Machado Motta, M.C.; Bou-Habib, D.C.; Savino, W. HTLV-1-infected thymic epithelial cells convey the virus to CD4[+] T lymphocytes. *Immunobiology* **2017**, *222*, 1053–1063. [CrossRef] [PubMed]

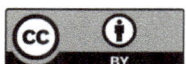

© 2020 by the authors. Licensee MDPI, Basel, Switzerland. This article is an open access article distributed under the terms and conditions of the Creative Commons Attribution (CC BY) license (http://creativecommons.org/licenses/by/4.0/).

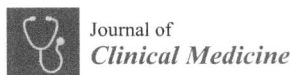

Review

Current State of Knowledge on Primary Sjögren's Syndrome, an Autoimmune Exocrinopathy

Dorian Parisis [1,2], Clara Chivasso [1], Jason Perret [1], Muhammad Shahnawaz Soyfoo [2] and Christine Delporte [1,*]

1. Laboratory of Pathophysiological and Nutritional Biochemistry, Université Libre de Bruxelles, 1070 Brussels, Belgium; dorian.parisis@ulb.be (D.P.); clara.chivasso@ulb.ac.be (C.C.); jason.perret@ulb.be (J.P.)
2. Department of Rheumatology, Erasme Hospital, Université Libre de Bruxelles, 1070 Brussels, Belgium; msoyfoo@ulb.ac.be
* Correspondence: christine.delporte@ulb.be; Tel.: +32-2-555-6210

Received: 25 June 2020; Accepted: 16 July 2020; Published: 20 July 2020

Abstract: Primary Sjögren's syndrome (pSS) is a chronic systemic autoimmune rheumatic disease characterized by lymphoplasmacytic infiltration of the salivary and lacrimal glands, whereby sicca syndrome and/or systemic manifestations are the clinical hallmarks, associated with a particular autoantibody profile. pSS is the most frequent connective tissue disease after rheumatoid arthritis, affecting 0.3–3% of the population. Women are more prone to develop pSS than men, with a sex ratio of 9:1. Considered in the past as innocent collateral passive victims of autoimmunity, the epithelial cells of the salivary glands are now known to play an active role in the pathogenesis of the disease. The aetiology of the "autoimmune epithelitis" still remains unknown, but certainly involves genetic, environmental and hormonal factors. Later during the disease evolution, the subsequent chronic activation of B cells can lead to the development of systemic manifestations or non-Hodgkin's lymphoma. The aim of the present comprehensive review is to provide the current state of knowledge on pSS. The review addresses the clinical manifestations and complications of the disease, the diagnostic workup, the pathogenic mechanisms and the therapeutic approaches.

Keywords: Sjögren's syndrome; autoimmune disease; physiopathology; treatment; diagnosis; review

1. Introduction

Sjögren's syndrome (SS) is a chronic systemic rheumatic disease characterized by lymphoplasmacytic infiltration of the exocrine glands—especially salivary and lachrymal glands—responsible for sicca syndrome and systemic manifestations. The dreaded complication of this dysregulated and unabated lymphocytic activation is the development of lymphoma. SS can be "primary" if it occurs alone (pSS) or "secondary" (sSS) when it is associated with another autoimmune disease [1].

First medical descriptions of SS date back to 1882 when the German Theodor Karl Gustav von Leber (1840–1917) described for the first time a dry inflammation of the ocular surface under the name of *"keratitis filamentosa"*. Ten years later, the Polish surgeon Jan Mikulicz-Radecki described the case of a man with swelling of the salivary and lacrimal glands, a clinical picture still called Mikulicz syndrome today. At the same time, several cases of patients with ocular and oral dryness were described, whether or not associated with the existence of rheumatism or gout. Dr. W. B. Hadden (1856–1893) described the improvement of xerostomia in one of these patients with the use of an alkaloid called pilocarpine [2]. Despite the involvement of these physicians in the first medical descriptions of SS, only two famous names have remained attached to the disease: Gougerot and Sjögren. Henri Gougerot (1881–1955) was a French dermatologist who described in 1925 three clinical cases characterized by generalized mucous dryness (eyes, mouth, nose, trachea and vagina) associated with atrophy of the salivary glands (SG). He was the first to describe that xerostomia and ocular dryness are part of a larger sicca syndrome resulting from dysfunction of the exocrine glands or their autonomic innervation. In France, the term "Gougerot(-Sjögren) syndrome" is often used to describe pSS. Henrik Samuel Conrad Sjögren (1899–1986) was a Swedish ophthalmologist who was mainly interested in the dryness of the ocular surface. With his wife, Maria Hellgren, daughter of a well-known oculist, he described keratoconjunctivitis sicca (KCS)—distinct from vitamin A deficiency xerophthalmia—using Rose Bengal and methylene blue staining techniques. In 1933, in his PhD thesis, he described the cases of 19 women with KCS and 13 of whom had arthritis. He was therefore, the first to link KCS to a systemic disease beyond the field of ophthalmology. Unfortunately, his thesis was not successful, and he stopped his academic career but not his medical and scientific one. It was only in the years 1935–1943 that Sjögren's work was recognized and that the term "Sjögren's syndrome" has been used since. Finally, the autoimmune origin was recognized only in early 1960s [2]. Sjögren was awarded the title of "Doctor" in 1957 by the University of Gothenburg and the honorary title of "Professor" in 1961 by the Swedish Government. Henrik Sjögren died of pneumonia on 17 September 1986, several years after a disabling stroke [3–5].

2. Epidemiology

2.1. Prevalence

pSS affects 0.1% to 4.8% of the population with a female to male ratio of 9:1, depending on the cohort studied, classification criteria and methodology used [6,7]. Although pSS is considered a common disorder, its prevalence seems to be overestimated in some studies. Overall, 0.5–1% seems to be a commonly accepted estimate of the prevalence of pSS in the general population [7]. However according to a more recent meta-analysis of 7 studies, prevalence rate is 0.043% with a sex ratio of 10.72. The prevalence of pSS in Europe is higher than in Asia, 0.7122% and 0.045%. Sex ratio does not differ according to the geographic/ethnic origin of the populations studied [8].

2.2. Incidence

There is an overt heterogeneity of SS incidence among several studies. A meta-analysis reported an incidence rate of 6.92 per 100,000 person–years, with an overall average age of 56.2 years at diagnosis and an incidence rate ratio between women and men estimated at 9.29. Six Asian studies reported a relatively higher incidence ratio around 6 per 100,000 person–years. Both Slovenian and American studies reported an incidence ratio of 3.9 per 100,000 person–years. Finally, a Greek study estimated an incidence ratio between the two at 5.3 per 100,000 person–years. Data regarding the incidence of pSS in Africa, Oceania and South America are lacking [8].

3. Physiopathology of Sjögren's Syndrome

SS is considered as a multifactorial process originating from the interaction between genetic factors and exogenous and endogenous agents able to trigger an abnormal autoimmune response mediated in particular by T and B lymphocytes [9]. The inflammation sustains, perpetuates and amplifies tissue damage and leads to a progressive functional impairment of the affected organs and a chronic inflammatory environment. Three recurrent events are generally associated with SS: (1) a trigger phase induced by environmental factors under specific epigenetic factors, genetic predisposition and hormonal regulation; (2) the dysregulation of normal salivary gland epithelial cell (SGEC) function; (3) a chronic inflammation characterized by SG infiltration made of lymphocytic cells, lymphocytes B hyperactivity and autoantibodies production [10] (Figure 1).

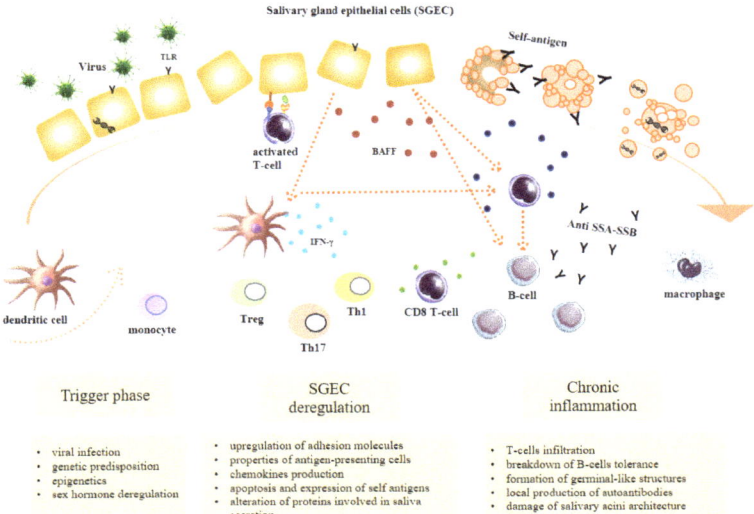

Figure 1. Overview of physiopathological mechanism underlying Sjögren's syndrome (SS). Environmental triggers, such as viral infections, genetic predispositions, epigenetics and sex hormone deregulation, cause the disruption of salivary gland epithelial cell (SGEC), the production of type I interferon (IFN) and other cytokines such as B cell Activating Factor of the tumour necrosis factor (TNF) Family (BAFF) [11] and the alteration of proteins involved in saliva secretion. Dendritic cells, as well as SGEC acquire the characteristics of antigen-presenting cells capable of processing viral and self-antigens, leading to the activation of autoreactive T and B cells. Autoreactive T cells induce tissue damage through the release of cytotoxic granules and cause the exposure of autoantigens on the surface of SGEC. In addition, activated B cells produce autoantibodies that induce SGEC apoptosis and create an inflammatory microenvironment. This complex mechanism triggers a self-perpetuating cycle of autoimmunity.

3.1. Trigger Phase

In SS pathogenesis, a trigger phase is induced by environmental factors such as viral infections combined with genetic predisposition, epigenetic factors and sex hormonal regulation (Figure 2).

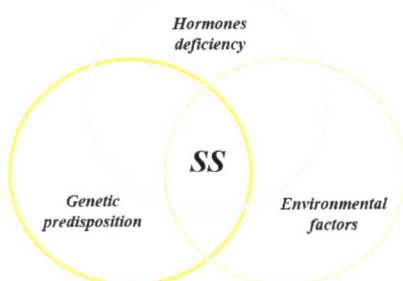

Figure 2. Factors involved in SS trigger phase.

3.1.1. Environmental Factors

According to the current physiopathogenic model of SS, environmental factors including viral infection lead to SGEC and Toll Like Receptors (TLRs) activation [12,13]. Primary viruses involved in SS induction include Epstein–Barr (EBV) viruses, Human T-lymphotropic virus type I (HTLVI), hepatitis virus C (HCV) and coxsackievirus [13].

EBV is a double stranded DNA virus appertaining to Herpesviridae family, with a strong tropism for B cells. EBV has often been associated with autoimmunity processes and diseases such as Rheumatoid Arthritis (RA), Systemic Lupus Erythematosus (SLE) and Multiple Sclerosis (MS) [14,15]. In addition, the high EBV load found in SG and lacrimal gland biopsies from SS patients as compared to controls [16,17] suggests its role in triggering the activation of the immune system. EBV is able to stimulate the production of proteins that mimic B cell receptor (BCR) and CD40 signalling and induce a strong B cell hyperactivity [18]. Recently, a correlation was established between past EBV infection and the presence of anti-Ro/SSA and anti-La/SSB autoantibodies in SS patients [19]. The RNA encoded by EBV binds TLR3 and induces the secretion of type I IFN and proinflammatory cytokines [20]. Another protein, the latent membrane protein 1 (LMP1) acting as a target for the EBV-induced cytotoxic T lymphocytes response may cause acini atrophy and SG lobule structure destruction observed in SS patients [21].

HTLV-1, a human endemic retrovirus in certain geographical areas such as Japan, has been reported to be present in SGEC [22]. In addition, epidemiologic studies revealed anti-HTLV-1 seropositivity in 23% of SS patients as compared to 3% in controls [23].

Coxsackie virus is a single stranded RNA virus belonging to the Picornaviridae family. A study has identified in SS patients a cross-reactivity between antibodies to the Ro60 epitope and 2B Coxsackie protein sharing 87% sequence homology [24]. However, these data remain controversial [25].

The role of HCV, a single stranded RNA small virus belonging to Flaviviridae family, has been examined in the initial triggering phase of SS. Clinical studies have shown that patients with HCV infection present sicca symptomatology, positive ocular tests, SG lymphocytic infiltration, and autoantibodies [26]. Therefore, HCV-associated SS (patients with HCV fulfilling SS 2002 classification criteria) is indistinguishable from pSS. On this basis, HCV chronic infection should be considered as an exclusion criterion for pSS as HCV infection could participate to SS development in a subset of patients.

Despite possible involvement of viral infection in SS, the most common antiviral drugs do not seem to show real benefit in the treatment of SS [26]. Indeed, as a viral infection may likely trigger onset of the disease, later antiviral treatment may manage a persistent infection but have no effect on the ongoing disease that may no longer be dependent on the presence of the initial viral infection.

3.1.2. Genetic Predisposition

Genetic predisposition to SS plays a role in the trigger phase of the disease. A strong association between human leucocyte antigen (HLA)-DR and HLA-DQ alleles belonging to the group of major histocompatibility genes (MHC) class II genes and SS was observed throughout different populations including Caucasian, Japanese and Chinese populations [27]. All discovered haplotypes are in strong linkage disequilibrium, causing difficulties in establishing which of them contain the locus that confers the risk. SS patients with HLA-DQ1/HLA-DQ2 alleles display more severe autoimmune disease than patients with any other allelic combination at HLA-DQ [28]. In addition to the HLA system, most recent studies have focused their attention on polymorphic genes that code for molecules physiologically involved in apoptosis such as Fas and Fas ligand (FasL). Using MRL/lpr-murine model, a retrotransposon inserted in Fas gene was identified as playing a role in cell apoptosis and induction of progressive sialadenitis [29,30]. Fas/FasL gene polymorphisms have also been found in SS patients [31] but have not clearly been identified as disease-determining factors. Ro52 gene encoding the 52-kd Ro autoantigen display single nucleotide polymorphism (SNP) located 13bp upstream of exon 4 identified as significantly associated with the presence of anti-Ro 52kD autoantibodies in SS patients [32]. Numerous additional genes including IL-10 [33], TNF alpha [34], alpha chain of the IL-4 receptor [35], IRF5, STAT4 [36] and CXCL13 [37] also display a gene polymorphism possibly associated with SS as well. Recent studies carried out in several SS cohorts of different ethnicity have revealed additional candidate genes probably associated with the risk to develop the lymphoma in SS patients.

The presence of a polymorphism in the tumour necrosis factor alpha induced protein 3 (TNFAIP3) gene is associated with the risk to develop the non-Hodkin's lymphoma in a SS Caucasian cohort [38–40]. In addition, two polymorphisms of methylene-tetrapholate reductase (MTHFR) gene are considered risk factors for lymphoma in SS patients [41]. While gene polymorphism plays an indisputable role in the triggering phase of SS, the individual contribution of each genetic factor remains to be assessed [42].

3.1.3. Epigenetic Factors

Several studies have analysed the contribution of epigenetics to SS and auto-antibodies production [43]. The epigenetic processes more closely linked to the disease are DNA methylation, miRNA, circular mRNA and long non-coding RNA function.

DNA methylation is a mechanism that consists in the addition of a methyl group from a methyl donor S-adenosylmethionine (SAM) to cytosine residues in the context of the CpG dinucleotide catalysed by DNA methyltransferases (DNMTs). In general, the addition of a methyl group onto DNA is associated with gene silencing due to a structural modification of chromatin. DNA methylation is one of most important mechanisms used by different type of cells to change their genetic expression such as the transition from naïve steady to effector B- and T-cells. An epigenome-wide analysis has identified several genes and epigenetic modification probably associated with SS [44]. The most frequent modification observed is the demethylation of several sites in SS patients' genome. Labial SG DNA methylation is significantly reduced in SS patients as compared to the control subjects. This defect was conserved when the SGEC were primarily cultured. Apparently, the SGEC from SS patients were associated with a 7-fold decrease in DNMT1 and a 2-fold increase in demethylating partner Gadd45-alpha expression. This demethylation process was also associated in part with the infiltration of SG by B cells and the pathology severity [45]. Different studies have also reported a link between demethylating drugs and SS. In fact, mice receiving an oral administration of hydralazine or isoniazid (demethylating agents) for several weeks develop a pathology similar to SS in terms of immunological features and autoantibodies production. The signs of SS pathology disappeared after discontinuation of the drug [46]. A recent study conducted in CD19 + B cells and minor SG of SS patients has also identified a hypomethylation site on interferon (IFN)-regulated genes which induces an increase of IFN response activation normally observed in SS disease [47]. In addition, DNA demethylation of the pro-apoptotic death associated protein kinase (DAP-kinase) gene [48] and the runt-related transcription factor (RUNX1) gene in CD4 + T cells [49] have been associated with non-Hodgkin B cell lymphoma predisposition in SS. In conclusion, the genome methylation analysis represents a useful tool to identify links between epigenetic modifications in various cell types related to SS.

miRNAs are small endogenous non-coding RNAs that regulate gene-expression transcriptionally and post-transcriptionally. Interestingly, miR-17-92 cluster, is downregulated [50] and associated with a lymphoproliferative disease and autoimmunity [51,52] in SG of SS patients. Another study has shown increased levels of miR-146a that regulates the inflammatory response, inducing the repression of IRAK1 and the increase of TRAF6 expression which, in turn, promote NF-κB expression in the peripheral mononuclear cells of SS patients [53]. Aberrations in microRNA expression are often observed in various autoimmune diseases and for this reason they could be used as a potential diagnostic or prognostic biomarkers. Furthermore, the small size of mature miRNA offers a high level of stability that renders them useful in disease follow-up using paraffin embedded samples stored for long periods of time [54,55].

Circular RNA (circRNA) consist in a class of RNA generated after an alternative splicing process of pre-mRNA named "backsplicing", in which a downstream 5' donor links an upstream 3' acceptor throughout a 3' → 5' phosphodiester bond. circRNAs are divided in three subgroups: exonic circRNAs (ecircRNAs), intronic circRNAs (ciRNAs) and exon-intron circRNAs (EIciRNAs) [56]. Recent studies have observed that circRNA could be involved in development of autoimmune diseases such as RA, MS, SLE and SS [57]. A microarray analysis has identified 234 differentially expressed circRNAs between SS patients and healthy controls, whereby 2 are significantly upregulated and 3 downregulated in SS.

Functional analysis has also shown that these circRNAs are related to arthritis and the presence of autoantibodies [58]. All this data taken into account, we can conclude that circRNAs could be used as biomarkers for a potentially valuable diagnostic tool for SS disease, but supplementary investigations assessing which of them is the most specific of pathology are necessary.

Long non-coding RNAs (lncRNA) are a novel class of functional non-translated RNAs with a length of over 200 nucleotides. Several studies revealed a strong link between lncRNAs and the immune responses [59]. The expression analysis of lncRNAs in SS patients has shown lncRNAs LINC00657, LINC00511 and CTD-2020K17.1 potentially associated with the disease. These 3 lncRNAs target different genes involved in B cell physiology and malignancy, including IL15, WDR5, GNAI2, LTßR, CBX8, BAK1, BAX ext [60]. IL15 and WDR5 play an important role in B cell proliferation and differentiation; GNAI2 regulates B cell trafficking to the lymph nodes [61]; LTßR and CBX8 are involved in GC formation in inflamed tissues [62,63], and BAK1 and BAX are overexpressed in B cell lymphoma [64]. These results illustrate an important role of lncRNAs in multiple processes and the understanding of their modulation and function could provide deeper insight into the pathogenesis of SS and facilitate the identification of novel therapeutic strategies.

3.1.4. Sex Hormones Deregulation and X-Chromosome Linked Factors

Nine out of ten SS patients are women and generally during menopause [65]. The strong predisposition of women to develop SS clearly demonstrates the role of sex hormones as a risk factor of the disease. In a recent case-control study, pSS in women was associated with lower oestrogen exposure and lower cumulative menstrual cycling time compared to sicca controls. Conversely, an increasing oestrogen exposure was negatively associated with development of pSS [66]. Finally, an effect of X chromosome per se is also evoked since men with Klinefelter's syndrome have a higher risk of developing pSS—20 times higher—compared to healthy men, despite normal sex hormone levels [67,68]. Similarly, the association between pSS and mixed connective tissue disease has been reported in a 16-year-old Japanese patient with trisomy X [69].

Androgens suppress the inflammation and enhance the function of lacrimal glands in female SS mouse models (MRL/MpJ-Tnfrsf6lpr[MRL/lpr]) [70]. The androgens could help maintaining acini structure in healthy SG, while their reduction observed in SS patients could cause a decrease in integrin expression and probably a dysregulation of acini architecture [71]. SS patients present low levels of androgen hormones both in the bloodstream and in SG [72]. In Klinefelter's syndrome associated SS and SLE, correction of hypogonadism by testosterone therapy for 60 days leads to remission in one case-series report [73].

Healthy ovariectomized C57BL/6 mice display an exocrinopathy with autoimmune characteristics similar to SS including SG focal adenitis, lacrimal glands lesions, Ro/SSA, La/SSB and α-fodrin autoantibodies [74]. Similarly to ovariectomized mice, both mice rendered deficient in aromatase, an enzyme important in the biosynthesis of oestrogens, as well as mice that received an aromatase inhibitor develop a lymphoproliferative autoimmune disease resembling SS [75,76]. How oestrogen deficiency promotes autoimmune lesions remains unclear. However, one putative explanation could be that oestrogen deficiency stimulates SGEC to secrete IFN-α and IL-8, and to express MHC class II, enabling them to act as antigen-presenting cells. Oestrogen deficiency is responsible for RbAp48 overexpression, which induces p53-mediated apoptosis in exocrine glands [77]. In another study, transgenic mice overexpressing RbAp48 develop SS-like exocrinopathy characterized by an increased propensity to apoptosis and the acquisition of an active immunocompetent role by epithelial cells, producing IFN-γ and IL-18 [78]. In primary cultures of human SG cells, pre-treatment with 7β-estradiol impede IFNγ-induced upregulation of ICAM-1 in control group but not in pSS group. These data suggest a protective role of oestrogens on epithelial activation and the existence of a deficient estrogenic responsiveness in pSS [79]. Not surprisingly, the use of aromatase inhibitors in the treatment of breast cancer is associated with arthralgia or even authentic SS [80–82].

Humans and other primates, secrete large amount of sex steroid precursors, such as dehydroepiandrosterone (DHEA) and DHEA-sulphate precursors, metabolic intermediates in the biosynthesis of androgens and oestrogens. According to tissue needs, the prohormones are directly processed within tissues. DHEA is present in low concentrations in patients with SS as compared to age-matched healthy controls [83]. Several studies have shown that human MSG possess an organized intracrine machinery capable to convert DHEA(-sulphate) pro-hormone to its active metabolites, dihydrotestosterone (DHT) and 17β-oestradiol [84] (Figure 3). However, the non-functionality of this enzymatic machinery in MSG from SS patients could account for the diminished local concentrations of DHT and androgen-regulated biomarker Cysteine-Rich Secretory Protein 3 (CRISP-3) in SS patients [85].

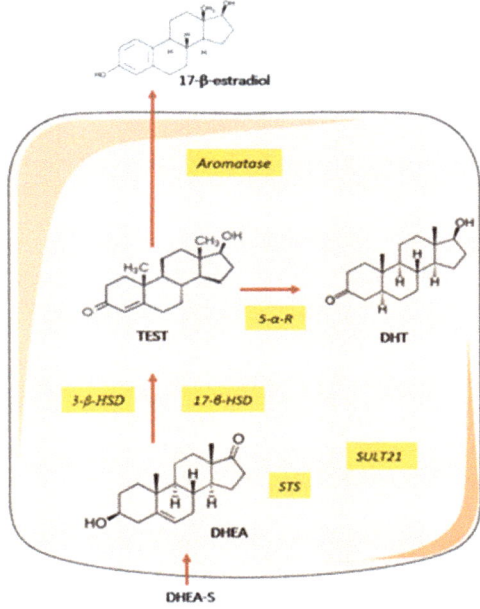

Figure 3. Intracrine steroidogenic machinery in healthy acinar cells. The figure shows the conversion of dehydroepiandrosterone (DHEA) to active sex steroids. STS: steroid sulphatase, SULT2B1: sulfotransferase 2B1, HSD: hydroxy steroid dehydrogenase, 5-α-R: 5α-reductase, TEST: testosterone, DHT: dihydrotestosterone. DHEA-S: DHEA-sulphate.

Taken together, these data suggest that women affected by SS at menopause, when the levels of testosterone produced by the ovaries has already declined, may be particularly vulnerable to androgen deficiency because the only source of DHT in SG is dependent on local conversion of DHEA. Whereas in men, the level of systemic androgens produces by gonads may satisfy the specific needs of SG, not requiring the intermediate metabolite.

3.2. SGEC Deregulation

3.2.1. Upregulation of Adhesion Molecules

According to recent observations, several SS pathogenic models could explain the role of SGEC in glandular damage. The current SS pathogenic model is the "autoimmune epithelitis". This model considers SGEC as a crucial player in the initial triggering phase of the disease [86]. SGEC from SS patients express significantly higher levels of TLRs mRNA levels, including TLR-1, TLR-2, TLR-3 and TLR-4 as compared to control SGEC [87]. Under physiological conditions, TLRs are activated by the recognition of pathogen-associated molecular patterns (PAMPs) derived from microorganisms and endogenous mediators of inflammation known as danger-associated molecular patterns (DAMPs) [88]. TLR signalling pathway acts as link between innate and adaptive immunity in autoimmune diseases. Indeed, upon activation, TLRs recruit adapter proteins in order to propagate the intracellular signal that results in the transcription of genes involved in inflammation, immune regulation, cell survival and proliferation and subsequent activation of the immune system. TLR signalling in SGEC upregulates several molecules such as MHC class I and class II, costimulatory molecules such as B7.1 (CD80) and B7.2 (CD86) and adhesion molecules 1 (ICAM-1) [89].

3.2.2. Antigen-Presenting Cell Properties

The expression of MHC class I, MHC class II, costimulatory molecules and adhesion molecules on SGECs empower them to present antigen to T cells (acting as non-professional antigen presenting cells).

3.2.3. Chemokines Production

The activation of Interferon Regulatory Factor (IRF) and nuclear factor kappa-light-chain-enhancer of activated B cells (NFkB) pathways increases the production of inflammatory cytokines, including type I IFN, tumour necrosis factor-α (TNF-α), interleukin(IL)-1, IL-6 and BAFF [90].

3.2.4. Apoptosis and Expression of Self-Antigens

In addition to chemokines production, the ribonucleoproteins, normally hidden from the immune system, are exposed on the cell surface. In particular, the expression of antigen Ro/SSA and La/SSB proteins on apoptotic SGEC promotes the initiation of autoimmunity.

3.2.5. Alteration of Proteins Involved in Saliva Secretion

Apoptosis of the acinar epithelial cells and altered expression and distribution of proteins involved in saliva secretion has been proposed as possible mechanisms responsible for the impairment of secretory function of SS SG. For example, an increase in AQP3 expression was observed at the apical membrane of acinar cell of SG from SS [91], while AQP1 [92] and AQP4 [93] expression was decreased in myoepithelial cells. Rituximab treatment, used in SS patients to deplete B cells, increases AQP1 protein expression in myoepithelial cell and induces an improvement of saliva flow [94]. These data could suggest a crucial role to AQP1 in saliva secretion. However, AQP1-null mice model has shown that this protein is not essential for saliva production [95]. Nevertheless, one cannot exclude a compensatory effect in such mouse models, whereby other AQPs could be alternatively used. In contrast, AQP5 is today considered the most important protein involved in saliva secretion [96]. Under physiological conditions, AQP5 translocates from the intracellular vesicular compartments to the apical membrane of SG acinar cells after activation of muscarinic and adrenergic receptors [97]. In SS patients and SS mice models, aberrant localization of AQP5 has been observed [98], which is predominately basolateral instead of apical [99–101]. The reason why the AQP5 localization is altered is still unknown but several hypotheses have been proposed.

The presence of autoantibodies against M3 receptor could impair its activation and block the translocation signal normally sent to AQP5 [102]. Another possible mechanism could be the alteration of protein–protein interactions between AQP5 and its partner proteins [103]. Prolactin inducible protein (PIP) is a known AQP5 protein partner in lacrimal glands in mice models. Aberrant binding of PIP to the c-terminal domain of AQP5 impairs AQP5 trafficking to the apical membrane of epithelial cells [104]. Lastly, the inflammatory environment that characterizes SS disease could also directly or indirectly be involved in these modifications [105,106]. IFN-γ for example, contributes to SS pathogenesis inducing SG apoptosis and expression of several chemoattractant cytokines and enhancing the antigen presenting function of epithelial cells [107–109]. IFN-γ administration leads to increased production of anti-M3R antibody, which affect the SG secretory function in response to an adequate stimulus [110]. Neutralization of IFN-γ in anti-programmed death ligand 1 (PDL1)-treated non-obese diabetic (NOD)/ShiLtJ mice improves AQP5 expression and saliva secretion [111]. TNF-α is another pro-inflammatory cytokine that is increased in SS [112]. Elevated TNF-α levels in both serum and SG has been observed in SS patients compared to controls [113]. In human SG acinar cells, TNF-α treatment down-regulates the expression of AQP5 [114]. The injection of antibodies against TNF-α in NOD mice reduces SG inflammatory foci and increases AQP5 protein expression [115]. It seems clear that correct expression, trafficking and localization of AQP5 are essential to overcome the impaired salivary secretion process and the combination of inflammation, antibodies production, protein–protein interaction and salivary epithelial cells deregulation are probably involved in the hypofunction of SG of SS patients.

3.3. Chronic Inflammation

3.3.1. T-Cell Infiltration

In the early stages of SS, the lymphocytic infiltrates, present in SG from SS patients, are constituted by a vast majority (>75%) of T lymphocytes being mostly CD4 T cells [116]. However, saliva from SS patients contains greater Th1 cytokines than saliva from controls [109,117], including IL-1β, IL-6, tumour necrosis factor (TNF)-α, and IFN-γ [118]. Th2-derived cytokines, such as IL-10 and IL-4, were also found in greater quantity in SG tissue from SS patients than in controls [119]. The two T cell responses are in a dynamic balance with a predominance of Th1 activity in patients suffering from SS [120]. In patients with SS, the activated T cells respond to an intense antigenic stimulus, such as the recognition of Ro and La autoantigens expressed on blebs of apoptotic cells [121], which induces a proliferative response [122]. Therefore, T-cell recognition of self-antigens and their subsequent activation are crucial for the cascade of events leading to the development of SS pathology. T cells may proliferate locally in SG or be re-directed by chemokines from the circulation to the glands. Two chemokines involved in the attraction of T-cells in SS SG are CXCL9 and CXCL10 [123]. In SS SG, T cells are likely to be involved in the disruption of the glandular architecture throughout the apoptosis mechanism mediated by FasL pathway [124], by a direct cytotoxic activity involving the release of perforin and/or secretion of cytokines and by the activation of B cells [125]. Th17 cells represent another subpopulation of T-cells strongly activated in SS patients [126]. In general, Th17 plays an important physiological role in mucosal defence in healthy individuals. In SS patients, the activated Th17 cells promote inflammation by secreting IL-6, IL-17, IL-21, IL-22 and IL-23 [127–129]. Follicular helper T cells have been shown to play an important role in lymphoid follicle formation and ectopic germinal centre formation in SS SG [130]. During pathology, SGEC induce activation and differentiation of T helper to T follicular helper by the release of IL6 and ICOS ligand expression. The activated follicular cells in turn secrete IL-21 cytokine which mediates B cell maturation and proliferation [131]. In conclusion, the combined activation of T-cell subtypes creates an optimal environment for detrimental B cell activation and the breakdown of tolerance.

3.3.2. Breakdown of B Cells Tolerance

Under physiological condition, B cells originate in the bone marrow from haematopoietic stem cells and during their development undergo several stages of selection because of a large portion of self-reactive and polyreactive B cell are normally generated [132]. The first checkpoint removes the polyreactive B cells in the bone marrow (central tolerance checkpoint), the second in the periphery ensures that only a small amount of self-reactive, and polyreactive mature naïve B cells survive. Finally, a third tolerance checkpoint called pre-germinal centre checkpoint, excludes self-reactive naïve B cells from entering B cell follicles [133].

A recent study has revealed the existence of deficiencies in both early and late B cell tolerance checkpoints in patients with SS. Indeed, the accumulation of circulating autoreactive naïve B cells in SS suggests an impairment of the autoreactive B cell clearance during the early peripheral tolerance checkpoints and an increased frequency of autoreactive unswitched and switched memory B cells reveals a possible impairment also in pre- and/or post-germinal centre tolerance checkpoints [134]. These observations have also been made in patients with SLE, RA and type 1 diabetes [135,136]. B cell depletion using anti-CD20 antibodies in Id3 knockout mice model leads to a significant histological improvement associated with a recovery of saliva secretory function and corroborate the hypothesis that B cells could play an important role in SS disease [137].

B cell hyperactivity is an important hallmark of SS. Two cytokines have been shown to be fundamental in B cell survival and proliferation: B cell Activating Factor of the TNF Family (BAFF) and APRIL (A proliferating ligand) [138]. Once SG tissue infiltration is established, a large number of cells such as dendritic cells, monocytes and macrophages but also SGEC and T lymphocytes can secrete BAFF. BAFF overexpression has indeed been documented in SS as well as in other systemic autoimmune diseases and has been correlated with autoantibodies [139].

3.3.3. Formation of Germinal-Like Structures

Germinal centres (GCs) were described for the first time by Walther Flemming in 1884 [140]. GCs are specific region in secondary lymphoid tissues such lymph nodes and spleen. GCs provide the environment for proliferation of mature B cells, differentiation and mutation of their immunoglobulin variable-region gene segments during a process called somatic hypermutation, which generates a diversity of clones. Following this process, the cells migrate from the dark zone to the lighter zone of the lymphoid tissues, where the affinity of immunoglobulins is tested on follicular dendritic cells (FDC) and follicular helper T cells (TFH) cells presenting the antigens. The non-selected cells undergo apoptosis while the selected cells are stimulated by T cells to undergo class switch recombination and differentiation into antibody-producing plasma cells or memory B cells [141,142]. SG from SS patients can contain similar GC structures made of T, B, and plasma cells, macrophages, and follicular dendritic cells [143]. Given the strong similarity of SG GC with the lymphoid organ GC, the SG GC observed in SS patients were defined as ectopic GC-like structures, also known as "tertiary lymphoid organs" [144]. Several studies have reported the association between GCs and the immunopathological features of SS [145]. Other important studies have observed a 6.5- to 15.6-fold increased risk to develop non-Hodgkin lymphomas in SS with an elevated presence of GCs [146,147].

3.3.4. Local Production of Autoantibodies

The most common and studied antibodies in SS patients are those directed against the autoantigens Ro/SSA and La/SSB [148]. Anti-Ro, Anti-La, anti-SSA and anti-SSB were originally described as four antibodies directed against antigens expressed by salivary and lacrimal glands tissues from SS patients. Later, anti-Ro and anti-La were shown to be the same antibodies as anti-SSA and anti-SSB, respectively [149,150].

Ro antigen is constituted of two distinct Ro proteins of 52 and 60 kDa, with the latter binding to small cytoplasmic RNAs known as hY RNAs. The Ro52 protein, also known as TRIM21, is frequently targeted by SS antibodies, which makes it a useful diagnostic marker, but its function and why it becomes a target protein in a lot of rheumatic diseases is not completely understood. Ro52 is a member of the tripartite motif (TRIM) protein family, and it plays an important role in the ubiquitination of proteins. Several targets have been suggested as substrate of Ro52 activity, including various members of the IFN-regulatory factor (IRF) transcription factor family. The most speculated hypothesis attributes to Ro52 a role of IFN negative regulator. Indeed, in a Ro52-null mouse, the lack of ubiquitination mediated by Ro52 leads to an aberrant expression of type I IFNs and proinflammatory cytokines, such as IL-6, IL-12, IL-23, and TNF-α [151]. La/SSB antigen is a 48 kDa phosphorylated protein located in the nucleus and the cytoplasm. La/SSB binds to many RNA molecules newly synthesized by RNA polymerase III [152]. These two antibodies are detected in 50% to 70% of primary SS patients, but the anti-La/SSB alone is observed in only 2% of patients [153,154].

In most cases, anti-Ro/SSA and anti-La/SSB are correlated with severe dysfunction of the exocrine glands, associated with parotid gland enlargement and large number of lymphocytic infiltrates in the MSG [155,156].

Other antibodies believed to be pathogenic in SS are anti-centromere antibodies (ACA), anti-citrullinated protein antibodies (ACPA), anti-carbonic anhydrase II antibodies, anti-aquaporin-5, anti-muscarinic receptor 3 (anti-M3R) and anti-fodrin antibodies. ACA are directed against six antigens associated with the centromere (complex of kinetochore proteins). The incidence of ACA antibody ranges from 3.7% to 4% [157,158]. ACPA are directed against fibrin and fibrinogen, vimentine and alpha-enolase (CEP-1). In general, ACPA antibodies are the marker most observed in rheumatoid arthritis but are usually present in low concentrations in pSS as well, in about 3–22% of cases [159]. Anti-carbonic anhydrase II antibodies have been detected in 12.5–20.8% of SS patients and also play a pathogenic role in renal tubular acidosis (RTA) [160,161]. In fact, immunization of mice with human carbonic anhydrase II resulted in autoimmune sialadenitis, production of anti-carbonic-anhydrase-II antibodies and urinary acidification defect [162,163]. Anti-AQP5 antibodies were observed to be associated with serologic and histopathological features of SS [164]. Anti-M3R antibodies are present in serum of up to 90% of subjects with SS [165]. Antibodies against alpha-fodrin are detected in serum samples from patients with primary or secondary SS, especially in patients with sicca symptoms. However, anti-alpha-fodrin antibodies do not represent a sensitive nor a specific serological marker of SS [166]. Other novel tissue-specific autoantibodies are currently under investigation: autoantibodies against salivary protein 1 (SP-1), parotid secretory protein (PSP) and carbonic anhydrase 6 have been described in pSS and non-pSS patients with chronic pain, which may help to understand and diagnose early pSS and pSS-associated widespread pain syndrome in the future [167]. Anti-cofilin-1, anti-alpha-enolase and anti-RGI2 antibodies are associated with pSS MALT lymphoma [168]. Other autoantibodies have also been described to be more frequently found in pSS patients and variously associated with the clinical and biological characteristics of the disease [168]. Table 1 summarizes the novel autoantibodies that have been detected in pSS patients.

Table 1. Rapid overview of original publications describing novel autoantibodies in pSS.

Autoantigen Targeted by Autoantibody	Number of Patients (N Total/Pooled)					Autoantibody Prevalence (% of Total)				Clinical Associations
	pSS	pSS MALT	Sicca	FM Sicca	Ctrl	pSS	pSS MALT	Sicca	FM Sicca	Ctrl	
Salivary protein 1 (SP1)	270	–	29	151	148	46.3	–	75.9	45.7	27	Early disease, low focus-score, SSA−/SSB− [169–173]
Carbonic anhydrase 6 (CA6)	13	–	–	151	23	53.8	–	–	7.3	4.3	Found in non-pSS dry eye and fibromyalgia with sicca syndrome [167,174,175]
Parotid secretory protein (PSP)	13	–	–	151	23	15.4	–	–	11.3	4.3	
Interferon-inducible protein-16	250	–	–	–	255	37.2	–	–	–	2.7	High focus-score and GC, hypery, ANA > 1:320 [176]
Mouse double minute 2 (MDM2)	100	–	–	–	74	21	–	–	–	5.4	⬇ disease duration, ESSDAI, ⬇ focus-score, anaemia, thrombocytopenia, SSB+ [177]
Nuclear autoantigen 14 kDa (NA-14)	204	–	–	–	144	12.7	–	–	–	0	⬇ IgA level, ANA < 1:320, ANA−, shorter disease duration [178,179]
Stathmin-4	72	–	–	–	128	15	–	–	–	5	Polyneuropathy, vasculitis [180]
Poly(U)-binding splicing factor 60 kDa	84	–	–	–	38	30	–	–	–	5.3	Asian or African descent, ANA+, RF+, hypery, SSA+, SSB+ [181]
NR2	66	–	–	–	99	20	–	–	–	7.6	⬇ memory function, ⬇ depression rate [182]
	50	–	–	–	–	12 *	–	–	–	–	⬇ hippocampal grey matter [183]
TRIM38	235	–	–	–	50	10	–	–	–	4	⬇ ocular stain scores, ⬇ Schirmer's test, focus-score ≥ 3, SSA+, RF+, hypery [184]
Saccharomyces cerevisiae	104	–	–	–	–	5	–	–	–	–	Triple Ro52+/Ro60+/La+, hypocomplementemia, cutaneous involvement [185]
Calponin-3	209	–	–	–	46	11	–	–	–	2.2	Peripheral neuropathy [186]
Ganglionic acetylcholine receptor	39	–	–	–	39	23	–	–	–	0	Autonomic neuropathy [187]
Aquaporin-4	109	–	–	–	–	10	–	–	–	–	NMOSD overlap [188]
Aquaporin-5	112	–	–	–	53	73	–	–	–	32	Low resting salivary flow [164]
Other aquaporins (1, 3, 8, 9)	34	–	–	–	–	38	–	–	–	–	⬇ ocular stain scores [189]
P-selectin	70	–	–	–	35	21	–	–	–	0	Low platelet count [190]
Carbamylated proteins	123	–	–	–	172	28.5	–	–	–	3.5	⬇ total IgG, IgM, RF+, β2-microglobulin, ⬇ focus-score and GC [191,192]
Moesin	50	–	–	–	50	42	–	–	–	4	[193]
Cofilin-1	50	20	–	–	50	76	80	–	–	18	Association with pSS lymphoma [194]
Alpha-enolase	50	20	–	–	50	82	90	–	–	26	IgA isotype of anti-Ro/SSA
Rho GDP-dissociation inhibitor 2	50	20	–	–	50	86	90	–	–	26	ACPA+ and high urine pH for anti-alpha-enolase [195]

* = antibody positivity in cerebrospinal fluid; Sicca = non-pSS Sicca syndrome; FM = fibromyalgia with non-pSS sicca syndrome similar to "Sicca Asthenia Polyalgia" syndrome; Ctrl = healthy controls; hypery = hypergammaglobulinemia; ANA = antinuclear antibodies; GC = germinal centre; SSA and SSB = anti-Ro/SSA (Ro52 and/or Ro60) and anti-La/SSB; ESSDAI = Eular Sjögren Syndrome Disease Activity Index; RF+ = rheumatoid factor positivity; NMOSD = Neuromyelitis Optica Spectrum Disorder; ACPA+ = anti-citrullinated protein antibodies positivity; ⬆ = increase(d)/higher; ⬇ = decrease(d)/lower; "−" = negativity.

3.3.5. Damage of Salivary Acini Architecture

One of the pathomorphological characteristics of SG from SS patients is the presence of focal infiltration made of lymphocytic cells. The focus infiltrate is defined as the "focus score" and "focus score = 1" is a group of 50 or more lymphocytes per 4 mm^2 of tissue [196]. SG infiltration is normally associated with destruction and fragmentation of the glandular tissue, acinar hyperplasia and replacement of acinar cells with fatty or fibrotic infiltrations [197]. These events lead to a deep modification and impaired function of the glandular tissue. An architectural disorganization of the epithelial cells has been described in the pSS: detachment of the basement membrane, alterations of the apical microvilli and disorganization of the tight junctions separating the apical and basolateral poles [198]. Several studies have shown that SS labial SG (LSG) display significant increase in proteolytic activity of matrix metalloproteinases (MMPs) and higher expression of MMP-3 and MMP-9 exclusively in acinar and ductal cells [199]. Some of the cytokines synthesized by the inflammatory cells, acinar and ductal cells of SS LSG can induce increased MMPs expression [108,200]. In turn, high MMPs expression triggers a high level of remodelling activity in the basal lamina that enhances the vulnerability of SGEC to direct contact with cytotoxic inflammatory cells [201]. The disorganisation of the basal lamina of acini and ducts of LSG from patients with SS is the most frequent modification observed that positively correlates with the number of inflammatory cells within the gland.

4. Clinical Manifestations

Although often reduced to its sicca syndrome due to its tropism for glandular tissue, pSS remains a systemic disease that can affect virtually all organs. These clinical manifestations can be due to various mechanisms: dryness secondary to exocrinopathy, autoimmune epithelitis with periepithelial lymphocytic infiltration of target organs, associated organ-specific autoimmunity with specific autoantibodies, systemic manifestations linked to the presence of immune complexes or cryoglobulinemia and clonal lymphocytic expansion. Three-quarters of pSS patients will have at least one extraglandular manifestation, ranging from mild inflammatory arthralgia to life-threatening manifestations. The clinical manifestations can occur at diagnosis or during follow-up, even after more than 10 years, which must justify careful monitoring of patients. In general, the manifestations due to lymphocytic infiltration around an epithelium of a target organ have a stable and indolent course (e.g., sicca syndrome, renal tubular acidosis, pulmonary involvement) while the autoimmune disorders linked to immune complexes or autoantibodies have a more unpredictable course, with flares and remissions.

4.1. General Manifestations

More than half of pSS patients report disabling fatigue and non-restful sleep [202], partly related to poor sleep quality due to dryness, night pain and an increased prevalence of obstructive sleep apnoea [203]. Low-grade fever is found in 6% to 41% of pSS patients [204], while periodic fever is found more anecdotally [204]. Weight loss and night sweats may also be due to the systemic activity of the disease, autonomic involvement or lymphoma development. B symptoms—the triad of fever, night sweating and weight loss classically described in lymphomas—are found only in 15% of low-grade lymphomas associated with pSS [205].

4.2. Ocular Manifestations

Dry eye is a classic manifestation of pSS, part of the sicca syndrome affecting more than 95% of pSS patients. Patients can report inability to tear, foreign-body sensation, conjunctival inflammation, eye fatigue and decreased visual acuity. Ocular dryness can be complicated by keratoconjunctivitis sicca, blepharitis, bacterial keratitis or corneal ulcer [206]. Uveitis, episcleritis and orbital pseudotumor are rare but possible systemic manifestations [207].

4.3. Stomatologic Manifestations

Lymphocytic infiltration of SG generates exocrinopathy with hyposialia responsible for soreness, adherence of food to the mucosa, dysphagia, difficulties in speaking or eating, dental caries, tooth loss, periodontal involvement, lip dryness and nonspecific ulcerations and aphthae [206,208]. Oral candidiasis and angular cheilitis are mycotic complications related to the loss of antimicrobial action of saliva [209]. Parenchymal involvement can be complicated by recurrent parotid enlargement of infectious, lithiasic, inflammatory or lymphomatous origin [210]. SG may be the site of bilateral multicystic parotid masses and lymphoma.

4.4. Musculoskeletal Manifestations

Joint inflammatory manifestations are, after sicca syndrome, the most frequent manifestations of pSS (50% of patients) [211]. Patients may have arthralgia with inflammatory characteristics (morning stiffness > 30 min) or less frequently true symmetric polysynovitis mimicking rheumatoid arthritis (RA). Joint involvement of the pSS is generally moderate (<5 affected joints) and preferentially affects the small joints of the hands and upper limbs [211,212]. Joint involvement is conventionally non-erosive—except in case of an overlap with RA—but can be deforming (Jaccoud arthropathy) [211]. More rarely, pSS can be responsible for myositis. Finally, widespread pain is frequent—nearly 50% of pSS patients—resembling primary fibromyalgia [213,214].

4.5. Neurological Manifestations

Neurological manifestations of pSS are relatively frequent (18–45% of patients) and affect both the central and peripheral (sensitivomotor and autonomic included) nervous systems, with a higher prevalence of peripheral manifestations [215].

The peripheral manifestations are polymorphic and can be differentiated according to electromyographic examinations in mixed polyneuropathy, axon sensory polyneuropathy, sensory ataxic neuronopathy, axon sensorimotor polyneuropathy, pure sensory neuronopathy, mononeuritis multiplex or rarely chronic demyelinating polyradiculoneuropathy. The mechanisms mentioned are mainly lymphocytic infiltration of the dorsal root ganglia (for sensory ganglioneuronopathy), vasculitic lesions of the vasa nervorum and/or the presence of axon-specific autoantibodies. The cranial nerves can also be involved, essentially the trigeminal nerve by involvement of the Gasser ganglion (associated or not with a more extensive ganglionopathy) and the facial nerve (uni- or bilateral paralysis). The other cranial nerves are affected anecdotally. Finally, damage to non-myelinated fibres can be responsible of autonomic neuropathy or small-fibre neuropathy.

In the central nervous system, pSS may be responsible for encephalic or spinal manifestations, with stroke-like or Multiple Sclerosis-like damage secondary to cerebral vasculitis. Some demyelinating manifestations combining myelitis and optic neuritis are part of an associated neuromyelitis optica spectrum disorder (NMOSD), a condition linked to the presence of anti-aquaporin 4 autoantibodies. Neuro-pSS can also manifest as a recurrent aseptic lymphocytic meningitis. Rarely, the association of upper and lower motor neuron diseases resulting in an amyotrophic lateral sclerosis-like syndrome has been described during pSS.

Finally, cognitive dysfunction ("brain frog"), restless leg syndrome and psychiatric abnormalities are classically linked to pSS, but it is not clear whether these manifestations are reactive or directly linked to the pathophysiology of the disease.

4.6. Pulmonary Manifestations

The prevalence of clinically significant lung disease in pSS is 9–20% although subclinical manifestations can be found in more than 50% of patients by CT-scan or bronchoalveolar lavage findings. pSS exocrinopathy also affects the lower airways causing coughing, tracheobronchitis sicca, bronchial hyperresponsiveness (mimicking late-onset asthma), cylindrical bronchiectasis and bronchiolitis (mainly follicular bronchiolitis). This involvement of the small airway epithelium is rarely responsible for an obstructive ventilatory syndrome (11–14%) but can be complicated by recurrent pulmonary infections or atelectasis [216,217].

Nonspecific interstitial pneumonia (NSIP) and usual interstitial pneumonia (UIP) are the most frequent interstitial lung diseases (ILD) patterns during pSS, corresponding to 45% and 16% of cases respectively. Lymphocytic interstitial pneumonitis (LIP) arrives in 3rd position (15% of ILD cases) and can be considered as a more specific benign diffuse lymphoproliferative disorder of pSS, probably starting from the follicular bronchiolitis. It must be differentiated from pulmonary lymphoma, which is found in 2% of pSS-ILD. Other patterns such as organizing pneumonitis are less frequent (11%) or even rare such as pulmonary amyloidosis, alveolar haemorrhage, Langerhans' histiocytosis, cavitary lung disease and/or combined pulmonary fibrosis and emphysema syndrome. However, presence of multifocal cysts on CT-scan should raise clinical suspicion for pSS-ILD [211,216,217].

Pleural involvement is rare. In fact, pSS manifests by pleurisy only in less than one percent of cases [207]. Shrinking lung syndrome occurs in extremely rare cases in pSS patients [218–223].

4.7. Dermatological Manifestations

Cutaneous involvement in pSS is relatively common and multiple manifestations are described such as xeroderma, eyelid dermatitis, annular erythema/subacute cutaneous lupus-like lesions and vascular purpura (caused by cutaneous vasculitis, urticarial vasculitis, cryoglobulinemia or hypergammaglobulinemic purpura of Waldenström) [211]. More rarely pSS can be responsible for cutaneous ulcer, livedo, erythema nodosum, panniculitis, amyloidosis or granuloma annulare [209].

4.8. Cardiovascular Manifestations

Raynaud phenomenon is the most frequent vascular manifestation, affecting 15% of patients [207]. Fortunately, cardiac manifestations such as pericarditis, pulmonary hypertension and cardiomyopathy are very rare, affecting <1% of pSS patients, respectively [207]. Cardiac rhythm disturbances have been described, secondary to ionic disorders, dysautonomia or direct impairment of the electrical conduction system of the heart [224,225].

4.9. Oeso-Gastrointestinal Manifestations

Dysphagia is a frequent complaint in pSS patients generally related to inadequate lubrication of the upper aerodigestive tract and food bolus resulting from hyposalivation. Oesophageal dysmobility is also mentioned in certain cases, explaining the lack of correlation between xerostomia and dysphagia [226,227]. Dyspepsia is frequent, occurring in 23% of pSS patients, and often linked to chronic atrophic gastritis where inflammatory infiltrates similar to those of the SG are found following tissue histological examination. Antibodies against parietal cells or intrinsic factor can be found, but pernicious anaemia remains rare [226]. Manifestations such as diffuse abdominal pain, diarrhoea or malabsorption can occur as part of a protein losing enteropathy or in case of overlap with Celiac disease [226,227]. Interestingly, pSS patients with Primary Biliary Cirrhosis overlap (PBC) are at higher risk of developing duodenal ulcers (85% of cases) [226]. The digestive tract can be the site of acute and serious complications in the context of cryoglobulinaemic vasculitis.

4.10. Pancreatic and Hepatobiliary Manifestations

The pancreas being an exocrine gland, it is not surprising to find cases of acute pancreatitis, chronic pancreatitis or pancreatic insufficiency in 0–7% of pSS patients. Moreover, 25% to 33% prevalence of chronic pancreatitis-like morphologic changes suggest that there are many asymptomatic cases [226]. Hepatomegaly is found in 10–20% of patients. Liver tests are disrupted in 10–50% of patients, usually mildly and with no particular clinical significance. pSS can be associated with Primary Biliary Cirrhosis (PBC)—another autoimmune epithelitis—or with autoimmune hepatitis (AH). Pseudolymphoma has been described to occur in liver like it may occur in salivary or lacrimal glands [226,227].

4.11. Uronephrologic Manifestations

Schematically, renal involvement linked to pSS can be divided into 3 groups: (1) tubulointerstitial nephritis linked to autoimmune epithelitis characterized by peritubular lymphocyte infiltration, (2) glomerulonephritis associated with immune complexes and (3) disorders linked to the presence of specific autoantibodies. According to different cohorts, about 5% of pSS patients have a renal involvement. However, this figure seems clearly underestimated if occult tubular involvement is systematically assessed [211,228].

Tubular involvement can be associated with dysfunction of any part of the renal tubule and can be responsible for polyuropolydypsic syndrome, low molecular weight proteinuria, aminoaciduria, euglycemic glycosuria, acidosis with normal anion gap, hypokalaemia that may be complicated by paralysis or disturbed heart rhythm, hypophosphoremia linked to increased phosphate excretion that may be complicated by osteomalacia, nephrocalcinosis or the formation of recurrent kidney stones [228,229]. More anecdotally, acquired Gitelman or Bartter syndrome has been described, possibly linked to the presence of specific autoantibodies targeting transporters (ie NaCl co-transporter in Gitelman syndrome) [228,230]. Glomerular disease occurs later in the history of the disease and most often corresponds to a mesangioproliferative glomerulonephritis (MPGN) caused by the deposition of immune complexes, usually cryoglobulinemia, which should be looked for [211,228].

Interstitial cystitis is a chronic inflammatory disease of the bladder that can be found in pSS patients. This rare manifestation is characterized by complaints such as pollakiuria, lower abdominal pain, urinary urgency, painful micturition, haematuria and dysuria [231]. Interstitial cystitis can be complicated by bilateral hydronephrosis and obstructive renal failure [231].

4.12. Haematological Manifestations

Anaemia is present in 20% of pSS cases, usually normochromic normocytic, of various mechanisms: anaemia of chronic disease or haemolytic, more rarely secondary to aplastic or pernicious anaemia or myelodysplastic syndrome [232,233]. Leukopenia is found in 15% of patients and most often corresponds to lymphocytopenia. Agranulocytosis is rare. Thrombocytopenia is found in 15% of patients, of peripheral origin, whether or not involved in Evans syndrome [232,233]. Rare cases of Thrombotic Thrombocytopenic Purpura (TTP) [234–236] and Hemophagocytic lymphohistiocytosis (HLH) [237] have been described.

Reactive multiple lymphadenopathy is possible, statistically associated with the presence of synovitis [212]. The intense stimulation of B cells explains the occurrence of hypergammaglobulinemia, hyperviscosity syndrome, monoclonal gammapathy, cryoglobulinemia and amyloidosis [232,238]. The formation of immune complexes leads to complement fraction consumption.

CD4-Lymphocytopenia is mainly found in anti-Ro-SSA positive patients and is associated with an increased risk of non-Hodgkin's lymphoma (NHL) [232]. NHL has a prevalence of 4.3% in pSS patients [205]. Schematically, pSS-associated NHL can be divided into two main categories: the first has an indolent course and is dominated by the extranodal marginal zone (MZ) B cell lymphomas of MALT-type, and the second corresponds to the high-grade lymphomas such as de novo or secondary diffuse large B cell lymphoma (DLBCL). In pSS patients, MALT lymphomas are indolent diseases characterized by a good performance status, small tumour burden and infrequent B symptoms. They are preferably located in one or more extranodal sites such as SG, stomach, nasopharynx, lung, liver, kidney, orbit and skin [205]. It is interesting to note that almost all of these sites are organs involved in autoimmune epithelitis. Locoregional nodal involvement can be observed while bone marrow infiltration is rare. DLBCL are aggressive and have a poor prognosis. A certain proportion of them probably come from a transformation from a low-grade lymphoma. NHL mainly occurs in pSS patients with cryoglobulinemia, palpable purpura and C4 fraction consumption [205].

4.13. Ear–Nose–Throat (ENT) Manifestations

ENT complaints are common (40–50%) in pSS patients but objective fibroscopic abnormalities are less frequent (20%) [239]. Exocrinopathy can generate rhinitis sicca—reported by about 40% of pSS patients—which is a source of discomfort, nasal crusting, sinusitis, epistaxis or smell and taste disorders [240]. pSS patients are more likely to develop laryngopharyngeal reflux (LPR) because oesophageal involvement impairs anti-reflux mechanisms. LPR—in addition to pharyngitis sicca—manifests itself through various ENT complaints such as dysphonia, throat pain, chronic throat clearing or Eustachian tube dysfunction [241].

As with other systemic vasculitides, pSS may be responsible for sensorineural hearing loss or chondritis [242], responding to corticosteroid treatments. In an appealing way, pSS is associated with a sensorineural hearing loss in a significant proportion of patients, mainly affecting high frequencies, but whose clinical impact is not obvious [243].

4.14. Gynaecological and Obstetrical Manifestations

pSS does not have a negative impact on fertility, but chronic pain and vaginal dryness can be the cause of dyspareunia having a negative impact on the sexuality of female patients [244]. During pregnancy, pSS can be responsible for two rare but classic manifestations: autoimmune congenital heart block and neonatal lupus [245–247]. These two manifestations are linked to the transplacental passage of anti-Ro/SSA autoantibodies. Congenital heart block occurs in 2% of anti-Ro/SSA positive pregnancies but with a 10 to 20% risk of recurrence in subsequent pregnancies. More rarely, neonatal lupus can be associated with endocardial fibroelastosis, valvular malformations or septal defects. Neonatal lupus—affecting one fifth of anti-Ro/SSA positive pregnancies—is characterized by an erythematous rash and photosensitivity that can be associated with hepatic, haematological and neurological involvement. Compared with healthy pregnancy, patients with pSS had significantly higher chance of pregnancy loss or neonatal death. However, there were no significant associations between pSS and premature birth, spontaneous or artificial abortion or stillbirth [248]. These data should be taken with caution because they are based on a limited number of heterogeneous—and not necessarily recent—studies.

5. Diagnosis Workup

5.1. Diagnosis Versus Classification Criteria

Faced with one or more compatible manifestations, the diagnosis of pSS must be evoked and investigated. Making a diagnosis is the basis of medical care. For the patient, it represents the end of questioning and diagnostic wandering. For the physician, the diagnosis makes it possible to clarify the management. Finally, for the researcher, the diagnosis makes it possible to create homogeneous groups around a consensus definition. Unfortunately, there is no single diagnostic test to confirm the diagnosis of pSS. Due to its protean and willingly insidious presentation, pSS is sometimes difficult to recognize and may delay diagnosis by more than 10 years. Sicca syndrome, fatigue and unspecific musculoskeletal pain can be wrongly taken for manifestations of age, anxio-depression or perimenopause in people with pSS. Systemic manifestations can sometimes precede sicca syndrome, resulting in an "occult pSS" [249]. For these various reasons, the gold standard for individual diagnosis of pSS remains the opinion of an expert clinician. To allow the study of the disease in groups of pSS patients, several consensuses have defined classification criteria allowing a common definition of what pSS is. The 3 most recent sets of classification criteria are presented in Table 2. By definition, classification criteria are specific but may lack sensitivity and should not be used blindly as diagnostic criteria but as a guide in clinical practice.

Table 2. Modern pSS Classification Criteria—comparisons of items, definitions and diagnosis performance compared to experts' opinions.

Domain	AECG Classification Criteria (2002) [250]		SICCA Classification Criteria (2012) [251]		ACR-EULAR Classification Criteria (2016) [252]	
	Item Definition	Value	Item Definition	Value	Item Definition	Value
Subjective eye dryness	≥1/3 specific questions	minor	/	–	/	–
Subjective oral dryness	≥1/3 specific questions	minor	/	–	/	–
Ocular signs	Schirmer (≤5 mm/5 min) OR Van Bijsterveld ≥ 4	minor	OSS ≥3	1	Schirmer (<5 mm/5 min) OSS ≥ 5 OR Van Bijsterveld ≥ 4	1 / 1
SG dysfunction	UWSF (≤1.5 mL/15 min) OR Compatible parotid sialography OR Anormal salivary scintigraphy	minor	/	–	UWSF (≤0.1 mL/min)	1
MSGB	Focus-score ≥ 1	Major	Focus-score ≥ 1	1	Focus-score ≥ 1	3
Auto antibodies	Anti-Ro/SSA or Anti-La/SSB	Major	Anti-Ro/SSA or Anti-La/SSB OR RF(+) with ANA(+) ≥1:320	1	Anti-Ro/SSA	3
pSS definition	4 out of 6 with ≥ 1 Major (or 3 out of 4 objectives findings)		pSS signs and/or symptoms with ≥2/3 criteria		Sicca or ESSDAI manifestation with a total score ≥ 4	
Exclusions criteria	- Past head and neck radiation - Hepatitis C infection - AIDS - Pre-existing lymphoma - Sarcoidosis - Graft-versus-host disease - Current use of anticholinergic drugs		- Past head and neck radiation - Hepatitis C infection - AIDS - Sarcoidosis - Graft-versus-host disease		- Past head and neck radiation - Hepatitis C infection - AIDS - Pre-existing lymphoma - Sarcoidosis - Graft-versus-host disease - Amyloidosis - IgG4-related disease - Current use of anticholinergic drugs	
Sensitivity	93.5%		92.5%		96%	
Specificity	94.0%		95.4%		95%	

AECG = American European Consensus Group, SICCA = Sjögren's International Collaborative Clinical Alliance, ACR-EULAR = American College of Rheumatology—European League Against Rheumatism, UWSF = unstimulated whole saliva flow, RF = rheumatoid factor, ANA = antinuclear antibodies, ESSDAI = EULAR Sjögren's syndrome disease activity index.

5.2. Sicca Syndrome and Glandular Assessment

The investigation for objective dysfunction of the salivary and lacrimal glands is useful for the diagnosis and symptomatic management of the patient. Anatomical or functional imaging can be used to assess changes in the major SG during pSS.

The evaluation of dry eyes requires a simple ophthalmological examination. The Schirmer test consists of positioning a small strip of filter paper inside the inferior fornix of each eye. The eyes are then closed for 5 min. After this time, the strips are removed, and the amount of tears absorbed by capillarity is measured in millimetres from the edge of the strip in contact with the ocular surface. Dryness is significant if ≤5 mm/5 min. The evaluation then continues with the evaluation of the stability of the tear film by the Break-up Time (BUT) and the search for conjunctival or corneal lesions linked to dryness (keratoconjunctivitis sicca). These various tests use the slit lamp and the ocular instillation of dyes. BUT is measured by placing a drop of fluorescein in each eye and measuring the time during which the coloured tear film uniformly covers the ocular surface, before the appearance of dry spots. A tear BUT test of less than 10 s (averaged over 3 testings') is considered pathological but is not specific of pSS manifestations. Finally, damage to the conjunctiva and cornea is highlighted by ocular surface staining techniques (fluorescein and lissamine green) [253]. The anomalies are scored using standardized scores: van Bijsterveld scale or the SICCA Ocular Staining Score (OSS). Respective cut-offs of ≥4 and ≥5 correspond to pathological situations suggestive of pSS. Those tests are more specific of pSS than Schirmer and Break-up time tests. Rose Bengal dye is no longer used because of its poor tolerance and local toxicity.

The evaluation of hyposalivation can be easily performed by sialometry. In its simplest form, sialometry consists of measuring the Unstimulated Whole Salivary Flow rate (UWSF) and the Stimulated Whole Salivary Flow rate (SWSF). UWSF is performed by asking the patient—fasted for minimum 2 h—to passively drain all the saliva produced in a tared jar for 15 min. The jar is then weighed and the saliva volume estimated. UWSF less than 0.1 mL/min is considered pathological (normal range 0.3–0.4 mL/min). UWSF represents a minor classification criterion. SWSF is measured in the presence of mechanical stimulation. SWSF can be measured using the Saxon test or Gum test protocols. Saxon test is performed by asking the patient to chew for 2 min a tared compress which will then be weighed. Gum test is performed as USWF, but in this case, the patient chews chewing gum and then spits saliva in a container. A diagnosis of hyposalivation is made if SWSF is ≤0.5–0.7 mL/min (normal range 1.5–2.0 mL/min). It is also possible to measure the salivary flow specific to each major SG by aspiration or cannulation. However, these techniques are of little use to the rheumatologist and especially uncomfortable for the patient.

Radiosialography is an X-ray imaging technique requiring the retrograde injection of a contrast solution into the excretory ducts of the major SG. This technique indirectly highlights glandular damage by studying changes in the "tree structure" of the excretory ducts [254]. Given the invasive nature and the complications of this technique, it has been abandoned in favour of other non-invasive techniques.

SG scintigraphy (SGS) studies the uptake, the concentration and the basal or stimulated secretion of a radioactive tracer by the parotid and submandibular glands following an infusion of Technethium-99 pertechnetate. SGS interpretation is mainly based on Schall's classification [255], a qualitative score classifying anomalies in 4 grades—from grade 1 (normal) to grade 4 (the total absence of uptake and mouth activity). With ≥3 as cut-off, sensitivity and specificity are 54–87% and 78–98%, respectively [256]. Salivary scintigraphy is one of the classification criteria of 2002 for pSS but has disappeared from the most recent classification criteria of 2016. An abnormal scintigraphy makes it possible to objectify a dysfunction of the SG but does not allow etiological diagnosis as no image is specific of pSS. However, it may be of interest for treatment: if the examination shows SG with normal uptake but with a major dysfunction of excretion (possibly due to an autonomic disorder), the patient could benefit from a sialagogue treatment. In case of a scintigraphy demonstrating no uptake of the tracer, the parenchyma is probably totally destroyed and a sialagogue treatment will be useless.

Ultrasound is a simple, non-invasive way to assess the parenchyma of parotid and submandibular glands for diagnostic and prognostic evidence for pSS. Mode-B ultrasound using a high frequency linear probe allows characterization of size, homogeneity, presence of hypo-/anechoic areas, hyperechoic bands and clearness of SG borders. These different items were included in several diagnostic scores [257]. The OMERACT group, in an attempt to standardize, developed in 2019 a semi-quantitative scoring (0–3) based on the presence of hypoechoic/anechoic zones within the parenchyma of the parotid and submandibular glands [258]. A score ≥ 2 is abnormal and suggestive of pSS. At present, SG ultrasound (SGUS) is not part of classification criteria but may well be in the future [259]. Unfortunately, correlations between histological abnormalities (lymphocytic infiltration, diseased parenchyma or ductal ectasia/cysts) and SGUS lesions have not been corroborated [254]. SGUS scores improvement after treatment with Rituximab prove that part of the abnormalities are correlated with the disease activity and not only damage accrual [260,261]. To date, there is currently insufficient evidence to use SGUS as a prognostic or treatment response factor. Thanks to its high spatial and contrast resolution, low cost and accessibility, SGUS has replaced MRI in the diagnosis of the pSS patient.

5.3. Labial Minor SG Biopsy

The minor SG biopsy (MSGB) is a simple procedure that can be performed with little equipment. Several biopsy techniques have been described in the literature [262,263]. After disinfection, the reappearance of small drops of saliva makes it possible to identify the accessory SG at the level of the lateral third of the lower lip. The mucosa above these glands is anesthetized with an injection of lidocaine. The mucosa is then opened with a scalpel over 5–10 mm and the glands removed with forceps. The individualization and extraction of the glands is made easier by the hydrodissection that occurs during local anaesthesia and by the eversion of the lip. Lobules are herniated towards the surface of the wound by the application of pressure—digital or instrumental—on the external part of the lip. For quality concerns, the removal of 4–6 glands—allowing the study of minimum 8 mm^2 of glands—is recommended [264]. A parotid biopsy is only exceptionally performed because technically more complex with a theoretical risk of damage to the facial nerve, for a diagnostic contribution identical to MSGB based on focus-score. On the other hand, the detection of lymphoepithelial lesions and early stage lymphomas—having a prognostic value—is more frequent/easier to detect on parotid biopsies [263].

The central element of MSGB pathology is the presence of clusters of more than 50 mononuclear cells (mainly lymphocytes) called foci. These foci in periductal or perivascular areas adjacent to normal acini are counted, reported to the area investigated and expressed as a Chisholm–Mason score [265] or a Focus-score [266]. Compared to the initial descriptions of those scores, some experts recommend counting all foci, including those associated with areas of fibrosis or atrophy, for fear of changing the Focus-score [264]. The Focus-score corresponds to the average number of foci per 4 mm^2 of gland. It goes from 0 to 12, 12 corresponding by convention to the coalescence of the foci. The Chisholm score ranks chronic sialadenitis from 0 to 4. Grade 0 corresponds in the absence of infiltration; grade 1 corresponds to a slight infiltration of mononuclear cells, however not forming a focus; grade 2 corresponds to the presence of an infiltrate of mononuclear cells organizing in foci but whose density is <1 focus per 4 mm^2; grades 3 and 4 correspond to the presence of 1 or > 1 focus per 4 mm^2, respectively. The presence of focal sialadenitis characterized by a Focus-score ≥ 1 (Chisholm grade ≥ 3) is a major diagnostic argument for pSS and is included in the different classification criteria. Due to its sensitivity and specificity >80% and its significant positive predictive value [267], the presence of a chronic focal sialadenitis (Focus-score ≥ 1) is particularly useful in the diagnosis of early pSS, even with specific manifestations and autoantibodies negativity [249].

Although not part of the classification criteria, other anomalies can be described: fibrosis, acinar atrophy, ectasia or metaplasia of the excretory ducts, histiocytic granulomas, presence of germinal centre-like structures, lymphoepithelial or myoepithelial sialadenitis (LESA/MESA) [268,269]. LESA/MESA are characterized by lymphocytic infiltration of ducts and basal cell hyperplasia, resulting in a multilayered epithelium. In addition, pathology allows differential diagnosis with sarcoidosis, IgG4-related disease, amyloidosis and lymphoma. Finally, MSGB provides information on the patient's prognosis: a Focus-score ≥3 and the presence of germinal centre-like structures or LESA/MESA are associated with more severe disease and an increased frequency of local and systemic manifestations, including lymphoma. For this reason, we recommend doing MSGB even if the diagnosis can be made based on anti-Ro/SSA positivity with objective sicca syndrome.

The parotid biopsy has fallen somewhat into disuse due to the ease of performing a minor SG biopsy with equivalent diagnostic performance. On the other hand, the possible discrepancies with MSGB [270,271], the possibility of early detection of lesions associated with a poor prognosis, the possibility of biopsying the same gland again to monitor the disease and the possibility of correlating it with SGUS semiology make parotid biopsy a tool that would need to be reassessed in the future [263].

5.4. Antinuclear Antibodies (ANA) Profile

The other major element in the diagnosis of pSS is the presence of anti-Ro/SSA and/or anti-La/SSB autoantibodies. The Ro/La system is a heterogeneous antigenic complex, composed by three different proteins (52kDa Ro, 60kDa Ro and La) and four small RNAs particles [272]. The search for antinuclear antibodies (ANA) by Immunofluorescence (IF) on HEp-2/HeLa cells is therefore an important element in the diagnosis of pSS. ANA is positive in 70% of pSS patients, usually with a fine speckled fluorescence [273]. Anti-Ro/SSA and/or anti-La/SSB autoantibodies are identified in 50–90% and 25–60% of patients, respectively [274]. It should be borne in mind that the Hep-2 cells do not sufficiently express Ro/SSA antigen, explaining the fact that 10% of patients anti-Ro/SSA-positive in ELISA have negative ANA in IF on HEp-2 cells [274]. Therefore, in case of suspicion of pSS, it is necessary to request the anti-Ro/SSA antibodies identification by ELISA, even in the presence of a negative ANA IF screening. Two types of anti-Ro/SSA autoantibodies can be differentiated: anti-Ro52 and anti-Ro60 [272]. Anti-Ro52/SSA have no specific ANA fluorescence staining pattern (might even exhibit a cytoplasmic pattern [274]), is precipitin negative and is not detected by ELISAs based on natural SSA/Ro. Ro52+ Ro60+ patients are likely to have pSS while Ro52+ Ro60- patients are not [275]. Isolated anti-Ro52/SSA positivity is statistically linked to primary myositis and systemic sclerosis. On the other hand, anti-Ro52/SSA and anti-La/SSB have the highest relative risks of congenital heart block in offspring from anti-Ro/SSA positive patients because these two antigens are expressed in foetal cardiac tissue from the 18th to 24th week [272]. Anti-La/SSB is mainly found in the presence of an anti-Ro/SSA, evoking a mechanism of epitope spreading. In only 2–3% of cases, pSS patients present with an isolated Anti-La/SSB antibody [276,277]. The presence of another ANA pattern or the identification of "atypical" ANAs can allow the identification of a secondary SS, an overlap with another systemic disease or a specific pSS subgroup [159]. The prognostic implication of these antibodies is discussed in the prognosis section.

5.5. Blood Workup

In addition to ANA testing, the initial blood workup for suspected autoimmune systemic disease includes a complete blood count; a coagulation profile with antiphospholipid panel; urea/creatinine dosage and urine sediment and 24-h urine protein or urine protein/creatinine levels; $Na^+/K^+/HCO_3^-/Cl^-$/Uric Acid levels to investigate renal tubulopathy; hepatic enzymes levels; creatine phosphokinase (CPK) to investigate myositis; C3/C4/CH50 levels, Rheumatoid Factor (RF), Cyclic Citrullinated Peptide (CCP) antibodies, Coombs test; serum protein electrophoresis and total IgG, IgM and IgA levels to investigate presence of polyclonal hypergammaglobulinemia and/or monoclonal gammapathy; HCV serology; VDRL/TPHA; free T4 levels, TSH, anti-thyroid peroxidase, anti-thyroglobulin, anti-mitochondrial, anti-smooth muscle, anti-gastric parietal cell antibodies in case of associated auto-immune diseases. Hypergammaglobulinemia and lymphopenia are classically described during pSS. Their presence may be an additional argument, but their diagnostic performance is not known.

5.6. Sjögren's Syndrome Differential Diagnosis

Classically all disorders manifested clinically by sicca symptoms, glandular enlargement and/or rheumatic/systemic manifestations fall under the differential diagnosis of pSS (Table 3). However, a rational and pragmatic approach often leads to the correct diagnosis [278].

5.7. Primary versus Secondary Sjögren's Syndrome

It is classic in medical nosology to describe the isolated and idiopathic form of a disorder as "primary" and to qualify as "secondary" the forms associated with specific causes or entities. SS is no exception. Historically, this dichotomy differentiated pSS patients from patients suffering from RA complicated by sicca syndrome. Subsequently, "secondary SS" (sSS) extended to other connective tissue diseases (e.g., SLE and Systemic Sclerosis (SScl)) and autoimmune diseases (e.g., primary biliary cirrhosis, thyroiditis and vasculitis) [279]. This nomenclature has also been indirectly "ratified" in AECG Classification Criteria from 2002 [250], classifying as "sSS" patients with another well-defined major connective tissue disease and at least one dry symptom (ocular or buccal) and 2 out of 3 signs of exocrine dysfunction (MSGB, SG signs or ocular signs in Table 2).

Table 3. Differential diagnosis of Sjögren's syndrome (non-exhaustive list).

	Sicca Symptoms Complex	Glandular Involvement	Articular Involvement	Systemic Involvement
Xerogenic medications	X	–	–	–
Aromatase inhibitors	(X)	–	X	(X) pSS-like
Age-related dryness	X	–	–	–
Metabolic sialadenosis	–	X	–	–
Non-SS dry eye diseases	X	–	–	–
Head and neck irradiation	X	–	–	–
Sarcoïdosis	X	X	X	X
Hyperlipoproteinemia (II, IV, V type)	X	X	(X)	–
Chronic Graft vs. Host disease	X	X	X	X
Primary lymphoma	X	X	–	(X)
Amyloïdosis	X	X	(X)	(X) Renal, purpura
Viral chronic sialadenitis (HCV, HIV, HTLV-1)	X	(X)	X	X
Other chronic Non-specific sialadenitis	X	X Usually unilateral	–	–
Diabetes Mellitus	X	(X) Sialadenosis	(X) Cheiroarthropathy	(X) Neuropathy
Haemochromatosis	X	(X)	X CPPD	(X)
Other connective tissue disease	X	–	X	X
Rheumatoid arthritis	(X)	–	X	(X)
Granulomatosis with polyangiitis	X	(X)	X	X
IgG4-related disease (Mikulicz syndrome)	X	X	(X)	(X)
Anxiety, fibromyalgia	X	–	(X)	–
Checkpoint inhibitors	X	(X)	X	X

In light of current data, this dichotomy seems obsolete and should be reviewed. While polyautoimmunity and overlap syndromes are currently recognized, one can wonder why SS is still considered a second-class disorder.

Based on the examination of salivary gland biopsies of 34 RA patients with sicca symptoms, two phenotypes can be differentiated [280]. One group of patients presented a phenotype characterized by mild salivary gland lesions and negative autoantibody. Histologically, minor SG biopsies display increased prevalence of antigen-presenting cells and CD8+ T cells, decreased presence of B cells, and "non-activated" epithelial cells (based on the expression of HLA-DR and co-stimulation proteins D80/B7.1). A second group of patients presented a phenotype characterized by glandular manifestations and/or auto-antibodies positivity. Their minor SG biopsies demonstrated CD80/B7.1 overexpression and low frequency of S100+ cells, correlated with the positivity of anti-Ro/SSA autoantibodies and/or focus score ≥ 1. Both groups had an historical RA-sSS and an RA-pSS overlap, respectively. In this study, compared to RA patients without sicca symptoms, RA-sicca patients statistically present more Raynaud's phenomenon, SG enlargement, palpable purpura and renal, lung and liver involvement. They displayed more frequent ANA, anti-Ro/SSA autoantibodies and RF positivity. The published data do not allow us to know if these manifestations are over-represented in the second group.

From a serohistological point of view, there is no difference in terms of anti-Ro/SSA positivity, anti-La/SSB positivity and SG infiltration between a pSS alone and an sSS associated with a SLE [281] or SScl [282]. It therefore seems more like an overlap than a so-called sSS. On the other hand, as for RA patients, SS overlap modifies the associated clinical phenotype. Compared with SLE-alone patients, patients with SLE-SS overlap are older and had a higher frequency of Raynaud's phenomenon, anti-Ro/SSA positivity, anti-La/SSB positivity and rheumatoid factor. They also had a significantly lower frequency of renal involvement, lymphadenopathy and thrombocytopenia [281]. Compared with SScl-alone patients, patients with SScl-SS overlap seem less at risk of serious complications from SScl namely lung fibrosis, pulmonary artery hypertension and scleroderma renal crisis [282].

To summarize, "secondary SS" is to be banned from our vocabulary [283] or—at a pinch—redefined very restrictively for some exocrine involvement occurring in rheumatoid arthritis not corresponding to a real SS, if such an entity exists. Moreover, "secondary SS" has disappeared from the classification criteria of 2012 and 2016. The patient has or does not have (p)SS, which may or not be associated with other autoimmune diseases, reflecting common etiopathogenic pathways. In this way, the clinician avoids three pitfalls: (1) minimizing the SS-related symptoms, which decrease the quality of life of the patients; (2) forgetting that overlap may change the clinical phenotype and (3) forgetting the risk of lymphoma. Unfortunately, pSS overlap syndromes had been under-recognized, under-researched and possibly under-treated in the past because of the historical label of "secondary SS" and their exclusions from the majority of clinical trials [284]. Their management is therefore based on the clinician's expertise, patient choices, best evidence and practice for the management of all associated diseases. To better individualize pSS in the future, it would be necessary to be able to move from a clinical definition to a molecular or even epigenetic signature.

6. Prognosis

Once the pSS diagnosis is made, treatment and medical decisions will be based on the expected course of the disease and its impact on the patient's life. This burden can be summarized in "5D": Death (mortality), Disease activity, Damage accrual, Discomfort (pain and sicca symptoms) and Disability. To assess the effect of therapeutic interventions on the natural history and functional repercussions of the disease, scores that can be used as clinical outcomes in trials have been developed.

6.1. Death

Although overall pSS mortality is low and similar to the general population [285], a subgroup of patients will have a poorer vital prognosis. The excess mortality observed in such subgroup of patients is generally attributed to the development of lymphoma or to uncommon but severe visceral involvement. The leading causes of mortality in pSS patients are cardiovascular events, followed by solid-organ and lymphoid malignancies and infections [285]. Risk factors associated with increased mortality are advanced age at diagnosis, male sex, parotid enlargement, abnormal parotid scintigraphy, extraglandular involvement, vasculitis, anti-SSB positivity, low C3 and C4 and cryoglobulinaemia [285].

pSS is associated with increased risks of overall cancer (pooled RR 1.17 to 1.88), non-Hodgkin lymphoma (NHL) (pooled RR 8.53 to 18.99) and thyroid cancer (pooled RR 1.14 to 4.03) [286,287]. Biomarkers associated with the development of lymphoma are mainly signs associated with exuberant B cell proliferation and immune-complex production [288–290]: parotid swelling, Focus-Score ≥3, germinal centre-like lesions, skin vasculitis or palpable purpura, complement consumption (Low C3, C4 or CH50), presence of cryoglobulinemia or monoclonal paraproteinemia, rheumatoid factor, increased β-2 microglobulin, lymphocytopenia, hypoglobulinemia, lymphadenopathy or splenomegaly and head and neck irradiation.

6.2. Disease Activity

Disease activity may be defined as the functional or structural changes in an organ related to inflammatory burden of the disease and are reversible under treatment. As in other inflammatory diseases, disease activity can fluctuate over time and progress between relapses and remissions. A significant proportion of pSS patients—nearly 50–70%—display a systemic manifestation at the time of glandular onset or within 6 months, mainly lymphadenopathy/splenomegaly, non-erosive arthritis and neurologic involvement [291]. The long-term study of the Antonius Nieuwegein Sjögren (ANS) cohort revealed that, within 10 years of diagnosis, 30.7% of the 140 patients included in this study developed an associated extraglandular or autoimmune manifestation such as polyneuropathy, interstitial lung disease, arthritis, discoid or subacute cutaneous lupus erythematosus (LE) and Hashimoto's disease [292]. The presence of cryoglobulinemia is associated with an increased risk of developing a systemic manifestation [211,292]. On the other hand, presenting widespread pain seems to be a "protective phenotype" [292].

Currently the European League Against Rheumatism (EULAR) SS disease activity index (ESSDAI) score has been used to quantify the inflammatory systemic activity of the disease. Within ESSDAI, clinical or biological manifestations are classified as "low" (1 point), "moderate" (2 points) or "high activity" (3 points) in 12 domains. To calculate the ESSDAI score, the value of the highest level of activity for each domain is multiplied by the domain weight (1 to 6) and then added together. The maximum theoretical ESSDAI score is 123. Minimal clinically important improvement was defined as an improvement of at least three points. More recently, ClinESSDAI score, a variant of the ESSDAI score without the biological domain, has also been used [293] (Table 4).

Table 4. Common damage, burden and activity scores for clinical monitoring of pSS patients.

	EULAR Sjögren's Syndrome Disease Activity Index	EULAR Sjögren's Syndrome Patient Reported Index	Sjögren's Syndrome Disease Damage Index	Sjögren's Syndrome Damage Index
Abbreviation	ESSDAI	ESSPRI	SSDDI	SSDI
First description	Seror et al. [294]	Seror et al. [295]	Vitali et al. [296]	Barry et al. [297]
Year	2010	2011	2007	2008
Type	Activity index	PRO	Damage index	Damage index
Domains (n)	12	1	6	9
Items (n)	44	3	9	27
Items scoring	0 to 3	VAS (0–10)	1, 2 or 5	1
Domain weight	1 to 6	1	1	1
Calculation	Sum	Mean	Sum	Sum
Score range	0–123	0–10	0–16	0–27
Clinically significant threshold	<5 Low ≥5, ≤13 moderate ≥14 high	≥5/10 is an unsatisfactory symptom state	-	-
Minimal clinically important difference	≥3 points improvement	≥1 point or ≥15% improvement	-	-

VAS = visual analogue scale, PRO = patient reported outcome.

However, it should be borne in mind that (clin) ESSDAI score does not investigate all of the possible events related to pSS. Out of 6331 patients included in the international register "The Big Data Sjögren Project Consortium" [207], 1641 patients (26%) had at least one non-ESSDAI systemic manifestation on a predefined list of 26 organ-specific features not currently included in the ESSDAI classification. Patients with non-ESSDAI manifestations are patients with higher systemic activity than patients without non-ESSDAI manifestations (mean ESSDAI 10.3 vs. 5.5, $p < 0.001$).

Patients with significant systemic activity are generally patients with early onset disease, antinuclear antibodies (ANA) positivity with a higher frequency of anti-Ro/SSA (with or without anti-La/SSB), low C3, low C4 and cryoglobulinemia [154,276,277,298]. Children of anti-Ro/SSA positive mothers are at risk of specific neonatal complications such as neonatal lupus and congenital heart block [277]. Paradoxically, patients with higher disease activity are less disabled by sicca syndrome or widespread pain [276,277]. Conversely, patients with late-onset seronegative disease will mainly present a more disabling sicca syndrome but fewer systemic manifestations linked to the activity of the disease [277]. Finally, isolated anti-La/SSB positivity occurs in only 3% of pSS patients and is associated with an intermediate phenotype between Ro/SSA positive- and seronegative patients [277]. Thus, systemic complications could appear many years after initial pSS diagnosis and justify long-term surveillance, especially in cryoglobulinemia or "high risk" phenotype patients.

The immunological profile of pSS highlights the presence of atypical ANA—12% of cases [299]—or other specific autoantibodies. A subset of pSS patients with anti-centromere positivity develops a clinical phenotype overlapping between SS and systemic sclerosis with a higher age, more frequent Raynaud's phenomenon and keratoconjonctivitis sicca and a lower proportion of anti-Ro/SSA and anti-La/SSB, rheumatoid factor, leukocytopenia and hypergammaglobulinemia [159,299]. In most cases, a minority of these patients appear to progress to an authentic systemic sclerosis. Anti-Cyclic Citrullinated Peptides (anti-CCP) positivity—present in 3–10% of patients—is associated with a greater frequency of joint manifestations or with overlap with rheumatoid arthritis (RA) [159,277]. The presence of anti-mitochondrial antibodies (1.7–13%) and anti-smooth muscle/anti-liver kidney microsomal antibodies (30–62%) is associated with overlap with primary biliary cirrhosis and autoimmune hepatitis [159].

6.3. Damage Accrual

Disease damage may be defined as the addition over time of irreversible functional or structural changes resulting from disease activity, iatrogenic treatments or co-morbidities.

Two scores exist to quantify damage related to pSS: SS Disease Damage Index (SSDDI) [296] and SS Damage Index (SSDI) [297]. SSDDI is composed of a list of 18 irreversible damages affecting 6 organ-domains (oral, ocular, neurologic, pleuropulmonary, renal and lymphoproliferative), divided into 9 items weighted for severity. SSDI is an unweighted checklist of 27 items divided into 3 lists: ocular damage, oral damage and systemic damage. Systemic damage is further subclassified into 7 areas: neurological, renal, pulmonary, cardiovascular, gastrointestinal, musculoskeletal and malignancy (Table 4).

In a retrospective study using 148 pSS patients attending the UCLH Sjögren's clinic followed for 10 years, Krylova et al. revealed that 28.3%, 36.7% and 45% of patients displayed SSDI damage (excluding oral damage that was not assessed in the study) after 1, 5 and 10 years of disease, respectively [300]. Items most involved are in the ocular domain, parotid swelling and malignancy. These results suggested that pSS patients accumulate less damage—calculated on different scores—over time than lupus patients, who have a greater inflammatory burden and use of immunosuppressive treatments [300].

Another retrospective study using 155 pSS patients showed that the total increase of patients with damage was 28% after 1 year, 44% after 3 years, 74% after 5 years and 83% at 10 years, with a good correlation between SSDDI and SSDI [301]. More specifically, teeth loss and/or caries, salivary flow impairment, corneal ulcers and tear flow impairment were reported in 49.5%, 34%, 22.6% and 11% of patients, respectively. Unsurprisingly, systemic damage—observed in 13.5% of patients—was correlated with basal ESSDAI, low C4 and lymphopenia. In the same way, persistent SG swelling—detected in 14% of patients—was associated with (bio)markers of systemic activity and B cell proliferation (lower age at diagnosis, anti-Ro/SSA positivity, cryoglobulinemia, low C4, hypergammaglobulinemia and lymphopenia). Lymphoproliferative disorders were detected in 4.5% and malignancy in 9% of cases at 10 years post-diagnosis [301].

6.4. Discomfort and Disability

SS can be disabling and associated with significant functional status impairment related to oral and/or ocular dryness, systemic activity, pain, fatigue and daytime somnolence, anxiety and depression symptoms [302–304]. Objective assessments of sicca syndrome correlated poorly with symptoms and remain generally stable over time [305]. Besides the associated symptoms, sicca syndrome also has a negative impact on smell, taste, pruritus, voice, swallowing and sexual function [306,307]. Fatigue and pain are both correlated with reduced quality of life and psychological distress [307]. Patients with widespread pain—34.9% of the cohort—were more frequently negative for anti-La/SSB, more frequently seronegative for all autoantibodies (ANA/SSA/SSB/RF) and had statistically fewer extraglandular manifestations in a Dutch study including 83 patients [308]. Another Italian study on 100 pSS patients demonstrated a prevalence of widespread pain of 22%, a phenotype statistically associated with fewer systemic and immunological manifestations (hypergammaglobulinemia, rheumatoid factor, focus-score ≥ 1) [309]. A subset of pSS patients therefore seem to develop a clinical phenotype with lower visceral involvement but with significant morbidity linked to glandular manifestations and a significant psychosomatic burden [302,310], bringing them closer to the notion of "Sicca Asthenia Polyalgia (SAP) Syndrome" [311–313]. At diagnosis, one in 4 patients is unable to work. This figure increases to more than 1 in 3 at 1 year. Work disability at 2 years is 40% and is related to fibromyalgia pattern, age and incapacity for work at diagnosis [314]. pSS has a high individual and societal cost, especially due to dental cost, symptomatic therapies and disease compensation [307].

EULAR SS Patient Reported Index (ESSPRI) is a consensus index calculated as the mean of 3 visual analogue scales (VAS)—self-assessment of dryness, (limb) pain and fatigue—allowing easy measurement of patients' symptoms in pSS [295]. By convention, patient-acceptable symptom state was defined by an ESSPRI <5/10 and the minimal clinically important improvement by a decrease of at least one point or 15%. The ESSPRI score is correlated with the Patient Global Assessment [PGA] [295] and with more complex and time-consuming scores such as the Profile of Fatigue and Discomfort [PROFAD] [295], Sicca Symptoms Inventory [SSI] [295], Health Assessment Questionnaire [HAQ] [315], Short Form 36 health survey [SF-36] [302], time trade-off values [TTO] and EuroQol5D VAS [316,317]. Very interestingly, a study using baseline data from 120 patients included in the TEARS study revealed that—even if there is a small correlation between ESSPRI and ESSDAI—ESSPRI is the only determinant associated with the quality of life score SF-36 in a multivariate model [318]. The ESSPRI score is therefore a good clinical screening and monitoring tool as well as a good surrogate endpoint to study the effectiveness of therapeutic interventions on pSS associated "Sicca Asthenia Polyalgia" Syndrome (Table 4).

It is therefore important, a fortiori in mild cases with low activity score but disabling sicca syndrome, to focus on improving the quality of life of patients through attentive and multimodal symptomatic management and to offer a multidisciplinary management program for the most disabled.

7. Therapeutic

Despite a better understanding of its pathophysiology, treatment of SS remains disappointing and essentially palliative. Systemic activity is treated by immunosuppressant drugs, based on scarce evidence. Manifestations linked to damage caused by local or systemic activity of pSS should be identified because they are by definition irreversible and cannot therefore be improved by immunosuppressive treatments. In the last 5 years, pSS management has been addressed by guidelines from EULAR [210], British Society of Rheumatology and National Institute for Health and Care Excellence (NICE) [319], Brazilian Society of Rheumatology [320], Research Team for Autoimmune Diseases [321] and Sjögren's Syndrome Foundation [322]. The main principles for care are summarized below.

7.1. Sicca Syndrome and Non-Visceral Manifestations

Despite the dysimmune origin of the disease, no immunosuppressive treatment has demonstrated sufficient efficacy associated with a satisfactory risk–benefit balance in the treatment of sicca syndrome and non-visceral aspecific manifestations (non-inflammatory widespread chronic pain, fatigue). Treatment is mainly focused on symptom management and prevention or treatment of complications resulting from exocrinopathy (Table 5).

Therapeutic approach to oral dryness must be driven by baseline objective and subjective severity of hyposialia and xerostomia. To this end, current guidelines recommend evaluating baseline SG function by measuring unstimulated (UWSF) and stimulated salivary flow (SWSF) or using salivary scintigraphy. Subjective xerostomia impact is captured by a simple Visual Analogue Scale, as part of the ESSPRI score. EULAR guidelines propose an algorithmic approach to the management of dry mouth: patients with an UWSF < 0.1 mL/min are categorized based on their SWSF as mild (>0.7 mL/min), moderate (0.1–0.7 mL/min) or severe dysfunction (<0.1 mL/min). Self-care advice and non-pharmacological stimulation are proposed to mild cases as first line therapy [210]. Pharmacological stimulation (pilocarpine per os or as a mouthwash, cevimeline per os) is the treatment of choice in moderate cases (with residual SG function) or in mild dysfunction patients who failed to respond to basic recommendations, in addition to first line therapy. Saliva substitutes are reserved for patients with no residual function or as a third line treatment in non-responding patients.

Table 5. Current treatment for sicca-related manifestations.

	Salivary Gland Involvement	Lachrymal Gland Involvement	Skin and Vaginal Mucosa Involvement
Self-Care	- Environment humidification - Elimination of offending drugs - Avoidance of caffeine, alcohol - Avoidance of tobacco - Excellent oral hygiene - Limit acidic and sugar intake - Limit eating between meals - Chew xylitol-containing gum	- Environment humidification - Elimination of offending drugs - Excellent ocular hygiene	
Conserve		- Scleral contact lenses	
Replace	- Salivary substitutes	- Artificial tears - Liposomal spray - Autologous serum drops	- Vaginal lubricants - Topical oestrogen
Stimulate	- Mechanical stimulants (gums) - Pilocarpine PO - Pilocarpine mouthwash - Cevimeline PO - Choleretic (anetholtrithione) - Mucolytic (NAC, bromhexine) - Electrostimulation	- Pilocarpine 5 mg q6h PO - Pilocarpine eye drops - Cevimeline 30 mg q8h - Lid hygiene with hot pad - Diquafosol eye drops (Japan) - Rebamipide eye drops (Japan)	- Pilocarpine 5 mg q6h PO - Cevimeline 30 mg q8h
Complications Prevention and Management	- Fluoride mouthwash - Chlorhexidine mouth bath In case of candida infection - Oral nystatin - Fluco-/Itraconazole In case of glands swelling - Exclude stone or infection - Massaging major glands	- NSAID or glucocorticoid drops - Calcineurin inhibitors drops - Lifitegrast eye drops - Botulinium toxin treatment - Corneal grafting - Doxycycline PO	

The stomatological complications of exocrinopathy affecting the SG are cavities formation, periodontal disease, candida infections and glandular swellings linked to abscess or to a lithiasic disease. It is therefore strongly recommended that patient adopts impeccable dental hygiene and be evaluated at least 2 times per year by a dental professional. Local fluoride-based treatments can be administrated. Candida simple infection (visible white plaques) are treated with Nystatin mouthwash for 7 days. One-week prophylactic treatment may be repeated every 8 weeks in the event of recurrence. Erythematous infection of tongue or oral cavity is treated with Fluconazole 50 mg for 10 days. Angular cheilitis is treated with Miconazole topically on each side of the mouth for 2 weeks. Presence of abscess or lithiasic involvement can be treated with antibiotic treatment and stomatologist involvement is indicated. If no infectious or mechanical cause is found in case of gland swelling, a distinction must be made between primary neoplasia, systemic activity of the disease (as scored in ESSDAI, treated by glucocorticoid in loco by sialendoscopy, per os or intra-muscular) and the appearance of a lymphomatous complication.

The management of dry eyes must also be guided by the objective and subjective severity of keratoconjunctivitis sicca (KCS), resulting from damage to corneal and conjunctival epithelium secondary to accelerated tear-film break-up and hyperosmolar tear composition. EULAR guidelines propose an algorithmic approach based on Ocular Staining Score (OSS) score and Ocular Surface Disease Index (OSDI) questionnaire to classify patients as non-severe or severe KCS [210]. The British Society of Rheumatology recommended a classification into 3 categories (mild, moderate and severe dry eyes) based on the Schirmer's test, Break Up Time (BUT) and ocular staining [319]. First line therapy for all patients with dry eyes is the instillation of preservative-free artificial tears containing methylcellulose or hyaluronate, and ointment at night. In DREAM studies, use of supplements of n-3 fatty acids for 12 month and beyond does not improve OSDI, staining scores, BUT or Schirmer test compared to olive oil in dry eyes patients [323,324]. Although these treatments are not associated with an improvement in objective parameters, substantial subjective improvement in both groups suggests that daily olive oil teaspoon should be used in dry eye management [325]. Although the origin of the dryness is the decrease in the production of tears, a dysfunction of the Meibomian glands can also be associated and must be treated by daily eyelid massage with hot pad or liposomal spray to reconstitute the lipid layer preventing the evaporation of the tear film. In patients with persistent Meibomian inflammation and blepharitis, doxycycline 50 mg once daily for a minimum of 3 months is effective as a metallomatrix proteinase inhibitor. In case of refractory case of severe KCS, local treatment using NSAID-, glucocorticoid- or cyclosporin-containing eyedrops can be used under the strict supervision of an ophthalmologist. Rescue therapies by serum eye drops, oral or topical muscarinic agonists, lifitegrast-containing eyedrops or lacrimal plugs insertion must be evaluated in specialized settings.

Only two Disease Modifying Anti-Rheumatic Drug (DMARDs) have demonstrated a significant effect on sicca syndrome: Methotrexate in a small uncontrolled trial [326], and Mizoribine (a Japanese DMARD) in 2 cohort studies [327,328]. With regard to biological therapies, infliximab, etanercept, belimumab and tocilizumab have failed to demonstrate a favourable effect on exocrine glandular function in their respective RCTs. "Abatacept Sjögren Active Patients" (ASAP) proof-of-concept trial on abatacept showed a significant improvement in ESSPRI and BUT, but not on SWSF while another trial showed no effect on ESSPRI and SWSF. Some randomized trials, but not all, find an improvement in exocrine function and dryness with rituximab. In TEARS study, a study using 120 patients, aims for a >30% improvement in at least 2 VAS in 4 (fatigue, pain, dryness and PGA) at 6–16–24 weeks, primary endpoint is only reached at week 6, and this effect is no longer found thereafter. Dryness VAS is statistically different from the placebo group from week 6 to 24, but no group achieved a clinically significant decrease. The other large trial, TRACTISS, studying the effect of rituximab on 133 patients with a primary endpoint of >30% improvement oral dryness and fatigue VAS at 48w, did not show significant improvements in any outcome measure, except unstimulated salivary flow. However, this intervention does not seem cost-effective. The clinical significance of those differences remains to be determined and is interpreted according to the various guidelines. Only the Sjögren's Syndrome Foundation proposes to use rituximab as rescue therapy for sicca syndrome [322].

In pSS patients, complaints regarding general non-specific symptoms (non-inflammatory musculoskeletal pain and fatigue) mimicking a fibromyalgia picture are common and can be challenging for the clinician. In this context, differential diagnosis is important. Non-specific manifestation of another condition (e.g., hypothyroidism, hypocortisolism, osteoarthritis, depression, neoplasia) or resulting from a misleading manifestation linked to the systemic activity of the disease (e.g., myositis, inflammatory arthralgia or arthritis, hypokalaemia or osteomalacia due to tubular involvement, small fibre neuropathy or lymphoma) must be ruled out. When no secondary cause is identified, this fibromyalgia-like presentation can be treated as such [329]. These can be quantified and monitored using the ESSPRI score or standardized scores such as the Profile of Fatigue and the Brief Pain Inventory. Education and management according to the biopsychosocial model of chronic pain, lifestyle adaptation, sleep management strategies and the practice of moderate physical activity are the cornerstones of the management of fatigue and pain. Many patients report benefit from joining a SS support group. If drug treatment is necessary, it will consist of the prescription of conventional painkillers (short-term acetaminophen or NSAID). Antidepressants and anticonvulsants may be considered as co-analgesic medications in chronic musculoskeletal or neuropathic pain, keeping in mind the anticholinergic effect of these drugs, which can worsen sicca syndrome. Opioids are not suitable treatments for chronic pain patients. DHEA supplementation is not recommended.

As a rule of thumb, systemic immunomodulatory drugs should not be used to treat non-specific systemic manifestations because evidence is scarce. In currently available biotherapies, abatacept and belimumab failed to demonstrate an effect on fatigue and pain VAS. Data on rituximab are conflicting: 3 RCTs showed an improvement in fatigue VAS, results not found in the large TRACTISS trial. A phase 2 RCT on a total of 17 patients failed to demonstrate >20% improvement of fatigue VAS at 24 weeks, fatigue VAS improvement at 24w or >30% improvement of fatigue VAS at 24w. The authors only report a statistically significant improvement in fatigue VAS in treated group compared to baseline, while the placebo group did not reach a statistically significant difference [330]. In two other studies, patients with early pSS and active disease treated with RTX displayed a significant improvement in fatigue VAS compared to placebo from different time points post-treatment [331,332]. All RCTs have shown that rituximab is not associated with an improvement in pain VAS. An RCT investigating the effect of anakinra on fatigue, although not reaching its primary endpoint, shows a significant improvement in VAS fatigue [333]. Off-label use of DMARD or biological treatments, even as a rescue therapy, is currently not mainstream recommendation in this indication. However, some guidelines suggest a trial of hydroxychloroquine in patients with recurrent musculoskeletal complaints or fatigue, mainly based on "experience-based medicine". In its 2015 guidelines, Sjögren's Syndrome Committee of Brazilian Society of Rheumatology highlighted the possibility of using rituximab as rescue therapy for fatigue (but not sicca syndrome) management [320].

7.2. Systemic Manifestations

Management of visceral manifestations linked to disease systemic activity is currently based only on rare randomized controlled trials, cohort studies or case-reports [334]. Treatment regimens are often borrowed from systemic lupus erythematosus (SLE), rheumatoid arthritis (RA), mixed cryoglobulinemia or idiopathic organ-specific autoimmune disease management.

Therapeutic regimen must be tailored to organ specific involvement and severity of the disorder. This approach requires organ-by-organ examination of disease activity and pre-existing damage. To this end, ESSDAI score may be used as a guide but does not take into count all the systemic manifestations of pSS [210]. As a rule of thumb, systemic immunosuppressive therapy will only be offered to patients with moderate or severe organ activity (as define in ESSDAI score) or moderate overall systemic activity (ESSDAI ≥5) [210]. Organ manifestation classified as mild usually requires only self-care advice, local treatment or pain relief medication (NSAID for inflammatory arthralgia or co-analgesic for neuropathic pain). In case of treatment failure, low-dose corticosteroid treatment and/or conventional DMARD may be considered depending on clinical manifestation.

In cases requiring immunosuppressive therapy, an induction/remission biphasic regimen is recommended for the rapid control of organ damage and the preservation of its function [210]. Corticosteroid therapy is an almost essential treatment for moderate to severe systemic manifestations. To date, no steroid-free regimen has been studied in pSS and 95% of the published regimens include corticosteroid therapy, alone or in combination with an immunosuppressant [210]. When immunosuppressive therapy is prescribed, it is usually a conventional broad-spectrum immunosuppressant used as a cortisone-sparing or as a remission-inducing agent: hydroxychloroquine, methotrexate, other conventional DMARDs (leflunomide, salazopirine), mycophenolate mofetil or cyclosporine. As there are no head-to-head comparisons, the choice of immunosuppressant is mainly based on the clinician's experience and on the therapeutic regimens used in idiopathic or lupus-related disorders (HCQ and MTX in skin and articular involvement, AZA, CyA or MMF in pulmonary or renal involvement). Severe life- or organ-threatening manifestations (central nervous system involvement, glomerulonephritis), generally require an aggressive regimen including methylprednisolone pulse-therapy combined with an alkylating agent (usually cyclophosphamide IV or PO, more rarely chlorambucil) as remission-inducing agents. IVIG at immunomodulatory doses are used in neuropathies or myositis. Biological therapies (mainly rituximab) generally come only in the third line as rescue therapies. The exception to this rule concerns the manifestations associated with cryoglobulinemia where rituximab is proposed as an immunosuppressant of choice, in combination with corticosteroid therapy or even plasmapheresis in life-threatening cases. As with other autoimmune diseases, corticosteroid therapy should be reasoned with a tapering regimen guaranteeing the shortest possible exposure to supraphysiological doses while maintaining remission. Complications of chronic corticosteroid therapy must be addressed proactively.

Hydroxychloroquine is commonly used as first line DMARD for moderate systemic manifestations mainly affecting the skin and joints. Its use is mainly based on the similarities between pSS and SLE, as pSS is sometimes considered as "lupus of mucous membranes". As opposed to SLE, the evidence for its use in systemic manifestations of pSS does not actually exist, and its use is completely empirical. The first—JOQUER trial—attempting to demonstrate the effect of hydroxychloroquine over 24 weeks failed to reach the primary endpoint (30% or greater reduction between weeks 0 and 24 in scores on 2 of 3 VAS (dryness, pain, and fatigue)) [335]. In a more recent RCT performed over 2 weeks, no effect of hydroxychloroquine was seen on BUT test, Schirmer test, corneal staining score or OSDI score [336]. While those RCT have not been designed to investigate the effect of the drug on systemic manifestations of the disease, and the number of patients was small, hypergammaglobulinemia statistically improved significantly [335,336].

7.3. pSS-Associated Lymphoma

The occurrence of lymphoma is a complication that must be screened clinically, especially in patients at risk (see above). Any appearance of a firm, painless glandular swelling must be investigated if it does not disappear spontaneously. The exams of choice to detect lymphoma are an MRI of the major SG and a CT of chest, abdomen and pelvis for staging or a PET scan to investigate the entire body in a single examination. pSS patients with lymphoma require personalized treatment provided by an oncohematologist according to the histological type, the extent of the involvement and the systemic manifestations.

7.4. Obstetrical Considerations

Ideally, pSS patients of childbearing age should benefit from a preconception consultation aimed at reviewing their treatment and their serological profile (anti-Ro/SSA, anti-La/SSB and antiphospholipid panel). Low-dose aspirin can be considered to promote placental implantation [319]. Anti-Ro/SSA positive mothers should be followed regularly by foetal ultrasound in a specialized centre [210,319]. Prophylactic treatment of neonatal atrioventricular block with hydroxychloroquine may be offered, since this drug is compatible with pregnancy [210]. If a conduction disorder appears on a follow-up ultrasound, rescue therapy with glucocorticoid with or without IVIG may be attempted [210]. In the event of atrioventricular block at birth, a pacemaker must be quickly implanted.

7.5. Targeted Therapies: Revolution or Disillusion?

Targeted therapies have revolutionized Rheumatology in recent years, especially in chronic inflammatory rheumatism—such as in RA—and, to a lesser extent, systemic diseases such as SLE and vasculitis. In terms of pSS, many targeted therapies have been tested or are currently in the pipeline. Unfortunately, a revolution like the one known in the field of RA has not yet occurred. These targeted drugs are shown in Figure 4 and summarized in Tables 6–12.

Given their predominant role in the production of autoantibodies, germinal centres and the evolution towards lymphoma, B cell depletion is one of the therapeutic mechanisms studied in pSS (Tables 6–8). In addition to the mixed results of the anti-CD20 Rituximab RCTs, other targeted drugs have been studied. Epratuzumab, an anti-CD22 B cell depleting therapy studied in SLE patients had a positive effect on the systemic activity of SLE patients with Sjögren syndrome in a post-hoc analysis of EMBODY trial [337]. However, an RCT should be designed to assess the effect of the therapy on both ESSDAI and ESSPRI in pSS patients. Other B cell depletion strategies aiming at blocking the BAFF pathway showed a positive effect on the ESSDAI and ESSPRI scores at 28–52 weeks [338,339]. However, the confirmation of these promising results against a placebo is necessary. Other strategies targeting BAFF pathway are also under investigation: a TACI-antibody fusion protein called RC18, rituximab + belimumab combo therapy, Tibulizumab—a dual anti-BAFF (belimumab) and anti-IL-17 antibody (Ixekizumab)—and Ianalumab (anti-BAFF receptor). The results of these different studies are expected during 2020. B cell targeting drugs by Bruton tyrosine kinase inhibitor (4 molecules), LTßR fusion protein, PI3Kδ inhibitor (3 molecules) and Cathepsin S inhibitor are currently being evaluated with inconclusive results to date. Bortezomib, a proteasome inhibitor used for the treatment of multiple myeloma, has been successfully used in 2 cases of refractory pSS reports but has never been studied on a larger scale [236,340].

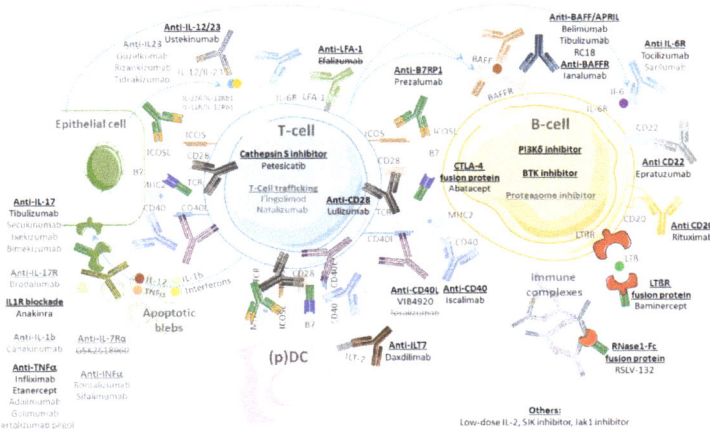

Figure 4. Synoptic view of targeted drugs (being) studied in pSS. Therapeutic classes are in bold. Biotherapies and small molecules are in black if they have been the subject of one or more trials in pSS or in grey if they exist but have not been tested in pSS. Names in strikethrough are drugs whose development has been stopped because of unacceptable side effects or because of portfolio prioritization.

T-cells play a central role in the modulation and polarization of the local autoimmune reaction within lymphocyte infiltrates in the exocrine glands. They are also used as therapeutic target by biotherapies interfering with the T-cell co-stimulation (Table 9). To date, there is no convincing result to recommend these treatments in pSS, but most studies targeting the CD40-ligand (CD154)/CD40 pathway are in progress. Therapies targeting T-cell trafficking, such as Fingolimod or Natalizumab, have not been studied in pSS.

With regard to anti-cytokine targeted therapies, RCTs using anti-TNF (infliximab and etanercept) and anti-IL6 receptor (tocilizumab) are negative (Table 11). Anakinra demonstrated a statistically significant decrease in fatigue VAS, without however reaching its primary clinical endpoint. The development of GSK2618960—an anti-IL-7Rα biotherapy—was stopped by the company due to the prioritization of their portfolio. So far, only one RCT studying the effect of Ustekinumab—an anti-IL-12/IL-23 antibody—on ESSDAI score at week 24 as primary endpoint is expected to give results in 2022 [341].

In a phase II trial, Filgotinib—a Jak1 inhibitor—and Lanraplenib—a SIK inhibitor—failed to demonstrate a significant effect on the ESSDAI and ESSPRI scores [342]. Finally, innovative therapies targeting plasmacytoid dendritic cells, immune complexes by RNase1-Fc fusion protein or the induction of T-reg cells by low-dose IL-2 injections are being evaluated. These various therapies are reviewed in Table 12.

Table 6. B cell targeted drugs in pSS part 1: monoclonal antibodies directed against B cell specific Cluster of Differentiation (CD).

DRUG	TRIAL (Reference)	Inclusion Criteria	Number of Subjects Drg	Number of Subjects Ctrl	Age (Years)	Disease Duration (Years)	Mean ESSDAI	Primary Outcome	Results	Effects (Statistically Significant) Sicca Syndrome	Fibro-Like	Systemic
Rituximab Anti-CD20	NCT00363350 Phase I/II [343]	AECG criteria RF+ and SSa and/or SSb+ SWS >0.15 mL/min	20	10	43 ±11	5.25 ±4.17	8 (4–13)	SWS ⇧ at 48w	met	SWS/UWS ⇧ LG test ⇧ Schirmer = BUT =	SF36 ⇧ MFI ⇧	Vasculitis ⇧
	Phase III [330]	AECG criteria SSa and/or SSb+ F-VAS ≥5/10	8	9	51 (22–64)	7.25 (1–18)	na	⇧ > 20% of F-VAS at 24w; F-VAS at 24w; ⇧ >30% of F-VAS at 24w	not met not met not met	UWS = Schirmer =	F-VAS ⇧ PROFAD ⇧ P-VAS ⇧ Soc-SF36 ⇧	Glandular ⇧
	Phase III [332]	AECG criteria SSa and/or SSb+ Disease duration ≤ 2y 2/5 of [PhGA >50 mm or ESSDAI ≥ 6 or subESSPRI ≥ 5]	19	22	40 (27–53)	1 (1–2)	20 (6–41)	ΔESSDAI until 120W	met from 24w to 120w	D-VAS ⇧ Schirmer ⇧ UWS ⇧	P-VAS = F-VAS ⇧	ESSDAI ⇧
	NCT00740948 Phase III TEARS [331]	AECG criteria with 2/4 VAS ≥ 5/10 for PhGA, pain, fatigue and dryness AND biologically active OR 1 extra-glandular manifestation or parotid gland enlargement.	63	57	52.9 ± 13.3	4.6 ± 4.8	10 ± 6.9	⇧ 30% of at least 2/4 VAS at 6-16-24w	met at 6w not met at 16-24w	D-VAS ⇧ Schirmer =	P-VAS = F-VAS ⇧	ESSDAI = Glandular = Articular =
	Phase III TRACTISS [344]	pSS with SSa+ UWS >0 mL/min F-VAS and D-VAS >5/10	67	66	54 ± 11.5	5.7 ± 5.4	5.7 ± 4.5	⇧ 30% D-VAS and F-VAS at 48w	not met	UWS ⇧ ESSPRI = D-VAS =	F-VAS = SF36 = PROFAD =	ESSDAI =
Epratuzumab Anti-CD22	Post-hoc Phase I/II EMBODY [337]	SLE with SSa+ and SS diagnosis	31 + 41	40	46.4 ± 12.3	5.1 (0–34)	na	BICLA at 48w ΔBILAG at 48w ΔSLEDAI at 48w ΔPhGA at 48w	met met not met not met	na	na	BILAG ⇧

AECG = American European Consensus Group, Drg = drug/treatment group, Ctrl = control group, Fibro-like = fibromyalgia-like symptoms such as fatigue and widespread pain, FR+ = presence of rheumatoid factor, SSa/SSb = anti-Ro/SSa and anti-La/SSb, SWS = stimulated whole saliva flow, UWS = unstimulated whole saliva flow, LG test = lissamine green test, BUT = break-up time, SF36 = Short Form 36 health survey score, Soc-SF36 = social component of SF36 score, Phys-SF36 = physical component of SF36 score, MFI = Multidimensional Fatigue Inventory score, F-VAS = fatigue visual analogue scale, Schirmer = Schirmer test, P-VAS = Pain visual analogue scale, PROFAD = Profile of Fatigue and Discomfort, DSST = Digit Symbol Substitution Test, ESSDAI = EULAR SS disease activity index, D-VAS = dryness visual analogue scale, PhGA = physician global activity visual analogue scale, subESSPRI = P-VAS, D-VAS or F-VAS, BILAG = British Isles Lupus Assessment Group index, BICLA = BILAG-based Combined Lupus Assessment, ESSPRI = EULAR SS Patient Reported Index, SAEs = serious adverse effects, SGUS = salivary gland ultrasound, Ig = immunoglobulin, ⇧ = decrease/increase, Δ = difference.

Table 7. B cell targeted drugs in pSS part 2: BAFF/APRIL system targeted therapies.

DRUG	TRIAL (References)	Inclusion Criteria	Number of Subjects Drg	Number of Subjects Ctrl	Age (Years)	Disease Duration (Years)	Mean ESSDAI	Primary Outcome	Results	Effects (Statistically Significant) Sicca Syndrome	Fibro-Like	Systemic
Belimumab Anti-BAFF	NCT01160666 NCT01008982 Phase II BELISS [338,339]	AECG criteria SSa and/or SSb+ AND systemic complication OR B cell activation OR early disease (≤5 years)	30	-	49.5 ±6.5	5.7 ±5.6	8.8 ±7.4	◊ of 2/5 VAS at 28w - ≥ 30% D-VAS; - ≥ 30% F-VAS; - ≥ 30% P-VAS; - ≥ 30% PhGA; - ≥ 25% B cell markers	60% response	ESSPRI ◊ D-VAS ◊ UWS ◊ Schirmer =	ESSPRI ◊ P-VAS = F-VAS = SF36 =	ESSDAI ◊ Glandular ◊
		Follow-up of previous study	15	-	40.2 ±11.8	5.9 ±5.7	3.8 ±3.1	Idem between 28-52w	86.7% Stable response	ESSPRI ◊ D-VAS ◊ UWS = Schirmer =	ESSPRI ◊ P-VAS = F-VAS = Phys-SF36 ◊	ESSDAI ◊ Glandular ◊ Articular ◊ Biologic ◊
RCt8 TACI-Igfusion protein	NCT04078386 Phase II [45]	AECG criteria SSa+ ESSDAI ≥ 5	30		?	?	?	ΔESSDAI at 24w	December 2020	Secondary endpoint	Secondary endpoint	Primary endpoint
Rituximab Anti-CD20 + Belimumab Anti-BAFF	NCT02631538 Phase II [46]	AECG criteria SSa and/or SSb+ ESSDAI ≥ 5 UWS >0 mL/min D-VAS ≥ 5/10	70		?	?	?	SAEs at 104w AESIs at 104w	Study completed on June 2020	Secondary endpoint	na	Secondary endpoint
Tibulizumab (LY3090106) Anti-BAFF + Anti-IL-17	NCT02614716 Phase I [47]	AECG criteria SSa and/or SSb+	32		?	?	?	SAEs at 197d	Not published	na	na	na
Ianalumab (VAY736) Anti-BAFFR	NCT02149420 Phase II [48]	AECG criteria ANA ≥1:160 SSa and/or SSb+ ESSDAI ≥ 6 UWS >0 mL/min	6+12	9	50.5 ±12.16	?	12.5 (6,31)	ΔESSDAI at 12w	not met	D-VAS ◊	SF-36 = MFI ◊ F-VAS ◊	ESSDAI = Articular ◊
	NCT02962895 Phase II [49]	AECG criteria SSa+ ESSDAI ≥ 6 (from 7 domains only)	195		?	?	?	Change in multi-dimensional disease activity at 24w	Study completed on June 2020	Secondary endpoint	Secondary endpoint	Primary endpoint

Table 8. B cell targeted drugs in pSS part 3: drugs targeting other B cells survival and function pathways.

DRUG	TRIAL (Reference)	Inclusion Criteria	Number of Subjects Drg	Number of Subjects Ctrl	Age (Years)	Disease Duration (Years)	Mean ESSDAI	Primary Outcome	Results	Effects (Statistically Significant) Sicca Syndrome	Fibro-Like	Systemic
LOU064 BTK inhibitor	NCT04035668 Phase II LOUiSSe [350]	2016 ACR/EULAR criteria SSa and/or SSb+ ESSDAI ≥ 6 UWS >0 mL/min	252		?	?	?	ΔESSDAI at 24w	Estimated Study Completion on January 2023	Secondary endpoint	Secondary endpoint	Secondary endpoint
Tirabrutinib (GS-4059) BTK inhibitor	NCT03100942 Phase II [342]	AECG criteria SSa and/or SSb+ ESSDAI ≥ 4	38	37	55.8 ± 10.06	?	10.4 ± 5.36	Protocol-Specified Response Criteria at 12w	not met	ESSPRI =	ESSPRI =	ESSDAI =
BMS-986142 BTK inhibitor	NCT02843659 Phase II [351]	2016 ACR/EULAR criteria SSa and/or SSb+ ESSDAI ≥ 6 UWS >0 mL/min	5+6	7	51.2 ± 11.41	?	?	ΔESSDAI at 12w	Not published	Secondary endpoint	Secondary endpoint	Secondary endpoint
Branebrutinib BTK inhibitor	NCT04186871 Phase II [352]	2016 ACR/EULAR criteria Moderate to severe pSS	?	?	?	?	?	Protocol-Specified Response Criteria at 24w	Estimated Study Completion on June 2022	na	na	Primary endpoint
Baminercept LTβ-R fusion protein	NCT01552681 Phase II [353]	2016 ACR/EULAR criteria UWS >0.1 mL/min ≥ 1 non-life-threatening systemic manifestation(s)	33	19	52.0 ± 11.0	?	3.1 ± 3.4	ΔSWS at 24w	not met	D-VAS = Schirmer ◊ UWS =	F-VAS =	ESSDAI =
Parsaclisib (INCB050465) PI3Kδ inhibitor	NCT03627065 Phase II [354]	AECG criteria SGUS score > 2 SSa and/or SSb+ ESSDAI ≥ 6 Oral dryness score ≥ 5.	10		?	?	?	ΔSGUS score at 12w	Not published	na	na	na
Seletalisib (UCB5857) PI3Kδ inhibitor	NCT02610543 Phase II [355]	AECG criteria FAN ≥ 1:160 SSa and/or SSb+ ESSDAI ≥ 6	13	14	?	?	?	ΔESSDAI at 12w	not met	ESSPRI = SWSF = Schirmer =	na	ESSDAI =
Leniolisib (CDZ173) PI3Kδ inhibitor	NCT02775916 Phase II [356]	pSS diagnosis SSa and/or SSb+ ESSDAI ≥ 6, ESSPRI ≥ 5 SWS > 0.1 mL/min	20	10	47.3 ± 13.07	?	?	ΔESSDAI at 12w SAEs at 12w	not met	ESSPRI =	SF-36 = MFI =	na

Table 9. T-cell targeted drugs in pSS: co-stimulation receptors or ligands inhibition.

DRUG	TRIAL	Inclusion Criteria	Number of Subjects Drg	Number of Subjects Ctrl	Age (Years)	Disease Duration (Years)	Mean ESSDAI	Primary Outcome	Results	Effects (Statistically Significant) Sicca Syndrome	Fibro-Like	Systemic
Abatacept CTLA-4 Ig fusion protein	NCT02915159 Phase III [357]	2016 ACR/EULAR criteria SSa+ ESSDAI ≥ 5	92	95	52 ± 12.9	?	9.4 ± 4.3	ΔESSDAI at 169d	Not met	ESSPRI = SWS =	ESSPRI =	ESSDAI = DAS28 ◇
	Phase I/II ASAP [358]	AECG criteria and ESSDAI ≥ 6 Disease duration ≤ 5 years SWS ≥ 0.10 mL/min SSa and/or SSb+ or FR+ Proven by parotid gland biopsy.	15	-	43 (32–51)	11 (7–36)	11 (8–14)	ΔESSDAI at 24–48w	met	ESSPRI ◇ SWS/UWS = Schirmer = BUT ◇	ESSPRI ◇	ESSDAI ◇
	NCT02067910 Phase III ASAPIII [359]	AECG criteria and ESSDAI ≥ 5 Time from diagnosis ≤ 7 years	40	39	49 ± 16	8 (4–14)	?	ΔESSDAI at 24w	Not met	ESSPRI ◇ FSFI ◇ DVAS = UWS = Schirmer =	Fatigue =	ESSDAI = Articular ◇
Iscalimab (CFZ533) Anti-CD40	NCT02291029 Phase IIa [360]	AECG criteria and ESSDAI ≥ 6 SSA+ OR FR+ and FAN ≥ 1:320 SWS ≥ 0 mL/min	8+21	4+11	51.3 ± 13.5	?	10.7 ± 4.6	SAEs at 12w	safe	ESSPRI = UWS ◇ Schirmer =	MFI = SF-36 =	ESSDAI ◇ Articular ◇
	NCT03905525 Phase II TWINSS [361]	2016 ACR/EULAR criteria SSa+ SWS > 0.01 mL/min, P1: ESSDAI ≥ 5 or P2 ESSPRI ≥ 5.	260		?	?	?	ΔESSDAI at 24w in P1 ΔESSPRI at 24w in P2	Estimated Study Completion on June 2022	Included endpoint	Included endpoint	Included endpoint
VIB4920 MEDI4920 Anti-CD40L	NCT04129164 Phase II [362]	P1: ESSDAI ≥ 5 P2: ESSDAI < 5 et ESSPRI ≥ 5	174		?	?	?	ΔESSDAI 169d in P1 ΔESSPRI at 169d in P2	Estimated Study Completion on April 2022	Included endpoint	Included endpoint	Included endpoint
Prezalumab (AMG557) (MEDI5872) Anti-B7RP1	NCT02334306 Phase IIa [363]	AECG criteria and ESSDAI ≥ 5 SSa and/or SSb+ FR+, cryoglobulinemia or hypergammaglobulinemia	16	16	50.7 ± 13	?	?	ΔESSDAI at 99d	Not met	ESSPRI =	ESSPRI =	ESSDAI =
Lulizumab (BMS-931699) Anti-CD28	NCT02843659 Phase II [51]	2016 ACR/EULAR criteria SSa and/or SSb+ ESSDAI ≥ 5 USW > 0.01 mL/min	5+6	7	51.2 ± 11.41	?	?	ΔESSDAI at 12w	Not published	Secondary endpoint	Secondary endpoint	Primary endpoint

Table 10. T-cell targeted drugs in pSS: therapies preventing autoantigen presentation.

DRUG	TRIAL (Reference)	Inclusion Criteria	Number of Subjects Drg	Number of Subjects Ctrl	Age (Years)	Disease Duration (Years)	Mean ESSDAI	Primary Outcome	Results	Effects (Statistically Significant) Sicca Syndrome	Fibro-Like	Systemic
Petesicatib RO5459072 Cathepsin S Inhibitor	NCT02701985 Phase IIa [364]	AECG criteria SSa and/or SSb+ ESSDAI ≥ 5 ESSPRI ≥ 5 USW > 0.0 mL/min Oral D-VAS ≥ 5/10	38	37	52.2 ± 12.5	?	?	ΔESSDAI ≥ 3 at 12w	Not met	ESSPRI =	ESSPRI = SF36 =	ESSDAI =
Efalizumab Anti-LFA-1	NCT00344448 Phase II [365]	AECG criteria SSa and/or SSb+	6	3	53 ± 11.2	?	?	Protocol-specified composite score at 12w	Early termination due to serious side effect in other trial			

Table 11. Anti-cytokine targeted drugs in pSS.

DRUG	TRIAL	Inclusion Criteria	Number of Subjects Drg	Number of Subjects Ctrl	Age (Years)	Disease Duration (Years)	Mean ESSDAI	Primary Outcome	Results	Effects (Statistically Significant) Sicca Syndrome	Fibro-Like	Systemic
Anakinra IL1R antagonist protein	NCT00683345 Phase II [333]	AECG criteria 18–80 years Western European descent No depression or comorbidity	13	13	55 (36–80)	5 (1–17)	?	Group-wise comparison of the fatigue scores at 4w	not met	na	F-VAS ⋄	na
Tocilizumab Anti-IL-6R	NCT01782235 Phase I/II ETAP [366]	AECG criteria ESSDAI ≥ 5	55	55	50.9 (26–76)	?	11.5 (5–25)	ΔESSDAI ≥ 3 at 12W without new item without ⋄ ≥1/10 PGA	not met	ESSPRI = Schirmer =	ESSPRI =	ESSDAI = Articular ⋄
Infliximab Anti-TNF	Phase III TRIPSS [367]	AECG criteria 2/3 D-VAS, F-VAS, P-VAS ≥ 5/10	54	49	54.4 ± 10.4	4.0 ± 5.5	na	⋄ 30% in 2/3 D-VAS, F-VAS, P-VAS at 10–22w	not met	SWS = Schirmer =	SF-36 =	SJC = TJC =
Etanercept TNFR-Ig fusion protein	NCT00001954 Phase II [368]	1986 and AECG criteria Elevated ESR or IgG levels	14	14	55.5 (46, 59)	?	na	⋄ 20% in 2/3 pSS domains (protocol-specified)	not met	D-VAS = Schirmer = VB = SWS =	na	na
Ustekinumab Anti-IL-12/IL-23 (p40 subunit)	NCT04093531 Phase I [341]	2016 ACR/EULAR criteria	15	-	?	?	?	ΔESSDAI at 24W	Estimated Study Completion on December 2021	na	Secondary endpoint	Primary endpoint
GSK2618960 anti-IL-7Rα	NCT03239600 Phase II [369]	AECG criteria SWS >0.1 mL/min ⋄ Ig or FR+ or ANA ≥ 1:320 D-VAS ≥ 5/10 or Schirmer < 10 mm	0	-	-	-	-	SAEs at 27w	Withdraw The study is stopped for Portfolio prioritization			

Table 12. Miscellaneous targeted drugs in pSS.

| DRUG | TRIAL (Reference) | Inclusion Criteria | Number of Subjects | | Age (years) | Disease Duration (Years) | Mean ESSDAI | Primary Outcome | Results | Effects (Statistically Significant) | | | |
			Drg	Ctrl						Sicca Syndrome	Fibro-Like	Systemic	
Daxdilimab VIB7734 Anti-ILT7	NCT03817424 Phase I [370]	Unspecified	?	?	?	?	SAEs at 169d AESIs at 169d	June 2020	na	na	na	na	
Filgotinib Jak1 inhibitor	NCT03100942 Phase II [342]	AECG criteria SSa and/or SSb+ ESSDAI ≥ 4	38	37	52.2 ± 10.54	?	10.2 ± 6.23	Protocol-Specified Response Criteria at 12w	not met	ESSPRI =	ESSPRI =	ESSDAI =	
Lanraplenib (GS-9876) SIK inhibitor	NCT03100942 Phase II [342]	AECG criteria SSa and/or SSb+ ESSDAI ≥ 4	38	37	56.2 ± 9.72	?	10.5 ± 4.89	Protocol-Specified Response Criteria at 12w	not met	ESSPRI =	ESSPRI =	ESSDAI =	
RSLV-132 RNase1-Fc fusion protein	NCT03247686 Phase II [371]	AECG criteria SSA+ Interferon signature	22	8	?	?	?	Interferon gene expression at day99	Not published	ESSPRI =	mPRO-F ⇩ DSST ⇩ FACIT-F = ESSPRI =	ESSDAI =	
Low-dose IL-2 T-reg induction	NCT01988506 Phase II Transreg [372]	pSS diagnosis	84–132		?	?	?	T-reg percentage	Estimated Study Completion on February 2022	na	na	na	

8. Conclusions

pSS is a multifaceted disease combining pleiomorphic systemic autoimmune manifestations, glandular manifestations, a frequently added psychosomatic component and the possible progression to non-Hodgkin lymphoma. Its management has two complementary facets: improving the quality of life of patients by tackling dryness, fatigue and chronic pain symptomatically in a multidisciplinary way and treating systemic manifestations to prevent damage, which will worsen the vital and functional prognosis. Although we understand more and more its pathophysiology, many questions remain unanswered, and its treatment remains disappointing compared to other autoimmune diseases. pSS therefore remains a vast field of investigation where much fundamental and clinical research remains to be done. Ten take-home messages:

1. SS is characterized by lymphoplasmacytic infiltration of exocrine glands. The cause of SS is complex and influenced by a combination of genetic, epigenetic, hormonal and environmental factors.
2. The pathogenic mechanisms remain unclear. However, the immune system-mediated loss of glands function, specifically of salivary and lacrimal glands, certainly explains the common symptoms of dry mouth and dry eyes. In this inflammatory environment, T-cells mediate a direct destruction of glandular tissue and B-cell activation, leading to the production of autoantibodies. More than 20 autoantibodies could be involved in SS, but the most commonly used for SS diagnosis are anti-Ro/SSA and anti-La/SSB.
3. Although often reduced to its sicca syndrome due to its tropism for glandular tissue, pSS remains a systemic disease that can affect virtually all organs. These clinical manifestations can be due to various mechanisms: dryness secondary to exocrinopathy, autoimmune epithelitis with periepithelial lymphocytic infiltration of target organs, autoimmunity and clonal lymphocytic expansion.
4. Due to its protean and willingly insidious presentation, pSS is sometimes difficult to recognize and may delay diagnosis by more than 10 years. Classification criteria are used to create cohorts for study purposes and should not be used blindly as diagnostic criteria but as a guide in clinical practice. For these various reasons, the gold standard for individual diagnosis of pSS remains the opinion of an expert clinician.
5. From a serohistological point of view, so-called "secondary Sjögren's syndrome" in SLE and SScl patients does not differ from pSS. It is therefore preferable to forget this historical dichotomy. In this way, the clinician avoids three pitfalls: (1) minimizing the SS-related symptoms, which decrease the quality of life of the patients; (2) forget that overlap may change the clinical phenotype and (3) forget the risk of lymphoma.
6. Although overall pSS mortality is low and similar to the general population, a subgroup of patients will have a poorer vital prognosis linked to cardiovascular events, solid-organ and lymphoid malignancies and infections. Biomarkers associated with the development of MALT lymphoma are mainly signs associated with exuberant B cell proliferation and immune-complex production.
7. The impact of pSS can be assessed according to three clinical dimensions: "sicca asthenia polyalgia" complex, inflammatory disease activity and structural damage. They are assessed by the ESSPRI, ESSDAI and SSD(D)I scores, respectively. Even in the absence of florid systemic manifestations, pSS can be disabling and associated with significant functional status impairment related to oral and/or ocular dryness, systemic activity, pain, fatigue and daytime somnolence, anxiety and depression symptoms.
8. The treatment of manifestations linked to the "sicca asthenia polyalgia" complex mainly involves symptomatic measures and rehabilitation. To date, no immunosuppressant has demonstrated a favourable risk–benefit balance in this indication.
9. The treatment of manifestations related to inflammatory disease activity is currently based on scarce evidence. Therapeutic regimen must be tailored to organ specific involvement and severity of the disorder. Mild manifestations will be treated with hydroxychloroquine or local corticosteroids while moderate to severe systemic involvement will require the use of systemic

corticosteroid therapy, combined or not with a broad-spectrum immunosuppressant. Rituximab will only be used as a third line, except in cases of cryoglobulinemia where it is the treatment of choice.
10. Despite targeted therapies having revolutionized rheumatology in recent years and the impressive number of molecules tested so far in pSS, a revolution like the one known in the field of RA has not yet occurred.

Author Contributions: D.P., C.C., J.P., M.S.S. and C.D. contributed to the writing of the review. All authors have read and agreed to the published version of the manuscript.

Funding: This research was funded the EU H2020 contract HarmonicSS (H2020-SC1-2016-RTD/731944), Fonds Erasme, Fonds de la Recherche Scientifique—FNRS (grant J.0053.20). DP is a Research Fellow of the Fonds de la Recherche Scientifique—FNRS.

Acknowledgments: The authors thank Bahija Jellouli for her secretarial help.

Conflicts of Interest: The authors declare no conflicts of interest.

Abbreviations

ACA	Anti-centromere antibodies
ACPA	Anti-citrullinated protein antibodies
ACR	American College of Rheumatology
AECG	American European Consensus Group
AH	Autoimmune Hepatitis
ANA	Antinuclear antibodies
anti-M3R	Anti-muscarinic receptor 3
APRIL	A proliferation-inducing ligand
ASAP	"Abatacept Sjögren Active Patients" study
AZA	Azathioprine
BAFF	B cell Activating Factor
BCR	B cell receptor
BUT	Break-up Time
CCP	Cyclic Citrullinated Peptide
circRNA	Circular RNA
ciRNAs	Intronic circRNAs
ClinESSDAI	Clinical ESSDAI variant
CPK	Creatine phosphokinase
CRISP-3	Cysteine-Rich Secretory Protein 3 ()
CT-scan	Computerized tomography
CyA	Ciclosporin A
DAMPS	Danger-associated molecular patterns
DAP-kinase	Pro-apoptotic death associated protein kinase
DHEA	Dehydroepiandrosterone
DHT	Dihydrotestosterone
DLBCL	Diffuse large B cell lymphoma
DMARD	Disease Modifying Anti-Rheumatic Drug
DNMTs	DNA methyltransferases
DREAM	"Dry Eye Assessment and Management" study
EBV	Epstein-Barr virus
ecircRNAs	Exonic circRNAs
EIciRNAs	Exon-intron circRNAs
ELISA	Enzyme-linked immunosorbent assay
ENT	Ear-Nose-Throat
ESSDAI	EULAR Sjögren's syndrome disease activity index
ESSPRI	EULAR Sjögren's Syndrome Patient Reported Index
EULAR	European League Against Rheumatism
FASl	Fas ligand

FDC	Follicular dendritic cells	
GCs	Germinal centres	
HCQ	Hydroxychloroquine	
HCV	Hepatitis C virus	
HLH	Hemophagocytic lymphohistiocytosis	
HTLV1	Human T-lymphotropic virus type I	
ICAM-1	InterCellular Adhesion Molecule 1	
IF	Immunofluorescence	
IFN	Interferon	
IgG,A,M	Immunoglobulin G, A and M	
IL-	Interleukin	
ILD	Interstitial lung disease(s)	
IRF	Interferon Regulatory Factor	
IV	Intravenous therapy	
IVIG	Intravenous Immunoglobulin	
KCS	Keratoconjunctivitis sicca	
LEMA	Myoepithelial sialadenitis	
LESA	lymphoepithelial sialadenitis	
LIP	Lymphocytic interstitial pneumonitis	
LMP1	Latent membrane protein 1	
lncRNA	Long non-coding RNAs	
LPR	Laryngopharyngeal reflux	
LSG	Labial SG	
MALT	mucosa-associated lymphoid tissue	
MHC	Major histocompatibility genes	
MMF	Mycophenolate mofetil	
MMP	Matrix metalloproteinases	
MPGN	Mesangioproliferative glomerulonephritis	
MRI	Magnetic Resonance Imaging	
MS	Multiple Sclerosis	
MSGB	Minor salivary gland biopsy	
MTX	Methotrexate	
NAC	N-acetylcystein	
NFkB	Nuclear factor kappa-light-chain-enhancer of activated B cells	
NHL	Non-Hodgkin's lymphoma	
NICE	National Institute for Health and Care Excellence	
NMOSD	Neuromyelitis optica spectrum disorder	
NOD	Non-obese diabetic	
NSAID	Nonsteroidal anti-inflammatory drugs	
NSIP	Nonspecific interstitial pneumonia	
OMERACT	Outcome Measures in Rheumatology group	
OSDI	Ocular Surface Disease Index	
OSS	Ocular Staining Score	
PAMPs	Pathogen-associated molecular patterns	
PBC	Primary Biliary Cirrhosis	
PDC	Plasmacytoid dendritic cells	
PDL1	Programmed death ligand 1	
PET scan	Positron emission tomography	
PGA	Patient Global Assessment	
PIP	Prolactin inducible protein	
PO	per os	
PSP	Parotid secretory protein	
pSS	Primary Sjögren's Syndrome	
pSS-ILD	pSS-related interstitial lung disease	
q6h, q8h	Every 6 h, every 8 h	
RA	Rheumatoid Arthritis	

RCT	Randomized controlled trial
RF	Rheumatoid Factor
RTA	Renal tubular acidosis
RTX	Rituximab
RX1	Runt-related transcription factor
SAM	Methyl donor S-adenosylmethionine
SAP	Sicca Asthenia Polyalgia
SF-36	Short Form 36 health survey
SG	Salivary Gland
SGS	Salivary glands scintigraphy
SGUS	Salivary glands ultrasound
SICCA	Sjögren's International Collaborative Clinical Alliance
SLE	Systemic lupus erythematosus
SNP	Single nucleotide polymorphism
SP-1	Salivary protein 1
SSDDI	Sjögren's Syndrome Disease Damage Index
SSDI	Sjögren's Syndrome Damage Index
sSS	Secondary Sjögren's Syndrome
SWSF	Stimulated Whole Salivary Flow rate
TACI	Transmembrane Activator and CAML Interactor
TEARS	"Tolerance and efficacy of rituximab in primary Sjögren syndrome" trial
Tfh	Follicular helper T cells
TLRs	Toll Like Receptors
TNF-α	Tumour necrosis factor-α
TPHA	Treponema Pallidum Hemagglutinations Assay
TRACTISS	"TRial of Anti-B-Cell Therapy In patients with primary Sjögren's Syndrome" trial
TSH	Thyroid-stimulating hormone
TTP	Thrombotic Thrombocytopenic Purpura
UCLH	University College London Hospitals
UIP	Usual interstitial pneumonia
UWSF	Unstimulated Whole Saliva Flow rate
VAS	Visual analogue scales
VDRL	Venereal Disease Research Laboratory

References

1. Fox, R.I. Sjögren's syndrome. *Lancet* **2005**, *366*, 321–331. [CrossRef]
2. Gerli, R.; Bartoloni, E.; Alunno, A. (Eds.) *Sjögren's Syndrome: Novel Insights in Pathogenic, Clinical, and Therapeutic Aspects*; Elsevier: Amsterdam, The Netherlands; Academic Press: Cambridge, MA, USA, 2016; ISBN 978-0-12-803604-4.
3. Ghafoor, M. Sjögren's Before Sjögren: Did Henrik Sjögren (1899–1986) Really Discover Sjögren's Disease? *J. Maxillofac. Oral Surg.* **2012**, *11*, 373–374. [CrossRef] [PubMed]
4. Murube, J. Henrik Sjögren, 1899–1986. *Ocul. Surf.* **2010**, *8*, 2–7. [CrossRef]
5. Wollheim, F.A. Henrik Sjögren and Sjögren's syndrome. *Scand. J. Rheumatol. Suppl.* **1986**, *61*, 11–16.
6. Binard, A.; Devauchelle-Pensec, V.; Fautrel, B.; Jousse, S.; Youinou, P.; Saraux, A. Epidemiology of Sjögren's syndrome: Where are we now? *Clin. Exp. Rheumatol.* **2007**, *25*, 1–4.
7. Mavragani, C.P.; Moutsopoulos, H.M. The geoepidemiology of Sjögren's syndrome. *Autoimmun. Rev.* **2010**, *9*, A305–A310. [CrossRef]
8. Qin, B.; Wang, J.; Yang, Z.; Yang, M.; Ma, N.; Huang, F.; Zhong, R. Epidemiology of primary Sjögren's syndrome: A systematic review and meta-analysis. *Ann. Rheum. Dis.* **2015**, *74*, 1983–1989. [CrossRef]
9. Delaleu, N.; Jonsson, M.V.; Appel, S.; Jonsson, R. New concepts in the pathogenesis of Sjögren's syndrome. *Rheum. Dis. Clin. N. Am.* **2008**, *34*, 833–845. [CrossRef]
10. Konttinen, Y.T.; Käsnä-Ronkainen, L. Sjögren's syndrome: Viewpoint on pathogenesis. One of the reasons I was never asked to write a textbook chapter on it. *Scand. J. Rheumatol. Suppl.* **2002**, *116*, 15–22. [CrossRef]

11. Mitsias, D.I.; Kapsogeorgou, E.K.; Moutsopoulos, H.M. Sjögren's syndrome: Why autoimmune epithelitis? *Oral Dis.* **2006**, *12*, 523–532. [CrossRef]
12. Igoe, A.; Scofield, R.H. Autoimmunity and infection in Sjögren's syndrome. *Curr. Opin. Rheumatol.* **2013**, *25*, 480–487. [CrossRef] [PubMed]
13. Björk, A.; Mofors, J.; Wahren-Herlenius, M. Environmental factors in the pathogenesis of primary Sjögren's syndrome. *J. Intern. Med.* **2020**, *287*, 475–492. [CrossRef] [PubMed]
14. Ascherio, A.; Munger, K.L. Epstein-barr virus infection and multiple sclerosis: A review. *J. Neuroimmune Pharmacol.* **2010**, *5*, 271–277. [CrossRef] [PubMed]
15. Toussirot, E.; Roudier, J. Epstein-Barr virus in autoimmune diseases. *Best Pract. Res. Clin. Rheumatol.* **2008**, *22*, 883–896. [CrossRef] [PubMed]
16. Saito, I.; Servenius, B.; Compton, T.; Fox, R.I. Detection of Epstein-Barr virus DNA by polymerase chain reaction in blood and tissue biopsies from patients with Sjogren's syndrome. *J. Exp. Med.* **1989**, *169*, 2191–2198. [CrossRef] [PubMed]
17. Mariette, X.; Gozlan, J.; Clerc, D.; Bisson, M.; Morinet, F. Detection of Epstein-Barr virus DNA by in situ hybridization and polymerase chain reaction in salivary gland biopsy specimens from patients with Sjögren's syndrome. *Am. J. Med.* **1991**, *90*, 286–294. [CrossRef]
18. Dimitriou, I.; Xanthou, G.; Kapsogeorgou, E.; Abu-Helu, R.; Moutsopoulos, H.; Manoussakis, M. High spontaneous CD40 expression by salivary gland epithelial cells in Sjogren's syndrome: Possible evidence for intrinsic activation of epithelial cells. *Arthritis Res.* **2001**, *3*, P018. [CrossRef]
19. Kivity, S.; Arango, M.T.; Ehrenfeld, M.; Tehori, O.; Shoenfeld, Y.; Anaya, J.-M.; Agmon-Levin, N. Infection and autoimmunity in Sjogren's syndrome: A clinical study and comprehensive review. *J. Autoimmun.* **2014**, *51*, 17–22. [CrossRef]
20. Iwakiri, D.; Zhou, L.; Samanta, M.; Matsumoto, M.; Ebihara, T.; Seya, T.; Imai, S.; Fujieda, M.; Kawa, K.; Takada, K. Epstein-Barr virus (EBV)-encoded small RNA is released from EBV-infected cells and activates signaling from Toll-like receptor 3. *J. Exp. Med.* **2009**, *206*, 2091–2099. [CrossRef]
21. Murray, R.J.; Wang, D.; Young, L.S.; Wang, F.; Rowe, M.; Kieff, E.; Rickinson, A.B. Epstein-Barr virus-specific cytotoxic T-cell recognition of transfectants expressing the virus-coded latent membrane protein LMP. *J. Virol.* **1988**, *62*, 3747–3755. [CrossRef]
22. Nakamura, H.; Takahashi, Y.; Yamamoto-Fukuda, T.; Horai, Y.; Nakashima, Y.; Arima, K.; Nakamura, T.; Koji, T.; Kawakami, A. Direct Infection of Primary Salivary Gland Epithelial Cells by Human T Lymphotropic Virus Type I in Patients With Sjögren's Syndrome. *Arthritis Rheumatol.* **2015**, *67*, 1096–1106. [CrossRef] [PubMed]
23. Terada, K.; Katamine, S.; Eguchi, K.; Moriuchi, R.; Kita, M.; Shimada, H.; Yamashita, I.; Iwata, K.; Tsuji, Y.; Nagataki, S. Prevalence of serum and salivary antibodies to HTLV-1 in Sjögren's syndrome. *Lancet* **1994**, *344*, 1116–1119. [CrossRef]
24. Stathopoulou, E.A.; Routsias, J.G.; Stea, E.A.; Moutsopoulos, H.M.; Tzioufas, A.G. Cross-reaction between antibodies to the major epitope of Ro60 kD autoantigen and a homologous peptide of Coxsackie virus 2B protein. *Clin. Exp. Immunol.* **2005**, *141*, 148–154. [CrossRef]
25. Gottenberg, J.-E.; Pallier, C.; Ittah, M.; Lavie, F.; Miceli-Richard, C.; Sellam, J.; Nordmann, P.; Cagnard, N.; Sibilia, J.; Mariette, X. Failure to confirm coxsackievirus infection in primary Sjögren's syndrome. *Arthritis Rheum.* **2006**, *54*, 2026–2028. [CrossRef] [PubMed]
26. Flores-Chávez, A.; Carrion, J.A.; Forns, X.; Ramos-Casals, M. Extrahepatic manifestations associated with Chronic Hepatitis C Virus Infection. *Rev. Espanola Sanid. Penit.* **2017**, *19*, 87–97. [CrossRef]
27. Kang, H.I.; Fei, H.M.; Saito, I.; Sawada, S.; Chen, S.L.; Yi, D.; Chan, E.; Peebles, C.; Bugawan, T.L.; Erlich, H.A. Comparison of HLA class II genes in Caucasoid, Chinese, and Japanese patients with primary Sjögren's syndrome. *J. Immunol. 1950* **1993**, *150*, 3615–3623.
28. Kerttula, T.O.; Collin, P.; Polvi, A.; Korpela, M.; Partanen, J.; Mäki, M. Distinct immunologic features of Finnish Sjögren's syndrome patients with HLA alleles DRB1*0301, DQA1*0501, and DQB1*0201. Alterations in circulating T cell receptor gamma/delta subsets. *Arthritis Rheum.* **1996**, *39*, 1733–1739. [CrossRef]
29. Mountz, J.D.; Zhou, T.; Su, X.; Wu, J.; Cheng, J. The role of programmed cell death as an emerging new concept for the pathogenesis of autoimmune diseases. *Clin. Immunol. Immunopathol.* **1996**, *80*, S2–S14. [CrossRef]

30. Adachi, M.; Watanabe-Fukunaga, R.; Nagata, S. Aberrant transcription caused by the insertion of an early transposable element in an intron of the Fas antigen gene of lpr mice. *Proc. Natl. Acad. Sci. USA* **1993**, *90*, 1756–1760. [CrossRef]
31. Bolstad, A.I.; Wargelius, A.; Nakken, B.; Haga, H.J.; Jonsson, R. Fas and Fas ligand gene polymorphisms in primary Sjögren's syndrome. *J. Rheumatol.* **2000**, *27*, 2397–2405.
32. Nakken, B.; Jonsson, R.; Bolstad, A.I. Polymorphisms of the Ro52 gene associated with anti-Ro 52-kd autoantibodies in patients with primary Sjögren's syndrome. *Arthritis Rheum.* **2001**, *44*, 638–646. [CrossRef]
33. Hulkkonen, J.; Pertovaara, M.; Antonen, J.; Lahdenpohja, N.; Pasternack, A.; Hurme, M. Genetic association between interleukin-10 promoter region polymorphisms and primary Sjögren's syndrome. *Arthritis Rheum.* **2001**, *44*, 176–179. [CrossRef]
34. Qin, B.; Wang, J.; Liang, Y.; Yang, Z.; Zhong, R. The association between TNF-α, IL-10 gene polymorphisms and primary Sjögren's syndrome: A meta-analysis and systemic review. *PLoS ONE* **2013**, *8*, e63401. [CrossRef] [PubMed]
35. Ramos-Casals, M.; Font, J.; Brito-Zeron, P.; Trejo, O.; García-Carrasco, M.; Lozano, F. Interleukin-4 receptor alpha polymorphisms in primary Sjögren's syndrome. *Clin. Exp. Rheumatol.* **2004**, *22*, 374.
36. Imgenberg-Kreuz, J.; Rasmussen, A.; Sivils, K.; Nordmark, G. Genetics and epigenetics in primary Sjögren's syndrome. *Rheumatology* **2019**. [CrossRef]
37. Traianos, E.Y.; Locke, J.; Lendrem, D.; Bowman, S.; Hargreaves, B.; Macrae, V. Serum CXCL13 levels are associated with lymphoma risk and lymphoma occurrence in primary Sjögren's syndrome. *Rheumatol. Int.* **2020**, *40*, 541–548. [CrossRef]
38. Ben-Eli, H.; Gomel, N.; Aframian, D.J.; Abu-Seir, R.; Perlman, R.; Ben-Chetrit, E.; Mevorach, D.; Kleinstern, G.; Paltiel, O.; Solomon, A. SNP variations in IL10, TNFα and TNFAIP3 genes in patients with dry eye syndrome and Sjogren's syndrome. *J. Inflamm.* **2019**, *16*, 6. [CrossRef]
39. Nocturne, G.; Tarn, J.; Boudaoud, S.; Locke, J.; Miceli-Richard, C.; Hachulla, E.; Dubost, J.J.; Bowman, S.; Gottenberg, J.E.; Criswell, L.A.; et al. Germline variation of TNFAIP3 in primary Sjögren's syndrome-associated lymphoma. *Ann. Rheum. Dis.* **2016**, *75*, 780–783. [CrossRef]
40. Nezos, A.; Gkioka, E.; Koutsilieris, M.; Voulgarelis, M.; Tzioufas, A.G.; Mavragani, C.P. TNFAIP3 F127C Coding Variation in Greek Primary Sjogren's Syndrome Patients. *J. Immunol. Res.* **2018**, *2018*, 6923213. [CrossRef]
41. Fragkioudaki, S.; Nezos, A.; Souliotis, V.L.; Chatziandreou, I.; Saetta, A.A.; Drakoulis, N.; Tzioufas, A.G.; Voulgarelis, M.; Sfikakis, P.P.; Koutsilieris, M.; et al. MTHFR gene variants and non-MALT lymphoma development in primary Sjogren's syndrome. *Sci. Rep.* **2017**, *7*, 7354. [CrossRef]
42. Nezos, A.; Mavragani, C.P. Contribution of Genetic Factors to Sjögren's Syndrome and Sjögren's Syndrome Related Lymphomagenesis. *J. Immunol. Res.* **2015**, *2015*, 754825. [CrossRef] [PubMed]
43. Arvaniti, P.; Le Dantec, C.; Charras, A.; Arleevskaya, M.A.; Hedrich, C.M.; Zachou, K.; Dalekos, G.N.; Renaudineau, Y. Linking genetic variation with epigenetic profiles in Sjögren's syndrome. *Clin. Immunol.* **2020**, *210*, 108314. [CrossRef]
44. Konsta, O.D.; Thabet, Y.; Le Dantec, C.; Brooks, W.H.; Tzioufas, A.G.; Pers, J.-O.; Renaudineau, Y. The contribution of epigenetics in Sjögren's Syndrome. *Front. Genet.* **2014**, *5*, 71. [CrossRef] [PubMed]
45. Thabet, Y.; Le Dantec, C.; Ghedira, I.; Devauchelle, V.; Cornec, D.; Pers, J.-O.; Renaudineau, Y. Epigenetic dysregulation in salivary glands from patients with primary Sjögren's syndrome may be ascribed to infiltrating B cells. *J. Autoimmun.* **2013**, *41*, 175–181. [CrossRef] [PubMed]
46. Cannat, A.; Seligmann, M. Induction by isoniazid and hydrallazine of antinuclear factors in mice. *Clin. Exp. Immunol.* **1968**, *3*, 99–105.
47. Imgenberg-Kreuz, J.; Sandling, J.K.; Almlöf, J.C.; Nordlund, J.; Signér, L.; Norheim, K.B.; Omdal, R.; Rönnblom, L.; Eloranta, M.-L.; Syvänen, A.-C.; et al. Genome-wide DNA methylation analysis in multiple tissues in primary Sjögren's syndrome reveals regulatory effects at interferon-induced genes. *Ann. Rheum. Dis.* **2016**, *75*, 2029–2036. [CrossRef]
48. Toso, A.; Aluffi, P.; Capello, D.; Conconi, A.; Gaidano, G.; Pia, F. Clinical and molecular features of mucosa-associated lymphoid tissue (MALT) lymphomas of salivary glands. *Head Neck* **2009**, *31*, 1181–1187. [CrossRef]

49. Altorok, N.; Coit, P.; Hughes, T.; Koelsch, K.A.; Stone, D.U.; Rasmussen, A.; Radfar, L.; Scofield, R.H.; Sivils, K.L.; Farris, A.D.; et al. Genome-wide DNA methylation patterns in naive CD4+ T cells from patients with primary Sjögren's syndrome. *Arthritis Rheumatol.* **2014**, *66*, 731–739. [CrossRef]
50. Alevizos, I.; Illei, G.G. MicroRNAs in Sjögren's syndrome as a prototypic autoimmune disease. *Autoimmun. Rev.* **2010**, *9*, 618–621. [CrossRef]
51. Mendell, J.T. miRiad roles for the miR-17-92 cluster in development and disease. *Cell* **2008**, *133*, 217–222. [CrossRef]
52. Xiao, C.; Srinivasan, L.; Calado, D.P.; Patterson, H.C.; Zhang, B.; Wang, J.; Henderson, J.M.; Kutok, J.L.; Rajewsky, K. Lymphoproliferative disease and autoimmunity in mice with increased miR-17-92 expression in lymphocytes. *Nat. Immunol.* **2008**, *9*, 405–414. [CrossRef] [PubMed]
53. Zilahi, E.; Tarr, T.; Papp, G.; Griger, Z.; Sipka, S.; Zeher, M. Increased microRNA-146a/b, TRAF6 gene and decreased IRAK1 gene expressions in the peripheral mononuclear cells of patients with Sjögren's syndrome. *Immunol. Lett.* **2012**, *141*, 165–168. [CrossRef] [PubMed]
54. Liu, A.; Tetzlaff, M.T.; Vanbelle, P.; Elder, D.; Feldman, M.; Tobias, J.W.; Sepulveda, A.R.; Xu, X. MicroRNA expression profiling outperforms mRNA expression profiling in formalin-fixed paraffin-embedded tissues. *Int. J. Clin. Exp. Pathol.* **2009**, *2*, 519–527. [PubMed]
55. Howe, K. Extraction of miRNAs from Formalin-Fixed Paraffin-Embedded (FFPE) Tissues. *Methods Mol. Biol.* **2017**, *1509*, 17–24. [CrossRef] [PubMed]
56. Zhou, Z.; Sun, B.; Huang, S.; Zhao, L. Roles of circular RNAs in immune regulation and autoimmune diseases. *Cell Death Dis.* **2019**, *10*, 1–13. [CrossRef]
57. Xia, X.; Tang, X.; Wang, S. Roles of CircRNAs in Autoimmune Diseases. *Front. Immunol.* **2019**, *10*. [CrossRef]
58. Su, L.-C.; Xu, W.-D.; Liu, X.-Y.; Fu, L.; Huang, A.-F. Altered expression of circular RNA in primary Sjögren's syndrome. *Clin. Rheumatol.* **2019**, *38*, 3425–3433. [CrossRef]
59. Roy, S.; Awasthi, A. Emerging roles of noncoding RNAs in T cell differentiation and functions in autoimmune diseases. *Int. Rev. Immunol.* **2019**, *38*, 232–245. [CrossRef]
60. Dolcino, M.; Tinazzi, E.; Vitali, C.; Del Papa, N.; Puccetti, A.; Lunardi, C. Long Non-Coding RNAs Modulate Sjögren's Syndrome Associated Gene Expression and Are Involved in the Pathogenesis of the Disease. *J. Clin. Med.* **2019**, *8*, 1349. [CrossRef]
61. Han, S.-B.; Moratz, C.; Huang, N.-N.; Kelsall, B.; Cho, H.; Shi, C.-S.; Schwartz, O.; Kehrl, J.H. Rgs1 and Gnai2 regulate the entrance of B lymphocytes into lymph nodes and B cell motility within lymph node follicles. *Immunity* **2005**, *22*, 343–354. [CrossRef]
62. Coca, A.; Sanz, I. Updates on B-cell immunotherapies for systemic lupus erythematosus and Sjogren's syndrome. *Curr. Opin. Rheumatol.* **2012**, *24*, 451–456. [CrossRef] [PubMed]
63. Béguelin, W.; Teater, M.; Gearhart, M.D.; Calvo Fernández, M.T.; Goldstein, R.L.; Cárdenas, M.G.; Hatzi, K.; Rosen, M.; Shen, H.; Corcoran, C.M.; et al. EZH2 and BCL6 Cooperate to Assemble CBX8-BCOR Complex to Repress Bivalent Promoters, Mediate Germinal Center Formation and Lymphomagenesis. *Cancer Cell* **2016**, *30*, 197–213. [CrossRef] [PubMed]
64. Bai, M.; Skyrlas, A.; Agnantis, N.J.; Kamina, S.; Tsanou, E.; Grepi, C.; Galani, V.; Kanavaros, P. Diffuse large B-cell lymphomas with germinal center B-cell-like differentiation immunophenotypic profile are associated with high apoptotic index, high expression of the proapoptotic proteins bax, bak and bid and low expression of the antiapoptotic protein bcl-xl. *Mod. Pathol.* **2004**, *17*, 847–856. [CrossRef] [PubMed]
65. Yang, L.; Wei, W.; He, X.; Xie, Y.; Kamal, M.A.; Li, J. Influence of Hormones on Sjögren's Syndrome. *Curr. Pharm. Des.* **2018**, *24*, 4167–4176. [CrossRef] [PubMed]
66. McCoy, S.S.; Sampene, E.; Baer, A.N. Sjögren's Syndrome is Associated With Reduced Lifetime Sex Hormone Exposure: A Case-Control Study. *Arthritis Care Res.* **2019**, acr.24014. [CrossRef] [PubMed]
67. Harris, V.M.; Sharma, R.; Cavett, J.; Kurien, B.T.; Liu, K.; Koelsch, K.A.; Rasmussen, A.; Radfar, L.; Lewis, D.; Stone, D.U.; et al. Klinefelter's syndrome (47,XXY) is in excess among men with Sjögren's syndrome. *Clin. Immunol.* **2016**, *168*, 25–29. [CrossRef] [PubMed]
68. Seminog, O.O.; Seminog, A.B.; Yeates, D.; Goldacre, M.J. Associations between Klinefelter's syndrome and autoimmune diseases: English national record linkage studies. *Autoimmunity* **2015**, *48*, 125–128. [CrossRef]
69. Fujimoto, M.; Ikeda, K.; Nakamura, T.; Iwamoto, T.; Furuta, S.; Nakajima, H. Development of mixed connective tissue disease and Sjögren's syndrome in a patient with trisomy X. *Lupus* **2015**, *24*, 1217–1220. [CrossRef]

70. Morthen, M.K.; Tellefsen, S.; Richards, S.M.; Lieberman, S.M.; Rahimi Darabad, R.; Kam, W.R.; Sullivan, D.A. Testosterone Influence on Gene Expression in Lacrimal Glands of Mouse Models of Sjögren Syndrome. *Investig. Ophthalmol. Vis. Sci.* **2019**, *60*, 2181–2197. [CrossRef]
71. Porola, P.; Laine, M.; Virtanen, I.; Pöllänen, R.; Przybyla, B.D.; Konttinen, Y.T. Androgens and Integrins in Salivary Glands in Sjögren's Syndrome. *J. Rheumatol.* **2010**, *37*, 1181–1187. [CrossRef]
72. Taiym, S.; Haghighat, N.; Al-Hashimi, I. A comparison of the hormone levels in patients with Sjogren's syndrome and healthy controls. *Oral Surg. Oral Med. Oral Pathol. Oral Radiol. Endod.* **2004**, *97*, 579–583. [CrossRef] [PubMed]
73. Bizzarro, A.; Valentini, G.; Martino, G.D.; Daponte, A.; De Bellis, A.; Iacono, G. Influence of Testosterone Therapy on Clinical and Immunological Features of Autoimmune Diseases Associated with Klinefelter's Syndrome. *J. Clin. Endocrinol. Metab.* **1987**, *64*, 32–36. [CrossRef] [PubMed]
74. Ishimaru, N.; Arakaki, R.; Watanabe, M.; Kobayashi, M.; Miyazaki, K.; Hayashi, Y. Development of autoimmune exocrinopathy resembling Sjögren's syndrome in estrogen-deficient mice of healthy background. *Am. J. Pathol.* **2003**, *163*, 1481–1490. [CrossRef]
75. Iwasa, A.; Arakaki, R.; Honma, N.; Ushio, A.; Yamada, A.; Kondo, T.; Kurosawa, E.; Kujiraoka, S.; Tsunematsu, T.; Kudo, Y.; et al. Aromatase Controls Sjögren Syndrome–Like Lesions through Monocyte Chemotactic Protein-1 in Target Organ and Adipose Tissue–Associated Macrophages. *Am. J. Pathol.* **2015**, *185*, 151–161. [CrossRef]
76. Shim, G.-J.; Warner, M.; Kim, H.-J.; Andersson, S.; Liu, L.; Ekman, J.; Imamov, O.; Jones, M.E.; Simpson, E.R.; Gustafsson, J.-A. Aromatase-deficient mice spontaneously develop a lymphoproliferative autoimmune disease resembling Sjogren's syndrome. *Proc. Natl. Acad. Sci. USA* **2004**, *101*, 12628–12633. [CrossRef]
77. Ishimaru, N.; Arakaki, R.; Omotehara, F.; Yamada, K.; Mishima, K.; Saito, I.; Hayashi, Y. Novel Role for RbAp48 in Tissue-Specific, Estrogen Deficiency-Dependent Apoptosis in the Exocrine Glands. *Mol. Cell. Biol.* **2006**, *26*, 2924–2935. [CrossRef]
78. Ishimaru, N.; Arakaki, R.; Yoshida, S.; Yamada, A.; Noji, S.; Hayashi, Y. Expression of the retinoblastoma protein RbAp48 in exocrine glands leads to Sjögren's syndrome–like autoimmune exocrinopathy. *J. Exp. Med.* **2008**, *205*, 2915–2927. [CrossRef]
79. Manoussakis, M.N.; Tsinti, M.; Kapsogeorgou, E.K.; Moutsopoulos, H.M. The salivary gland epithelial cells of patients with primary Sjögren's syndrome manifest significantly reduced responsiveness to 17β-estradiol. *J. Autoimmun.* **2012**, *39*, 64–68. [CrossRef]
80. Laroche, M.; Borg, S.; Lassoued, S.; De Lafontan, B.; Roché, H. Joint pain with aromatase inhibitors: Abnormal frequency of Sjögren's syndrome. *J. Rheumatol.* **2007**, *34*, 2259–2263.
81. Shanmugam, V.K.; McCloskey, J.; Elston, B.; Allison, S.J.; Eng-Wong, J. The CIRAS study: A case control study to define the clinical, immunologic, and radiographic features of aromatase inhibitor-induced musculoskeletal symptoms. *Breast Cancer Res. Treat.* **2012**, *131*, 699–708. [CrossRef]
82. Guidelli, G.M.; Martellucci, I.; Galeazzi, M.; Francini, G.; Fioravanti, A. Sjögren's syndrome and aromatase inhibitors treatment: Is there a link? *Clin. Exp. Rheumatol.* **2013**, *31*, 653–654. [PubMed]
83. Laine, M.; Porola, P.; Udby, L.; Kjeldsen, L.; Cowland, J.B.; Borregaard, N.; Hietanen, J.; Ståhle, M.; Pihakari, A.; Konttinen, Y.T. Low salivary dehydroepiandrosterone and androgen-regulated cysteine-rich secretory protein 3 levels in Sjögren's syndrome. *Arthritis Rheum.* **2007**, *56*, 2575–2584. [CrossRef] [PubMed]
84. Konttinen, Y.T.; Fuellen, G.; Bing, Y.; Porola, P.; Stegaev, V.; Trokovic, N.; Falk, S.S.I.; Liu, Y.; Szodoray, P.; Takakubo, Y. Sex steroids in Sjögren's syndrome. *J. Autoimmun.* **2012**, *39*, 49–56. [CrossRef]
85. Spaan, M.; Porola, P.; Laine, M.; Rozman, B.; Azuma, M.; Konttinen, Y.T. Healthy human salivary glands contain a DHEA-sulphate processing intracrine machinery, which is deranged in primary Sjögren's syndrome. *J. Cell. Mol. Med.* **2009**, *13*, 1261–1270. [CrossRef] [PubMed]
86. Moutsopoulos, H.M.; Kordossis, T. Sjögren's syndrome revisited: Autoimmune epithelitis. *Br. J. Rheumatol.* **1996**, *35*, 204–206. [CrossRef] [PubMed]
87. Spachidou, M.P.; Bourazopoulou, E.; Maratheftis, C.I.; Kapsogeorgou, E.K.; Moutsopoulos, H.M.; Tzioufas, A.G.; Manoussakis, M.N. Expression of functional Toll-like receptors by salivary gland epithelial cells: Increased mRNA expression in cells derived from patients with primary Sjögren's syndrome. *Clin. Exp. Immunol.* **2007**, *147*, 497–503. [CrossRef] [PubMed]
88. Chen, J.-Q.; Szodoray, P.; Zeher, M. Toll-Like Receptor Pathways in Autoimmune Diseases. *Clin. Rev. Allergy Immunol.* **2016**, *50*, 1–17. [CrossRef] [PubMed]

89. Spachidou, M.; Kapsogeorgou, E.; Bourazopoulou, E.; Moutsopoulos, H.; Manoussakis, M. Cultured salivary gland epithelial cells from patients with primary Sjögren's syndrome and disease controls are sensitive to signaling via Toll-like receptors 2 and 3: Upregulation of intercellular adhesion molecule-1 expression. *Arthritis Res. Ther.* **2005**, *7*, P154. [CrossRef]
90. Iwanaszko, M.; Kimmel, M. NF-κB and IRF pathways: Cross-regulation on target genes promoter level. *BMC Genom.* **2015**, *16*, 307. [CrossRef]
91. Ichiyama, T.; Nakatani, E.; Tatsumi, K.; Hideshima, K.; Urano, T.; Nariai, Y.; Sekine, J. Expression of aquaporin 3 and 5 as a potential marker for distinguishing dry mouth from Sjögren's syndrome. *J. Oral Sci.* **2018**, *60*, 212–220. [CrossRef]
92. Beroukas, D.; Hiscock, J.; Gannon, B.J.; Jonsson, R.; Gordon, T.P.; Waterman, S.A. Selective down-regulation of aquaporin-1 in salivary glands in primary Sjögren's syndrome. *Lab. Investig. J. Tech. Methods Pathol.* **2002**, *82*, 1547–1552. [CrossRef] [PubMed]
93. Sisto, M.; Lorusso, L.; Ingravallo, G.; Nico, B.; Ribatti, D.; Ruggieri, S.; Lofrumento, D.D.; Lisi, S. Abnormal distribution of AQP4 in minor salivary glands of primary Sjögren's syndrome patients. *Autoimmunity* **2017**, *50*, 202–210. [CrossRef] [PubMed]
94. Ring, T.; Kallenbach, M.; Praetorius, J.; Nielsen, S.; Melgaard, B. Successful treatment of a patient with primary Sjögren's syndrome with Rituximab. *Clin. Rheumatol.* **2006**, *25*, 891–894. [CrossRef] [PubMed]
95. Hua, Y.; Ying, X.; Qian, Y.; Liu, H.; Lan, Y.; Xie, A.; Zhu, X. Physiological and pathological impact of AQP1 knockout in mice. *Biosci. Rep.* **2019**, *39*. [CrossRef]
96. Verkman, A.S.; Yang, B.; Song, Y.; Manley, G.T.; Ma, T. Role of water channels in fluid transport studied by phenotype analysis of aquaporin knockout mice. *Exp. Physiol.* **2000**, *85*, 233S–241S. [CrossRef]
97. Hosoi, K.; Yao, C.; Hasegawa, T.; Yoshimura, H.; Akamatsu, T. Dynamics of Salivary Gland AQP5 under Normal and Pathologic Conditions. *Int. J. Mol. Sci.* **2020**, *21*, 1182. [CrossRef]
98. Delporte, C.; Bryla, A.; Perret, J. Aquaporins in Salivary Glands: From Basic Research to Clinical Applications. *Int. J. Mol. Sci.* **2016**, *17*, 166. [CrossRef]
99. Steinfeld, S.; Cogan, E.; King, L.S.; Agre, P.; Kiss, R.; Delporte, C. Abnormal distribution of aquaporin-5 water channel protein in salivary glands from Sjögren's syndrome patients. *Lab. Investig. J. Tech. Methods Pathol.* **2001**, *81*, 143–148. [CrossRef]
100. Soyfoo, M.S.; De Vriese, C.; Debaix, H.; Martin-Martinez, M.D.; Mathieu, C.; Devuyst, O.; Steinfeld, S.D.; Delporte, C. Modified aquaporin 5 expression and distribution in submandibular glands from NOD mice displaying autoimmune exocrinopathy. *Arthritis Rheum.* **2007**, *56*, 2566–2574. [CrossRef]
101. Yoshimura, S.; Nakamura, H.; Horai, Y.; Nakajima, H.; Shiraishi, H.; Hayashi, T.; Takahashi, T.; Kawakami, A. Abnormal distribution of AQP5 in labial salivary glands is associated with poor saliva secretion in patients with Sjögren's syndrome including neuromyelitis optica complicated patients. *Mod. Rheumatol.* **2016**, *26*, 384–390. [CrossRef]
102. Lee, B.H.; Gauna, A.E.; Perez, G.; Park, Y.; Pauley, K.M.; Kawai, T.; Cha, S. Autoantibodies against Muscarinic Type 3 Receptor in Sjögren's Syndrome Inhibit Aquaporin 5 Trafficking. *PLoS ONE* **2013**, *8*. [CrossRef] [PubMed]
103. Roche, J.V.; Törnroth-Horsefield, S. Aquaporin Protein-Protein Interactions. *Int. J. Mol. Sci.* **2017**, *18*, 2255. [CrossRef] [PubMed]
104. Ohashi, Y.; Tsuzaka, K.; Takeuchi, T.; Sasaki, Y.; Tsubota, K. Altered distribution of aquaporin 5 and its C-terminal binding protein in the lacrimal glands of a mouse model for Sjögren's syndrome. *Curr. Eye Res.* **2008**, *33*, 621–629. [CrossRef]
105. Soyfoo, M.S.; Konno, A.; Bolaky, N.; Oak, J.S.; Fruman, D.; Nicaise, C.; Takiguchi, M.; Delporte, C. Link between inflammation and aquaporin-5 distribution in submandibular gland in Sjögren's syndrome? *Oral Dis.* **2012**, *18*, 568–574. [CrossRef] [PubMed]
106. Soyfoo, M.S.; Bolaky, N.; Depoortere, I.; Delporte, C. Relationship between aquaporin-5 expression and saliva flow in streptozotocin-induced diabetic mice? *Oral Dis.* **2012**, *18*, 501–505. [CrossRef]
107. Jin, J.-O.; Yu, Q. T Cell-Associated Cytokines in the Pathogenesis of Sjögren's Syndrome. *J. Clin. Cell. Immunol.* **2013**, *S1*. [CrossRef] [PubMed]
108. Fox, R.I.; Kang, H.I.; Ando, D.; Abrams, J.; Pisa, E. Cytokine mRNA expression in salivary gland biopsies of Sjögren's syndrome. *J. Immunol. 1950* **1994**, *152*, 5532–5539.

109. Boumba, D.; Skopouli, F.N.; Moutsopoulos, H.M. Cytokine mRNA expression in the labial salivary gland tissues from patients with primary Sjögren's syndrome. *Br. J. Rheumatol.* **1995**, *34*, 326–333. [CrossRef]
110. Sumida, T.; Tsuboi, H.; Iizuka, M.; Hirota, T.; Asashima, H.; Matsumoto, I. The role of M3 muscarinic acetylcholine receptor reactive T cells in Sjögren's syndrome: A critical review. *J. Autoimmun.* **2014**, *51*, 44–50. [CrossRef]
111. Zhou, J.; Jin, J.-O.; Kawai, T.; Yu, Q. Endogenous programmed death ligand-1 restrains the development and onset of Sjögren's syndrome in non-obese diabetic mice. *Sci. Rep.* **2016**, *6*, 1–12. [CrossRef]
112. Arce-Franco, M.; Dominguez-Luis, M.; Pec, M.K.; Martínez-Gimeno, C.; Miranda, P.; Alvarez de la Rosa, D.; Giraldez, T.; García-Verdugo, J.M.; Machado, J.D.; Díaz-González, F. Functional effects of proinflammatory factors present in Sjögren's syndrome salivary microenvironment in an in vitro model of human salivary gland. *Sci. Rep.* **2017**, *7*, 1–12. [CrossRef] [PubMed]
113. Kang, E.H.; Lee, Y.J.; Hyon, J.Y.; Yun, P.Y.; Song, Y.W. Salivary cytokine profiles in primary Sjögren's syndrome differ from those in non-Sjögren sicca in terms of TNF-α levels and Th-1/Th-2 ratios. *Clin. Exp. Rheumatol.* **2011**, *29*, 970–976. [PubMed]
114. Yamamura, Y.; Motegi, K.; Kani, K.; Takano, H.; Momota, Y.; Aota, K.; Yamanoi, T.; Azuma, M. TNF-α inhibits aquaporin 5 expression in human salivary gland acinar cells via suppression of histone H4 acetylation. *J. Cell. Mol. Med.* **2012**, *16*, 1766–1775. [CrossRef] [PubMed]
115. Zhou, J.; Kawai, T.; Yu, Q. Pathogenic role of endogenous TNF-α in the development of Sjögren's-like sialadenitis and secretory dysfunction in non-obese diabetic mice. *Lab. Investig.* **2017**, *97*, 458–467. [CrossRef] [PubMed]
116. Fox, R.I.; Adamson, T.C.; Fong, S.; Young, C.; Howell, F.V. Characterization of the phenotype and function of lymphocytes infiltrating the salivary gland in patients with primary Sjogren syndrome. *Diagn. Immunol.* **1983**, *1*, 233–239. [PubMed]
117. Roescher, N.; Tak, P.P.; Illei, G.G. Cytokines in Sjögren's syndrome. *Oral Dis.* **2009**, *15*, 519–526. [CrossRef]
118. Fox, R.I.; Kang, H.I. Pathogenesis of Sjögren's syndrome. *Rheum. Dis. Clin. N. Am.* **1992**, *18*, 517–538.
119. Bertorello, R.; Cordone, M.P.; Contini, P.; Rossi, P.; Indiveri, F.; Puppo, F.; Cordone, G. Increased levels of interleukin-10 in saliva of Sjögren's syndrome patients. Correlation with disease activity. *Clin. Exp. Med.* **2004**, *4*, 148–151. [CrossRef]
120. Youinou, P.; Pers, J.-O. Disturbance of cytokine networks in Sjögren's syndrome. *Arthritis Res. Ther.* **2011**, *13*, 227. [CrossRef]
121. Ohlsson, M.; Jonsson, R.; Brokstad, K.A. Subcellular redistribution and surface exposure of the Ro52, Ro60 and La48 autoantigens during apoptosis in human ductal epithelial cells: A possible mechanism in the pathogenesis of Sjögren's syndrome. *Scand. J. Immunol.* **2002**, *56*, 456–469. [CrossRef]
122. Davies, M.L.; Taylor, E.J.; Gordon, C.; Young, S.P.; Welsh, K.; Bunce, M.; Wordsworth, B.P.; Davidson, B.; Bowman, S.J. Candidate T cell epitopes of the human La/SSB autoantigen. *Arthritis Rheum.* **2002**, *46*, 209–214. [CrossRef]
123. Hasegawa, H.; Inoue, A.; Kohno, M.; Muraoka, M.; Miyazaki, T.; Terada, M.; Nakayama, T.; Yoshie, O.; Nose, M.; Yasukawa, M. Antagonist of interferon-inducible protein 10/CXCL10 ameliorates the progression of autoimmune sialadenitis in MRL/lpr mice. *Arthritis Rheum.* **2006**, *54*, 1174–1183. [CrossRef] [PubMed]
124. Kong, L.; Ogawa, N.; Nakabayashi, T.; Liu, G.T.; D'Souza, E.; McGuff, H.S.; Guerrero, D.; Talal, N.; Dang, H. Fas and Fas ligand expression in the salivary glands of patients with primary Sjögren's syndrome. *Arthritis Rheum.* **1997**, *40*, 87–97. [CrossRef] [PubMed]
125. Ibrahem, H.M. B cell dysregulation in primary Sjögren's syndrome: A review. *Jpn. Dent. Sci. Rev.* **2019**, *55*, 139–144. [CrossRef] [PubMed]
126. Verstappen, G.M.; Corneth, O.B.J.; Bootsma, H.; Kroese, F.G.M. Th17 cells in primary Sjögren's syndrome: Pathogenicity and plasticity. *J. Autoimmun.* **2018**, *87*, 16–25. [CrossRef]
127. Katsifis, G.E.; Rekka, S.; Moutsopoulos, N.M.; Pillemer, S.; Wahl, S.M. Systemic and local interleukin-17 and linked cytokines associated with Sjögren's syndrome immunopathogenesis. *Am. J. Pathol.* **2009**, *175*, 1167–1177. [CrossRef]
128. Sonnenberg, G.F.; Nair, M.G.; Kirn, T.J.; Zaph, C.; Fouser, L.A.; Artis, D. Pathological versus protective functions of IL-22 in airway inflammation are regulated by IL-17A. *J. Exp. Med.* **2010**, *207*, 1293–1305. [CrossRef]

129. Lavoie, T.N.; Stewart, C.M.; Berg, K.M.; Li, Y.; Nguyen, C.Q. Expression of interleukin-22 in Sjögren's syndrome: Significant correlation with disease parameters. *Scand. J. Immunol.* **2011**, *74*, 377–382. [CrossRef]
130. Monteiro, R.; Martins, C.; Barcelos, F.; Nunes, G.; Lopes, T.; Borrego, L.-M. Follicular helper and follicular cytotoxic T cells in primary Sjögren's Syndrome: Clues for an abnormal antiviral response as a pathogenic mechanism. *Ann. Med.* **2019**, *51*, 42. [CrossRef]
131. Saito, M.; Otsuka, K.; Ushio, A.; Yamada, A.; Arakaki, R.; Kudo, Y.; Ishimaru, N. Unique Phenotypes and Functions of Follicular Helper T Cells and Regulatory T Cells in Sjögren's Syndrome. *Curr. Rheumatol. Rev.* **2018**, *14*, 239–245. [CrossRef]
132. Scheid, J.F.; Mouquet, H.; Kofer, J.; Yurasov, S.; Nussenzweig, M.C.; Wardemann, H. Differential regulation of self-reactivity discriminates between IgG+ human circulating memory B cells and bone marrow plasma cells. *Proc. Natl. Acad. Sci. USA* **2011**. [CrossRef] [PubMed]
133. Mouquet, H.; Nussenzweig, M.C. Polyreactive antibodies in adaptive immune responses to viruses. *Cell. Mol. Life Sci.* **2012**, *69*, 1435–1445. [CrossRef] [PubMed]
134. Corsiero, E.; Sutcliffe, N.; Pitzalis, C.; Bombardieri, M. Accumulation of self-reactive naïve and memory B cell reveals sequential defects in B cell tolerance checkpoints in Sjögren's syndrome. *PLoS ONE* **2014**, *9*, e114575. [CrossRef] [PubMed]
135. Samuels, J.; Ng, Y.-S.; Coupillaud, C.; Paget, D.; Meffre, E. Impaired early B cell tolerance in patients with rheumatoid arthritis. *J. Exp. Med.* **2005**, *201*, 1659–1667. [CrossRef]
136. Mietzner, B.; Tsuiji, M.; Scheid, J.; Velinzon, K.; Tiller, T.; Abraham, K.; Gonzalez, J.B.; Pascual, V.; Stichweh, D.; Wardemann, H.; et al. Autoreactive IgG memory antibodies in patients with systemic lupus erythematosus arise from nonreactive and polyreactive precursors. *Proc. Natl. Acad. Sci. USA* **2008**, *105*, 9727–9732. [CrossRef]
137. Hayakawa, I.; Tedder, T.F.; Zhuang, Y. B-lymphocyte depletion ameliorates Sjögren's syndrome in Id3 knockout mice. *Immunology* **2007**, *122*, 73–79. [CrossRef]
138. Baff and April: A Tutorial on B Cell Survival. PubMed NCBI. Available online: https://www.ncbi.nlm.nih.gov/pubmed/12427767 (accessed on 2 April 2020).
139. Pers, J.-O.; Daridon, C.; Devauchelle, V.; Jousse, S.; Saraux, A.; Jamin, C.; Youinou, P. BAFF overexpression is associated with autoantibody production in autoimmune diseases. *Ann. N. Y. Acad. Sci.* **2005**, *1050*, 34–39. [CrossRef]
140. Nieuwenhuis, P.; Opstelten, D. Functional anatomy of germinal centers. *Am. J. Anat.* **1984**, *170*, 421–435. [CrossRef]
141. Maeda, T.; Wakasawa, T.; Shima, Y.; Tsuboi, I.; Aizawa, S.; Tamai, I. Role of polyamines derived from arginine in differentiation and proliferation of human blood cells. *Biol. Pharm. Bull.* **2006**, *29*, 234–239. [CrossRef]
142. Meyer-Hermann, M. A mathematical model for the germinal center morphology and affinity maturation. *J. Theor. Biol.* **2002**, *216*, 273–300. [CrossRef]
143. Jonsson, M.V.; Skarstein, K. Follicular dendritic cells confirm lymphoid organization in the minor salivary glands of primary Sjögren's syndrome. *J. Oral Pathol. Med.* **2008**, *37*, 515–521. [CrossRef] [PubMed]
144. Jonsson, M.V.; Skarstein, K.; Jonsson, R.; Brun, J.G. Serological implications of germinal center-like structures in primary Sjögren's syndrome. *J. Rheumatol.* **2007**, *34*, 2044–2049.
145. Salomonsson, S.; Jonsson, M.V.; Skarstein, K.; Brokstad, K.A.; Hjelmström, P.; Wahren-Herlenius, M.; Jonsson, R. Cellular basis of ectopic germinal center formation and autoantibody production in the target organ of patients with Sjögren's syndrome. *Arthritis Rheum.* **2003**, *48*, 3187–3201. [CrossRef] [PubMed]
146. Johnsen, S.J.; Brun, J.G.; Gøransson, L.G.; Småstuen, M.C.; Johannesen, T.B.; Haldorsen, K.; Harboe, E.; Jonsson, R.; Meyer, P.A.; Omdal, R. Risk of non-Hodgkin's lymphoma in primary Sjögren's syndrome: A population-based study. *Arthritis Care Res.* **2013**, *65*, 816–821. [CrossRef] [PubMed]
147. Theander, E.; Henriksson, G.; Ljungberg, O.; Mandl, T.; Manthorpe, R.; Jacobsson, L.T.H. Lymphoma and other malignancies in primary Sjögren's syndrome: A cohort study on cancer incidence and lymphoma predictors. *Ann. Rheum. Dis.* **2006**, *65*, 796–803. [CrossRef]
148. Nardi, N.; Brito-Zerón, P.; Ramos-Casals, M.; Aguiló, S.; Cervera, R.; Ingelmo, M.; Font, J. Circulating auto-antibodies against nuclear and non-nuclear antigens in primary Sjögren's syndrome: Prevalence and clinical significance in 335 patients. *Clin. Rheumatol.* **2006**, *25*, 341–346. [CrossRef]
149. Jones, B. Lacrimal and salivary precipitating antibodies in Sjögren's syndrome. *Lancet* **1958**, *272*, 773–776. [CrossRef]

150. Anderson, J.R.; Gray, K.; Beck, J.S.; Kinnear, W.F. Precipitating autoantibodies in Sjögren's syndrome. *Lancet* **1961**, *278*, 456–460. [CrossRef]
151. Espinosa, A.; Dardalhon, V.; Brauner, S.; Ambrosi, A.; Higgs, R.; Quintana, F.J.; Sjöstrand, M.; Eloranta, M.L.; Ní Gabhann, J.; Winqvist, O.; et al. Loss of the lupus autoantigen Ro52/Trim21 induces tissue inflammation and systemic autoimmunity by disregulating the IL-23-Th17 pathway. *J. Exp. Med.* **2009**, *206*, 1661–1671. [CrossRef]
152. Keene, J.D. Molecular structure of the La and Ro autoantigens and their use in autoimmune diagnostics. *J. Autoimmun.* **1989**, *2*, 329–334. [CrossRef]
153. Elkon, K.B.; Gharavi, A.E.; Hughes, G.R.; Moutsoupoulos, H.M. Autoantibodies in the sicca syndrome (primary Sjögren's syndrome). *Ann. Rheum. Dis.* **1984**, *43*, 243–245. [CrossRef] [PubMed]
154. Baer, A.N.; McAdams DeMarco, M.; Shiboski, S.C.; Lam, M.Y.; Challacombe, S.; Daniels, T.E.; Dong, Y.; Greenspan, J.S.; Kirkham, B.W.; Lanfranchi, H.E.; et al. The SSB-positive/SSA-negative antibody profile is not associated with key phenotypic features of Sjögren's syndrome. *Ann. Rheum. Dis.* **2015**, *74*, 1557–1561. [CrossRef] [PubMed]
155. Manoussakis, M.N.; Pange, P.J.; Moutsopulos, H.M. The autoantibody profile in Sjögren's syndrome. *Ter. Arkh.* **1988**, *60*, 17–20. [PubMed]
156. Mavragani, C.P.; Tzioufas, A.G.; Moutsopoulos, H.M. Sjögren's syndrome: Autoantibodies to cellular antigens. Clinical and molecular aspects. *Int. Arch. Allergy Immunol.* **2000**, *123*, 46–57. [CrossRef]
157. Bournia, V.-K.K.; Diamanti, K.D.; Vlachoyiannopoulos, P.G.; Moutsopoulos, H.M. Anticentromere antibody positive Sjögren's Syndrome: A retrospective descriptive analysis. *Arthritis Res. Ther.* **2010**, *12*, R47. [CrossRef]
158. Salliot, C.; Gottenberg, J.-E.; Bengoufa, D.; Desmoulins, F.; Miceli-Richard, C.; Mariette, X. Anticentromere antibodies identify patients with Sjögren's syndrome and autoimmune overlap syndrome. *J. Rheumatol.* **2007**, *34*, 2253–2258.
159. Bournia, V.-K.; Vlachoyiannopoulos, P.G. Subgroups of Sjögren syndrome patients according to serological profiles. *J. Autoimmun.* **2012**, *39*, 15–26. [CrossRef]
160. Kyriakidis, N.C.; Kapsogeorgou, E.K.; Tzioufas, A.G. A comprehensive review of autoantibodies in primary Sjögren's syndrome: Clinical phenotypes and regulatory mechanisms. *J. Autoimmun.* **2014**, *51*, 67–74. [CrossRef]
161. Takemoto, F.; Hoshino, J.; Sawa, N.; Tamura, Y.; Tagami, T.; Yokota, M.; Katori, H.; Yokoyama, K.; Ubara, Y.; Hara, S.; et al. Autoantibodies against carbonic anhydrase II are increased in renal tubular acidosis associated with Sjogren syndrome. *Am. J. Med.* **2005**, *118*, 181–184. [CrossRef]
162. Nishimori, I.; Bratanova, T.; Toshkov, I.; Caffrey, T.; Mogaki, M.; Shibata, Y.; Hollingsworth, M.A. Induction of experimental autoimmune sialoadenitis by immunization of PL/J mice with carbonic anhydrase II. *J. Immunol. 1950* **1995**, *154*, 4865–4873.
163. Takemoto, F.; Katori, H.; Sawa, N.; Hoshino, J.; Suwabe, T.; Sogawa, Y.; Nomura, K.; Nakanishi, S.; Higa, Y.; Kanbayashi, H.; et al. Induction of anti-carbonic-anhydrase-II antibody causes renal tubular acidosis in a mouse model of Sjögren's syndrome. *Nephron Physiol.* **2007**, *106*, p63–p68. [CrossRef] [PubMed]
164. Jeon, S.; Lee, J.; Park, S.-H.; Kim, H.-D.; Choi, Y. Associations of Anti-Aquaporin 5 Autoantibodies with Serologic and Histopathological Features of Sjögren's Syndrome. *J. Clin. Med.* **2019**, *8*, 1863. [CrossRef] [PubMed]
165. Clinical Associations of Autoantibodies to Human Muscarinic Acetylcholine Receptor 3 (213–228) in Primary Sjögren's Syndrome. PubMed NCBI. Available online: https://www.ncbi.nlm.nih.gov/pubmed/?term=10.1093%2Frheumatology%2Fkeh672 (accessed on 2 April 2020).
166. Sordet, C.; Gottenberg, J.E.; Goetz, J.; Bengoufa, D.; Humbel, R.-L.; Mariette, X.; Sibilia, J. Anti-α-fodrin autoantibodies are not useful diagnostic markers of primary Sjögren's syndrome. *Ann. Rheum. Dis.* **2005**, *64*, 1244–1245. [CrossRef] [PubMed]
167. Applbaum, E.; Lichtbroun, A. Novel Sjögren's autoantibodies found in fibromyalgia patients with sicca and/or xerostomia. *Autoimmun. Rev.* **2019**, *18*, 199–202. [CrossRef] [PubMed]
168. Martín-Nares, E.; Hernández-Molina, G. Novel autoantibodies in Sjögren's syndrome: A comprehensive review. *Autoimmun. Rev.* **2019**, *18*, 192–198. [CrossRef] [PubMed]
169. De Langhe, E.; Bossuyt, X.; Shen, L.; Malyavantham, K.; Ambrus, J.L.; Suresh, L. Evaluation of Autoantibodies in Patients with Primary and Secondary Sjogren's Syndrome. *Open Rheumatol. J.* **2017**, *11*, 10–15. [CrossRef]

170. Jin, Y.; Li, J.; Chen, J.; Shao, M.; Zhang, R.; Liang, Y.; Zhang, X.; Zhang, X.; Zhang, Q.; Li, F.; et al. Tissue-Specific Autoantibodies Improve Diagnosis of Primary Sjögren's Syndrome in the Early Stage and Indicate Localized Salivary Injury. *J. Immunol. Res.* **2019**, *2019*, 1–8. [CrossRef]
171. Suresh, L.; Malyavantham, K.; Shen, L.; Ambrus, J.L. Investigation of novel autoantibodies in Sjogren's syndrome utilizing Sera from the Sjogren's international collaborative clinical alliance cohort. *BMC Ophthalmol.* **2015**, *15*, 38. [CrossRef]
172. Shen, L.; Suresh, L.; Lindemann, M.; Xuan, J.; Kowal, P.; Malyavantham, K.; Ambrus, J.L. Novel autoantibodies in Sjogren's syndrome. *Clin. Immunol.* **2012**, *145*, 251–255. [CrossRef]
173. Xuan, J.; Wang, Y.; Xiong, Y.; Qian, H.; He, Y.; Shi, G. Investigation of autoantibodies to SP-1 in Chinese patients with primary Sjögren's syndrome. *Clin. Immunol.* **2018**, *188*, 58–63. [CrossRef]
174. Everett, S.; Vishwanath, S.; Cavero, V.; Shen, L.; Suresh, L.; Malyavantham, K.; Lincoff-Cohen, N.; Ambrus, J.L. Analysis of novel Sjogren's syndrome autoantibodies in patients with dry eyes. *BMC Ophthalmol.* **2017**, *17*, 20. [CrossRef] [PubMed]
175. Hubschman, S.; Rojas, M.; Kalavar, M.; Kloosterboer, A.; Sabater, A.L.; Galor, A. Association Between Early Sjögren Markers and Symptoms and Signs of Dry Eye. *Cornea* **2020**, *39*, 311–315. [CrossRef] [PubMed]
176. Uchida, K.; Akita, Y.; Matsuo, K.; Fujiwara, S.; Nakagawa, A.; Kazaoka, Y.; Hachiya, H.; Naganawa, Y.; Oh-Iwa, I.; Ohura, K.; et al. Identification of specific autoantigens in Sjögren's syndrome by SEREX. *Immunology* **2005**, *116*, 53–63. [CrossRef] [PubMed]
177. Liu, Y.; Liao, X.; Wang, Y.; Chen, S.; Sun, Y.; Lin, Q.; Shi, G. Autoantibody to MDM2: A potential serological marker of primary Sjogren's syndrome. *Oncotarget* **2017**, *8*, 14306–14313. [CrossRef] [PubMed]
178. Nozawa, K.; Ikeda, K.; Satoh, M.; Reeves, W.H.; Stewart, C.M.; Li, Y.-C.; Yen, T.J.; Rios, R.M.; Takamori, K.; Ogawa, H.; et al. Autoantibody to NA14 is an independent marker primarily for Sjogren's syndrome. *Front. Biosci. Landmark Ed.* **2009**, *14*, 3733–3739. [CrossRef] [PubMed]
179. Uomori, K.; Nozawa, K.; Ikeda, K.; Doe, K.; Yamada, Y.; Yamaguchi, A.; Fujishiro, M.; Kawasaki, M.; Morimoto, S.; Takamori, K.; et al. A re-evaluation of anti-NA-14 antibodies in patients with primary Sjögren's syndrome: Significant role of interferon-γ in the production of autoantibodies against NA-14. *Autoimmunity* **2016**, *49*, 347–356. [CrossRef]
180. Duda, S.; Witte, T.; Stangel, M.; Adams, J.; Schmidt, R.E.; Baerlecken, N.T. Autoantibodies binding to stathmin-4: New marker for polyneuropathy in primary Sjögren's syndrome. *Immunol. Res.* **2017**, *65*, 1099–1102. [CrossRef]
181. Fiorentino, D.F.; Presby, M.; Baer, A.N.; Petri, M.; Rieger, K.E.; Soloski, M.; Rosen, A.; Mammen, A.L.; Christopher-Stine, L.; Casciola-Rosen, L. PUF60: A prominent new target of the autoimmune response in dermatomyositis and Sjögren's syndrome. *Ann. Rheum. Dis.* **2016**, *75*, 1145–1151. [CrossRef]
182. Tay, S.H.; Fairhurst, A.-M.; Mak, A. Clinical utility of circulating anti-N-methyl-d-aspartate receptor subunits NR2A/B antibody for the diagnosis of neuropsychiatric syndromes in systemic lupus erythematosus and Sjögren's syndrome: An updated meta-analysis. *Autoimmun. Rev.* **2017**, *16*, 114–122. [CrossRef]
183. Lauvsnes, M.B.; Beyer, M.K.; Kvaløy, J.T.; Greve, O.J.; Appenzeller, S.; Kvivik, I.; Harboe, E.; Tjensvoll, A.B.; Gøransson, L.G.; Omdal, R. Association of hippocampal atrophy with cerebrospinal fluid antibodies against the NR2 subtype of the N-methyl-D-aspartate receptor in patients with systemic lupus erythematosus and patients with primary Sjögren's syndrome. *Arthritis Rheumatol.* **2014**, *66*, 3387–3394. [CrossRef]
184. Wolska, N.; Rybakowska, P.; Rasmussen, A.; Brown, M.; Montgomery, C.; Klopocki, A.; Grundahl, K.; Scofield, R.H.; Radfar, L.; Stone, D.U.; et al. Brief Report: Patients With Primary Sjögren's Syndrome Who Are Positive for Autoantibodies to Tripartite Motif-Containing Protein 38 Show Greater Disease Severity. *Arthritis Rheumatol.* **2016**, *68*, 724–729. [CrossRef] [PubMed]
185. Alunno, A.; Bistoni, O.; Carubbi, F.; Valentini, V.; Cafaro, G.; Bartoloni, E.; Giacomelli, R.; Gerli, R. Prevalence and significance of anti-saccharomyces cerevisiae antibodies in primary Sjögren's syndrome. *Clin. Exp. Rheumatol.* **2018**, *36*, 73–79. [PubMed]
186. Birnbaum, J.; Hoke, A.; Lalji, A.; Calabresi, P.; Bhargava, P.; Casciola-Rosen, L. Brief Report: Anti-Calponin 3 Autoantibodies: A Newly Identified Specificity in Patients With Sjögren's Syndrome. *Arthritis Rheumatol.* **2018**, *70*, 1610–1616. [CrossRef]
187. Mukaino, A.; Nakane, S.; Higuchi, O.; Nakamura, H.; Miyagi, T.; Shiroma, K.; Tokashiki, T.; Fuseya, Y.; Ochi, K.; Umeda, M.; et al. Insights from the ganglionic acetylcholine receptor autoantibodies in patients with Sjögren's syndrome. *Mod. Rheumatol.* **2016**, *26*, 708–715. [CrossRef] [PubMed]

188. Birnbaum, J.; Atri, N.M.; Baer, A.N.; Cimbro, R.; Montagne, J.; Casciola-Rosen, L. Relationship Between Neuromyelitis Optica Spectrum Disorder and Sjögren's Syndrome: Central Nervous System Extraglandular Disease or Unrelated, Co-Occurring Autoimmunity?: Relationship Between Sjögren's Syndrome and NMOSD. *Arthritis Care Res.* **2017**, *69*, 1069–1075. [CrossRef] [PubMed]
189. Tzartos, J.S.; Stergiou, C.; Daoussis, D.; Zisimopoulou, P.; Andonopoulos, A.P.; Zolota, V.; Tzartos, S.J. Antibodies to aquaporins are frequent in patients with primary Sjögren's syndrome. *Rheumatology* **2017**, *56*, 2114–2122. [CrossRef] [PubMed]
190. Hu, Y.-H.; Zhou, P.-F.; Long, G.-F.; Tian, X.; Guo, Y.-F.; Pang, A.-M.; Di, R.; Shen, Y.-N.; Liu, Y.-D.; Cui, Y.-J. Elevated Plasma P-Selectin Autoantibodies in Primary Sjögren Syndrome Patients with Thrombocytopenia. *Med. Sci. Monit.* **2015**, *21*, 3690–3695. [CrossRef]
191. Bergum, B.; Koro, C.; Delaleu, N.; Solheim, M.; Hellvard, A.; Binder, V.; Jonsson, R.; Valim, V.; Hammenfors, D.S.; Jonsson, M.V.; et al. Antibodies against carbamylated proteins are present in primary Sjögren's syndrome and are associated with disease severity. *Ann. Rheum. Dis.* **2016**, *75*, 1494–1500. [CrossRef]
192. Pecani, A.; Alessandri, C.; Spinelli, F.R.; Priori, R.; Riccieri, V.; Di Franco, M.; Ceccarelli, F.; Colasanti, T.; Pendolino, M.; Mancini, R.; et al. Prevalence, sensitivity and specificity of antibodies against carbamylated proteins in a monocentric cohort of patients with rheumatoid arthritis and other autoimmune rheumatic diseases. *Arthritis Res. Ther.* **2016**, *18*, 276. [CrossRef]
193. Zhang, Y.; Hussain, M.; Yang, X.; Chen, P.; Yang, C.; Xun, Y.; Tian, Y.; Du, H. Identification of Moesin as a Novel Autoantigen in Patients with Sjögren's Syndrome. *Protein Pept. Lett.* **2018**, *25*, 350–355. [CrossRef]
194. Cui, L.; Elzakra, N.; Xu, S.; Xiao, G.G.; Yang, Y.; Hu, S. Investigation of three potential autoantibodies in Sjogren's syndrome and associated MALT lymphoma. *Oncotarget* **2017**, *8*, 30039–30049. [CrossRef] [PubMed]
195. Nezos, A.; Cinoku, I.; Mavragani, C.P.; Moutsopoulos, H.M. Antibodies against citrullinated alpha enolase peptides in primary Sjogren's syndrome. *Clin. Immunol.* **2017**, *183*, 300–303. [CrossRef] [PubMed]
196. Segerberg-Konttinen, M.; Konttinen, Y.T.; Bergroth, V. Focus score in the diagnosis of Sjögren's syndrome. *Scand. J. Rheumatol. Suppl.* **1986**, *61*, 47–51. [PubMed]
197. Bodeutsch, C.; de Wilde, P.C.; Kater, L.; van Houwelingen, J.C.; van den Hoogen, F.H.; Kruize, A.A.; Hené, R.J.; van de Putte, L.B.; Vooijs, G.P. Quantitative immunohistologic criteria are superior to the lymphocytic focus score criterion for the diagnosis of Sjögren's syndrome. *Arthritis Rheum.* **1992**, *35*, 1075–1087. [CrossRef]
198. Barrera, M.J.; Bahamondes, V.; Sepúlveda, D.; Quest, A.F.G.; Castro, I.; Cortés, J.; Aguilera, S.; Urzúa, U.; Molina, C.; Pérez, P.; et al. Sjögren's syndrome and the epithelial target: A comprehensive review. *J. Autoimmun.* **2013**, *42*, 7–18. [CrossRef]
199. Pérez, P.; Goicovich, E.; Alliende, C.; Aguilera, S.; Leyton, C.; Molina, C.; Pinto, R.; Romo, R.; Martinez, B.; González, M.J. Differential expression of matrix metalloproteinases in labial salivary glands of patients with primary Sjögren's syndrome. *Arthritis Rheum.* **2000**, *43*, 2807–2817. [CrossRef]
200. Sun, D.; Emmert-Buck, M.R.; Fox, P.C. Differential cytokine mRNA expression in human labial minor salivary glands in primary Sjögren's syndrome. *Autoimmunity* **1998**, *28*, 125–137. [CrossRef]
201. Molina, C.; Alliende, C.; Aguilera, S.; Kwon, Y.-J.; Leyton, L.; Martínez, B.; Leyton, C.; Pérez, P.; González, M.-J. Basal lamina disorganisation of the acini and ducts of labial salivary glands from patients with Sjögren's syndrome: Association with mononuclear cell infiltration. *Ann. Rheum. Dis.* **2006**, *65*, 178–183. [CrossRef]
202. Ng, W.-F.; Bowman, S.J. Primary Sjogren's syndrome: Too dry and too tired. *Rheumatology* **2010**, *49*, 844–853. [CrossRef]
203. Hackett, K.L.; Gotts, Z.M.; Ellis, J.; Deary, V.; Rapley, T.; Ng, W.-F.; Newton, J.L.; Deane, K.H.O. An investigation into the prevalence of sleep disturbances in primary Sjögren's syndrome: A systematic review of the literature. *Rheumatology* **2017**, *56*, 570–580. [CrossRef]
204. Wang, H.-C.; Chang, K.; Lin, C.-Y.; Chen, Y.-H.; Lu, P.-L. Periodic fever as the manifestation of primary Sjogren's syndrome: A case report and literature review. *Clin. Rheumatol.* **2012**, *31*, 1517–1519. [CrossRef] [PubMed]
205. Voulgarelis, M.; Moutsopoulos, H.M. Mucosa-associated lymphoid tissue lymphoma in Sjögren's syndrome: Risks, management, and prognosis. *Rheum. Dis. Clin. N. Am.* **2008**, *34*, 921–933. [CrossRef] [PubMed]
206. Kassan, S.S.; Moutsopoulos, H.M. Clinical manifestations and early diagnosis of Sjögren syndrome. *Arch. Intern. Med.* **2004**, *164*, 1275–1284. [CrossRef]

207. Retamozo, S.; Acar-Denizli, N.; Rasmussen, A.; Horváth, I.F.; Baldini, C.; Priori, R.; Sandhya, P.; Hernandez-Molina, G.; Armagan, B.; Praprotnik, S.; et al. Systemic manifestations of primary Sjögren's syndrome out of the ESSDAI classification: Prevalence and clinical relevance in a large international, multi-ethnic cohort of patients. *Clin. Exp. Rheumatol.* **2019**, *37*, 97–106. [PubMed]
208. López-Pintor, R.M.; Fernández Castro, M.; Hernández, G. Oral involvement in patients with primary Sjögren's syndrome. Multidisciplinary care by dentists and rheumatologists. *Reumatol. Clin.* **2015**, *11*, 387–394. [CrossRef] [PubMed]
209. Generali, E.; Costanzo, A.; Mainetti, C.; Selmi, C. Cutaneous and Mucosal Manifestations of Sjögren's Syndrome. *Clin. Rev. Allergy Immunol.* **2017**, *53*, 357–370. [CrossRef] [PubMed]
210. Ramos-Casals, M.; Brito-Zerón, P.; Bombardieri, S.; Bootsma, H.; De Vita, S.; Dörner, T.; Fisher, B.A.; Gottenberg, J.-E.; Hernandez-Molina, G.; Kocher, A.; et al. EULAR recommendations for the management of Sjögren's syndrome with topical and systemic therapies. *Ann. Rheum. Dis.* **2020**, *79*, 3–18. [CrossRef]
211. Ramos-Casals, M.; Brito-Zerón, P.; Seror, R.; Bootsma, H.; Bowman, S.J.; Dörner, T.; Gottenberg, J.-E.; Mariette, X.; Theander, E.; Bombardieri, S.; et al. Characterization of systemic disease in primary Sjögren's syndrome: EULAR-SS Task Force recommendations for articular, cutaneous, pulmonary and renal involvements. *Rheumatology* **2015**, *54*, 2230–2238. [CrossRef]
212. Mirouse, A.; Seror, R.; Vicaut, E.; Mariette, X.; Dougados, M.; Fauchais, A.-L.; Deroux, A.; Dellal, A.; Costedoat-Chalumeau, N.; Denis, G.; et al. Arthritis in primary Sjögren's syndrome: Characteristics, outcome and treatment from French multicenter retrospective study. *Autoimmun. Rev.* **2019**, *18*, 9–14. [CrossRef]
213. Vitali, C.; Del Papa, N. Pain in primary Sjögren's syndrome. *Best Pract. Res. Clin. Rheumatol.* **2015**, *29*, 63–70. [CrossRef]
214. Atzeni, F.; Cazzola, M.; Benucci, M.; Di Franco, M.; Salaffi, F.; Sarzi-Puttini, P. Chronic widespread pain in the spectrum of rheumatological diseases. *Best Pract. Res. Clin. Rheumatol.* **2011**, *25*, 165–171. [CrossRef]
215. Alunno, A.; Carubbi, F.; Bartoloni, E.; Cipriani, P.; Giacomelli, R.; Gerli, R. The kaleidoscope of neurological manifestations in primary Sjögren's syndrome. *Clin. Exp. Rheumatol.* **2019**, *37*, 192–198.
216. Flament, T.; Bigot, A.; Chaigne, B.; Henique, H.; Diot, E.; Marchand-Adam, S. Pulmonary manifestations of Sjögren's syndrome. *Eur. Respir. Rev.* **2016**, *25*, 110–123. [CrossRef] [PubMed]
217. Hatron, P.-Y.; Tillie-Leblond, I.; Launay, D.; Hachulla, E.; Fauchais, A.L.; Wallaert, B. Pulmonary manifestations of Sjögren's syndrome. *Presse Med. 1983* **2011**, *40*, e49–e64. [CrossRef] [PubMed]
218. Tavoni, A.; Vitali, C.; Cirigliano, G.; Frigelli, S.; Stampacchia, G.; Bombardieri, S. Shrinking lung in primary Sjögren's syndrome. *Arthritis Rheum.* **1999**, *42*, 2249–2250. [CrossRef]
219. Singh, R.; Huang, W.; Menon, Y.; Espinoza, L.R. Shrinking lung syndrome in systemic lupus erythematosus and Sjogren's syndrome. *J. Clin. Rheumatol.* **2002**, *8*, 340–345. [CrossRef] [PubMed]
220. Langenskiöld, E.; Bonetti, A.; Fitting, J.W.; Heinzer, R.; Dudler, J.; Spertini, F.; Lazor, R. Shrinking lung syndrome successfully treated with rituximab and cyclophosphamide. *Respiration* **2012**, *84*, 144–149. [CrossRef]
221. Blanco Pérez, J.J.; Pérez González, A.; Guerra Vales, J.L.; Melero Gonzalez, R.; Pego Reigosa, J.M. Shrinking Lung in Primary Sjogrën Syndrome Successfully Treated with Rituximab. *Arch. Bronconeumol.* **2015**, *51*, 475–476. [CrossRef] [PubMed]
222. Baenas, D.F.; Retamozo, S.; Pirola, J.P.; Caeiro, F. Shrinking lung syndrome and pleural effusion as an initial manifestation of primary Sjögren's syndrome. Síndrome de pulmón encogido y derrame pleural como manifestación inicial de síndrome de Sjögren primario. *Rheumatol. Clin.* **2020**, *16*, 65–68. [CrossRef]
223. Uslu, S.; Köken Avşar, A.; Erez, Y.; Sarı, İ. Shrinking Lung Syndrome in Primary Sjögren Syndrome. *Balk. Med. J.* **2020**. [CrossRef]
224. Liang, M.; Bao, L.; Xiong, N.; Jin, B.; Ni, H.; Zhang, J.; Zou, H.; Luo, X.; Li, J. Cardiac arrhythmias as the initial manifestation of adult primary Sjögren's syndrome: A case report and literature review. *Int. J. Rheum. Dis.* **2015**, *18*, 800–806. [CrossRef] [PubMed]
225. Sung, M.J.; Park, S.-H.; Kim, S.-K.; Lee, Y.-S.; Park, C.-Y.; Choe, J.-Y. Complete atrioventricular block in adult Sjögren's syndrome with anti-Ro autoantibody. *Kor. J. Intern. Med.* **2011**, *26*, 213–215. [CrossRef] [PubMed]
226. Popov, Y.; Salomon-Escoto, K. Gastrointestinal and Hepatic Disease in Sjogren Syndrome. *Rheum. Dis. Clin. N. Am.* **2018**, *44*, 143–151. [CrossRef] [PubMed]
227. Ebert, E.C. Gastrointestinal and hepatic manifestations of Sjogren syndrome. *J. Clin. Gastroenterol.* **2012**, *46*, 25–30. [CrossRef] [PubMed]

228. Evans, R.; Zdebik, A.; Ciurtin, C.; Walsh, S.B. Renal involvement in primary Sjögren's syndrome. *Rheumatology* **2015**, *54*, 1541–1548. [CrossRef] [PubMed]
229. Geng, Y.; Zhao, Y.; Zhang, Z. Tubulointerstitial nephritis-induced hypophosphatemic osteomalacia in Sjögren's syndrome: A case report and review of the literature. *Clin. Rheumatol.* **2018**, *37*, 257–263. [CrossRef]
230. Gu, X.; Su, Z.; Chen, M.; Xu, Y.; Wang, Y. Acquired Gitelman syndrome in a primary Sjögren syndrome patient with a SLC12A3 heterozygous mutation: A case report and literature review. *Nephrology* **2017**, *22*, 652–655. [CrossRef]
231. Darrieutort-Laffite, C.; André, V.; Hayem, G.; Saraux, A.; Le Guern, V.; Le Jeunne, C.; Puéchal, X. Sjögren's syndrome complicated by interstitial cystitis: A case series and literature review. *Joint Bone Spine* **2015**, *82*, 245–250. [CrossRef]
232. Manganelli, P.; Fietta, P.; Quaini, F. Hematologic manifestations of primary Sjögren's syndrome. *Clin. Exp. Rheumatol.* **2006**, *24*, 438–448.
233. Ramos-Casals, M.; Font, J.; Garcia-Carrasco, M.; Brito, M.-P.; Rosas, J.; Calvo-Alen, J.; Pallares, L.; Cervera, R.; Ingelmo, M. Primary Sjögren syndrome: Hematologic patterns of disease expression. *Medicine* **2002**, *81*, 281–292. [CrossRef]
234. Yamashita, H.; Takahashi, Y.; Kaneko, H.; Kano, T.; Mimori, A. Thrombotic thrombocytopenic purpura with an autoantibody to ADAMTS13 complicating Sjögren's syndrome: Two cases and a literature review. *Mod. Rheumatol.* **2013**, *23*, 365–373. [CrossRef] [PubMed]
235. Xu, X.; Zhu, T.; Wu, D.; Zhang, L. Sjögren's syndrome initially presented as thrombotic thrombocytopenic purpura in a male patient: A case report and literature review. *Clin. Rheumatol.* **2018**, *37*, 1421–1426. [CrossRef] [PubMed]
236. Sun, R.; Gu, W.; Ma, Y.; Wang, J.; Wu, M. Relapsed/refractory acquired thrombotic thrombocytopenic purpura in a patient with Sjögren syndrome: Case report and review of the literature. *Medicine* **2018**, *97*, e12989. [CrossRef]
237. García-Montoya, L.; Sáenz-Tenorio, C.N.; Janta, I.; Menárguez, J.; López-Longo, F.J.; Monteagudo, I.; Naredo, E. Hemophagocytic lymphohistiocytosis in a patient with Sjögren's syndrome: Case report and review. *Rheumatol. Int.* **2017**, *37*, 663–669. [CrossRef] [PubMed]
238. Hernandez-Molina, G.; Faz-Munoz, D.; Astudillo-Angel, M.; Iturralde-Chavez, A.; Reyes, E. Coexistance of Amyloidosis and Primary Sjögren's Syndrome: An Overview. *Curr. Rheumatol. Rev.* **2018**, *14*, 231–238. [CrossRef] [PubMed]
239. Freeman, S.R.M.; Sheehan, P.Z.; Thorpe, M.A.; Rutka, J.A. Ear, Nose, and Throat Manifestations of Sjögren's Syndrome: Retrospective Review of a Multidisciplinary Clinic. *J. Otolaryngol.* **2005**, *34*, 20. [CrossRef] [PubMed]
240. Midilli, R.; Gode, S.; Oder, G.; Kabasakal, Y.; Karci, B. Nasal and paranasal involvement in primary Sjogren's syndrome. *Rhinol. J.* **2013**, *51*, 265–267. [CrossRef] [PubMed]
241. Belafsky, P.C.; Postma, G.N. The laryngeal and esophageal manifestations of Sjögren's syndrome. *Curr. Rheumatol. Rep.* **2003**, *5*, 297–303. [CrossRef]
242. Rodriguez, M.A.; Tapanes, F.J.; Stekman, I.L.; Pinto, J.A.; Camejo, O.; Abadi, I. Auricular chondritis and diffuse proliferative glomerulonephritis in primary Sjogren's syndrome. *Ann. Rheum. Dis.* **1989**, *48*, 683–685. [CrossRef]
243. Tumiati, B. Hearing Loss in the Sjogren Syndrome. *Ann. Intern. Med.* **1997**, *126*, 450. [CrossRef]
244. Isik, H.; Isik, M.; Aynioglu, O.; Karcaaltincaba, D.; Sahbaz, A.; Beyazcicek, T.; Harma, M.I.; Demircan, N. Are the women with Sjögren's Syndrome satisfied with their sexual activity? *Rev. Bras. Reumatol. Engl. Ed.* **2017**, *57*, 210–216. [CrossRef] [PubMed]
245. Capone, C.; Buyon, J.P.; Friedman, D.M.; Frishman, W.H. Cardiac Manifestations of Neonatal Lupus: A Review of Autoantibody-associated Congenital Heart Block and its Impact in an Adult Population. *Cardiol. Rev.* **2012**, *20*, 72–76. [CrossRef]
246. Picone, O.; Alby, C.; Frydman, R.; Mariette, X. Sjögren syndrome in Obstetric and Gynecology: Literature review. *J. Gynecol. Obstet. Biol. Reprod.* **2006**, *35*, 169–175. [CrossRef]
247. Costedoat-Chalumeau, N.; Amoura, Z.; Villain, E.; Cohen, L.; Fermont, L.; Le Thi Huong, D.; Vauthier, D.; Georgin-Lavialle, S.; Wechsler, B.; Dommergues, M.; et al. Prise en charge obstétricale des patientes à risque de « lupus néonatal ». *J. Gynécologie Obstétrique Biol. Reprod.* **2006**, *35*, 146–156. [CrossRef]

248. Upala, S.; Yong, W.C.; Sanguankeo, A. Association between primary Sjögren's syndrome and pregnancy complications: A systematic review and meta-analysis. *Clin. Rheumatol.* **2016**, *35*, 1949–1955. [CrossRef]
249. Brito-Zerón, P.; Theander, E.; Baldini, C.; Seror, R.; Retamozo, S.; Quartuccio, L.; Bootsma, H.; Bowman, S.J.; Dörner, T.; Gottenberg, J.-E.; et al. Early diagnosis of primary Sjögren's syndrome: EULAR-SS task force clinical recommendations. *Expert Rev. Clin. Immunol.* **2016**, *12*, 137–156. [CrossRef]
250. Vitali, C.; Bombardieri, S.; Jonsson, R.; Moutsopoulos, H.M.; Alexander, E.L.; Carsons, S.E.; Daniels, T.E.; Fox, P.C.; Fox, R.I.; Kassan, S.S.; et al. Classification criteria for Sjögren's syndrome: A revised version of the European criteria proposed by the American-European Consensus Group. *Ann. Rheum. Dis.* **2002**, *61*, 554–558. [CrossRef]
251. Shiboski, S.C.; Shiboski, C.H.; Criswell, L.A.; Baer, A.N.; Challacombe, S.; Lanfranchi, H.; Schiødt, M.; Umehara, H.; Vivino, F.; Zhao, Y.; et al. American College of Rheumatology classification criteria for Sjögren's syndrome: A data-driven, expert consensus approach in the Sjögren's International Collaborative Clinical Alliance cohort. *Arthritis Care Res.* **2012**, *64*, 475–487. [CrossRef]
252. Shiboski, C.H.; Shiboski, S.C.; Seror, R.; Criswell, L.A.; Labetoulle, M.; Lietman, T.M.; Rasmussen, A.; Scofield, H.; Vitali, C.; Bowman, S.J.; et al. 2016 American College of Rheumatology/European League Against Rheumatism Classification Criteria for Primary Sjögren's Syndrome: A Consensus and Data-Driven Methodology Involving Three International Patient Cohorts. *Arthritis Rheumatol.* **2017**, *69*, 35–45. [CrossRef]
253. Begley, C.; Caffery, B.; Chalmers, R.; Situ, P.; Simpson, T.; Nelson, J.D. Review and analysis of grading scales for ocular surface staining. *Ocul. Surf.* **2019**, *7*, 208–220. [CrossRef]
254. Baldini, C.; Zabotti, A.; Filipovic, N.; Vukicevic, A.; Luciano, N.; Ferro, F.; Lorenzon, M.; De Vita, S. Imaging in primary Sjögren's syndrome: The "obsolete and the new". *Clin. Exp. Rheumatol.* **2018**, *36*, 215–221. [PubMed]
255. Schall, G.L.; Anderson, L.G.; Wolf, R.O.; Herdt, J.R.; Tarpley, T.M.; Cummings, N.A.; Zeiger, L.S.; Talal, N. Xerostomia in Sjögren's syndrome. Evaluation by sequential salivary scintigraphy. *JAMA* **1971**, *216*, 2109–2116. [CrossRef]
256. Vinagre, F.; Santos, M.J.; Prata, A.; da Silva, J.C.; Santos, A.I. Assessment of salivary gland function in Sjögren's syndrome: The role of salivary gland scintigraphy. *Autoimmun. Rev.* **2009**, *8*, 672–676. [CrossRef] [PubMed]
257. Zhou, M.; Song, S.; Wu, S.; Duan, T.; Chen, L.; Ye, J.; Xiao, J. Diagnostic accuracy of salivary gland ultrasonography with different scoring systems in Sjögren's syndrome: A systematic review and meta-analysis. *Sci. Rep.* **2018**, *8*, 17128. [CrossRef] [PubMed]
258. Jousse-Joulin, S.; Milic, V.; Jonsson, M.V.; Plagou, A.; Theander, E.; Luciano, N.; Rachele, P.; Baldini, C.; Bootsma, H.; Vissink, A.; et al. Is salivary gland ultrasonography a useful tool in Sjögren's syndrome? A systematic review. *Rheumatology* **2016**, *55*, 789–800. [CrossRef]
259. Nimwegen, J.F.; Mossel, E.; Delli, K.; Ginkel, M.S.; Stel, A.J.; Kroese, F.G.M.; Spijkervet, F.K.L.; Vissink, A.; Arends, S.; Bootsma, H. Incorporation of Salivary Gland Ultrasonography Into the American College of Rheumatology/European League Against Rheumatism Criteria for Primary Sjögren's Syndrome. *Arthritis Care Res.* **2020**, *72*, 583–590. [CrossRef] [PubMed]
260. Fisher, B.A.; Everett, C.C.; Rout, J.; O'Dwyer, J.L.; Emery, P.; Pitzalis, C.; Ng, W.-F.; Carr, A.; Pease, C.T.; Price, E.J.; et al. Effect of rituximab on a salivary gland ultrasound score in primary Sjögren's syndrome: Results of the TRACTISS randomised double-blind multicentre substudy. *Ann. Rheum. Dis.* **2018**, *77*, 412–416. [CrossRef] [PubMed]
261. Jousse-Joulin, S.; Devauchelle-Pensec, V.; Cornec, D.; Marhadour, T.; Bressollette, L.; Gestin, S.; Pers, J.O.; Nowak, E.; Saraux, A. Brief Report: Ultrasonographic Assessment of Salivary Gland Response to Rituximab in Primary Sjögren's Syndrome: Ultrasonographic response to Rituximab in primary SS. *Arthritis Rheumatol.* **2015**, *67*, 1623–1628. [CrossRef]
262. Varela-Centelles, P.; Seoane-Romero, J.-M.; Sánchez-Sánchez, M.; González-Mosquera, A.; Diz-Dios, P.; Seoane, J. Minor salivary gland biopsy in Sjögren's syndrome: A review and introduction of a new tool to ease the procedure. *Med. Oral Patol. Oral Cirugia Bucal* **2014**, *19*, e20–e23. [CrossRef]
263. Spijkervet, F.K.L.; Haacke, E.; Kroese, F.G.M.; Bootsma, H.; Vissink, A. Parotid Gland Biopsy, the Alternative Way to Diagnose Sjögren Syndrome. *Rheum. Dis. Clin. N. Am.* **2016**, *42*, 485–499. [CrossRef]

264. Fisher, B.A.; Jonsson, R.; Daniels, T.; Bombardieri, M.; Brown, R.M.; Morgan, P.; Bombardieri, S.; Ng, W.-F.; Tzioufas, A.G.; Vitali, C.; et al. Standardisation of labial salivary gland histopathology in clinical trials in primary Sjögren's syndrome. *Ann. Rheum. Dis.* **2017**, *76*, 1161–1168. [CrossRef] [PubMed]
265. Chisholm, D.M.; Mason, D.K. Labial salivary gland biopsy in Sjogren's disease. *J. Clin. Pathol.* **1968**, *21*, 656–660. [CrossRef] [PubMed]
266. Greenspan, J.S.; Daniels, T.E.; Talal, N.; Sylvester, R.A. The histopathology of Sjögren's syndrome in labial salivary gland biopsies. *Oral Surg. Oral Med. Oral Pathol.* **1974**, *37*, 217–229. [CrossRef]
267. Guellec, D.; Cornec, D.; Jousse-Joulin, S.; Marhadour, T.; Marcorelles, P.; Pers, J.-O.; Saraux, A.; Devauchelle-Pensec, V. Diagnostic value of labial minor salivary gland biopsy for Sjögren's syndrome: A systematic review. *Autoimmun. Rev.* **2013**, *12*, 416–420. [CrossRef]
268. Campos, J.; Hillen, M.R.; Barone, F. Salivary Gland Pathology in Sjögren's Syndrome. *Rheum. Dis. Clin. N. Am.* **2016**, *42*, 473–483. [CrossRef]
269. Barone, F.; Campos, J.; Bowman, S.; Fisher, B.A. The value of histopathological examination of salivary gland biopsies in diagnosis, prognosis and treatment of Sjögren's Syndrome. *Swiss Med. Wkly.* **2015**, *145*, w14168. [CrossRef]
270. Pijpe, J.; Kalk, W.W.I.; van der Wal, J.E.; Vissink, A.; Kluin, P.M.; Roodenburg, J.L.N.; Bootsma, H.; Kallenberg, C.G.M.; Spijkervet, F.K.L. Parotid gland biopsy compared with labial biopsy in the diagnosis of patients with primary Sjogren's syndrome. *Rheumatology* **2006**, *46*, 335–341. [CrossRef]
271. Marx, R.E.; Hartman, K.S.; Rethman, K.V. A prospective study comparing incisional labial to incisional parotid biopsies in the detection and confirmation of sarcoidosis, Sjögren's disease, sialosis and lymphoma. *J. Rheumatol.* **1988**, *15*, 621–629.
272. Franceschini, F.; Cavazzana, I. Anti-Ro/SSA and La/SSB antibodies. *Autoimmunity* **2005**, *38*, 55–63. [CrossRef]
273. Tzioufas, A.G.; Tatouli, I.P.; Moutsopoulos, H.M. Autoantibodies in Sjögren's syndrome: Clinical presentation and regulatory mechanisms. *Presse Med. 1983* **2012**, *41*, e451–e460. [CrossRef]
274. Trevisani, V.F.M.; Pasoto, S.G.; Fernandes, M.L.M.S.; Lopes, M.L.L.; de Magalhães Souza Fialho, S.C.; Pinheiro, A.C.; dos Santos, L.C.; Appenzeller, S.; Fidelix, T.; Ribeiro, S.L.E.; et al. Recommendations from the Brazilian society of rheumatology for the diagnosis of Sjögren's syndrome (Part I): Glandular manifestations (systematic review). *Adv. Rheumatol.* **2019**, *59*, 58. [CrossRef]
275. Robbins, A.; Hentzien, M.; Toquet, S.; Didier, K.; Servettaz, A.; Pham, B.-N.; Giusti, D. Diagnostic Utility of Separate Anti-Ro60 and Anti-Ro52/TRIM21 Antibody Detection in Autoimmune Diseases. *Front. Immunol.* **2019**, *10*, 444. [CrossRef]
276. Kontny, E.; Lewandowska-Poluch, A.; Chmielińska, M.; Olesińska, M. Subgroups of Sjögren's syndrome patients categorised by serological profiles: Clinical and immunological characteristics. *Reumatologia* **2018**, *56*, 346–353. [CrossRef] [PubMed]
277. Brito-Zerón, P.; Retamozo, S.; Ramos-Casals, M. Phenotyping Sjögren's syndrome: Towards a personalised management of the disease. *Clin. Exp. Rheumatol.* **2018**, *36*, 198–209.
278. Cornec, D.; Saraux, A.; Jousse-Joulin, S.; Pers, J.O.; Boisramé-Gastrin, S.; Renaudineau, Y.; Gauvin, Y.; Roguedas-Contios, A.M.; Genestet, S.; Chastaing, M.; et al. The Differential Diagnosis of Dry Eyes, Dry Mouth, and Parotidomegaly: A Comprehensive Review. *Clin. Rev. Allergy. Immunol.* **2015**, *49*, 278–287. [CrossRef] [PubMed]
279. Moutsopoulos, H.M.; Chused, T.M.; Mann, D.L.; Klippel, J.H.; Fauci, A.S.; Frank, M.M.; Lawley, T.J.; Hamburger, M.I. Sjögren's syndrome (Sicca syndrome): Current issues. *Ann. Intern. Med.* **1980**, *92*, 212–226. [CrossRef] [PubMed]
280. Fragoulis, G.E.; Fragkioudaki, S.; Reilly, J.H.; Kerr, S.C.; McInnes, I.B.; Moutsopoulos, H.M. Analysis of the cell populations composing the mononuclear cell infiltrates in the labial minor salivary glands from patients with rheumatoid arthritis and sicca syndrome. *J. Autoimmun.* **2016**, *73*, 85–91. [CrossRef] [PubMed]
281. Manoussakis, M.N.; Georgopoulou, C.; Zintzaras, E.; Spyropoulou, M.; Stavropoulou, A.; Skopouli, F.N.; Moutsopoulos, H.M. Sjögren's syndrome associated with systemic lupus erythematosus: Clinical and laboratory profiles and comparison with primary Sjögren's syndrome. *Arthritis Rheum.* **2004**, *50*, 882–891. [CrossRef]
282. Salliot, C.; Mouthon, L.; Ardizzone, M.; Sibilia, J.; Guillevin, L.; Gottenberg, J.E.; Mariette, X. Sjogren's syndrome is associated with and not secondary to systemic sclerosis. *Rheumatology* **2007**, *46*, 321–326. [CrossRef]

283. Rojas-Villarraga, A.; Amaya-Amaya, J.; Rodriguez-Rodriguez, A.; Mantilla, R.D.; Anaya, J.M. Introducing polyautoimmunity: Secondary autoimmune diseases no longer exist. *Autoimmune Dis.* **2012**, *2012*, 254319. [CrossRef] [PubMed]
284. Kollert, F.; Fisher, B.A. Equal rights in autoimmunity: Is Sjögren's syndrome ever 'secondary'? *Rheumatology* **2020**, *59*, 1218–1225. [CrossRef] [PubMed]
285. Singh, A.G.; Singh, S.; Matteson, E.L. Rate, risk factors and causes of mortality in patients with Sjögren's syndrome: A systematic review and meta-analysis of cohort studies. *Rheumatology* **2016**, *55*, 450–460. [CrossRef] [PubMed]
286. Liang, Y.; Yang, Z.; Qin, B.; Zhong, R. Primary Sjogren's syndrome and malignancy risk: A systematic review and meta-analysis. *Ann. Rheum. Dis.* **2014**, *73*, 1151–1156. [CrossRef] [PubMed]
287. Zintzaras, E.; Voulgarelis, M.; Moutsopoulos, H.M. The risk of lymphoma development in autoimmune diseases: A meta-analysis. *Arch. Intern. Med.* **2005**, *165*, 2337–2344. [CrossRef] [PubMed]
288. Jonsson, M.V.; Theander, E.; Jonsson, R. Predictors for the development of non-Hodgkin lymphoma in primary Sjögren's syndrome. *Presse Med. 1983* **2012**, *41*, e511–e516. [CrossRef] [PubMed]
289. Nishishinya, M.B.; Pereda, C.A.; Muñoz-Fernández, S.; Pego-Reigosa, J.M.; Rúa-Figueroa, I.; Andreu, J.-L.; Fernández-Castro, M.; Rosas, J.; Loza Santamaría, E. Identification of lymphoma predictors in patients with primary Sjögren's syndrome: A systematic literature review and meta-analysis. *Rheumatol. Int.* **2015**, *35*, 17–26. [CrossRef]
290. Papageorgiou, A.; Voulgarelis, M.; Tzioufas, A.G. Clinical picture, outcome and predictive factors of lymphoma in Sjögren syndrome. *Autoimmun. Rev.* **2015**, *14*, 641–649. [CrossRef]
291. Hernandez-Molina, G.; Michel-Peregrina, M.; Bermúdez-Bermejo, P.; Sánchez-Guerrero, J. Early and late extraglandular manifestations in primary Sjögren's syndrome. *Clin. Exp. Rheumatol.* **2012**, *30*, 455.
292. Ter Borg, E.J.; Kelder, J.C. Development of new extra-glandular manifestations or associated auto-immune diseases after establishing the diagnosis of primary Sjögren's syndrome: A long-term study of the Antonius Nieuwegein Sjögren (ANS) cohort. *Rheumatol. Int.* **2017**, *37*, 1153–1158. [CrossRef]
293. Seror, R.; Meiners, P.; Baron, G.; Bootsma, H.; Bowman, S.J.; Vitali, C.; Gottenberg, J.-E.; Theander, E.; Tzioufas, A.; De Vita, S.; et al. Development of the ClinESSDAI: A clinical score without biological domain. A tool for biological studies. *Ann. Rheum. Dis.* **2016**, *75*, 1945–1950. [CrossRef]
294. Seror, R.; Ravaud, P.; Bowman, S.J.; Baron, G.; Tzioufas, A.; Theander, E.; Gottenberg, J.-E.; Bootsma, H.; Mariette, X.; Vitali, C. EULAR Sjögren's syndrome disease activity index: Development of a consensus systemic disease activity index for primary Sjögren's syndrome. *Ann. Rheum. Dis.* **2010**, *69*, 1103–1109. [CrossRef] [PubMed]
295. Seror, R.; Ravaud, P.; Mariette, X.; Bootsma, H.; Theander, E.; Hansen, A.; Ramos-Casals, M.; Dörner, T.; Bombardieri, S.; Hachulla, E.; et al. EULAR Sjögren's Syndrome Patient Reported Index (ESSPRI): Development of a consensus patient index for primary Sjögren's syndrome. *Ann. Rheum. Dis.* **2011**, *70*, 968–972. [CrossRef] [PubMed]
296. Vitali, C.; Palombi, G.; Baldini, C.; Benucci, M.; Bombardieri, S.; Covelli, M.; Del Papa, N.; De Vita, S.; Epis, O.; Franceschini, F.; et al. Sjögren's syndrome disease damage index and disease activity index: Scoring systems for the assessment of disease damage and disease activity in Sjögren's syndrome, derived from an analysis of a cohort of Italian patients. *Arthritis Rheum.* **2007**, *56*, 2223–2231. [CrossRef] [PubMed]
297. Barry, R.J.; Sutcliffe, N.; Isenberg, D.A.; Price, E.; Goldblatt, F.; Adler, M.; Canavan, A.; Hamburger, J.; Richards, A.; Regan, M.; et al. The Sjogren's Syndrome Damage Index—A damage index for use in clinical trials and observational studies in primary Sjogren's syndrome. *Rheumatology* **2008**, *47*, 1193–1198. [CrossRef] [PubMed]
298. Quartuccio, L.; Baldini, C.; Bartoloni, E.; Priori, R.; Carubbi, F.; Corazza, L.; Alunno, A.; Colafrancesco, S.; Luciano, N.; Giacomelli, R.; et al. Anti-SSA/SSB-negative Sjögren's syndrome shows a lower prevalence of lymphoproliferative manifestations, and a lower risk of lymphoma evolution. *Autoimmun. Rev.* **2015**, *14*, 1019–1022. [CrossRef] [PubMed]
299. Fauchais, A.L.; Martel, C.; Gondran, G.; Lambert, M.; Launay, D.; Jauberteau, M.O.; Hachulla, E.; Vidal, E.; Hatron, P.Y. Immunological profile in primary Sjögren syndrome: Clinical significance, prognosis and long-term evolution to other auto-immune disease. *Autoimmun. Rev.* **2010**, *9*, 595–599. [CrossRef] [PubMed]
300. Krylova, L.; Isenberg, D. Assessment of patients with primary Sjogren's syndrome–outcome over 10 years using the Sjogren's Syndrome Damage Index. *Rheumatology* **2010**, *49*, 1559–1562. [CrossRef]

301. Baldini, C.; Ferro, F.; Pepe, P.; Luciano, N.; Sernissi, F.; Cacciatore, C.; Martini, D.; Tavoni, A.; Mosca, M.; Bombardieri, S. Damage Accrual In a Single Centre Cohort Of Patients With Primary Sjögren's Syndrome Followed Up For Over 10 Years. In *Sjögren's Syndrome: Clinical Aspects, Proceedings of the 2013 ACR/ARHP Annual Meeting, San Diego, CA, USA, 25–30 October 2013*; WILEY: Hoboken, NJ, USA, 2013.
302. Cho, H.J.; Yoo, J.J.; Yun, C.Y.; Kang, E.H.; Lee, H.-J.; Hyon, J.Y.; Song, Y.W.; Lee, Y.J. The EULAR Sjogren's syndrome patient reported index as an independent determinant of health-related quality of life in primary Sjogren's syndrome patients: In comparison with non-Sjogren's sicca patients. *Rheumatology* **2013**, *52*, 2208–2217. [CrossRef]
303. Hackett, K.L.; Newton, J.L.; Frith, J.; Elliott, C.; Lendrem, D.; Foggo, H.; Edgar, S.; Mitchell, S.; Ng, W.-F. Impaired functional status in primary Sjögren's syndrome. *Arthritis Care Res.* **2012**, *64*, 1760–1764. [CrossRef]
304. Zhang, Q.; Wang, X.; Chen, H.; Shen, B. Sjögren's syndrome is associated with negatively variable impacts on domains of health-related quality of life: Evidence from Short Form 36 questionnaire and a meta-analysis. *Patient Prefer. Adherence* **2017**, *11*, 905–911. [CrossRef]
305. Haldorsen, K.; Moen, K.; Jacobsen, H.; Jonsson, R.; Brun, J.G. Exocrine function in primary Sjögren syndrome: Natural course and prognostic factors. *Ann. Rheum. Dis.* **2008**, *67*, 949–954. [CrossRef]
306. Al-Ezzi, M.Y.; Pathak, N.; Tappuni, A.R.; Khan, K.S. Primary Sjögren's syndrome impact on smell, taste, sexuality and quality of life in female patients: A systematic review and meta-analysis. *Mod. Rheumatol.* **2017**, *27*, 623–629. [CrossRef] [PubMed]
307. Miyamoto, S.T.; Valim, V.; Fisher, B.A. Health-related quality of life and costs in Sjögren's syndrome. *Rheumatology* **2019**. [CrossRef] [PubMed]
308. Ter Borg, E.J.; Kelder, J.C. Lower prevalence of extra-glandular manifestations and anti-SSB antibodies in patients with primary Sjögren's syndrome and widespread pain: Evidence for a relatively benign subset. *Clin. Exp. Rheumatol.* **2014**, *32*, 349–353. [PubMed]
309. Ostuni, P.; Botsios, C.; Sfriso, P.; Punzi, L.; Chieco-Bianchi, F.; Semerano, L.; Grava, C.; Todesco, S. Fibromyalgia in Italian patients with primary Sjögren's syndrome. *Joint Bone Spine* **2002**, *69*, 51–57. [CrossRef]
310. Champey, J.; Corruble, E.; Gottenberg, J.; Buhl, C.; Meyer, T.; Caudmont, C.; Bergé, E.; Pellet, J.; Hardy, P.; Mariette, X. Quality of life and psychological status in patients with primary Sjögren's syndrome and sicca symptoms without autoimmune features. *Arthritis Rheum.* **2006**, *55*, 451–457. [CrossRef] [PubMed]
311. Mariette, X. Dry eyes and mouth syndrome or sicca, asthenia and polyalgia syndrome? *Rheumatology* **2003**, *42*, 914–915. [CrossRef]
312. Mavragani, C.P.; Skopouli, F.N.; Moutsopoulos, H.M. Increased Prevalence of Antibodies to Thyroid Peroxidase in Dry Eyes and Mouth Syndrome or Sicca Asthenia Polyalgia Syndrome. *J. Rheumatol.* **2009**, *36*, 1626–1630. [CrossRef]
313. Price, E.J. Dry eyes and mouth syndrome—A subgroup of patients presenting with sicca symptoms. *Rheumatology* **2002**, *41*, 416–422. [CrossRef]
314. Mandl, T.; Jørgensen, T.S.; Skougaard, M.; Olsson, P.; Kristensen, L.-E. Work Disability in Newly Diagnosed Patients with Primary Sjögren Syndrome. *J. Rheumatol.* **2017**, *44*, 209–215. [CrossRef]
315. Pertovaara, M.; Korpela, M. ESSPRI and other patient-reported indices in patients with primary Sjogren's syndrome during 100 consecutive outpatient visits at one rheumatological clinic. *Rheumatology* **2014**, *53*, 927–931. [CrossRef] [PubMed]
316. Lendrem, D.; Mitchell, S.; McMeekin, P.; Gompels, L.; Hackett, K.; Bowman, S.; Price, E.; Pease, C.T.; Emery, P.; Andrews, J.; et al. Do the EULAR Sjogren's syndrome outcome measures correlate with health status in primary Sjögren's syndrome? *Rheumatology* **2015**, *54*, 655–659. [CrossRef] [PubMed]
317. Koh, J.; Kwok, S.; Lee, J.; Son, C.; Kim, J.-M.; Kim, H.; Park, S.; Sung, Y.; Choe, J.; Lee, S.; et al. Pain, xerostomia, and younger age are major determinants of fatigue in Korean patients with primary Sjögren's syndrome: A cohort study. *Scand. J. Rheumatol.* **2017**, *46*, 49–55. [CrossRef] [PubMed]
318. Cornec, D.; Devauchelle-Pensec, V.; Mariette, X.; Jousse-Joulin, S.; Berthelot, J.; Perdriger, A.; Puéchal, X.; Le Guern, V.; Sibilia, J.; Gottenberg, J.; et al. Severe Health-Related Quality of Life Impairment in Active Primary Sjögren's Syndrome and Patient-Reported Outcomes: Data From a Large Therapeutic Trial. *Arthritis Care Res.* **2017**, *69*, 528–535. [CrossRef]
319. Price, E.J.; Rauz, S.; Tappuni, A.R.; Sutcliffe, N.; Hackett, K.L.; Barone, F.; Granata, G.; Ng, W.-F.; Fisher, B.A.; Bombardieri, M.; et al. The British Society for Rheumatology guideline for the management of adults with primary Sjögren's Syndrome. *Rheumatology* **2017**. [CrossRef]

320. Valim, V.; Trevisani, V.F.M.; Pasoto, S.G.; Serrano, E.V.; Ribeiro, S.L.E.; de Fidelix, T.S.A.; Vilela, V.S.; do Prado, L.L.; Tanure, L.A.; Libório-Kimura, T.N.; et al. Recommendations for the treatment of Sjögren's syndrome. *Rev. Bras. Reumatol.* **2015**, *55*, 446–457. [CrossRef]
321. Sumida, T.; Azuma, N.; Moriyama, M.; Takahashi, H.; Asashima, H.; Honda, F.; Abe, S.; Ono, Y.; Hirota, T.; Hirata, S.; et al. Clinical practice guideline for Sjögren's syndrome 2017. *Mod. Rheumatol.* **2018**, *28*, 383–408. [CrossRef]
322. Vivino, F.B.; Carsons, S.E.; Foulks, G.; Daniels, T.E.; Parke, A.; Brennan, M.T.; Forstot, S.L.; Scofield, R.H.; Hammitt, K.M. New Treatment Guidelines for Sjögren's Disease. *Rheum. Dis. Clin. N. Am.* **2016**, *42*, 531–551. [CrossRef]
323. The Dry Eye Assessment and Management Study Research Group. n−3 Fatty Acid Supplementation for the Treatment of Dry Eye Disease. *N. Engl. J. Med.* **2018**, *378*, 1681–1690. [CrossRef]
324. Hussain, M.; Shtein, R.M.; Pistilli, M.; Maguire, M.G.; Oydanich, M.; Asbell, P.A. The Dry Eye Assessment and Management (DREAM) extension study—A randomized clinical trial of withdrawal of supplementation with omega-3 fatty acid in patients with dry eye disease. *Ocul. Surf.* **2020**, *18*, 47–55. [CrossRef]
325. Asbell, P.A.; Maguire, M.G. Why DREAM should make you think twice about recommending Omega-3 supplements. *Ocul. Surf.* **2019**, *17*, 617–618. [CrossRef]
326. Skopouli, F.N.; Jagiello, P.; Tsifetaki, N.; Moutsopoulos, H.M. Methotrexate in primary Sjögren's syndrome. *Clin. Exp. Rheumatol.* **1996**, *14*, 555–558. [PubMed]
327. Nakayamada, S.; Saito, K.; Umehara, H.; Ogawa, N.; Sumida, T.; Ito, S.; Minota, S.; Nara, H.; Kondo, H.; Okada, J.; et al. Efficacy and safety of mizoribine for the treatment of Sjögren's syndrome: A multicenter open-label clinical trial. *Mod. Rheumatol.* **2007**, *17*, 464–469. [CrossRef] [PubMed]
328. Nakayamada, S.; Fujimoto, T.; Nonomura, A.; Saito, K.; Nakamura, S.; Tanaka, Y. Usefulness of initial histological features for stratifying Sjogren's syndrome responders to mizoribine therapy. *Rheumatology* **2009**, *48*, 1279–1282. [CrossRef] [PubMed]
329. MacFarlane, G.J.; Kronisch, C.; Dean, L.E.; Atzeni, F.; Häuser, W.; Fluß, E.; Choy, E.; Kosek, E.; Amris, K.; Branco, J.; et al. EULAR revised recommendations for the management of fibromyalgia. *Ann. Rheum. Dis.* **2017**, *76*, 318–328. [CrossRef] [PubMed]
330. Dass, S.; Bowman, S.J.; Vital, E.M.; Ikeda, K.; Pease, C.T.; Hamburger, J.; Richards, A.; Rauz, S.; Emery, P. Reduction of fatigue in Sjogren syndrome with rituximab: Results of a randomised, double-blind, placebo-controlled pilot study. *Ann. Rheum. Dis.* **2008**, *67*, 1541–1544. [CrossRef] [PubMed]
331. Devauchelle-Pensec, V.; Mariette, X.; Jousse-Joulin, S.; Berthelot, J.-M.; Perdriger, A.; Puéchal, X.; Le Guern, V.; Sibilia, J.; Gottenberg, J.-E.; Chiche, L.; et al. Treatment of Primary Sjögren Syndrome With Rituximab: A Randomized Trial. *Ann. Intern. Med.* **2014**, *160*, 233–242. [CrossRef]
332. Carubbi, F.; Cipriani, P.; Marrelli, A.; Benedetto, P.; Ruscitti, P.; Berardicurti, O.; Pantano, I.; Liakouli, V.; Alvaro, S.; Alunno, A.; et al. Efficacy and safety of rituximab treatment in early primary Sjögren's syndrome: A prospective, multi-center, follow-up study. *Arthritis Res. Ther.* **2013**, *15*, R172. [CrossRef]
333. Norheim, K.B.; Harboe, E.; Gøransson, L.G.; Omdal, R. Interleukin-1 Inhibition and Fatigue in Primary Sjögren's Syndrome—A Double Blind, Randomised Clinical Trial. *PLoS ONE* **2012**, *7*, e30123. [CrossRef]
334. Van der Heijden, E.H.M.; Kruize, A.A.; Radstake, T.R.D.J.; van Roon, J.A.G. Optimizing conventional DMARD therapy for Sjögren's syndrome. *Autoimmun. Rev.* **2018**, *17*, 480–492. [CrossRef]
335. Gottenberg, J.-E.; Ravaud, P.; Puéchal, X.; Le Guern, V.; Sibilia, J.; Goeb, V.; Larroche, C.; Dubost, J.-J.; Rist, S.; Saraux, A.; et al. Effects of Hydroxychloroquine on Symptomatic Improvement in Primary Sjögren Syndrome: The JOQUER Randomized Clinical Trial. *JAMA* **2014**, *312*, 249. [CrossRef] [PubMed]
336. Yoon, C.H.; Lee, H.J.; Lee, E.Y.; Lee, E.B.; Lee, W.-W.; Kim, M.K.; Wee, W.R. Effect of Hydroxychloroquine Treatment on Dry Eyes in Subjects with Primary Sjögren's Syndrome: A Double-Blind Randomized Control Study. *J. Kor. Med. Sci.* **2016**, *31*, 1127. [CrossRef] [PubMed]
337. Gottenberg, J.-E.; Dörner, T.; Bootsma, H.; Devauchelle-Pensec, V.; Bowman, S.J.; Mariette, X.; Bartz, H.; Oortgiesen, M.; Shock, A.; Koetse, W.; et al. Efficacy of Epratuzumab, an Anti-CD22 Monoclonal IgG Antibody, in Systemic Lupus Erythematosus Patients with Associated Sjögren's Syndrome: Post Hoc Analyses From the EMBODY Trials. *Arthritis Rheumatol.* **2018**, *70*, 763–773. [CrossRef] [PubMed]
338. Mariette, X.; Seror, R.; Quartuccio, L.; Baron, G.; Salvin, S.; Fabris, M.; Desmoulins, F.; Nocturne, G.; Ravaud, P.; De Vita, S. Efficacy and safety of belimumab in primary Sjögren's syndrome: Results of the BELISS open-label phase II study. *Ann. Rheum. Dis.* **2015**, *74*, 526–531. [CrossRef]

339. De Vita, S.; Quartuccio, L.; Seror, R.; Salvin, S.; Ravaud, P.; Fabris, M.; Nocturne, G.; Gandolfo, S.; Isola, M.; Mariette, X. Efficacy and safety of belimumab given for 12 months in primary Sjögren's syndrome: The BELISS open-label phase II study. *Rheumatology* **2015**. [CrossRef]
340. Jakez-Ocampo, J.; Atisha-Fregoso, Y.; Llorente, L. Refractory Primary Sjögren Syndrome Successfully Treated With Bortezomib. *JCR J. Clin. Rheumatol.* **2015**, *21*, 31–32. [CrossRef]
341. Shah, U. Pilot Trial of Ustekinumab for Primary Sjögren's Syndrome. 2020. Available online: clinicaltrials.gov (accessed on 9 July 2020).
342. Gilead Sciences. *Study to Assess Safety and Efficacy of Filgotinib, Lanraplenib and Tirabrutinib in Adults With Active Sjogren's Syndrome*; Clinical Trial Registration; Gilead Sciences, Inc.: Foster City, CA, USA, 2020.
343. Meijer, J.M.; Meiners, P.M.; Vissink, A.; Spijkervet, F.K.L.; Abdulahad, W.; Kamminga, N.; Brouwer, E.; Kallenberg, C.G.M.; Bootsma, H. Effectiveness of rituximab treatment in primary Sjögren's syndrome: A randomized, double-blind, placebo-controlled trial. *Arthritis Rheum.* **2010**, *62*, 960–968. [CrossRef]
344. Bowman, S.J.; Everett, C.C.; O'Dwyer, J.L.; Emery, P.; Pitzalis, C.; Ng, W.-F.; Pease, C.T.; Price, E.J.; Sutcliffe, N.; Gendi, N.S.T.; et al. Randomized Controlled Trial of Rituximab and Cost-Effectiveness Analysis in Treating Fatigue and Oral Dryness in Primary Sjögren's Syndrome: Rituximab for symptomatic fatigue and oral dryness in primary SS. *Arthritis Rheumatol.* **2017**, *69*, 1440–1450. [CrossRef]
345. RemeGen A Phase II Study of RC18, a Recombinant Human B Lymphocyte Stimulator Receptor: Immunoglobulin G (IgG) Fc Fusion Protein for Injection for the Treatment of Subjects with Primary Sjögren's Syndrome. 2019. Available online: clinicaltrials.gov (accessed on 20 May 2020).
346. GlaxoSmithKline A Randomized, Double Blind (Sponsor Open), Comparative, Multicenter Study to Evaluate the Safety and Efficacy of Subcutaneous Belimumab (GSK1550188) and Intravenous Rituximab Co-administration in Subjects With Primary Sjögren's Syndrome. 2020. Available online: clinicaltrials.gov (accessed on 9 July 2020).
347. Eli Lilly and Company A Multiple Ascending Dose Study to Evaluate the Safety, Tolerability, Pharmacokinetics, and Pharmacodynamics of LY3090106 in Subjects With Sjögren's Syndrome. 2018. Available online: clinicaltrials.gov (accessed on 20 May 2020).
348. Dörner, T.; Posch, M.G.; Li, Y.; Petricoul, O.; Cabanski, M.; Milojevic, J.M.; Kamphausen, E.; Valentin, M.-A.; Simonett, C.; Mooney, L.; et al. Treatment of primary Sjögren's syndrome with ianalumab (VAY736) targeting B cells by BAFF receptor blockade coupled with enhanced, antibody-dependent cellular cytotoxicity. *Ann. Rheum. Dis.* **2019**, *78*, 641–647. [CrossRef]
349. Novartis Pharmaceuticals Study of Safety and Efficacy of Multiple VAY736 Doses in Patients with Moderate to Severe Primary Sjogren's Syndrome (pSS). 2020. Available online: clinicaltrials.gov (accessed on 9 July 2020).
350. Novartis Pharmaceuticals An Adaptive Phase 2 Randomized Double-blind, Placebo-controlled Multi-center Study to Evaluate the Safety and Efficacy of Multiple LOU064 Doses in Patients With Moderate to Severe Sjögren's Syndrome (LOUiSSe). 2020. Available online: clinicaltrials.gov (accessed on 9 July 2020).
351. Bristol-Myers Squibb A Phase II, Randomized, Multi-Center, Double-Blind, Placebo Controlled Study to Evaluate the Efficacy and Safety of BMS-931699 (Lulizumab) or BMS-986142 in Subjects With Moderate to Severe Primary Sjögren's Syndrome. 2018. Available online: clinicaltrials.gov (accessed on 20 May 2020).
352. Bristol-Myers Squibb A Randomized, Placebo-Controlled, Double-Blind, Multicenter Study to Assess the Efficacy and Safety of Branebrutinib Treatment in Subjects With Active Systemic Lupus Erythematosus or Primary Sjögren's Syndrome, or Branebrutinib Treatment Followed by Open-label Abatacept Treatment in Subjects With Active Rheumatoid Arthritis. 2020. Available online: clinicaltrials.gov (accessed on 9 July 2020).
353. St.Clair, E.W.; Baer, A.N.; Wei, C.; Noaiseh, G.; Parke, A.; Coca, A.; Utset, T.O.; Genovese, M.C.; Wallace, D.J.; McNamara, J.; et al. Clinical Efficacy and Safety of Baminercept, a Lymphotoxin β Receptor Fusion Protein, in Primary Sjögren's Syndrome: Results From a Phase II Randomized, Double-Blind, Placebo-Controlled Trial. *Arthritis Rheumatol.* **2018**, *70*, 1470–1480. [CrossRef]
354. Incyte Corporation An Open-Label Phase 2 Study of INCB050465 in Participants With Primary Sjögren's Syndrome. 2020. Available online: clinicaltrials.gov (accessed on 20 May 2020).
355. Juarez, M.; Diaz, N.; Johnston, G.I.; Nayar, S.; Payne, A.; Helmer, E.; Cain, D.; Williams, P.; Ng, W.F.; Fisher, B.; et al. AB0458 a phase II randomised double-blind, placebo-controlled, proof of concept study of oral Seletalisib in patients with priary Sjögren's syndrome (PSS). *Ann. Rheum. Dis.* **2019**, *78*, 1692–1693.

356. Dörner, T.; Zeher, M.; Laessing, U.; Chaperon, F.; De Buck, S.; Hasselberg, A.; Valentin, M.-A.; Ma, S.; Cabanski, M.; Kalis, C.; et al. OP0250 A randomised, double-blind study to assess the safety, tolerability and preliminary efficacy of leniolisib (CDZ173) in patients with primary sjÖgren's syndrome. *Ann. Rheum. Dis.* **2018**, *77*, 174.
357. Baer, A.; Gottenberg, J.-E.; St.Clair, W.E.; Sumida, T.; Takeuchi, T.; Seror, R.; Foulks, G.; Nys, M.; Johnsen, A.; Wong, R.; et al. OP0039 Efficacy and safety of Abatacept in active primary Sjögren's syndrome: Results of a randomised placebo-controlled phase III trial. *Ann. Rheum. Dis.* **2019**, *78*, 89–90.
358. Meiners, P.M.; Vissink, A.; Kroese, F.G.M.; Spijkervet, F.K.L.; Smitt-Kamminga, N.S.; Abdulahad, W.H.; Bulthuis-Kuiper, J.; Brouwer, E.; Arends, S.; Bootsma, H. Abatacept treatment reduces disease activity in early primary Sjogren's syndrome (open-label proof of concept ASAP study). *Ann. Rheum. Dis.* **2014**, *73*, 1393–1396. [CrossRef] [PubMed]
359. Van Nimwegen, J.F.; Mossel, E.; van Zuiden, G.S.; Wijnsma, R.F.; Delli, K.; Stel, A.J.; van der Vegt, B.; Haacke, E.A.; Olie, L.; Los, L.I.; et al. Abatacept treatment for patients with early active primary Sjögren's syndrome: A single-centre, randomised, double-blind, placebo-controlled, phase 3 trial (ASAP-III study). *Lancet Rheumatol.* **2020**, *2*, e153–e163. [CrossRef]
360. Fisher, B.A.; Szanto, A.; Ng, W.-F.; Bombardieri, M.; Posch, M.G.; Papas, A.S.; Gergely, P. Assessment of the anti-CD40 antibody iscalimab in patients with primary Sjögren's syndrome: A multicentre, randomised, double-blind, placebo-controlled, proof-of-concept study. *Lancet Rheumatol.* **2020**, *2*. [CrossRef]
361. Novartis Pharmaceuticals A 48-week, 6-arm, Randomized, Double-blind, Placebo-controlled Multicenter Trial to Assess the Safety and Efficacy of Multiple CFZ533 Doses Administered Subcutaneously in Two Distinct Populations of Patients with Sjögren's Syndrome (TWINSS). 2020. Available online: clinicaltrials.gov (accessed on 9 July 2020).
362. Viela Bio A Phase 2 Randomized, Double-blind, Placebo-controlled, Proof of Concept Study to Evaluate the Efficacy and Safety of VIB4920 in Subjects With Sjögren's Syndrome (SS). 2020. Available online: clinicaltrials.gov (accessed on 9 July 2020).
363. Mariette, X.; Bombardieri, M.; Alevizos, I.; Moate, R.; Sullivan, B.; Noaiseh, G.; Kvarnström, M.; Rees, W.; Wang, L.; Illei, G. A Phase 2a Study of MEDI5872 (AMG557), a Fully Human Anti-ICOS Ligand Monoclonal Antibody in Patients with Primary Sjögren's Syndrome. In *Sjögren's Syndrome—Basic & Clinical Science Poster I, Proceedings of the 2019 ACR/ARP Annual Meeting, Atlanta, GA, USA, 8–13 November 2019*; WILEY: Hoboken, NJ, USA, 2019.
364. Hoffmann-La Roche A Multi-Center, Randomized, Double-Blind, Placebo-Controlled, Parallel Group Phase 2A Study to Assess the Efficacy of RO5459072 in Patients With Primary Sjogren's Syndrome. 2018. Available online: clinicaltrials.gov (accessed on 20 May 2020).
365. Gabor Illei, M. D A Randomized, Placebo Controlled, Proof of Concept, Study of Raptiva, a Humanized Anti-CD-11a Monoclonal Antibody, in Patients With Sjögren's Syndrome. 2015. Available online: clinicaltrials.gov (accessed on 20 May 2020).
366. Cacoub, P.; Felten, R.; Devauchelle-Pensec, V.; Duffau, P.; Hachulla, E.; Hatron, P.Y.; Salliot, C.; Perdriger, A.; Morel, J.; Mekinian, A.; et al. Inhibition du récepteur de l'interleukine-6 au cours du syndrome de Gougerot-Sjögren primaire: Essai randomisé multicentrique académique en double aveugle tocilizumab versus placebo (ETAP study). *Rev. Médecine Interne* **2019**, *40*, A33. [CrossRef]
367. Mariette, X.; Ravaud, P.; Steinfeld, S.; Baron, G.; Goetz, J.; Hachulla, E.; Combe, B.; Puéchal, X.; Pennec, Y.; Sauvezie, B.; et al. Inefficacy of infliximab in primary Sjögren's syndrome: Results of the randomized, controlled trial of remicade in primary Sjögren's syndrome (TRIPSS): Infliximab in Primary Sjögren's Syndrome. *Arthritis Rheum.* **2004**, *50*, 1270–1276. [CrossRef]
368. Sankar, V.; Brennan, M.T.; Kok, M.R.; Leakan, R.A.; Smith, J.A.; Manny, J.; Baum, B.J.; Pillemer, S.R. Etanercept in Sjögren's syndrome: A twelve-week randomized, double-blind, placebo-controlled pilot clinical trial: Randomized Controlled Pilot Study of Etanercept in SS. *Arthritis Rheum.* **2004**, *50*, 2240–2245. [CrossRef]
369. GlaxoSmithKline A Two Part Phase IIa Study, to Evaluate the Safety and Tolerability, Pharmacokinetics, Proof of Mechanism and Potential for Efficacy of an Anti-IL-7 Receptor-α Monoclonal Antibody (GSK2618960) in the Treatment of Primary Sjögren's Syndrome. 2018. Available online: clinicaltrials.gov (accessed on 20 May 2020).

370. Viela Bio A Phase 1 Randomized, Placebo-Controlled, Blinded, Multiple Ascending Dose Study to Evaluate VIB7734 in Systemic Lupus Erythematosus, Cutaneous Lupus Erythematosus, Sjogren's Syndrome, Systemic Sclerosis, Polymyositis, and Dermatomyositis. 2020. Available online: clinicaltrials.gov (accessed on 20 May 2020).
371. Fisher, B.; Barone, F.; Jobling, K.; Gallagher, P.; Macrae, V.; Filby, A.; Hulmes, G.; Milne, P.; Traianos, E.; Iannizzotto, V.; et al. OP0202 Effects of RSLV-132 on fatigue in patients with primary Sjögren's syndrome—Results of a phase II randomised double-blind, placebo-controlled proof of concept study. *Ann. Rheum. Dis.* **2019**, *78*, 177. [CrossRef]
372. Assistance Publique—Hôpitaux de Paris Induction of Regulatory t Cells by Low Dose il2 in Autoimmune and Inflammatory Diseases. 2020. Available online: clinicaltrials.gov (accessed on 9 July 2020).

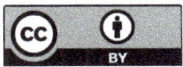

© 2020 by the authors. Licensee MDPI, Basel, Switzerland. This article is an open access article distributed under the terms and conditions of the Creative Commons Attribution (CC BY) license (http://creativecommons.org/licenses/by/4.0/).

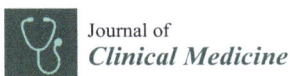

Review

Understanding the Complexity of Sjögren's Syndrome: Remarkable Progress in Elucidating NF-κB Mechanisms

Margherita Sisto *, Domenico Ribatti and Sabrina Lisi

Department of Basic Medical Sciences, Neurosciences and Sensory Organs (SMBNOS),
Section of Human Anatomy and Histology, University of Bari "Aldo Moro", 70124 Bari, Italy;
domenico.ribatti@uniba.it (D.R.); sabrina.lisi@uniba.it (S.L.)
* Correspondence: margherita.sisto@uniba.it; Tel.: +39-080-547-8315; Fax: +39-080-547-8327

Received: 3 July 2020; Accepted: 28 August 2020; Published: 31 August 2020

Abstract: Sjögren's syndrome (SS) is a systemic autoimmune inflammatory disease with a poorly defined aetiology, which targets exocrine glands (particularly salivary and lachrymal glands), affecting the secretory function. Patients suffering from SS exhibit persistent xerostomia and keratoconjunctivitis sicca. It is now widely acknowledged that a chronic grade of inflammation plays a central role in the initiation, progression, and development of SS. Consistent with its key role in organizing inflammatory responses, numerous recent studies have shown involvement of the transcription factor nuclear factor κ (kappa)-light-chain-enhancer of activated B cells (NF-κB) in the development of this disease. Therefore, chronic inflammation is considered as a critical factor in the disease aetiology, offering hope for the development of new drugs for treatment. The purpose of this review is to describe the current knowledge about the NF-κB-mediated molecular events implicated in the pathogenesis of SS.

Keywords: Sjögren's syndrome; NF-κB; inflammation

1. Introduction

The nuclear factor κ (kappa)-light-chain-enhancer of activated B cells (NF-κB) is a pleiotropic regulator of many cellular signalling pathways activated in response to a wide variety of stimuli linked to inflammation. Once activated, this B cell enhancer plays an important role in the pathogenesis of several inflammatory autoimmune diseases, including Sjögren's syndrome (SS) [1]. SS presents lymphocytic infiltration of the salivary glands (SGs) and lachrymal glands as the characteristic hallmark resulting in chronic inflammation. A dry mouth and dry eyes, resulting in keratoconjunctivitis sicca and xerostomia, are common complaints in SS [2]. NF-κB is a family of DNA-binding proteins that regulates many cellular processes, notably the immune response and inflammation, influencing the transcription of a broad array of pro-inflammatory cytokines [3]. NF-κB is ubiquitously expressed in SGs, and the constitutive NF-κB activation observed in primary SS (pSS) is associated with NF-κB release and nuclear translocation of NF-κB, to focal infiltrated lymphocytes and the acinar epithelium of patients with pSS, to regulate the pro-inflammatory gene transcriptions [4]. However, the role of NF-κB in pSS remains to be clarified in detail. This article provides an update on the current state of knowledge about the relationship between NF-κB-molecular pathway activation in SGs and the chronic inflammation characterizing pSS, with the aim of providing a strong basis for a better understanding of the signal transduction pathways mediating the induction of NF-κB in pSS SGs, in order to allow this disease to be manipulated, to gain therapeutic benefit.

2. Sjögren's Syndrome

The chronic inflammatory autoimmune disorder SS arises as primary SS (pSS) and, when linked with another underlying systemic autoimmune disorder, such as scleroderma, systemic lupus erythematosus (SLE), or rheumatoid arthritis (RA), is defined as secondary SS [5]. The evolution to non-Hodgkin's lymphoma occurs in a larger percentage of SS patients than in the normal population [6,7]. The clinical hallmarks of SS, keratoconjunctivitis sicca and xerostomia [2], can be confirmed by various objective tests highlighting significant functional impairment of the SGs and lachrymal glands [8]. The involvement of these glands is characterized by focal infiltrating lymphocytes that surround the ducts and, in some patients, extend and replace the secretory functional units. Although infiltration of the SGs by lymphocytes is a hallmark of SS [9,10], multiple cytokines are upregulated, even in the absence of lymphocytic infiltrates, and have a direct effect on SGs epithelial cells (SGEC). Interestingly, substantial new evidence supports the role of epithelia in the production of constitutive or inducible mediators of the innate and acquired immune responses. The picture that emerges shows intrinsically activated SGEC that induce and promote chronic inflammatory reactions [11]. For this reason, on the basis of clinical observation, pSS was defined as an "autoimmune epithelitis" [12]. Indeed, SGEC are capable of releasing many cytokines that result overexpressed and thus act as key molecules in chronic inflammation, contributing to both systemic and exocrine manifestations of pSS [13–29]. A number of explanations has been offered for the dysregulated cytokine network in pSS and, in the past, the presence of anti-Ro/SSA and anti-La/SSB antibodies was shown to be related to increased glandular and extra-glandular manifestations. Important findings provided evidence for a pathogenic role of autoantibodies, demonstrating that anti-Ro/SSA autoantibodies stimulate the production of pro-inflammatory cytokines such as IL-6 and IL-8 by human SGEC from healthy donors, promoting chronic inflammatory reactions [25]. Furthermore, pSS autoantibodies can promote the activation of the NF-κB pathway, leading to the overexpression of multiple proangiogenic/pro-inflammatory factors. Indeed, inhibiting the NF-κB activity abrogated the release of these cytokines [25]. Starting from the initial studies carried out on autoantibodies, considerable progress has been made in identifying other possible molecular mechanisms implicated in the activation of NF-κB, which could explain the chronic inflammatory situation characteristic of SS. Accumulated data suggest that the multiple roles of NF-κB in pSS could be related to the dynamic context of dysregulated inflammatory factors observed in pSS.

3. NF-κB Transcription Factors

The family of NF-κB is composed of five members of proteins linking to DNA, (RelA, RelB, RelC, NFκ-B1, and NFκ-B2) that trigger a set of inflammatory downstream effectors after nuclear translocation, involved in a broad range of biological processes. Either a canonical or a non-canonical pathway can be responsible for their activation; the canonical pathway mediates inflammatory responses and leads to a rapid but transient NF-κB activation, while the non-canonical signalling is a slow, long-lasting pathway (see Figure 1). Typical inducers of the non-canonical NF-κB pathway are ligands of a subset of the tumour necrosis factor receptors (TNFR) superfamily involved in the differentiation of the immune system, as well as in secondary lymphoid organogenesis [30]. The NF-κB family members show homology through a 300 amino acid N-terminal DNA binding/dimerization domain, named the Rel homology domain (RHD). The RHD is a complex system where family members can constitute homodimers and heterodimers, which are normally kept inactive in the cytoplasm through interaction with inhibitory proteins of the IκB family (IκBs) [31]. The common regulatory step in both the canonical and non-canonical cascades is the activation of an IκB kinase (IKK) complex consisting of catalytic kinase subunits (IKKα and/or IKKβ) and the regulatory non-enzymatic scaffold protein NF-κB essential modulator (NEMO), also known as IKKγ [31]. NF-κB dimers are activated by IKK-mediated phosphorylation of IκBs, which triggers proteasomal IκBs degradation, liberating the dimers of NF-κB from the NF-κB-IκBs complex, that subsequently translocate to the nucleus, linking to κB enhancer elements of target genes [32] (Figure 1). Among the IκBs, the best characterized is IκBα, which requires degradation of the activity of IKK kinase. IκBα functions as a negative feedback loop to sequester NF-κB subunits, because NF-κB activation induces the expression of the IκBα gene, which terminates signalling unless a persistent activation signal is present [32].

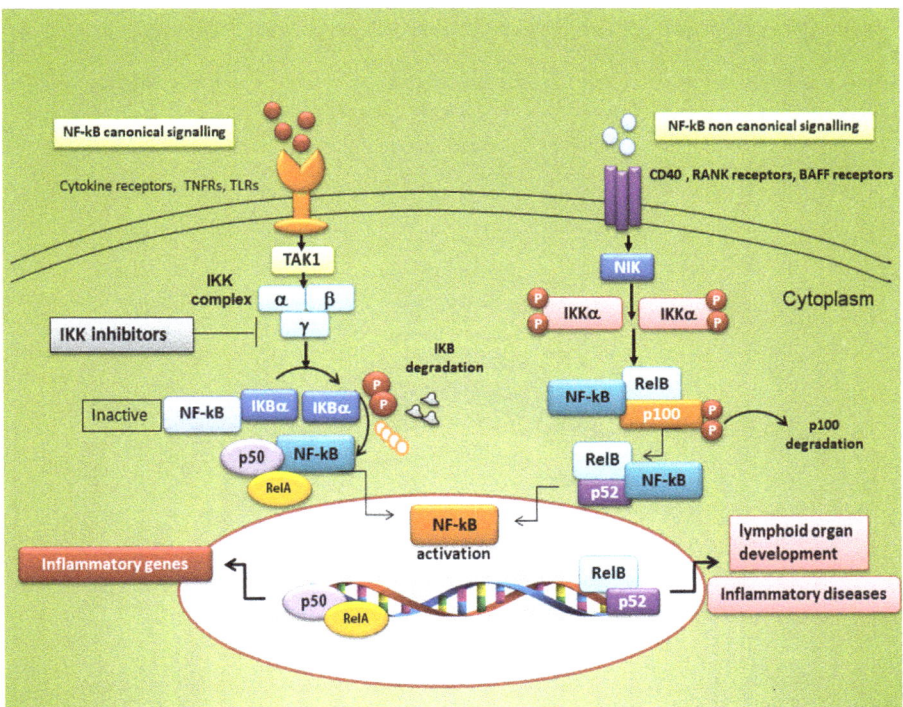

Figure 1. Canonical and non-canonical nuclear factor κ (kappa)-light-chain-enhancer of activated B cells (NF-κB) signalling pathways. The canonical NF-κB pathway starts with the activation of innate and adaptive immune receptors in response to various ligand molecules, which transfers the signal across the cell membrane causing the activation of the trimeric IκB kinase (IKK) complex, composed of catalytic (IKKα and IKKβ) and regulatory (IKKγ) subunits. The IKK complex phosphorylates IκBα and phosphorylated IκB undergo ubiquitylation and proteasomal degradation, allowing nuclear translocation of the RelA/p50 dimer of the NF-κB heterodimer. The non-canonical NF-κB pathway selectively responds to a subset of TNFR members that induce the activation of the NF-κB-inducing kinase (NIK). NIK phosphorylates and activates IKKα, which in turn phosphorylates carboxy-terminal serine residues of p100, triggering selective degradation of the C-terminal IκB-like structure of p100, and mediates the persistent activation of the RelB/p52 complex.

NF-κB is activated in every cell type and has a central role in inflammation. It is, therefore, fundamentally implicated in the molecular pathways that induce the transcription of pro-inflammatory genes [17,18,25,26,33,34]. NF-κB is highly activated in various inflammatory disorders and triggers the transcription of chemokines, cytokines, pro-inflammatory enzymes, adhesion proteins, and other factors to modulate the inflammatory response, such as metalloproteinases, Cox-2, and inducible nitric oxide synthase [35–37], although the mechanism is still unclear (a schematic representation of NF-κB activation is reported in Figure 2). In RA, NF-κB is highly expressed in the inflamed synovial stratum [38,39], where it enhances the engagement of inflammatory cells and pro-inflammatory cytokines production such as IL-1, IL-6, IL-8, and TNF-α [38,39]. Interestingly, recent evidence has shown that alterations in the modulation of NF-κB-dependent gene expression lead to a variety of other inflammatory and autoimmune disorders, neurological conditions and cancers [33,34]. In pSS, a correlation between NF-κB signalling and chronic inflammation has been demonstrated by various reports; nuclear translocation of NF-κB into focal infiltrated lymphocytes and into the acinar epithelium surrounding the infiltrates from SGs of patients with pSS was detected, while distal normal acini and ductal structures showed no nuclear translocation [1]. In addition, the non-canonical NF-κB p65 nuclear translocation has been induced in pSS SGEC by a range of molecular agents such as epidermal growth factor receptor (EGFR) and B-cell activator CD40 [40,41]. Furthermore, a downregulated gene and protein expression of IκBα was detected in pSS monocytes, contributing to an enhanced NF-κB activity. Finally, pSS autoantibodies can trigger the NF-κB signalling pathway, thus, contributing to exacerbate the inflammatory condition [13].

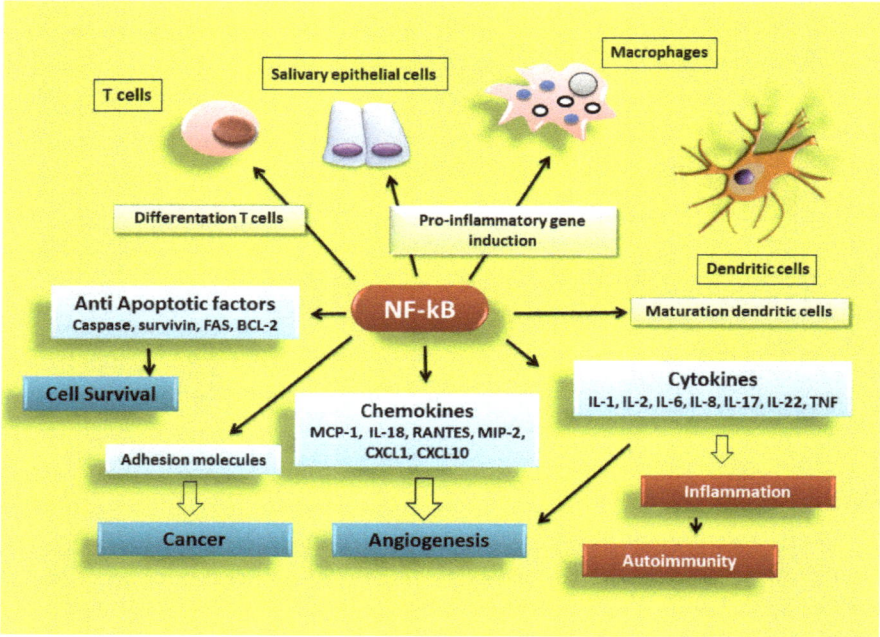

Figure 2. NF-κB signalling pathway dictates the inflammatory responses. After its activation, it can induce the transcription of a large number of genes including pro-inflammatory cytokines, chemokines, adhesion molecules, cell cycle regulatory molecules, anti-apoptotic proteins and angiogenic factors, and thereby regulate cell proliferation, apoptosis, morphogenesis, differentiation, angiogenesis, and inflammation. The regulation of inflammation, cell proliferation and apoptosis is central to the understanding of many diseases, such as autoimmune diseases and cancer.

Based on all these assumptions, that are extensively documented, we report a close review of the recent literature on the molecular mechanisms that check NF-κB activation in pSS and on the potential of new pharmacological interventions for optimizing pSS treatment regimes.

4. Small-Molecule Inhibitors of NF-κB in Sjögren's Syndrome

The modulation of the NF-κB pathways has frequently been described as "pro-inflammatory", largely due to the key role of NF-κB in the pro-inflammatory genes expression including cytokines, chemokines, and adhesion molecules [42,43]. Many findings demonstrated that epithelial cells in the glandular sites of patients affected by pSS are able to release factors that address the chemoattraction of lymphocytes and promote chronic inflammatory responses [12,15,16,24–26]. NF-κB pathway modulation was therefore investigated in pSS, highlighting a role in regulating the production of pro-inflammatory cytokines, leukocyte enrolment, or cell survival [17,18,25,26,44]. In pSS, the NF-κB activation cascade can be modulated at different levels [30]. Considering the correlation with the biopsy focus score, grade of infiltration and evaluated disease activity, phosphorylated IKKε, responsible for the degradation of IkB proteins, were significantly and positively correlated with NF-κB levels in pSS [4]. The levels of B-Cell Activating Factor (BAFF) and those of numerous pro-inflammatory cytokines, all regulated by NF-κB signalling, are augmented in pSS [45]. Nucleotide polymorphisms in NF-κB pathway genes have been linked with pSS [46], and a specific mutation in the Ikα-826T, one of the promoters of a member of the inhibitory IkB complex, was associated with susceptibility of pSS [47,48]. Numerous small molecule inhibitors of the NF-κB signalling pathways are currently commercially available for use, and NF-κB modulators are under study in clinical trials for pSS treatment [19,25,30,49–54]. Many preclinical studies have already analysed the role of NF-κB signalling in the glandular tissue in pSS. The pSS SGECs have been recognized to have an active NF-κB pathway. The phosphorylated forms of IKKε, IκBα, and NF-κB were expressed in the ductal cells in minor SGs derived from pSS patients [19]. By stimulating the Toll-Like Receptor 2 (TLR2) in SGECs, IL-2 production was induced through the NF-κB cascade in pSS SGECs [49–51]. SGECs treated with the anti-Ro/SSA autoantibodies isolated from pSS patients showed a progressive increase in constitutive NF-κB activation, and transfection of SGECs with IκBα in SGECs treated with anti-Ro/SSA led to a remarkable production of pro-inflammatory cytokines and an enhanced apoptosis [25]. Furthermore, recent findings showed that gene silencing of the natural NF-κB inhibitor TNF Alpha Induced Protein 3 (TNFAIP3) in keratin-14-positive epithelial cells, promoting the activation of the constitutive NF-κB cascade, induces the initial phases of pSS, leading to a reduced production of saliva and lymphocyte invasion in the SGs [52]. This effect is likely related to the calcium pathway in the acinar cells, since calcium signalling has an important role in NF-κB pathway activity [53,54]. A list of NF-κB small molecule inhibitors tested in pSS is reported in Table 1.

Table 1. List of NF-κB small molecules inhibitors tested or identified in primary SS (pSS).

Small Inhibitors of NF-kB in pSS	Study	References
Iguratimod	Clinical study	[30]
Syk-inihibitor-Gs-9876	Clinical study	[30]
IKKε	Pre-clinical study	[4,30]
IκBα	Pre-clinical study	[19,26,47,48]
anti-Ro/SSA autoantibodies	Pre-clinical study	[14,16,24,25]
TNFAIP3	Pre-clinical study	[17]
Calcium mobilization	Pre-clinical study	[53,54]

The Key Role of IκBα in NF-κB Modulation in pSS

Among the well-characterized regulators of NF-κB activation in SGEC, IκBα is particularly important for the pathogenesis of pSS. The concept that IκBα expression negatively regulates NF-κB DNA binding activity was demonstrated by the fact that reduced IκBα overlaps with nuclear translocation of the NF-κB and the appearance of NF-κB activity [55]. For SGs, adenoid cystic carcinoma of human SGs cell lines, stably transfected with the mutant IκBα expression vector (IκBαM) share an effectively cancelled constitutive and liposaccharide-induced NF-κB activity, concomitantly with a significantly diminished VEGF gene and protein expression. This effect leads to a lower endothelial cell mobility and, thus, might represent a promising anti-angiogenesis strategy in adenoid cystic carcinoma (ACC) therapy [56]. In pSS SGEC, abnormal levels of IκBα were detected in comparison with those in healthy subjects, showing a clear reduction of IκBα in salivary tissues from active pSS patients [19]. This was confirmed in biopsy specimens, where a moderate IκBα positive staining located in the cytoplasm of acini and ductal cells was revealed in healthy controls, whereas in pSS salivary gland biopsies the cytoplasmic positivity for IκBα was very weak [19]. All of this suggests that the production of proinflammatory cytokines occurs through the persistent activation of NF-κB signalling [17,18,25,26]. In addition, a reduced gene and protein expression of IκBα was demonstrated in monocytes from pSS patients in comparison with healthy subjects, suggesting that the reduced expression of this NF-κB inhibitor may reflect an increased inflammatory response [26]. Specifically, published data show that mutations in IκBα are linked to inflammatory autoimmune disorders. An 8-bp insertion in the promoter region of IκBα represents a protective factor against the development of primary progressive multiple sclerosis [57]. Klein et al. showed that IκBα polymorphisms might also be associated with Crohn's disease [58], SLE [59] and pSS [47,48]. In particular, mutant mice, that have defective IκBα expression, showed a shorter lifetime, hypersensitivity to septic shock and altered T cell development, all features of pSS [47,48]. Furthermore, overexpression of the NF-κB repressor, IκBα, determines an inhibitory effect on the production of STAT-4 protein, a transcription factor activated by interleukin 12 whose gene polymorphism was recently linked to pSS [60,61].

NF-κB signalling activation and termination is secured by various regulatory processes. In view of the well-characterized links between NF-κB and pSS disease, disentangling the complexity of NF-κB modulation is an essential goal in order to find effective, more specific therapeutic agents for the treatment of pSS.

5. Impaired NF-κB Signalling Activated by EDA-A1/EDAR in pSS Salivary Glands

In addition to its role in mediation inflammation, NF-κB is also essential for developing the epidermal derivatives, hair, nails, and SGs [62]; a series of molecular signals is now well defined, beginning with the binding of ectodysplasin (EDA-A1) to the EDA-receptor (EDAR), components of the tumour necrosis factor α (TNFα)-related signalling pathway [62]. EDA-A1 signalling is recognized as an important evolutionarily conserved pathway regulating the formation and patterning of vertebrate skin appendages, including SGs [63]. When these genes show mutations, a condition known as hypohidrotic (or anhidrotic) ectodermal dysplasia (HED/EDA) occurs [64]. The NF-κB pathway that mainly impinges on EDA-A1/EDAR-dependent SGs branching morphogenesis is the canonical NF-κB activation cascade [65].

Over the last years, great progress has been made in identifying the key molecular regulators controlling NF-κB activation, and a repertoire of crucial self-regulators ensuring the termination of NF-κB responses has been identified [66]. Interestingly, this well-orchestrated biological process may undergo alterations [33,34,67] and, consequently, deregulated NF-κB activation contributes to the autoimmune diseases pathogenesis, characterized by an intense inflammatory response [34,67]. As a matter of fact, NF-κB was demonstrated to play a salient role in the pathological development of pSS, correlated with the intense chronic inflammation findings in this disease [17,18,25,26,48]. In this context, several studies conducted on SGEC derived from pSS patients investigated the mechanism-of-action of the NF-κB cascade and performed target identification in the deregulated inflammatory situation. Recent findings demonstrated that EDA-A1 induces several genes involved in the synthesis of the NF-κB pathway molecules, including the feedback inhibitors IκBα and TNFAIP3. IκBα is known to be expressed in hair placodes and SGs [68], and TNFAIP3, a key negative feedback regulator of the NF-κB signalling cascade, plays a role in the EDA-A1, EDAR and EDAR-associated death domain (EDARADD) genes control, which results mutated in HED/EDA [69]. Therefore, recently, chemokines have been revealed as immediate target genes of the EDA/NF-κB pathway, leading to modulation of the multiple signalling pathways implicated in skin appendage development; when this scheme is deregulated, an inflammatory process may be induced [69]. Against this background, a recent study has investigated the EDA-A1 and EDAR genes and proteins expression in pSS SGs, showing that TNFAIP3 is deregulated in pSS SGEC. This results in an increased and excessive EDA-A1/EDAR gene and protein expression in pSS SGEC that determines a correlated high induction of NF-κB [70] (Figure 3). Furthermore, TNFAIP3 gene knockdown performed on healthy SGEC, through the application of the siRNA gene silencing technology, determined an over-activation of the EDA-A1/EDAR expression and consequently NF-κB nuclear translocation and activation [70] (Figure 3). The authors have shown that, in pSS SGEC, NF-κB is activated downstream of EDA-A1/EDAR signalling and after transfecting pSS SGEC with the mutated form of the regulatory protein IκBα, the EDA-A1/EDAR-NF-κB signalling pathway was affected in SGs, suggesting that the IκBα-dependent canonical NF-κB cascade was active in pSS SGEC [70]. This recent discovery suggests that the pathways involved in ectodermal development and inflammation may be fundamentally the same, but lead to target gene activation depending on the cell type and/or on the specific pathological condition features. The implication of the NF-κB pathway in development was a very surprising finding, because it is involved primarily in TNF-α receptors-mediated inflammation and immunity; now, the recurrent question is how cells can distinguish between the NF-κB pathway activation signals, as well as how specific target genes activation is precisely and independently controlled during developmental or inflammatory events.

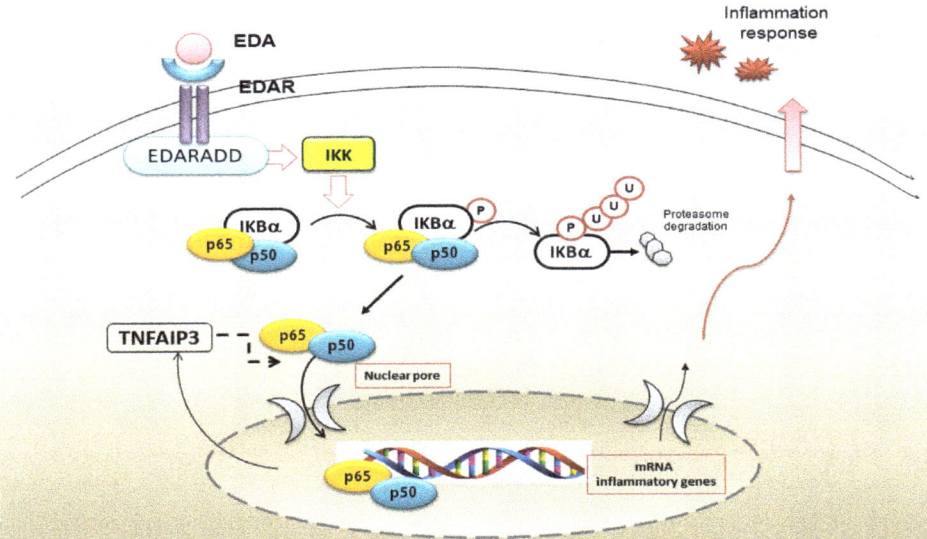

Figure 3. Schematic overview of the EDA/EDAR/canonical NF-κB pathway. The EDA isoform of the TNF-α family member Ectodysplasin interacts with its receptor EDAR leading to the recruitment of EDARADD (death domain adaptor); in turn, this complex activates the IKK complex. The IKK complex phosphorylates IκBα, that undergoes ubiquitylation and proteasomal degradation, inducing nuclear translocation of the NF-κB heterodimer RelA/p50 that triggers the transcription of pro-inflammatory genes, including those that encode the negative regulators IκBα and TNF-α-induced protein 3 (TNFAIP3). EDA: Ectodysplasin-A; EDAR: Ectodysplasin-A Receptor; EDARADD: Ectodysplasin-A receptor-associated associated death domain.

6. Toll-Like Receptor-Mediated NF-κB Activation in pSS

A large volume of recent evidence underlines the finding that the SGs epithelium is the major actor in the promotion and progression of the chronic inflammatory reactions observed in pSS, through the induction of pro-inflammatory cytokines and chemokines [8,71]. The innate immune system uses a diverse set of recognition receptors to activate the intracellular signalling pathway, such as Toll-like receptors (TLRs) molecules. Indeed, TLRs activation lead to the recruitment of adaptor proteins within the cytosol, that culminates in signal transduction resulting in the transcription of genes involved in chronic inflammation [72,73]. TLRs were initially identified as receptors important only in host defences, but it is now clear that the TLRs, for example TLR2 and TLR4, are crucial in autoimmunity development [74–76], as demonstrated in RA [74], SLE [77], multiple sclerosis [78], and inflammatory bowel diseases [79]. Studies comparing mice and humans revealed that numerous types of epithelial cells express TLRs, supporting the hypothesis that the epithelium represents the first line of defence of the innate immune system [80,81]. These observations were confirmed also in pSS; the induction of TLRs signalling in SGEC leads to the release of inflammatory mediators, including IL-6, IL-8, and TNF-α [72], which are critical mediators of the inflammatory processes of pSS. In addition, recent works have evidenced the important contribution of TLRs activation to the initiation and progression of the pSS pathogenesis. In particular, TLR2, TLR3, and TLR4 are expressed on the SGEC membrane [82], and in addition, immunohistochemical analyses of TLR2, 3 and 4 on labial SG tissue from pSS patients confirmed a significantly higher constitutive expression of these receptors, found in SG-infiltrating mononuclear cells as well as acinar cells and ductal SGEC, supporting the intrinsic epithelial activation in pSS [40]. TLR4, in particular, resulted highly expressed specifically in infiltrating mononuclear cells and in ductal and acinar cells [83,84] of pSS SGs, and receptor levels were correlated with the degree of glandular inflammation [83,84]. At the same time, investigations conducted on pSS peripheral blood mononuclear cell (PBMC) confirmed a dysregulation of TLR7, 8 and 9 molecules compared to controls, where TLR7 and 8 recognize single-stranded RNA [85], while TLR9 is activated by un-methylated CpG DNA [86]. This led to an altered recognition of DNA and RNA, eventually resulting in the development of pSS. [87].

Role of TLRs in the NF-κB-Mediated Inflammatory State in pSS

Several authors now agree that TLRs trigger an intracellular cascade of molecular events, which has, as its final step, NF-κB activation. Active NF-κB determines the transcription of inflammatory cytokine genes responsible for the exacerbation of inflammation [73]. Studies conducted on experimental animal models confirm that an intensely inflammatory microenvironment could be the basis of autoimmune diseases [88]. This scenario seems to be plausible also for pSS. A recent study reported that TLR-7 and its downstream signalling factors are strongly expressed in labial SG of pSS patients. The authors observed that TLR-7 downstream molecules are expressed in pSS SGEC after TLR-7 ligand stimulation in vitro, inducing the activation of the NF-κB pathway, which elicits the release of inflammatory factors such as IFN-α and IFN-γ [89]. Furthermore, Kwok et al. demonstrated an increased expression of TLR2, TLR4, and TLR6 in pSS SGs, in association with IL-17, IL-6, and IL-23 over-expression, factors that promote T helper17 (Th17) differentiation and amplification. The signalling pathway starts with TLR2 stimulation, which induces a cascade that involves the activation of TLR4 and TLR6. This determines the production of IL-17 and IL-23, which, as demonstrated by the authors, occurs through IκBα phosphorylation, the IL-6, signal transducer and activator of transcription 3 (STAT3), and NF-κB pathways [90]. However, the ligands that eventually activate TLR2 in the context of pSS are still doubtful and little known. Using peptidoglycan (PNG) as stimulus for TLR2 activation, an increased expression of immune mediators (ICAM-1, CD40, and MHC-1) was observed in SGECs derived from pSS patients and controls [82]. In a corroborative study using SGEC from pSS patients, TLR2 drove the NF-κB-dependent secretion of IL-15 [50,51] as confirmed using antibodies anti-TLR2 to block IL-15 secretion [50,51]. Furthermore, by using the dominant-negative inhibitory IκBα vector to inhibit NF-κB activation, TLR2-dependent IL-15 production was reduced, suggesting a transcriptional level control [50,51]. Therefore, this study underlines the importance of the TLR2/IL-15/ NF-κB pathway as a strong potential candidate for the therapeutic modulation of pSS, ameliorating both local and systemic pSS disease manifestations [50,51] A schematic representation of the TLR2 molecular pathway activation in pSS is reported in Figure 4.

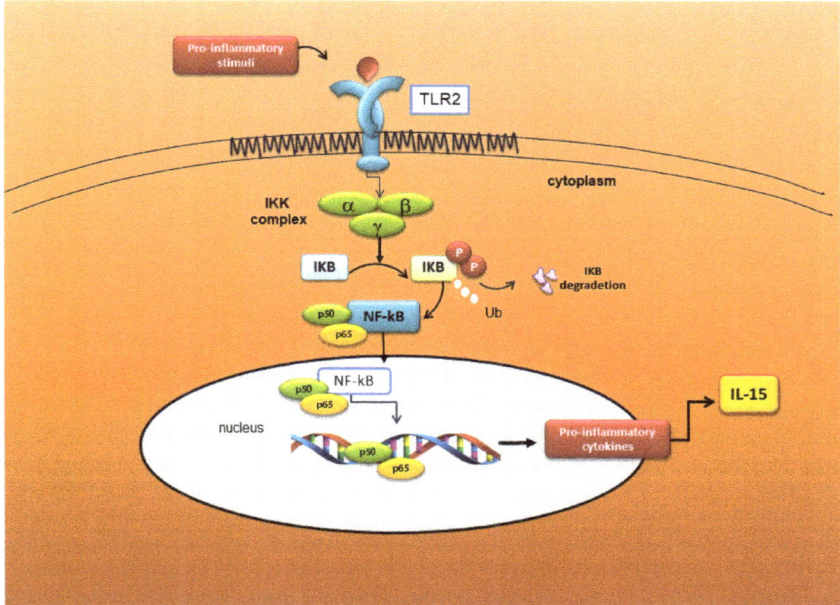

Figure 4. Schematic representation of the Toll-Like Receptor 2 (TLR2)/IL-15/NF-κB pathway in pSS SGEC. TLR2, in response to pro-inflammatory stimuli, activate the NF-κB pathway; in the nucleus, the active NF-κB promote IL-15 gene transcription; thus, incrementing inflammatory disorders in SGs of pSS patients.

7. Modulation of NF-κB Activation by the Anti CD-20 Monoclonal Antibody Rituximab

The management of pSS patients is essentially symptomatic, no curative agents for SS yet exist and demonstrations of the efficacy of systemic drugs are lacking. Given the key role of chronic B-cell activation in pSS, B-cell target therapies based on B-cell downregulation have been individuated as the first potential candidates. CD20's attractiveness as a therapeutic target derived from the growing understanding of the molecular basis for several properties related to its structure and its interaction networks [91]. CD20 is a non-glycosylated surface phosphoprotein, found on a variety of healthy and malignant B cells, whose function is probably involved in calcium influx [92,93]. CD20 expression appears early during B cell maturation but is lost during B-cell differentiation into plasma cells [94]. For many years, the function of CD20 in normal immune physiology remained poorly defined, based on few data demonstrating a role in the generation of the long-term humoral response [95].

Hypothetical Scenario Involving RTX as a Negative Regulator of the NF-κB Pathway in pSS

Rituximab (RTX), a mouse/human chimeric monoclonal antibody directed against CD20 antigen on B cells surface, represents a treatment for both pSS and SS-related malignant lymphoproliferative disease [96], whose efficacy has been investigated in the last decade, in the presence (or not) of a lymphoproliferative disorder [97–99], owing to its proven efficacy in other chronic inflammatory diseases, such as RA [100] and systemic vasculitis [101].

Recent experimental evidence demonstrated that in a co-culture system of pSS SGEC with pSS lymphocytes, RTX stimulation causes B cells depletion, leading to a drastically reduced transcription of pro-inflammatory mediator genes and protein secretion. This report suggests that B-lymphocytes regulate the cytokine and chemokine release by pSS SGEC because of their proximity in inflammatory areas. This intrinsic activation of SGEC exacerbates the inflammation, further modulating the release of inflammatory factors along post-translational pathways [102,103]. In this hypothetical scenario, a decisive role could be played by the inhibition of the constitutive activation of NF-κB. Treatment with RTX of pSS SGEC co-cultured with pSS B-lymphocytes, determines a lower NF-κB DNA binding activity in the SGEC, so inhibiting the pro-inflammatory genes transcription [102,103]. Now, RTX interferes with the constitutive activation of the NF-κB pathway through the modulation of Raf-1 kinase inhibitor protein (RKIP) expression [104], which acts directly by down-regulating IkB kinase (IKK) activity and indirectly by interfering with IKK activators [105]. RKIP is believed to play an important role in various inflammatory diseases and cancers [106] and results constitutively under-expressed in pSS SGEC [102]. These data suggest that RKIP could increase NF-κB activity, leading to the persistent chronic inflammatory condition characteristic of pSS. Therefore, the function of RTX as a negative regulator of the NF-κB pathway in pSS SGEC is based on the modulation of RKIP expression; RTX, in fact, up-regulates RKIP expression in pSS SGEC, and RTX-mediated RKIP induction diminishes the phosphorylation of the components of the NF-κB pathway [102] (Figure 5). Experimental RKIP gene silencing in pSS SGEC confirmed this hypothesis, leading to pro-inflammatory cytokine secretion by pSS SGEC, and preventing NF-κB inhibition. However, what is the effect of RTX on NF-κB relate to the B cells depletion, since literature indicates that treatment with RTX leads to an effective depletion of B cells in pSS patients? Evidence suggests that Fc/FcγR interactions are critical, as determined in both animal models and humans [107]. Data collected suggest that the formation of IgG immune complexes between B lymphocytes and RTX could engage specific FcγR on pSS SGEC, resulting in a decreased NF-κB activity and interruption of the NF-κB signalling pathway through the up-regulation of the RKIP protein [102] and engagement of the mitogen-activated protein kinase (MAP kinase) signalling [108]. A schematic model of RTX-mediated inhibition of the NF-κB pathway in pSS SGEC is reported in Figure 5.

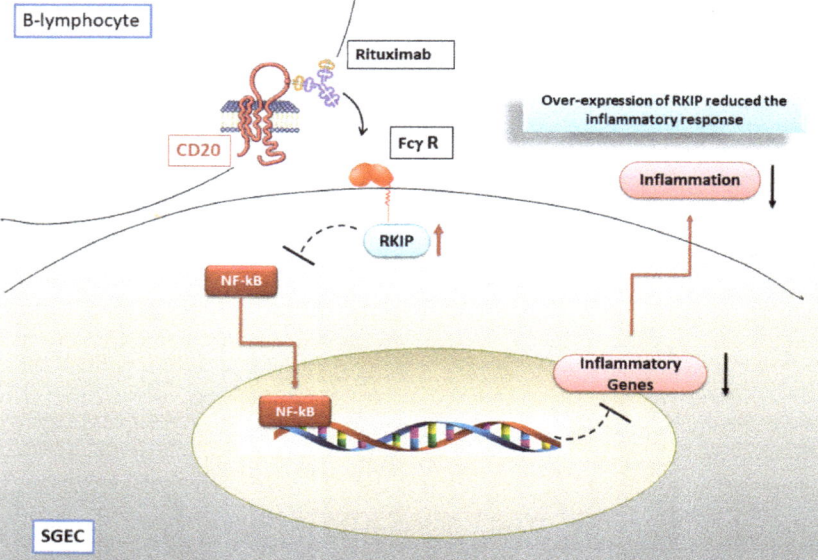

Figure 5. Rituximab (RTX) inhibits NF-κB signalling in pSS SGEC. The pSS SGs epithelial cells (SGEC) were found to express low levels of Raf-1 kinase inhibitor protein (RKIP). In a co-culture system with pSS B-lymphocytes, the FcγR-mediated interaction of RTX/CD20 induces the upregulation of RKIP expression, decreasing NF-κB activity, and, consequently, inhibiting the pro-inflammatory genes transcription.

8. Fine Modulation of NF-κB Activity by TNFAIP3

Numerous studies reported in this review clearly show that several cell types isolated from patients affected by autoimmune diseases show constitutively activated NF-κB transcription factors; there is considerable evidence of NF-κB activation in SGECs derived from pSS patients [17,18,25,26]. Dysregulation of NF-κB-dependent gene expression leads to a variety of autoimmune inflammatory conditions, cancer and neurological disorders [33,34]. Since NF-κB signalling activation is important for several cellular processes, not surprisingly, a tight modulation of this pathway is absolutely essential to trigger target genes. As reported above, among the small regulators of NF-κB activity, great attention has been paid, in the last years, to TNFAIP3, which is a negative feedback regulator of NF-κB activation via TNF-α signalling. Given its key role in the fine modulation of NF-κB pathway, it has been demonstrated that a dysregulated expression of TNFAIP3 protein contributes to chronic inflammation and tissue injury [109]. The importance of TNFAIP3 in reducing inflammation is underlined by the linking of TNFAIP3 genomic region polymorphisms with human autoimmune and inflammatory diseases, including RA [110], psoriasis [111], SLE [112], and type 1 diabetes [113]. Thus, TNFAIP3 has been considered as a crucial anti-inflammatory factor acting to limit prolonged inflammation. A presumed association of TNFAIP3 polymorphism with pSS syndrome has recently been reported [114]. Moreover, TNFAIP3 gene and protein expression levels resulted diminished in salivary tissue from active pSS, demonstrating that under-expression of this protein may reflect an enhanced inflammatory reaction.

Reduced TNFAIP3 Expression Levels in pSS Affect NF-κB Signalling

Recent investigations support an anti-inflammatory role of TNFAIP3, indeed, knockout mice for this gene evolve multiple organ inflammation [115], TNFAIP3 gene silencing in dendritic cells leads to the release of specific co-stimulatory factors, such as pro-inflammatory cytokines [116] and genetically TNFAIP3 deficient mice also show severe intestinal inflammation [115]. The reduced levels of TNFAIP3 observed in pSS, characterized by a remarkable inflammation of the SGs, may promote chronic invasive immune processes in these patients, triggering an initial abnormal inflammatory response. Several findings suggest that the reduction of TNFAIP3 expression levels could lead to the deregulation of NF-κB signalling in pSS patients who show a higher transcriptional activity of NF-κB than normal control subjects [17]. Since TNFAIP3 is a negative regulator of NF-κB signalling in human SGECs, its deregulation could be responsible for the persistent expression of NF-κB that occurs in pSS. This corroborates the notion that human SGECs play an essential role in coordinating the SGs inflammatory reactions to pro-inflammatory factors and suggests that the NF-κB pathway is crucial in these cells for modulating immune responses (see, for example, Figure 3) [17]. Since TNF-α contributes to tissue inflammation, a system mediated by TNF-α-dependent NF-κB activation, it is plausible to postulate that it may translocate the nucleus and promote the expression of inflammatory genes [117]. In accordance with this hypothesis, our recent findings have shown a higher expression of TNF-α in SGECs isolated from pSS patients [15], confirming the role of TNF-α as an inducer of TNFAIP3 protein expression. The enhanced NF-κB activity that occurs in human SGECs, following treatment of the epithelium with TNF-α, could be responsible for the paracrine progression of the inflammatory response shown in SS, inducing pro-inflammatory genes transcription. Therefore, because TNFAIP3 is affected in the negative regulation of NF-κB activation, the inactivity of TNFAIP3 protein was postulated to give rise to a constitutive activation of NF-κB contributing to marked inflammatory reactions. These hypotheses were demonstrated in TNFAIP3 knockdown experiments showing that TNFAIP3 gene silencing induces a constitutive activation of NF-κB in human healthy SGEC [17] (Figure 6) and in experiments conducted on TNFAIP3 knockout mice [115]. Mice with deficient TNFAIP3 are, in fact, hypersensitive to TNF-α and showed grave inflammation and severe damage in multiple organs. TNFAIP3-deficient cells are not able to terminate TNF-α-induced NF-κB responses and rapidly die due to TNF-α-mediated apoptosis [115].

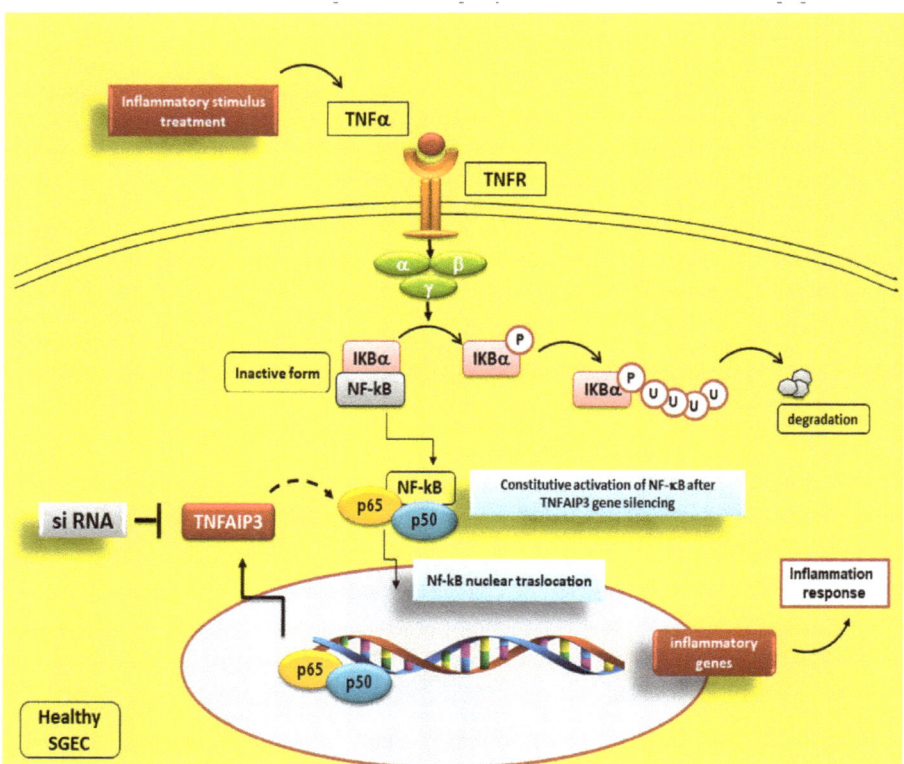

Figure 6. Effect of TNFAIP3 gene silencing in TNF-α stimulated healthy SGEC. This scheme shows how TNFAIP3 knockdown experiments induce a constitutive activation of NF-κB in human healthy SGEC, leading to a severe inflammatory response. siRNA: short interfering RNA; dashed line represents inhibition of the constitutive activation of NF-κB; solid line indicates activation.

9. Conclusions

In this review, we summarize the aberrant activation of NF-κB in pSS, clearly demonstrating that NF-κB has a crucial role in the pathogenesis of pSS, since it promotes chronic inflammation. NF-κB, through intrinsic SGEC activation, regulates sophisticated feedback circuits in pSS that comprise all elements of the cellular immune response. Since NF-κB and members of its signalling pathways regulate cellular activity from DNA transcription to translation into proteins, efficient and properly controlled NF-κB signalling is important during physiological immune homeostasis. In fact, the integrity of the signal triggered by NF-κB is essential in preventing the onset of pSS autoimmune disease. It is noteworthy that the significance of NF-κB activation in pSS suggests that inhibition of this signalling pathway could provide novel strategies for the prevention and treatment of the SGs dysfunction characterizing pSS. New future perspectives suggest, for example, the use of IKKε inhibitors for the treatment of pSS, repressing downstream NF-κB signalling activation. Furthermore, great attention is now being paid to the modulation of NF-κB activity and expression of NF-κB target genes through an IκBα-mediated negative feedback mechanism. Hopefully, as our understanding of the regulation of the NF-κB pathways increases, insights into a better design of drugs that can effectively target NF-κB for the prevention and treatment of pSS may be gained.

Author Contributions: All authors conceived of the presented idea and approved the final version of the manuscript. M.S. and S.L. collected the data reported in the study and take responsibility for their integrity. D.R. performed a critical reading of this review. All authors have read and agreed to the published version of the manuscript.

Funding: No external funding was involved in this review.

Acknowledgments: We are grateful to the professional scientific text editor M.V.C. Pragnell, B.A., for critical reading of the manuscript.

Conflicts of Interest: The authors declare no conflict of interest.

References

1. Wang, X.; Shaalan, A.; Liefers, S.; Coudenys, J.; Elewaut, D.; Proctor, G.B.; Bootsma, H.; Kroese, F.G.M.; Pringle, S. Dysregulation of NF-kB in glandular epithelial cells results in Sjögren's-like features. *PLoS ONE* **2018**, *13*, e0200212. [CrossRef]
2. Fox, P.C. Autoimmune Diseases and Sjögren's Syndrome. *Ann. N. Y. Acad. Sci.* **2007**, *1098*, 15–21. [CrossRef] [PubMed]
3. Oeckinghaus, A.; Ghosh, S. The NF-kappaB family of transcription factors and its regulation. *Cold Spring Harb. Perspect. Biol.* **2009**, *1*, a000034. [CrossRef] [PubMed]
4. Chen, W.; Lin, J.; Cao, H.; Xu, D.; Xu, B.; Xu, L.; Yue, L.; Sun, C.; Wu, G.; Qian, W. Local and Systemic IKKε and NF-κB Signaling Associated with Sjögren's Syndrome Immunopathogenesis. *J. Immunol. Res.* **2015**, *2015*, 534648. [CrossRef]
5. Cafaro, G.; Croia, C.; Argyropoulou, O.D.; Leone, M.C.; Orlandi, M.; Finamore, F.; Cecchettini, A.; Ferro, F.; Baldini, C.; Bartoloni, E. One year in review 2019: Sjögren's syndrome. *Clin. Exp. Rheumatol.* **2019**, *118*, 3–15.
6. Tzioufas, A.G.; Voulgarelis, M. Update on Sjögren's syndrome autoimmune epithelitis: From classification to increased neoplasias. *Best Pract. Res. Clin. Rheumatol.* **2007**, *21*, 989–1010. [CrossRef]
7. Papageorgiou, A.; Ziogas, D.C.; Mavragani, C.P.; Zintzaras, E.; Tzioufas, A.G.; Moutsopoulos, H.M.; Voulgarelis, M. Predicting the outcome of Sjogren's syndrome-associated non-hodgkin's lymphoma patients. *PLoS ONE* **2015**, *10*, e0116189. [CrossRef]
8. Voulgarelis, M.; Tzioufas, A.G. Current aspects of pathogenesis in Sjögren's syndrome. *Ther. Adv. Musculoskelet. Dis.* **2010**, *2*, 325–334. [CrossRef]
9. Fox, P.C.; Speight, P.M. Current concepts of autoimmune exocrinopathy: Immunologic mechanisms in the salivary pathology of Sjögren's syndrome. *Crit. Rev. Oral Biol. Med.* **1996**, *7*, 144–158. [CrossRef]
10. Humphreys-Beher, M.G.; Peck, A.B.; Dang, H.; Talal, N. The role of apoptosis in the initiation of the autoimmune response in Sjögren's syndrome. *Clin. Exp. Immunol.* **1999**, *116*, 383–387. [CrossRef]
11. Manoussakis, M.N.; Kapsogeorgou, E.K. The role of epithelial cells in the pathogenesis of Sjögren's syndrome. *Clin. Rev. Allergy Immunol.* **2007**, *32*, 225–230. [CrossRef]
12. Moutsopoulos, H.M. Sjögren's syndrome: Autoimmune epithelitis. *Clin. Immunol. Immunopathol.* **1994**, *72*, 162–165. [CrossRef] [PubMed]
13. Sisto, M.; Lisi, S.; Castellana, D.; Scagliusi, P.; D'Amore, M.; Caprio, S.; Scagliusi, A.; Acquafredda, A.A.; Panaro, M.A.; Mitolo, V. Autoantibodies from Sjögren's syndrome induce activation of both the intrinsic and extrinsic apoptotic pathways in human salivary gland cell line A-253. *J. Autoimmun.* **2006**, *27*, 38–49. [CrossRef]
14. Sisto, M.; Lisi, S.; Lofrumento, D.; D'Amore, M.; Scagliusi, P.; Mitolo, V. Autoantibodies from Sjögren's syndrome trigger apoptosis in salivary gland cell line. *Ann. N. Y. Acad. Sci.* **2007**, *1108*, 418–425. [CrossRef] [PubMed]
15. Sisto, M.; Lisi, S.; Lofrumento, D.D.; Caprio, S.; Mitolo, V.; D'Amore, M. TNF blocker drugs modulate human TNF-α-converting enzyme pro-domain shedding induced by autoantibodies. *Immunobiology* **2010**, *215*, 874–883. [CrossRef] [PubMed]
16. Sisto, M.; Lisi, S.; Lofrumento, D.D.; Ingravallo, G.; Mitolo, V.; D'Amore, M. Expression of pro-inflammatory TACE-TNF-α-amphiregulin axis in Sjögren's syndrome salivary glands. *Histochem. Cell Biol.* **2010**, *134*, 345–353. [CrossRef]

17. Sisto, M.; Lisi, S.; Lofrumento, D.D.; Ingravallo, G.; Maiorano, E.; D'Amore, M. A failure of TNFAIP3 negative regulation maintains sustained NF-κB activation in Sjögren's syndrome. *Histochem. Cell Biol.* **2011**, *135*, 615–625. [CrossRef]
18. Sisto, M.; Lisi, S.; Lofrumento, D.D.; D'Amore, M.; Frassanito, M.A.; Ribatti, D. Sjögren's syndrome pathological neovascularization is regulated by VEGF-A-stimulated TACE-dependent crosstalk between VEGFR2 and NF-κB. *Genes Immun.* **2012**, *13*, 411–420. [CrossRef]
19. Sisto, M.; Lisi, S.; Lofrumento, D.D.; Ingravallo, G.; De Lucro, R.; D'Amore, M. Salivary gland expression level of IκBα regulatory protein in Sjögren's syndrome. *J. Mol. Histol.* **2013**, *44*, 447–454. [CrossRef]
20. Sisto, M.; Lisi, S.; D'Amore, M.; Lofrumento, D.D. The metalloproteinase ADAM17 and the epidermal growth factor receptor (EGFR) signaling drive the inflammatory epithelial response in Sjögren's syndrome. *Clin. Exp. Med.* **2015**, *15*, 215–225. [CrossRef]
21. Lisi, S.; Sisto, M.; Soleti, R.; Saponaro, C.; Scagliusi, P.; D'Amore, M.; Saccia, M.; Maffione, A.B.; Mitolo, V. Fcgamma receptors mediate internalization of anti-Ro and anti-La autoantibodies from Sjögren's syndrome and apoptosis in human salivary gland cell line A-253. *J. Oral Pathol. Med.* **2007**, *36*, 511–523. [CrossRef] [PubMed]
22. Lisi, S.; Sisto, M.; Scagliusi, P.; Mitolo, V.; D'Amore, M. Sjögren's syndrome: Anti-Ro and anti-La autoantibodies trigger apoptotic mechanism in the human salivary gland cell line, A-253. *Panminerva Med.* **2007**, *49*, 103–108.
23. Lisi, S.; D'Amore, M.; Scagliusi, P.; Mitolo, V.; Sisto, M. Anti-Ro/SSA autoantibody-mediated regulation of extracellular matrix fibulins in human epithelial cells of the salivary gland. *Scand. J. Rheumatol.* **2009**, *38*, 198–206. [CrossRef] [PubMed]
24. Lisi, S.; Sisto, M.; Lofrumento, D.D.; Cucci, L.; Frassanito, M.A.; Mitolo, V.; D'Amore, M. Pro-inflammatory role of Anti-Ro/SSA autoantibodies through the activation of Furin-TACE-amphiregulin axis. *J. Autoimmun.* **2010**, *35*, 160–170. [CrossRef] [PubMed]
25. Lisi, S.; Sisto, M.; Lofrumento, D.D.; D'Amore, M. Sjögren's syndrome autoantibodies provoke changes in gene expression profiles of inflammatory cytokines triggering a pathway involving TACE/NF-κB. *Lab. Investig.* **2012**, *92*, 615–624. [CrossRef]
26. Lisi, S.; Sisto, M.; Lofrumento, D.D.; D'Amore, M. Altered IκBα expression promotes NF-κB activation in monocytes from primary Sjögren's syndrome patients. *Pathology* **2012**, *44*, 557–561. [CrossRef] [PubMed]
27. Lisi, S.; Sisto, M.; Lofrumento, D.D.; D'Amore, M.; De Lucro, R.; Ribatti, D. A potential role of the GRO-α/CXCR2 system in Sjögren's syndrome: Regulatory effects of pro-inflammatory cytokines. *Histochem. Cell Biol.* **2013**, *139*, 371–379. [CrossRef]
28. Lisi, S.; Sisto, M.; D'Amore, M.; Lofrumento, D.D.; Ribatti, D. Emerging avenues linking inflammation, angiogenesis and Sjögren's syndrome. *Cytokine* **2013**, *61*, 693–703. [CrossRef]
29. Lisi, S.; Sisto, M.; Ribatti, D.; D'Amore, M.; De Lucro, R.; Frassanito, M.A.; Lorusso, L.; Vacca, A.; Lofrumento, D.D. Chronic inflammation enhances NGF-β/TrkA system expression via EGFR/MEK/ERK pathway activation in Sjögren's syndrome. *J. Mol. Med.* **2014**, *92*, 523–537. [CrossRef]
30. Pringle, S.; Wang, X.; Bootsma, H.; Spijkervet, F.K.L.; Vissink, A.; Kroese, F.G.M. Small-molecule inhibitors and the salivary gland epithelium in Sjögren's syndrome. *Expert Opin. Investig. Drugs.* **2019**, *28*, 605–616. [CrossRef]
31. Hayden, M.S.; Ghosh, S. NF-κB, the first quarter-century: Remarkable progress and outstanding questions. *Genes Dev.* **2012**, *26*, 203–234. [CrossRef]
32. Sun, S.C.; Ganchi, P.A.; Ballard, D.W.; Greene, W.C. NF-κB controls expression of inhibitor IκBα: Evidence for an inducible autoregulatory pathway. *Science* **1993**, *259*, 1912–1915. [CrossRef]
33. Christman, J.W.; Sadikot, R.T.; Blackwell, T.S. The role of nuclear factor-kappa B in pulmonary diseases. *Chest* **2000**, *117*, 1482–1487. [CrossRef]
34. Yamamoto, Y.; Gaynor, R.B. Role of the NF-kB pathway in the pathogenesis of human disease states. *Curr. Mol. Med.* **2001**, *1*, 287–296. [CrossRef]
35. Li, Q.; Verma, I.M. NF-kappaB regulation in the immune system. *Nat. Rev. Immunol.* **2002**, *2*, 725–734. [CrossRef]
36. Kaltschmidt, B.; Widera, D.; Kaltschmidt, C. Signaling via NF-kappaB in the nervous system. *Biochim. Biophys. Acta* **2005**, *1745*, 287–299. [CrossRef]
37. Ledoux, A.C.; Perkins, N.D. NF-kappaB and the cell cycle. *Biochem. Soc. Trans.* **2014**, *42*, 76–81. [CrossRef]

38. Han, Z.; Boyle, D.L.; Manning, A.M.; Firestein, G.S. AP-1 and NF-kappa B regulation in rheumatoid arthritis and murine collagen-induced arthritis. *Autoimmunity* **1998**, *28*, 197–208. [CrossRef] [PubMed]
39. Makarov, S.S. NF-kappa B in rheumatoid arthritis: A pivotal regulator of inflammation, hyperplasia, and tissue destruction. *Arthritis Res.* **2001**, *3*, 200–206. [CrossRef]
40. Nakamura, H.; Kawakami, A.; Ida, H.; Koji, T.; Eguchi, K. EGF activates PI3K-Akt and NF-κB via distinct pathways in salivary epithelial cells in Sjögren's syndrome. *Rheumatol. Int.* **2007**, *28*, 127–136. [CrossRef]
41. Ping, L.; Ogawa, N.; Zhang, Y.; Sugai, S.; Masaki, Y.; Xiao, W. p38 mitogen-activated protein kinase and nuclear factor-kappaB facilitate CD40-mediated salivary epithelial cell death. *J. Rheumatol.* **2012**, *39*, 1256–1264. [CrossRef]
42. Barnes, P.; Karin, M. Nuclear Factor-κB: A Pivotal Transcription Factor in Chronic Inflammatory Diseases. *N. Engl. J. Med.* **1997**, *336*, 1066–1071. [CrossRef]
43. Tak, P.P.; Firestein, G.S. NF-kappaB: A key role in inflammatory diseases. *J. Clin. Investig.* **2001**, *107*, 7–11. [CrossRef]
44. Dale, E.; Davis, M.; Faustman, D.L. A role for transcription factor NF-κB in autoimmunity: Possible interactions of genes, sex, and the immune response. *Adv. Physiol. Educ.* **2006**, *30*, 152–158. [CrossRef]
45. Thompson, N.; Isenberg, D.A.; Jury, E.C.; Ciurtin, C. Exploring BAFF: Its expression, receptors and contribution to the immunopathogenesis of Sjögren's syndrome. *Rheumatology* **2016**, *55*, 1548–1555. [CrossRef]
46. Nordmark, G.; Wang, C.; Vasaitis, L.; Eriksson, P.; Theander, E.; Kvarnstrom, M.; Forsblad-d'Elia, H.; Jazebi, H.; Sjowall, C.; Reksten, T.R.; et al. Association of Genes in the NF-kappaB Pathway with Antibody-Positive Primary Sjogren's Syndrome. *Scand. J. Immunol.* **2013**, *78*, 447–454. [CrossRef]
47. Ou, T.T.; Lin, C.H.; Lin, Y.C.; Li, R.N.; Tsai, W.C.; Liu, H.W.; Yen, J.H. IkappaBalpha promoter polymorphisms in patients with primary Sjögren's syndrome. *J. Clin. Immunol.* **2008**, *28*, 440–444. [CrossRef]
48. Peng, B.; Ling, J.; Lee, A.J.; Wang, Z.; Chang, Z.; Jin, W.; Kang, Y.; Zhang, R.; Shim, D.; Wang, H.; et al. Defective feedback regulation of NF-kappaB underlies Sjogren's syndrome in mice with mutated kappaB enhancers of the IkappaBalpha promoter. *Proc. Natl. Acad. Sci. USA* **2010**, *107*, 15193–15198. [CrossRef]
49. Kwok, S.K.; Cho, M.L.; Her, Y.M.; Oh, H.J.; Park, M.K.; Lee, S.Y.; Woo, Y.J.; Ju, J.H.; Park, K.S.; Kim, H.Y.; et al. TLR2 ligation induces the production of IL-23/IL-17 via IL-6, STAT3 and NF-kB pathway in patients with primary Sjögren's syndrome. *Arthritis Res. Ther.* **2012**, *14*, R64. [CrossRef]
50. Sisto, M.; Lorusso, L.; Lisi, S. Interleukin-15 as a potential new target in Sjögren's syndrome-associated inflammation. *Pathology* **2016**, *48*, 602–607. [CrossRef]
51. Sisto, M.; Lorusso, L.; Lisi, S. TLR2 signals via NF-κB to drive IL-15 production in salivary gland epithelial cells derived from patients with primary Sjögren's syndrome. *Clin. Exp. Med.* **2017**, *17*, 341–350. [CrossRef] [PubMed]
52. Das, T.; Chen, Z.; Hendriks, R.W.; Kool, M. A20/Tumor Necrosis Factor α-Induced Protein 3 in Immune Cells Controls Development of Autoinflammation and Autoimmunity: Lessons from Mouse Models. *Front. Immunol.* **2018**, *9*, 104. [CrossRef] [PubMed]
53. Dawson, L.J.; Field, E.A.; Harmer, A.R.; Smith, P.M. Acetylcholine-evoked calcium mobilization and ion channel activation in human labial gland acinar cells from patients with primary Sjogren's syndrome. *Clin. Exp. Immunol.* **2001**, *124*, 480–485. [CrossRef] [PubMed]
54. Lilienbaum, A.; Israël, A. From calcium to NF-kappa B signaling pathways in neurons. *Mol. Cell. Biol.* **2003**, *23*, 2680–2698. [CrossRef] [PubMed]
55. Liu, T.; Zhang, L.; Joo, D.; Sun, S.C. NF-κB signaling in inflammation. *Sig. Transduct. Target Ther.* **2017**, *2*, 17023. [CrossRef]
56. Zhang, J.; Peng, B. NF-kappaB promotes iNOS and VEGF expression in salivary gland adenoid cystic carcinoma cells and enhances endothelial cell motility in vitro. *Cell Prolif.* **2009**, *42*, 150–161. [CrossRef]
57. Miterski, B.; Böhringer, S.; Klein, W.; Sindern, E.; Haupts, M.; Schimrigk, S.; Epplen, J.T. Inhibitors in the NFkappaB cascade comprise prime candidate genes predisposing to multiple sclerosis, especially in selected combinations. *Genes Immun.* **2002**, *3*, 211–219. [CrossRef]
58. Klein, W.; Tromm, A.; Folwaczny, C.; Hagedorn, M.; Duerig, N.; Epplen, J.T.; Schmiegel, W.H.; Griga, T. A polymorphism of the NFKBIA gene is associated with Crohn's disease patients lacking a predisposing allele of the CARD15 gene. *Int. J. Colorectal Dis.* **2004**, *19*, 153–156. [CrossRef]

59. Zubair, A.; Frieri, M. NF-κB and systemic lupus erythematosus: Examining the link. *J. Nephrol.* **2013**, *26*, 953–959. [CrossRef]
60. Gestermann, N.; Mekinian, A.; Comets, E.; Loiseau, P.; Puechal, X.; Hachulla, E.; Gottenberg, L.E.; Mariette, X.; Miceli-Richard, C. STAT4 is a confirmed genetic risk factor for Sjögren's syndrome and could be involved in type 1 interferon pathway signaling. *Genes Immun.* **2010**, *11*, 432438.
61. Palomino-Morales, R.J.; Diaz-Gallo, L.M.; Witte, T.; Anaya, J.M.; Martín, J. Influence of STAT4 polymorphism in primary Sjögren's syndrome. *J. Rheumatol.* **2010**, *37*, 1016–1019. [CrossRef] [PubMed]
62. Pispa, J.; Pummila, M.; Barker, P.A.; Thesleff, I.; Mikkola, M.L. Edar and Troy signalling pathways act redundantly to regulate initiation of hair follicle development. *Hum. Mol. Genet.* **2008**, *17*, 3380–3391. [CrossRef] [PubMed]
63. Mikkola, M.L. TNF superfamily in skin appendage development. *Cytokine Growth Factor Rev.* **2008**, *19*, 219–230. [CrossRef] [PubMed]
64. Headon, D.J.; Emmal, S.A.; Ferguson, B.M.; Tucker, A.S.; Justice, M.J.; Sharpe, P.T.; Zonana, J.; Overbeek, P.A. Gene defect in ectodermal dysplasia implicates a death domain adapter in development. *Nature* **2001**, *414*, 913–916. [CrossRef] [PubMed]
65. Melnick, M.; Jaskoll, T. Mouse submandibular gland morphogenesis: A paradigm for embryonic signal processing. *Crit. Rev. Oral Biol. Med.* **2000**, *11*, 199–215. [CrossRef] [PubMed]
66. Skaug, B.; Jiang, X.; Chen, Z.J. The role of ubiquitin in NF-kappaB regulatory pathways. *Annu. Rev. Biochem.* **2009**, *78*, 769–796. [CrossRef]
67. Yamamoto, Y.; Gaynor, R.B. Therapeutic potential of inhibition of the NF-kappaB pathway in the treatment of inflammation and cancer. *J. Clin. Investig.* **2001**, *107*, 135–142. [CrossRef]
68. Schmidt-Ullrich, R.; Aebischer, T.; Hulsken, J.; Birchmeier, W.; Klemm, U.; Scheidereit, C. Requirement of NF-kappaB/Rel for the development of hair follicles and other epidermal appendices. *Development* **2001**, *128*, 3843–3853.
69. Courtney, J.M.; Blackburn, J.; Sharpe, P.T. The Ectodysplasin and NFkappaB signalling pathways in odontogenesis. *Arch. Oral Biol.* **2005**, *50*, 159–163. [CrossRef]
70. Sisto, M.; Barca, A.; Lofrumento, D.D.; Lisi, S. Downstream activation of NF-κB in the EDA-A1/EDAR signalling in Sjögren's syndrome and its regulation by the ubiquitin-editing enzyme A20. *Clin. Exp. Immunol.* **2016**, *184*, 183–196. [CrossRef] [PubMed]
71. Ambrosi, A.; Wahren-Herlenius, M. Update on the immunobiology of Sjögren's syndrome. *Curr. Opin. Rheumatol.* **2015**, *27*, 468–475. [CrossRef]
72. Takeda, K.; Kaisho, T.; Akira, S. Toll-like receptors. *Annu. Rev. Immunol.* **2003**, *21*, 335–376. [CrossRef]
73. Kawai, T.; Akira, S. Signaling to NF-kB by Toll-like receptors. *Trends Mol. Med.* **2007**, *13*, 460–469. [CrossRef]
74. Brentano, F.; Kyburz, D.; Schorr, O.; Gay, R.; Gay, S. The role of Toll like receptor signaling in the pathogenesis of arthritis. *Cell Immunol.* **2005**, *233*, 90–96. [CrossRef]
75. Kanczkowski, W.; Ziegler, C.G.; Zacharowski, K.; Bornstein, S.R. Toll-like receptors in endocrine disease and diabetes. *NeuroImmunoModulation* **2008**, *15*, 54–60. [CrossRef]
76. Pisetsky, D.S. The role of innate immunity in the induction of autoimmunity. *Autoimmun. Rev.* **2008**, *8*, 69–72. [CrossRef]
77. Wu, Y.W.; Tang, W.; Zuo, J.P. Toll-like receptors: Potential targets for lupus treatment. *Acta Pharmacol. Sin.* **2015**, *36*, 1395–1407. [CrossRef]
78. Gooshe, M.; Aleyasin, A.R.; Abdolghaffari, A.H.; Rezaei, N. Toll like receptors: A new hope on the horizon to treat multiple sclerosis. *Expert Rev. Clin. Immunol.* **2014**, *10*, 1277–1279. [CrossRef]
79. Sipos, F.; Furi, I.; Constantinovits, M.; Tulassay, Z.; Muzes, G. Contribution of TLR signaling to the pathogenesis of colitis-associated cancer in inflammatory bowel disease. *World J. Gastroenterol.* **2014**, *20*, 12713–12721. [CrossRef]
80. Birchler, T.; Seibl, R.; Buchner, K.; Loeliger, S.; Seger, R.; Hossle, J.P.; Aguzzi, A.; Lauener, R.P. Human Toll-like receptor 2 mediates induction of the antimicrobial peptide human beta-defensin 2 in response to bacterial lipoprotein. *Eur. J. Immunol.* **2001**, *31*, 3131–3137. [CrossRef]
81. Hertz, C.J.; Wu, Q.; Porter, E.M.; Zhang, Y.J.; Weismüller, K.H.; Godowski, P.J.; Ganz, T.; Randell, S.H.; Modlin, R.L. Activation of Toll-like receptor 2 on human tracheobronchial epithelial cells induces the antimicrobial peptide human beta defensin-2. *J. Immunol.* **2003**, *171*, 6820–6826. [CrossRef]

82. Spachidou, M.P.; Bourazopoulou, E.; Maratheftis, C.I.; Kapsogeorgou, E.K.; Moutsopoulos, H.M.; Tzioufas, A.G.; Manoussakis, M.N. Expression of functional Toll-like receptors by salivary gland epithelial cells: Increased mRNA expression in cells derived from patients with primary Sjogren's syndrome. *Clin. Exp. Immunol.* **2007**, *147*, 497–503. [CrossRef]
83. Liu, Y.; Yin, H.; Zhao, M.; Lu, Q. TLR2 and TLR4 in Autoimmune Diseases: A Comprehensive Review. *Clin. Rev. Allerg. Immunol.* **2014**, *47*, 136–147. [CrossRef] [PubMed]
84. Kiripolsky, J.; Kramer, J.M. Current and Emerging Evidence for Toll-Like Receptor Activation in Sjögren's Syndrome. *J. Immunol. Res.* **2018**, *2018*, 1246818. [CrossRef] [PubMed]
85. Heil, F.; Hemmi, H.; Hochrein, H.; Franziska Ampenberger, F.; Kirschning, C.; Akira, S.; Lipford, G.; Wagner, H.; Bauer, S. Species-specific recognition of single-stranded RNA via toll-like receptor 7 and 8. *Science* **2004**, *303*, 1526–1529. [CrossRef] [PubMed]
86. Bauer, S.; Kirschning, C.J.; Häcker, H.; Redecke, V.; Hausmann, S.; Akira, S.; Wagner, H.; Lipford, G.B. Human TLR9 confers responsiveness to bacterial DNA via species-specific CpG motif recognition. *Proc. Natl. Acad. Sci. USA* **2001**, *98*, 9237–9242. [CrossRef]
87. Zheng, L.; Zhang, Z.; Yu, C.; Yang, C. Expression of Toll-like receptors 7, 8, and 9 in primary Sjogren's syndrome. *Oral Surg. Oral Med. Oral Pathol. Oral Radiol. Endodontol.* **2010**, *109*, 844–850. [CrossRef]
88. Rosenblum, M.D.; Remedios, K.A.; Abbas, A.K. Mechanisms of human autoimmunity. *J. Clin. Investig.* **2015**, *125*, 2228–2233. [CrossRef]
89. Shimizu, T.; Nakamura, H.; Takatani, A.; Umeda, V.; Horai, Y.; Kurushima, S.; Michitsuji, T.; Nakashima, Y.; Kawakami, A. Activation of Toll-like receptor 7 signaling in labial salivary glands of primary Sjögren's syndrome patients. *Clin. Exp. Immunol.* **2019**, *196*, 39–51. [CrossRef] [PubMed]
90. Flynn, C.M.; Garbers, Y.; Lokau, J.; Wesch, D.; Schulte, D.M.; Laudes, M.; Lieb, W.; Aparicio-Siegmund, S.; Garbers, C. Activation of Toll Like Receptor 2 (TLR2) induces interleukin-6 trans-signalling. *Sci. Rep.* **2019**, *9*, 7306. [CrossRef] [PubMed]
91. Nadler, L.M.; Ritz, J.; Hardy, R.; Pesando, J.M.; Schlossman, S.F.; Stashenko, P. A unique cell surface antigen identifying lymphoid malignancies of B cell origin. *J. Clin. Investig.* **1981**, *67*, 134–140. [CrossRef] [PubMed]
92. Cragg, M.S.; Walshe, C.A.; Ivanov, A.O.; Glennie, M.J. The biology of CD20 and its potential as a target for mAb therapy In: B cell trophic factors and B cell antagonism in autoimmune disease. *Curr. Dir. Autoimmun.* **2005**, *8*, 140–174.
93. Walshe, C.A.; Beers, S.A.; French, R.R.; Chan, C.H.T.; Johnson, P.W.; Packham, G.K.; Glennie, M.J.; Cragg, M.S. Induction of cytosolic calcium flux by CD20 is dependent upon B Cell antigen receptor signaling. *J. Biol. Chem.* **2008**, *283*, 16971–16984. [CrossRef]
94. Leandro, M.J. B-cell subpopulations in humans and their differential susceptibility to depletion with anti-CD20 monoclonal antibodies. *Arthritis Res. Ther.* **2013**, *15*, S3. [CrossRef]
95. Rehnberg, M.; Amu, S.; Tarkowski, A.; Bokarewa, M.J.; Brisslert, M. Short- and long-term effects of anti-CD20 treatment on B cell ontogeny in bone marrow of patients with rheumatoid arthritis. *Arthritis Res. Ther.* **2009**, *11*, R123. [CrossRef]
96. Polyak, M.J.; Li, H.; Shariat, N.; Deans, J.P. CD20 homo-oligomers physically associate with the B cell antigen receptor. *J. Biol. Chem.* **2008**, *283*, 18545–18552. [CrossRef]
97. Devauchelle-Pensec, V.; Pennec, Y.; Morvan, J.; Pers, J.O.; Daridon, C.; Jousse-Joulin, S.; Roudaut, A.; Jamin, C.; Renaudineau, Y.; Roué, I.Q.; et al. Improvement of Sjögren's syndrome after two infusions of rituximab (anti-CD20). *Arthritis Rheum.* **2007**, *57*, 310–317. [CrossRef]
98. Meijer, J.M.; Meiners, P.M.; Vissink, A.; Spijkervet, F.K.L.; Abdulahad, W.; Kamminga, N.; Brouwer, E.; Kallenberg, C.G.M.; Bootsma, H. Effectiveness of rituximab treatment in primary Sjögren's syndrome: A randomized, double-blind, placebo controlled trial. *Arthritis Rheum.* **2010**, *62*, 960–968. [CrossRef]
99. Abdulahad, W.H.; Meijer, J.M.; Kroese, F.G.; Meiners, P.M.; Vissink, A.; Spijkervet, F.K.; Kallenberg, C.G.; Bootsma, H. B cell reconstitution and T helper cell balance after rituximab treatment of active primary Sjogren's syndrome: A double-blind, placebo-controlled study. *Arthritis Rheum.* **2011**, *63*, 1116–1123. [CrossRef]
100. Edwards, J.C.; Szczepanski, L.; Szechinski, J.; Filipowicz-Sosnowska, A.; Emery, P.; Close, D.R.; Stevens, R.M.; Shaw, T. Efficacy of B-cell-targeted therapy with rituximab in patients with rheumatoid arthritis. *N. Engl. J. Med.* **2004**, *350*, 2572–2581. [CrossRef]

101. Stone, J.H.; Merkel, P.A.; Spiera, R.; Merkel, P.A.; Seo, P.; Spiera, R.; Langford, C.A.; Hoffman, G.S.; Kallenberg, C.G.M.; Clair, E.W.S.; et al. Rituximab versus cyclophosphamide for ANCA associated vasculitis. *N. Engl. J. Med.* **2010**, *363*, 221–232. [CrossRef]
102. Sisto, M.; Lisi, S.; D'Amore, M.; Lofrumento, D.D. Rituximab-mediated Raf kinase inhibitor protein induction modulates NF-κB in Sjögren syndrome. *Immunology* **2014**, *143*, 42–51. [CrossRef]
103. Lisi, S.; Sisto, M.; D'Amore, M.; Lofrumento, D.D. Co-culture system of human salivary gland epithelial cells and immune cells from primary Sjögren's syndrome patients: An in vitro approach to study the effects of Rituximab on the activation of the Raf-1/ERK1/2 pathway. *Int. Immunol.* **2015**, *27*, 183–194. [CrossRef]
104. Jazirehi, A.R.; Huerta-Yepez, S.; Cheng, G.; Bonavida, B. Rituximab (chimeric anti-CD20 monoclonal antibody) inhibits the constitutive nuclear factor-jB signalling pathway in non-Hodgkin's lymphoma B-cell lines: Role in sensitization to chemotherapeutic drug induced apoptosis. *Cancer Res.* **2005**, *65*, 264–276.
105. Zeng, L.; Imamoto, A.; Rosner, M.R. Raf kinase inhibitory protein (RKIP): A physiological regulator and future therapeutic target. *Expert Opin. Ther. Targets* **2008**, *12*, 1275–1287. [CrossRef]
106. Al-Mulla, F.; Bitar, M.S.; Taqi, Z.; Yeung, K.C. RKIP: Much more than Raf kinase inhibitory protein. *J. Cell Physiol.* **2013**, *228*, 1688–1702. [CrossRef]
107. Casey, E.; Bournazos, S.; Mo, G.; Mondello, P.; Tan, K.S.; Ravetch, J.V.; Scheinberg, D.A. A new mouse expressing human Fcγ receptors to better predict therapeutic efficacy of human anti-cancer antibodies. *Leukemia* **2018**, *32*, 547–549. [CrossRef]
108. Zhao, J.; Wenzel, S. Interactions of RKIP with Inflammatory Signaling Pathways critical reviews in oncogenesis. *Crit. Rev. Oncog.* **2014**, *19*, 497–504. [CrossRef]
109. Bedford, L.; Lowe, J.; Dick, L.; Mayer, R.J.; Brownell, J.E. Ubiquitin-like protein conjugation and the ubiquitin–proteasome system as drug targets. *Nat. Rev. Drug Discov.* **2011**, *10*, 29–46. [CrossRef]
110. Plenge, R.M.; Cotsapas, C.; Davies, L.; Price, A.L.; de Bakker, P.I.; Maller, J.; Pe'er, I.; Burtt, N.P.; Blumenstiel, B.; DeFelice, M.; et al. Two independent alleles at 6q23 associated with risk of rheumatoid arthritis. *Nat. Genet.* **2007**, *39*, 1477–1482. [CrossRef]
111. Nair, R.P.; Duffin, K.C.; Helms, C.; Ding, J.; Stuart, P.E.; Goldgar, D.; Gudjonsson, J.E.; Li, Y.; Tejasvi, T.; Feng, B.J.; et al. Genome-wide scan reveals association of psoriasis with IL-23 and NF-kappa B pathways. *Nat. Genet.* **2009**, *41*, 199–204. [CrossRef]
112. Graham, R.R.; Cotsapas, C.; Davies, L.; Hackett, R.; Lessard, C.J.; Leon, J.M.; Burtt, N.P.; Guiducci, C.; Parkin, M.; Gates, C.; et al. Genetic variants near TNFAIP3 on 6q23 are associated with systemic lupus erythematosus. *Nat. Genet.* **2008**, *40*, 1059–1061. [CrossRef] [PubMed]
113. Fung, E.Y.; Smyth, D.J.; Howson, J.M.; Cooper, J.D.; Walker, N.M.; Stevens, H.; Wicker, L.S.; Todd, J.A. Analysis of 17 autoimmune disease associated variants in type 1 diabetes identifies 6q23/TNFAIP3 as a susceptibility. *Genes Immun.* **2009**, *10*, 188–191. [CrossRef] [PubMed]
114. Musone, S.L.; Taylor, K.E.; Lu, T.T.; Nititham, J.; Ferreira, R.C.; Ortmann, W.; Shifrin, N.; Petri, M.A.; Kamboh, M.I.; Manzi, S.; et al. Multiple polymorphisms in the TNFAIP3 region are independently associated with systemic lupus erythematosus. *Nat. Genet.* **2008**, *40*, 1062–1064. [CrossRef] [PubMed]
115. Lee, E.G.; Boone, D.L.; Chai, S.; Libby, S.L.; Chien, M.; Lodolce, J.P.; Ma, A. Failure to regulate TNF-induced NF-kappa B and cell death responses in A20-deficient mice. *Science* **2000**, *289*, 2350–2354. [CrossRef]
116. Song, X.T.; Evel-Kabler, K.; Shen, L.; Rollins, L.; Huang, X.F.; Chen, S.Y. A20 is an antigen presentation attenuator, and its inhibition overcomes regulatory T cell-mediated suppression. *Nat. Med.* **2008**, *14*, 258–265. [CrossRef] [PubMed]
117. Heyninck, K.; Beyaert, R. A20 inhibits NF-kappa B activation by dual ubiquitin-editing functions. *Trends Biochem. Sci.* **2005**, *30*, 1–4. [CrossRef]

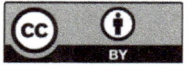

© 2020 by the authors. Licensee MDPI, Basel, Switzerland. This article is an open access article distributed under the terms and conditions of the Creative Commons Attribution (CC BY) license (http://creativecommons.org/licenses/by/4.0/).

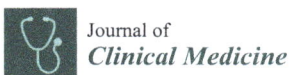 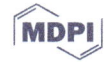

Review

Contributions of Major Cell Populations to Sjögren's Syndrome

Richard Witas [1,2,†], **Shivai Gupta** [1,†] **and Cuong Q. Nguyen** [1,2,3,*]

1. Department of Infectious Diseases and Immunology, College of Veterinary Medicine, University of Florida, Gainesville, FL 32608, USA; rwitas@ufl.edu (R.W.); shivai.gupta@ufl.edu (S.G.)
2. Department of Oral Biology and College of Dentistry, University of Florida, Gainesville, FL 32610, USA
3. Center of Orphaned Autoimmune Diseases, University of Florida, Gainesville, FL 32610, USA
* Correspondence: nguyenc@ufl.edu
† These authors contributed equally to this work.

Received: 18 August 2020; Accepted: 15 September 2020; Published: 22 September 2020

Abstract: Sjögren's syndrome (SS) is a female dominated autoimmune disease characterized by lymphocytic infiltration into salivary and lacrimal glands and subsequent exocrine glandular dysfunction. SS also may exhibit a broad array of extraglandular manifestations including an elevated incidence of non-Hodgkin's B cell lymphoma. The etiology of SS remains poorly understood, yet progress has been made in identifying progressive stages of disease using preclinical mouse models. The roles played by immune cell subtypes within these stages of disease are becoming increasingly well understood, though significant gaps in knowledge still remain. There is evidence for distinct involvement from both innate and adaptive immune cells, where cells of the innate immune system establish a proinflammatory environment characterized by a type I interferon (IFN) signature that facilitates propagation of the disease by further activating T and B cell subsets to generate autoantibodies and participate in glandular destruction. This review will discuss the evidence for participation in disease pathogenesis by various classes of immune cells and glandular epithelial cells based upon data from both preclinical mouse models and human patients. Further examination of the contributions of glandular and immune cell subtypes to SS will be necessary to identify additional therapeutic targets that may lead to better management of the disease.

Keywords: Sjögren's syndrome; autoimmunity; salivary gland; innate cells; adaptive cells

1. Introduction

Sjögren's syndrome (SS) is the second most common autoimmune disorder after rheumatoid arthritis (RA) [1]. Like systemic lupus erythematosus (SLE), SS is a chronic and systemic autoimmune disease [2]. While SS is most commonly associated with xerostomia, xeropthalmia, and lymphocytic infiltration into the exocrine glands, SS patients may present with gastrointestinal symptoms, fatigue, pulmonary problems, and experience a higher incidence of non-Hodgkin's B cell lymphoma (NHL) [2,3]. The lymphocytes that infiltrate into the exocrine glands can organize into focal structures in which germinal center-like formation is present in approximately 25% of primary SS patients [4], establishing a structure for local production of autoantibodies [4,5]. SS primarily affects women and features a highly skewed sex distribution (9:1) [6]. SS is a complex heterogenous disease that can present alone, referred to as primary SS (pSS), or as secondary SS with another autoimmune disease such as RA or SLE. While the adaptive immune cells like B and T cells have traditionally attracted the most interest due to their predominant presence in the exocrine glands and the immunological importance autoantibodies, increasing evidence shows that immune system dysfunction in SS incorporates cells of the innate immune system as well [7–12]. In this review, we aim to present the current state of knowledge on how the common cell types of the innate and adaptive immune systems contribute to SS as revealed by studies of human patients and animal models.

2. Disease Development

Like other autoimmune diseases, SS is considered a multifactorial disease where a susceptible genetic background requires an environmental factor trigger, such as viral infection [13], to initiate the development of disease. Genome wide association studies (GWAS) have identified several genetic risk factors for SS. Two GWAS in SS have been performed, one with patients of European descent, and another with Han Chinese patients [14,15]. Both studies identified alleles within human leukocyte antigen (HLA) Class II to be the most associated with SS, particularly alleles of the HLA-DR and HLA-DQ isotypes. While major histocompatibility complex (MHC) Class II alleles show the greatest association with SS, several non-MHC genes also possess a significant association. Many of these susceptibility genes, including *IRF5*, *STAT4*, and *IL12A* are involved in the regulation of the interferon (IFN) system [14,15]. The upregulation of IFN pathways and its stimulated genes are associated with the clinical symptoms of SS [16,17]. Over half of all pSS patients exhibit an IFN signature, and these patients typically present higher titers of anti–Sjögren's-syndrome-related antigen A (SSA/Ro) and anti–Sjögren's-syndrome-related antigen B (SSB/La) autoantibodies and higher disease activity as measured by the European League Against Rheumatism Disease Activity Index (ESSDAI) [18]. Additionally, an increased IFN gene signature in the salivary glands (SG) has been linked to poorer patient response to Rituximab, a chimeric mouse/human monoclonal antibody (mAb) therapy with binding specificity to CD20 [19]. Both Type I and type II IFN signatures have been detected for SS patients and genetic ablation of interferon α receptor 1 (IFNAR1), IFN-γ, or its receptor IFNγR prevent the onset of disease in the spontaneous SS models: the non-obese diabetic (NOD) mouse and it's derivative C57BL/6.NOD-*Aec1Aec2* [20–23]. The initial events activating the IFN system remain unclear, as does how the precise nature of how the IFN signature of SS mediates disease. Type I IFNs (T1-IFN) are driven by toll-like receptor (TLR) stimulation and while capable of being produced by all nucleated cell types, they are strongly associated with cells of the innate immune system, whereas Type II IFNs are largely produced by T cells, NK cells and macrophages [24,25]. The apparent necessity of IFNs in the SS disease process together with IFN regulatory risk genes in humans, indicates a role for cells of the innate immune system as well as the adaptive in the development of disease. Indeed, therapies targeting T1-IFN and the IFN pathway continue to be investigated in SS [26].

The insidious onset of SS, coupled with generalized symptoms, overlap with other autoimmune diseases, and the complex classification/diagnostic parameters contributes partially to a frequent delay in diagnosis [2]. Due to the challenges of identifying "pre-SS patients", understanding of the disease in humans has been limited to studying patients with advanced symptomatic disease. This deficit has contributed to a lack of understanding of pathological events preceding observable symptoms. Therefore, in an attempt to elucidate the early patho-immunological processes, many induced and spontaneous mouse models for SS have been developed and used to study disease progression [27]. These mouse models can differ greatly in their SS disease manifestations. For example, NOD mice develop well characterized salivary gland pathology with less lacrimal gland (LG) involvement, whereas thrombospondin-1 (TSP-1) deficient mice experience more severe LG disease [28]. These discrepancies between models mirror the heterogenous presentation of SS in human patients. Critically, the disease profile of individual mouse models can mimic that of subgroups of patients (IFN[+], IFN[−], etc.) thereby facilitating understanding of disease in these subgroups. Much of the work on spontaneous models has been done using the NOD mouse and its derivatives [29]. In studying SS progression in C57BL/6.NOD-*Aec1Aec2* mice, we were able to identify 3 distinct but overlapping phases of disease [27]. C57BL/6.NOD-*Aec1Aec2* mice develop SS symptoms temporally and phenotypically similar to NOD mice but without the presence of diabetes, making them an ideal candidate to study spontaneous pSS [30–32]. Phase 1 (0–8 weeks) is characterized by acinar epithelial cell death and delayed salivary gland (SG) morphogenesis. Phase 2 (8–16 weeks), where IFN stimulated genes become activated, coincides with migration of macrophages and dendritic cells (DCs), followed by CD4$^+$T and B220$^+$B lymphocytes, and the emergence of autoantibodies. Finally, in Phase 3 (16 weeks onward) there is overt clinical disease where a progressive measurable loss of exocrine gland function occurs. Disease development in C57BL/6.NOD-*Aec1Aec2* mice shares some similarities to other SS mouse models, even if different glands are targeted. For example, increased apoptosis was observed at 8 weeks in the LGs of TSP-1-deficient mice, which can also be seen in the SG of C57BL/6.NOD-*Aec1Aec2* mice. Additionally, TSP-1 mice displayed ocular surface damage at 12 weeks with an increase in SSA/Ro and SSB/La antibodies detected at 12–16 weeks. Finally, infiltrates primarily composed of CD4$^+$ T cells were discovered in the LGs of TSP-1-deficient mice with increased expression of Th1 and Th17 and related transcription factors. Similar observation was seen in the SG of C57BL/6.NOD-*Aec1Aec2* mice at similar age [28]. Together these findings offer insights as to how the aberrant activity of both innate and adaptive immune cells mediate the pathogenesis of SS.

3. Innate Immune Cells

3.1. Dendritic Cells

Considering that SS is characterized by overstimulation of the immune system and IFN signature, the role of DCs in SS has been the subject of considerable study [33]. DCs can be subdivided into three main types: conventional or myeloid DCs (mDCs), which are the most potent antigen presenting cells (APCs) of the immune system; plasmacytoid DCs (pDCs), the foremost IFN-α producing cell; and follicular dendritic cells (fDCs), which are not from the hematopoietic lineage and are critically involved in B cell development in germinal centers (GCs) [34,35]. DCs are one of the first cell types to infiltrate the minor SG of patients and submandibular glands of NOD mice [36,37]. Their prevalence is negatively correlated with lesion severity, whereas fDC frequency is unaffected by lesion severity. fDCs are organized into networks within GCs in severe lesions within the glands [38].

mDCs are cells of hematopoietic origin and include a number of tissue specific subtypes, such as Langerhan's cells. Immature DCs disseminate through the blood to inhabit peripheral tissues where they sample the local environment through endocytosis. DCs that have encountered antigen migrate to the secondary lymphoid tissue and develop into mature DCs [39]. They are unique in their capacity to both prime T cells and participate in peripheral tolerance [40]. Immature DCs have reduced frequency in primary and secondary SS patient blood, while mature DCs are found at increased frequency within the SGs [41,42]. DCs isolated from NOD mouse SGs lacked the expression of the regulatory chemokine receptor CCR5. The absence of CCR5 on DCs contributes to an increased expression of the T helper (Th) 1 cytokine IL-12, thereby enhancing the activity of the adaptive cellular response through Th1 cells and establishing a more proinflammatory environment [43]. Patient monocyte derived DCs (moDCs) were reported to express increased HLA-DR compared control moDCs, suggesting more antigen presenting activity. moDCs from SS patients secreted higher levels of IL-12p40 than moDCs from control patients both upon TLR7/8 stimulation [44] and under basal conditions [45].

pDCs are a rare subset of DC best known for their production of T1-IFN upon stimulation of TLR 7 and 9 [46]. pSS patients exhibit low levels of serum T1-IFN but have elevated levels in the minor SG (mSG) [47], and reduced circulating pDC within peripheral blood [48]. However, while diminished in number, pDCs of pSS patients present in peripheral blood expressed high levels of CD40 and CD86 [49]. Microarray analysis of mSGs biopsies showed significant activation of both T1 and T2-IFN pathways with elevated numbers of pDCs [50]. Analysis of pSS pDCS has revealed dysregulated miRNAs relating to apoptosis, antigen presentation, and cytokine production [51]. Furthermore, pDCs from pSS patients demonstrated increased pro-inflammatory cytokine production [52]. Finally, it has been suggested that pDC recognition of apoptotic cell debris drives the loss of immune tolerance in SS [7].

fDCs are stromal cells within GCs that lack MHC-II expression and instead present antigen-antibody complexes to B cells via complement and Fc receptors [35]. fDCs attract B cells with CXCL13 and promote positive and negative selection, isotype switching, and development of high affinity B cell receptors [53]. About 20–25% of SS patients develop ectopic GCs containing B cells, T cells, and fDC networks within the mSGs [54]. Expression of the enzyme activation-induced cytidine deaminase is critical for B cells to perform class switch recombination and somatic hypermutation, driving affinity maturation within GCs of secondary lymphoid organs. Proliferating B cells found within fDC networks in ectopic GCs express AID, indicating that these GCs are functional and a source of local antibody production and B cell expansion within the SGs of SS patients [55].

3.2. Macrophages

Macrophages are a broad variety of phagocytic cells of the innate immune system. Monocytes circulate within the blood and migrate to tissues where local signals can differentiate them into macrophages or DCs. While mDCs and pDCs are recognized as the master antigen presenting cells and T1-IFN producing cells respectively, macrophages also participate in both of these roles and are crucial for producing other pro-inflammatory cytokines, apoptotic corpse removal, and wound healing [56]. SS patient saliva contain high expression of the monocyte chemokine CCL2, and histological analysis of SS patient biopsies identified macrophages within infiltrates of mSGs biopsies [57,58]. Infiltrating macrophages in pSS patients were positively correlated with lesion severity [38] and IL-18, suggesting macrophage activation within the infiltrate [59]. Furthermore, high IL-18 expression by infiltrating macrophages correlated with lymphoma risk factors such as C4 hypocomplementemia and SG enlargement [59]. The polarization of macrophages remains unclear in SS. M1 polarization has been suggested to be more likely in part because proinflammatory cytokines B cell activating factor (BAFF), T1 IFN, IL-6, and IL-12, that are expressed by M1 macrophages, are detected at higher levels in SS patients [60]. Macrophage linked protease genes including cathepsins, matrix metalloproteases (MMPs), and carboxypeptidases were found to be upregulated in highly inflamed SGs biopsies from SS patients, suggesting a role for macrophages in orchestrating tissue destruction and aberrant repair processes in SS [61]. Further investigation revealed that IFN signaling drives plasmin expression by macrophages in SGs and promotes tissue destruction [62]. In addition, macrophage derived chitinases were highly expressed in mSG samples from pSS patients and were associated with disease severity [61]. While focal lymphocytic infiltration can occur in healthy individuals, negligible numbers of macrophages are observed in foci of healthy individuals [63].

Within the NOD mouse model for SS, macrophages have been observed to infiltrate the SGs early in disease development, and precede the arrival of B and T cells [32]. Both M1 and M2 macrophages have been observed in SGs of NOD mice [64]. Among the most important functions carried out by macrophages is the removal of the corpses of apoptotic cells, a process termed efferocytosis [65]. In the related autoimmune disease SLE, delayed removal of dead cells is believed to contribute to disease onset [66]. Delays in the uptake and disposal of dead cells can allow the corpse to progress to secondary necrosis where self-antigens can leak out and activate the immune system [67]. Considering the observation of increased apoptotic cells in the SGs of SS patients and mouse models, this concept has received some attention in SS [68,69]. Analysis of pSS patient monocytes revealed impaired phagocytosis of apoptotic cells and a corresponding defect in initiating immunosuppressive signaling in response to uptake [70]. Additional investigation into SS monocyte derived macrophages determined that SS patient macrophages suffered an intrinsic reduction in phagocytic ability, exacerbated by inhibitory IgG antibodies against apoptotic cells [71]. NOD mice, which have been employed as a model for secondary SS, display impaired efferocytosis by both bone marrow derived and peritoneal macrophages [72]. Our own observations confirm that this efferocytic defect is maintained in the SS C57BL/6.NOD-*Aec1Aec2* mouse model (unpublished data) and may be a result of defective signaling within the Tyro3, Axl, Mertk (TAM) receptor pathway [73].

3.3. Innate Lymphoid Cells (ILCs) and Natural Killer Cells (NK)

Innate lymphoid cells (ILCs) have received little attention in SS compared to other immune cells. However, ILCs have been observed in both human and mouse salivary gland [74,75]. Natural killer

(NK) cells are ILCs that arise from the same common lymphoid progenitor as B and T cells. NK cells have well characterized roles in the elimination of tumor cells and virally infected cells [76,77]. Yet, the role of NK cells in SS remains poorly understood. NK cells have been discovered within minor SG biopsy patients of SS patients, however the cells are rarer than DCs or macrophages [38]. Despite rarity with the SS lesion, NK cells incidence was found to be positively correlated to presence of rheumatoid factor (RF) and C4 levels in the sera [38]. NKp44$^+$ ILCs were found to be major producers of IL-22 in pSS patient SG, and infiltration of these cells into the SG correlated with SG inflammation [74]. Levels of NK cells in the blood of SS patients remain controversial. Szodoray et al. observed the percentage of NK cells to be increased in the peripheral blood of pSS patients [78]. In a separate study, the count of NK cells in the peripheral blood was found to be reduced in pSS patients with anti-SSA and SSB autoantibodies [79]. Greater concordance has been achieved in studies of NK activity in pSS, where NK cell activity was found to be reduced in pSS as well as SLE [80]. In addition, Izumi et al. detected decreased NK cells, decreased NK cell activity, and increased apoptotic NK cells in pSS patients [81]. Interestingly, there is evidence that NK cell contribution to SS is not through the traditionally explored lens of NK cells as killers, but rather through the regulatory capacity of NK cells [82,83]. In this study, Rusakiewicz et al. identified a new mechanism for NK involvement in SS where dysfunctional regulation by NK cells via *NCR3/Nkp30* permits over activation of DCs, facilitating activation of lymphocytes and systemic immunity [82].

3.4. Salivary Gland Epithelial Cells (SGECs)

SGECs are one of the targets of autoimmune attack in SS as exhibited by the aberrant apoptosis that occurs in the SG. However, further scrutiny into the role of SGECs has revealed that this class of cells is not merely the bystander target, but rather an active participant in the autoimmune response [84,85]. SGECs expressed high levels of HLA-DR, costimulatory molecules CD80 and CD86, and adhesion molecules, allowing them to perform as non-professional antigen presenting cells [86]. Additionally, SGECs have been identified to be sources of multiple chemokines and proinflammatory cytokines including CXCL12, CXCL13, IL-6, IL-7, IL-22, ICOSL, and BAFF [74,87–93]. Local expression of certain chemokines by SGEGs, including CXCL12 and CXCL13 is believed to contribute to the formation of ectopic GCs in the glands [89]. Furthermore, the Ro52 antigen has been detected in SGECs of pSS at higher levels than control patients, and is positively associated with the severity of inflammation [94]. Enhanced endoplasmic reticulum (ER) stress detected in the SGECs of pSS patients has been hypothesized to contribute to the production of proinflammatory cytokines from SGECs [95]. Co-culture experiments discovered that SGEC expression of ICOSL and IL-6 can differentiate naïve T cells into follicular T cells, demonstrating the ability of SGECs to influence lymphocytic organization in the SGs [91].

TLR 1, 2, 3, 4, and 7 are known to be expressed by SGECs [96–98]. Furthermore, TLR3 stimulation of the SG of New Zealand Black X New Zealand White (NZB/W) F1 mice was shown to reduce salivary flow in mice [99]. Separate studies observed that TLR3 stimulation induced apoptosis in SGECs, and SGECs from pSS patients were more susceptible to anoikis induced by TLR3 stimulation [100,101]. Additionally, pSS patients were found to overexpress the costimulatory molecule B7-H3 which was determined to be able to induce apoptosis of SGECs [102]. Stimulation of patient SGECs with TLR agonists dsRNA virus and poly I:C resulted in increased BAFF expression, further demonstrating the role of SGECs as regulators of the immune response [92]. The anti-inflammatory activity of peroxisome-proliferator-activated receptor-γ (PPARγ) was found to be reduced in SS patient derived SGECs, allowing for overactive NF-κB and IL-1β pathways [103]. TLR stimulation of the SGECs, presumably from a viral infection, represents a possible initiating event in the autoimmune cascade where increased cell death, and the release of inflammatory cytokines drive an escalating cycle of inflammation [84,85,104]. Overall, like macrophages and DCs, SGECs possess the ability to both produce various chemokines, inflammatory cytokines, and act as APCs, allowing them to exert a powerful influence guiding the behavior of lymphocytes within the SGs.

4. Adaptive Immune Cells

4.1. T cells

4.1.1. Th1 Cells

Th1 cells produce the inflammatory cytokines IFN-γ and TNF-α, and both of these cytokines regulate cell mediated immunity and activate macrophages, NK, and CD8$^+$T cells [105]. SS was originally considered a Th1 dominated autoimmune disorder, but it has gradually been observed that both Th1 and Th2 cells are drivers of the disease depending on the stage. Deciphering the specific roles of the Th1 subpopulation in the disease progression in SS has been a primary goal in understanding the disease [106]. IFN-γ has a significant effect on the organ development of SGs. *Ifnγ*$^{-/-}$ and NOD.*IfncR*$^{-/-}$ mice have been shown to be clinically asymptomatic for SS and indicate normal acinar cell proliferation and maturation [107,108]. It has been established that IFN-γ induces expression of glandular adhesion molecules including vascular cell adhesion molecule-1 (VCAM-1), α4β1 integrin, peripheral node addressin, L-selectin and LFA-1, which facilitate the influx of inflammatory cells into glands [108–110]. Further transcription signature analysis of the Th1 cell type suggests that the IFN-γ regulated cytokines CCL5, CCL8, CXCL9, CXCL13, and CXCL16 (an IFN-γ regulated chemokine) attract both NK and memory T cells [109]. IFN-γ plays an important role in the perpetuation of inflammation of SS as labial salivary gland primary cell cultures from patients indicate epithelial HLA-DR expression in 80% of cultures. IFN-γ can alter tight junction function and causes an increase of permeability across the epithelium [111]. The in-vitro exposure of acinar cells to IFN-γ causes alterations in tight junction components as observed in the SGs of patients with pSS [112]. It can induce Fas mediated apoptosis in SGEC cultures, ultimately contributing to epithelial cell damage and diminished saliva secretion [113]. Other proteins like IFN inducible guanylate binding protein 1 and CD45$^+$ cell infiltration are corelated and may be analyzed by the degree of CD45$^+$ infiltration in the major SGs of pSS patients [107]. CCL9 and CCL19 expression is up-regulated in the salivary (SG) and LGs (LG) of NOD and C57BL/6.NOD-*Aec1Aec2* mice during disease onset, inducing other potentially disease relevant genes such as *Epsti1* and *Ubd* that show enhanced activity in the LGs of male mice [109,114]. IL-7, known to cause increased production of IFN-γ and CXCR3 via upregulation of Th1 cells, has been shown to accelerate the development of SS [115]. Okamoto et al. have shown that IκB-ζ induction is necessary for Th17 cell differentiation and is important in experimental autoimmune encephalomyelitis [116]. Similarly, Okuma et al. have determined that the STAT3-IκB-ζ signaling pathway is essential for the development of SS-like disease, as the genetic deletion of the STAT3-IκB-ζ signaling pathway is sufficient for the development of SS-like disease, as enhanced apoptosis is observed after deletion of the pathway in SG tissue [117]. The epithelial cell-specific STAT3-deficient mice develop SS-like inflammation with impaired IκB-ζ expression in the LGs, activating Th1 cells [117]. The disruption of STAT3-mediated IκB-ζ induction elicits the activation of self-reactive lymphocytes that causes the spontaneous development of SS. The IκB-ζ-deficient epithelial cells accelerate apoptosis even without the involvement of lymphocytes [117]. STAT3 is widely expressed in different cells and is activated by an array of cytokines and growth factors [118,119]. It controls RORγt expression and Th17 development, but alternatively it has been found that epithelial deletion of STAT3 induced SS-like symptoms. IκB-ζ expression is significantly reduced in the LGs of STAT3-deficient mice, proving that STAT3 is required for the expression of IκB-ζ [117].

IL-18, another Th1 cytokine, has been detected in CD68$^+$ macrophages, ductal, and acinar cells of SGs of SS mice and is secreted at a significantly higher level in sera and the saliva of patients with SS and NOD mice [59,120,121]. It has been established that IL-18 produced by activated macrophages and T cells stimulates the inflammatory pathway within the glands [122].

4.1.2. Th2 Cells

Th2 cells mediate humoral immunity and are involved in allergic immune responses in the body [123]. Th2 cells play a critical role in sustaining B cell function and conversely, B cells regulate the maintenance and expansion of both IL-4 producing cell lineages [124]. Hyperactivity of B cells, specifically overproduction of autoantibodies is observed in SS patients. This activity is attributed by cytokines secreted by Th2 cells. Th2 cells are generated following priming of CD4$^+$ T cells by IL-4, resulting in the induction of the Th2 transcription factor GATA3. Th2 cells express a range of cytokines that influence B cell differentiation, eosinophil recruitment, and mucus production [125]. The signature cytokines produced by Th2 cells are IL-4, IL-5, and IL-13 but they can also produce IL-9, IL-10, IL-25, and amphiregulin [126]. Genetic ablation of IL-4 in NOD mice was able to restore normal levels of secretory function however, leukocytic infiltration and pathophysiological abnormalities in gland pathology persisted [127,128]. IL-4 has also been found to play a crucial function during the clinical manifestation of SS while having limited effect on the pathology associated with the preclinical disease. *Il4* KO mice do not produce IgG1 isotypic autoantibodies against the muscarinic acetylcholine receptor (M3R), a known autoantibody target in SS, indicating a critical role of IgG1 isotype switching in SS. Other antibodies such as IgG2a, IgG2b, IgG3, IgM, and IgA are produced against M3R [108] in both the *Il4* KO and NOD.B10-*H2^b* mouse models. The NOD.B10-*H2^b* mouse model has the *Stat6* gene knocked out that impairs the capability of IgG1 production against M3R [129]. Purified IgG fractions from NOD.B10-*H2b* mice were capable of reducing saliva secretions in normal C57BL/6 mice as opposed to fractions isolated from sera of NOD.B10-H2b. Stat6$^{-/-}$ mice that inhibited saliva flow rates when infused into naive C57BL/6 mice [129]. Thus, it is essential to note that IL-4, the primary cytokine produced by Th2 cells, plays a part in the isotype class switching to produce pathogenic IgG1 auto-antibodies highlighting the significance of the IL-4/Stat6 pathway.

4.1.3. Th17 Cells

The role of Th17 cells, has been studied extensively in the past decade in the pathogenesis of SS [130]. Both IL-6 and transforming growth factor (TGF)-β are required to induce naive murine CD4$^+$ T cells to develop into Th17 cells, which are characterized by the expression of retinoic acid receptor-related orphan receptor γ (RORγ)t. In humans, the differentiation of Th17 cells occurs by activation of T cell receptor (TCR) signaling in the presence of TGF-β and IL-6 or IL-21 stimulation [131]. Other critical cytokines that play a role in the progression of the disease include IL-22 and IL-23. IL-22 is derived primarily from natural killer cells, but it is also produced by Th17 cells, and it has been identified in the mSG tissue of pSS patients [74]. IL-23, while not required for differentiation of Th17 cells, is a cytokine that is necessary for their survival and maintenance [132]. Th17 cells produce IL-17A (referred to here as IL-17) and five other IL-17 members which have also been described that are termed as IL-17B, C, D, E (or IL-25), and F with conserved residues in the c-terminal region that form homodimers [133]. Local IL-17 protein production and mRNA levels, together with IL-6 and IL-23 mRNA, have been shown to increase with the progression of lesion severity in mSGs of pSS patients [134]. Th17 cells are the primary producers of IL-17A and IL17F and other cytokines such as TGFβ, IL-6, and IL-12, which have been detected in the plasma and saliva of pSS patients [134]. The nuclear receptor RORγt plays an indispensable role in the differentiation of Th17 cells as increased presence and activation indicates an increase in autoimmunity [135]. PBMCs from SS patients have the capacity to secrete IL-17 and IL-12 which skew naïve CD4$^+$ T cells to Th1 and Th17 cells respectively, thereby facilitating initiation of the auto-immune cascade [136]. IL-21 expression in SGs has also been associated with hypergammaglobulinemia and patients with primary SS [137]. Th17 cells display the CD4$^+$ CD161$^+$ phenotype in circulation and have been found to be increased at advanced stages of the disease [138]. There are other subsets of marker specific T cells that contribute to disease progression. CD4$^-$CD8$^-$ double negative T cells are a subset that is capable of producing IL-17 and has been correlated with more severe glandular infiltration and is present during the formation of GCs [139]. Another direct set of Th17 cells that secrete IL-17 consistently in the periductal infiltrates of all mSGs, has been identified with the level of expression directly correlating with the severity of glandular inflammation and as a result destruction of healthy gland tissue [134].

Other Th17 cytokines that include IL-17 and IL-23 expression in SGs cause an increase in Tbet expression in the pre-disease phase in the C57BL/6.NOD-*Aec1Aec2* model [140]. The systemic effect of IL-17 on sexual dimorphism has been elucidated by genetically ablating IL-17 in C57BL/6.NOD-*Aec1Aec2* mice. It has been observed that the elimination of IL-17 reduces sialadenitis more drastically in females than in males [141]. The TCR repertoires of Th1 and Th17 cells in SG infiltrates have been found to be restricted, with an increase in the number of pathogenic effector T cells in the glands with a sex-based selection bias of TCR repertoires [142]. Furthermore, it has been observed that transferring Th17 cells in IL-17 deficient mice, restores the SS disease phenotype, highlighting the key role of Th17 cells in the inflammatory cascade and subsequent disease progression [143].

The function of RORγt overexpression in naive $CD4^+$ T cells has been elucidated in RAG deficient mice showing the development of pSS phenotype upon transfer of RORγt-overexpressing $CD4^+$T cells that induce sialadenitis. The findings in IL-17-deficient mice therefore, suggest that IL-17 is essential for the development of sialadenitis [144]. Gene therapy studied in the C57BL/6.NOD-*Aec1Aec2* mice has explored the role of cytokines like IL-27. Induction of IL-27, a natural inhibitory cytokine of Th17 expression, was found to down-regulate or reverse SS in C57BL/6.NOD-*Aec1Aec2* mice via a recombinant adeno-associated virus (rAAV) 2-IL27 vector injection. Th1 activation and inhibitory activity of Th17 cells was observed [145].

M3R-reactive $CD3^+$ T cells play a pathogenic role in the development of murine autoimmune sialadenitis (MIS), which mimics SS [146]. M3R is the primary receptor subtype that promotes fluid secretion in salivary acinar cells. Both interferon IFN-γ and IL-17 are required for induction of SS in MIS, indicating that M3R-reactive Th1 and Th17 cells contribute to the pathogenesis of autoimmune sialadenitis. Thus, MIS is used to analyze the effectiveness of RORγt antagonists [147]. As mentioned, anti-M3R autoantibodies have been proposed to contribute to secretory dysfunction in SS. Iizuka et al. showed that transferring the M3R deficient splenocytes to RAG deficient mice lead to Th1 and Th17 infiltration in SGs and pSS like symptoms. Lymphocytic infiltration and destruction of epithelial cells in the SGs indicated that M3R reactive $CD3^+$ T cells played a pathogenic role in the development of autoimmune sialadenitis [146].

In the lacrimal glands, the lymphocytic infiltration and the presence of IL-17 can also be observed. IL-17 conjunctival mRNA and protein expression in tears is observed to be higher in pSS as compared to non-SS patients exhibiting dry eye disease [148], whereas percentages of peripheral IL-17-producing $CD4^+$ T cells are shown to be similar between pSS patients and controls. The importance of Th17 was further supported in animal models of SS. IL-2Rα (CD25) knockout mice develop autoimmunity and lymphoproliferative disorders and produce significantly higher levels of IL-6, TGF-β1, IL-23R, IL-17, IL-17F, IL-21, IL-10, and IFN-γ mRNA in the cornea and conjunctiva. This promotes autoimmune lacrimal-keratoconjunctivitis with symptoms closely resembling SS. Th-17 cells are shown to produce IL-17 that overlap with the peak severity of corneal epithelial disease [149]. A clinical trial using anti-IL-17 failed to improve dry eye in SS patients, which makes the role of Th17 cells in disease progression within LGs ambiguous [150].

4.1.4. T Regulatory Cells (Tregs)

Tregs possess suppressive activity towards autoreactive lymphocytes via either cell-cell contact or the release of soluble mediators including IL-10 and TGF-β. The commitment of a naïve T lymphocyte towards a Treg phenotype is dependent on a specific cytokine microenvironment and of the expression of the forkhead box protein P3 (FoxP3) transcription factor [151]. Understanding the role of Treg cells in SS pathogenesis has been complicated by studies reporting mixed and controversial results. The inconsistencies in results can be explained at least in part by the different strategies employed to assess Treg cells in the course of disease progression. Studies follow two approaches of either enumerating the proportion of circulating Treg cells according to the high surface expression of

CD25^{high} cells or combining surface expression with the co-expression of FoxP3, the most specific marker of Treg cells. An increase of circulating FoxP3$^+$ cells in pSS biopsies correlates with worse clinical disease has been observed as shown by Sarigul et al., similar to FoxP3$^+$ cells circulating in patients with RA [143,152,153]. Several studies report a reduction of peripheral blood Treg cells [78,154–157] and highlight an association between the reduction of these cells and exacerbated clinical symptoms. Szodoray et al. have proven that Treg cell reduction resulted in prevention of extra-glandular manifestations [78]. Contrary to these results, other groups report increased circulating Treg cells in pSS patients that show clinical symptoms, with no glandular manifestation and no serological features [152,158], and in a few cases CD4$^+$CD25^{high} cell percentages are similar in the peripheral blood of pSS patients and controls [153,159,160].

Disease activity does not influence the number of circulating Treg cells and the disease presents as either being a mild stable polyclonal hypergammaglobulinemia, as was the case for one group (inactive) or a more severe polyclonal hypergammaglobulinemia (active) [160], as was the case for another group. Other murine studies on Tregs in SS include the treatment of TSP1-KO mice with TSP1-derived peptide to prove attenuation of the clinical symptoms of SS-associated dry eye in TSP-1 deficient mice. This demonstrates that an increase in Treg cells, which reduce Th17 cells, can attenuate disease symptoms. TGF-β plays a pivotal role in differentiation for immunosuppressive FoxP3$^+$Tregs, where an increase is evident in biopsy specimens with mild and moderate inflammation which is disproportionate to escalating pro-inflammatory Th17 populations in advanced disease [134].

There is an increase in the frequency of CD4$^+$Foxp3$^+$ Tregs observed with age in the cervical lymph node (CLN), spleen, and LG of NOD.B10.H2b mice. These CD4$^+$CD25$^+$ cells lose suppressive ability, while maintaining expression of Foxp3 and producing IL-17 and IFN-γ. Furthermore, an increase of Foxp3$^+$IL-17$^+$ or Foxp3$^+$IFN-γ$^+$ cells was observed in the LG and LG-draining CLN of these mice [161]. The role of Tregs is uncertain because of a balance in between Tregs and Th17 cells [162]. Further soluble mediators, such as TGF-β, the level of which is increased in SGs of SS patients compared to controls, is required for both Treg and Th17 cell development [163,164].

4.1.5. T Follicular Helper Cells (Tfh)

T follicular helper (Tfh) cells are specialized providers of T cell help to B cells, and are essential for GC formation, affinity maturation, and the development of high affinity antibodies and memory B cells. Tfh cell differentiation is a multi-factorial process involving B cell lymphoma 6 (Bcl6) and other transcription factors that are usually upregulated in autoimmunity [165]. B cell depletion therapy by Rituximab has been used in patients with pSS, where it decreased the elevated levels of circulating Tfh cells and improved the symptoms of patients, illustrating the crucial role of the crosstalk between B cells and Tfh cells in pSS [166]. Tfh cell differentiation is driven by the transcription factor Bcl-6 and activates Tfh cells to express high levels of Inducible T-cell costimulator (ICOS) and Programmed cell death protein 1 (PD-1) [167]. Tfh cells are important in the formation of GCs and primarily show presence of CD84 as a cell surface marker. CD84$^+$ PD-1$^+$Bcl6$^+$ Tfh cells have been identified in organized structures with high focus scores and are in close proximity with Bcl6$^+$ B cells, suggesting an association with increased disease severity in SS [168]. Tfh cells facilitate T cell–dependent B cell responses, mainly by secretion of IL-21, a primary driver of B cell activation and differentiation towards plasma cells. Increased frequencies of Tfh cells have been associated with several autoimmune diseases [169,170]. Cohorts of Tfh cells have been defined where the frequencies of circulating Tfh (cTfh) cells, defined as CD4$^+$CD45RA$^-$CXCR5$^+$PD-1$^+$cells, and are increased in pSS patients. Tfh cells within glandular tissue cannot be easily identified due to overlapping CXCR5 expression with B cells. Detection by immunohistochemistry and quantification of these cells by flow cytometry is difficult because biopsies are processed into cell suspensions using enzymatic digestion, and in the process CXCR5 expression is lost [171]. The function of CXCR5 positive Tfh cells is thus directly related to the secretion of IL-21 mediating B cell maturation, proliferation, and GC formation.

4.1.6. Cytotoxic T Cells/ CD8+ T Lymphocytes (CTLs)

CTLs are best known for their destruction of virally infected and tumor cells. They produce the pro-inflammatory effector cytokines TNF-α or IFN-γ. The effector function of CD8+ T cells follows recognition by the T lymphocyte T-cell receptor of major histocompatibility complex class I (MHC I) molecules loaded with the relevant antigenic peptide, expressed at the surface of the target cells. Due to their lytic capacity, these cells represent key effectors in various autoimmune diseases [172]. Tissue resident memory CD8+ T cells act as mediators of SG damage in murine models of SS but the pathogenic significance of CD8+ T cells is unclear as limited studies have been performed to illuminate their role. CD8+ T cells have been observed within labial SGs infiltrates of patients with SS. They tend to colocalize with salivary duct epithelial cells and acinar cells, and they potentially produce pro-inflammatory cytokines. Infiltrating lymphocytes with a CD69+CD103+/− tissue-resident phenotype and increased IFN-γ production were prominent in the submandibular glands of p40−/−CD25−/− mice used as a murine model of SS, indicating initiation of the inflammatory pathway. This knockout mitigated symptoms and reduced progression of the disease, elucidating the role of CD8a in SS [173]. Subsequently, genetic ablation of IFNγ resulted in decreased CD8+ T cell infiltration and glandular tissue destruction. More importantly, depletion of CD8+ T cells fully protected mice against the pathologic manifestations of SS, even after the onset of disease [173]. A subset of these CD8+ T cells show an activated phenotype, as reflected in higher expression levels of HLA-DR where increased proportions of HLA-DR+ T cells are associated with higher disease severity [174]. Increased HLA-DR expression has been observed in both CD4+ and CD8+ T cells in the blood of patients that were positive for anti-SSA antibodies. The frequencies of HLA-DR-expressing activated CD4+ and CD8+ T cells in blood correlated with high ESSDAI scores [174]. Whole blood transcriptomic studies, serum proteomics, and peripheral immunophenotyping show a proportion of activated CD8+ T cells in blood that indicate an activated gene signature profile [175]. CXCR3 is necessary for the migration of CD8+ T cells into SGs [176]. High ESSDAI scores correspond to the activation of CD8+ T cells in lymphoid organs, CXCR3 upregulation, and consequent migration to the SGs [174]. Within the LGs and SGs of NOD mice, CD8 T cells proliferate, express an activated phenotype, and produced inflammatory cytokines. Transfer of purified CD8 T cells isolated from the cervical lymph nodes of NOD mice into NOD-severe combined immunodeficiency recipients resulted in inflammation of the LGs, but was not sufficient to cause inflammation of the SGs as observed in the study by Barr et al., demonstrating that CD8 T cells have a pathogenic role in LG autoimmunity [177].

Tissue auto-antigen responses and activated CD8+ T cells have not been well characterized in explaining autoimmune diseases like SS. Identifying human leukocyte antigen class I (HLA-I) binding peptide motifs gives insight to CD8+ T cells involved in pSS, but their role in pathogenicity and progression of the disease besides secretion of cytokines, primarily TNF-α, and IFN-γ is still unclear. New findings in the pathophysiology of CD8+ T cells in autoimmunity and a better understanding of their activation may provide opportunities for the development of targeted immunologic therapies in various autoimmune disorders.

4.2. B Cells

4.2.1. Marginal Zone B Cells

Marginal zone (MZ) B cells are a class of innate-like lymphocytes positioned in the marginal zone of the spleen, inhabiting a junction between the circulation and lymphoid follicle [178–180]. While some differences exist between human and mouse MZ B development and function, in both organisms the positioning of MZ B cells within the spleen allows them to act as antibody generating first responders against pathogens in the blood [178,181]. While MZ B cells occupy a critical niche between innate and adaptive immunity, MZ B cells expansion has been associated with autoimmunity and previous studies have determined that MZ B cells possess polyreactive BCRs that can be potentially be self-reactive [178,182–185]. Among the most serious complications of SS is the increased incidence of B cell lymphoma [3]. Investigation into the types of non-Hodgkin Lymphoma (NHL) tumors within a cohort of 58 pSS patients identified that the two most commonly occurring types of tumors were indolent extranodal MZ B-cell lymphoma of the mucosal associated lymphoid tissue (MALT) at 59%, and nodal MZ lymphoma at 15%, indicating the importance MZ B cells within the disease [186]. MZ-like B cells have been found to be increased in the SGs and peripheral blood of pSS patients [187].

Investigations in SS mouse models have provided additional clues regarding the role of MZ B cells in the disease process. Mice transgenic (tg) for BAFF are known to develop autoimmune symptoms similar to SLE and SS [188,189]. In order to study the role of MZ B cells in this model, Fletcher et al. generated BAFF tg mice lacking lymphotoxin-β (LTβ), as mice lacking LTβ will fail to develop MZ B cells [190]. The authors discovered that while the mice still developed nephritis, they did not develop severe sialadenitis associated with the SS phenotype, suggesting a critical role played by MZ B cells in this aspect of disease [190]. A separate study investigated the role of MZ B cells within the IL-14α transgenic mouse model (IL14αtg) [191]. Elimination of MZ B cells within the IL14atg model restored saliva flow rate, removed lymphocytic infiltrations into the SGs, and prevented formation of autoantibodies [191]. Considering that depletion of MZ B cells improves disease in two separate SS mouse models, targeted depletion of MZ B cells has attracted attention as a potential therapy. Ly9 (CD229) is a cell surface receptor highly expressed on MZ B cells, and anti-Ly9 has been demonstrated to selectively target and deplete MZ B cells [192]. Treatment of NOD.H-2^{h4} SS model mouse with anti-Ly9 reduced both SG and renal infiltration, and also decreased ANAs and RF [193]. Considering the overwhelming involvement of MZ B cells in NHLs of SS patients, anti-Ly9 antibodies likely represent the first of many strategies to target MZ B cells for depletion in SS.

4.2.2. Memory B Cells and Plasma B Cells

Memory B cells are the important cell type that is involved in SS pathogenesis due to their ability to maintain memory for a given antigen in the absence of constant antigen stimulation [194,195]. They are characterized by $CD27^+$ expression and BCR somatic hypermutation [196,197]. SS shows an increase in accumulation of $CD27^+$ memory B cells and plasma cells within the SGs infiltrate and the peripheral blood of patients. The glands show a distinct cytokine profile that includes adhesion molecules, cytokines, and B-cell chemokines CXCL13 and CXCL12 [88,90]. CXCL13 is the key cytokine responsible for the homing of B cells to the SGs. GC formation in the SGs is facilitated by CXCL13 secreted by Tfh and fDCs. Interaction with its corresponding receptor CXCR5 on B-cells regulates B-cell movement between different tissues. In the SGs, CXCL13 guides B cell entry into the follicles that causes lymphoid organization visualized in SG biopsies of SS [198–200]. CXCL13 over-expression in inflamed glands of patients with pSS plays the primary role in the recruitment of circulatory CXCR5 expressing $CD27^+$ memory B cells, attracting the subpopulation of peripheral $CD27^+$ memory B cells into the inflamed glands where they then reside [88,90].

Plasma B cells are terminally differentiated cells of the B lymphocyte lineage, the primary cell type that produces antibodies, and thus are drivers of antibody-mediated immunity [201]. They are maintained for extended periods, making them an essential component of immune memory and thus linking them closely to memory B cells from which they can differentiate [202]. BAFF, a member of the TNF family, is secreted by inflammatory cells and is needed for prolonged plasma cell survival and sustained Ig production by plasma B cells [203]. The glandular microenvironment is generally rich in BAFF, promoting accumulation of $CD27^+$ B memory cells resulting in more IgG producing plasma cells in the tissue [203–205]. BAFF has a role in B cell maturation, class switching, survival, and proliferation especially in advanced disease and is produced by SGEC, DC, macrophages, activated T cells, and also B cells [204]. Mice transgenic for BAFF possess increased numbers of mature B and effector T cells, and develop high levels of circulating immune complexes, glandular Ig deposition, and anti-DNA antibodies [189]. The patients of pSS have auto-reactive plasma B cell infiltrates that produce anti-SSA/Ro or anti-SSB/La autoantibodies. These infiltrates appear from the differentiation of $CD27^+$ memory B cells recruited from circulating blood and from B cells generated in ectopic SG GCs.

Other notable cytokines include CXCR3 and CXCR4, whose expression on activated B cells leads to the migration of the plasma cells to the site of inflammation and causes the attraction of lymphocytic cells to the SGs [206–211].

B-cell-targeted mAbs (see below), largely rely on two mAb Fc-dependent mechanisms: antibody-dependent cellular cytotoxicity (ADCC) and complement-dependent cytotoxicity (CDC).

Rituximab, a mouse/human chimeric IgG1 mAb, was the first B-cell targeting therapeutic antibody approved by the US Food and Drug Administration [212,213]. Ocrelizumab a second generation CD20 mAb(rhumAb 2H7v.16) is a humanized CD20 mAb, which binds a different but overlapping epitope from rituximab [214]. Furthermore B-cell survival, differentiation, and functional properties are tightly regulated by a variety of cytokines and chemokines. Targeting survival and differentiation factors with specific mAbs or fusion proteins is an alternative approach to targeting B-cell surface antigens for active cell depletion [215].

5. Conclusions

SS is a heterogeneous disease with a wide spectrum of severity. Both human and mouse studies of SS indicate an involvement of multiple cell types in producing local inflammation in pSS and SS-like disease as summarized in Table 1. The innate immune response is crucial for the pathogenesis of SS and is implicated in disease initiation, contributing to starting the immune cascade and guiding adaptive immune responses. The activation of innate immune cells is considered to be indicative of disease onset while T and B cell infiltrates indicate driving responses in more severe cases that is reflected in glandular tissue destruction. Both cellular and cytokine repertoires that mediate the skewing, activation, and differentiation of different cell types in peripheral blood and exocrine tissue initiate the epithelial cell activation and in turn the innate immune response as illustrated in Figure 1. This process ultimately leads to chronic autoimmune responses resulting from adaptive immune cells. To date, numerous studies have been performed to identify the cells relevant to autoimmune disease and to understand the individual contributions of all interacting cell types. As a result, comprehending contributions of individual cell types and their interactions is of great importance for elucidating disease pathogenesis and the development of effective therapeutic interventions.

Table 1. Immune cells and their functions involved in SS.

Cell Type	Immunity	Function	References
Dendritic cells	Innate	• mDC are increased in pSS SGs, pSS patient mDCs have increased IL-12p40 secretion and HLA-DR expression. • pDC identified in pSS SGs, pSS patient pDCs are decreased in circulation but show increased activation. • fDC can be organized into fDC networks within functional ectopic GC in the SGs.	[41,42,44]
Macrophages	Innate	• Macrophage infiltration correlates with disease severity in pSS. • Infiltrating macrophages express IL-18 and proteases allowing them to contribute to inflammation and tissue destruction. • pSS monocytes and SS mouse model macrophages display impaired efferocytosis.	[38,59,61]
Salivary gland epithelial cells (SGECs)	Innate	• SGECs can operate as non-professional APCs and as sources of multiple inflammatory cytokines. • SGECs are sensitive to TLR induced apoptosis. • Play a role in the organ development of SGs. They prevent normal acinar cell proliferation and maturation.	[86,101]
Th1 cells	Adaptive	• Secrete IFN-γ that induces expression of glandular adhesion molecules allow the influx of inflammatory cells into SGs. • In-vitro exposure of acinar cells to IFN-γ causes alterations in tight junction components as observed in the SGs of patients with pSS.	[97,108,109,112]

Table 1. *Cont.*

Cell Type	Immunity	Function	References
Th2 cells	Adaptive	• Secrete IL-4 that prevents secretory function. • Secretion of IL-4 causes formation of IgG1 isotypic autoantibodies against M3R indicating a critical role of IgG1, IgG2a, IgG2b, IgG3, IgM, and IgA isotype switching in SS. • *Stat6* gene also prevents IgG1 production against M3R and also plays a part in the isotype class switching.	[108,129,216]
Th17 cells	Adaptive	• They are stimulated by cytokines that play a role in the progression of the disease such as IL-22 and IL-23. • IL-22 is derived primarily from natural killer cells, is produced by Th17 cells, and it has been identified in the mSG tissue of pSS patients. • Th17 cells produce IL-17A (refer to as IL-17) and five other IL-17 members which have also been described that are termed as IL-17B, C, D, E (or IL-25), and F with conserved residues in the c-terminal region that form homodimers. • Local IL-17 protein production and mRNA levels, together with IL-6 and IL-23 mRNA, have been shown to increase with the progression of lesion severity in mSGs of pSS patients. • Conjunctival RORγT mRNA and protein expression in tears is observed to be higher in pSS as compared to non-SS patients exhibiting dry eye disease. • IL-21 expression in SGs has also been associated with hypergammaglobulinemia and patients with primary SS.	[133,134,152,155,163,217]
T regulatory cells (Tregs)	Adaptive	• Important for the induction and maintenance of peripheral tolerance therefore, they are key in preventing excessive immune responses in SS. • Suppressive activity towards autoreactive lymphocytes via either cell-cell contact or the release of soluble mediators that notably include IL-10 and TGF-β. • Reduction of peripheral blood Treg cells in humans that lead to exacerbated clinical symptoms of SS. Role of Tregs is uncertain because of a balance in between Tregs and Th17 cells.	[152,154,218,219]
T follicular helper cells (Tfh)	Adaptive	• Specialized providers of T cell help to B cells, marked increase of Bcl6 and other transcription factors that are usually upregulated in SS. • Important in the formation of GCs and primarily show presence of CD84 a cell surface marker, observed in SS. • The function of CXCR5 positive Tfh cells is directly related to the secretion of IL-21 mediating B cell maturation, proliferation, and GC formation. • They produce the pro-inflammatory effector cytokines TNF-α or IFN-γ.	[165,166]
Cytotoxic T cells/ CD8$^+$ T cells (CTLs)	Adaptive	• Tissue resident memory CD8$^+$ T cells act as mediators of SG damage in murine models of SS but the pathogenic significance of CD8$^+$ T cells is unclear as limited studies have been performed to illuminate their role. • Tend to colocalize with salivary duct epithelial cells and acinar cells, and produce pro-inflammatory cytokines.	[172]
Marginal Zone B cells	Adaptive	• Stimulated by BAFF. • MZ B cells within the IL14atg model drive reduced saliva flow rate, lymphocytic infiltrations into the SGs, and formation of autoantibodies. • Possess self-reactive BCRs that cause complications of SS and the increased incidence of B cell lymphoma.	[174,179,189,192,193]

Table 1. *Cont.*

Cell Type	Immunity	Function	References
Memory B cells	Adaptive	• Maintain memory for SS antigens in the absence of constant antigen stimulation. • CXCL13 is the key cytokine responsible for the homing of B cells to the SGs. • CD27+ memory B cells, attract the subpopulation of peripheral CD27+ memory B cells into the inflamed glands where they reside and cause inflammation. • The primary cell type that produces antibodies, and thus are drivers of antibody-mediated immunity. • BAFF primary cytokine produced, that has a role in B cell maturation, class switching, survival, and proliferation especially in advanced disease and is produced by SGEC, DC, macrophages, activated T cells, and also B cells • Cause the formation of GCs in SGs and work antagonistically to Tfr cells.	[88,167,194,195,220]
Plasma B cells	Adaptive	• B cells that produce SS auto-antibodies with specific BCRs against auto-antigens after differentiation from Memory B cells or circulating peripheral B cells.	[189,203,221]

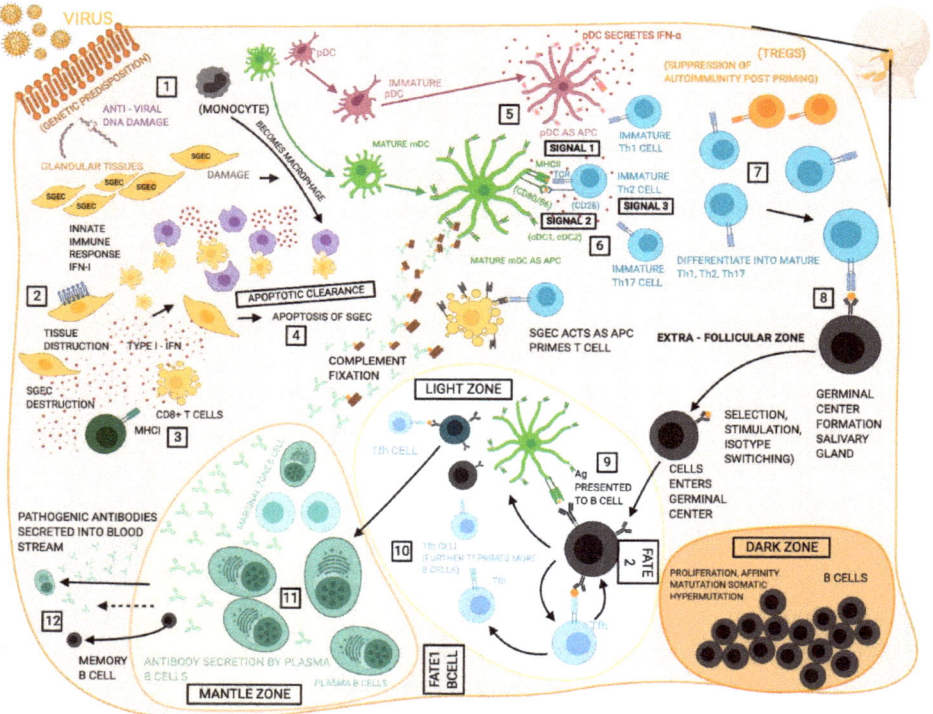

Figure 1. Proposed functions of different cell types in the pathogenesis of Sjögren's syndrome (SS). (1) The initiating events in the development of SS remain unclear, but evidence suggests the disease proceeds following an environmental trigger on a susceptible genetic background, likely a viral infection. (2) Salivary gland epithelia cells (SGECs) experience increased apoptosis and act as sources of inflammatory cytokines and chemokines within the salivary gland (SG). (3) CD8+ T cells are poorly understood in SS, but may contribute to tissue destruction in the glands. (4) Macrophages participate in tissue destruction through the release of proteases and cytokines and display reduced efferocytosis

allowing unremoved apoptotic cells to act as sources of self-antigen. (5) Type I interferon (T1-IFN) both initiates antiviral activity and exerts an activating effect on cells of the immune system. T1-IFN is produced by multiple cell types but is closely associated with plasmacytoid DCs (pDCs). (6) Myeloid dendritic cells (mDCs) are the dominant antigen presenting cells to T cells, however, macrophages and SGECs also participate. (7) Antigen presentation allows for activation of $CD8^+$ T cells and the Th1, Th2, and Th17 $CD4^+$ T cell subsets, which can then contribute to various aspects of the disease pathology. Th1 cells enter the glands and compose much of the early infiltrates and exacerbate the inflammatory environment with the production of type II interferon, while Th17 cells play an increasingly well recognized role in SS as sources of cytokines including IL-17. Conflicting evidence has caused the roles of regulatory T cells (Tregs) remain indistinct in SS. Th2 cells support the humoral autoimmune response through cytokines incusing IL-4. (8 and 9) T follicular helper (Tfh) cells support B cell development in germinal centers (GC) that include follicular dendritic cell (fDC) networks. Germinal centers exist in the spleen, but about 25% of SS patients develop ectopic germinal centers in the SG containing Tfh and fDC. B cells in the germinal center undergo proliferation, somatic hypermutation and affinity hypermutation in the dark zone of the germinal center. (10) B cells then proceed to germinal center selection by fDCs in the light zone and either leave the germinal center as memory B cells or antibody producing plasma cells (Fate 1), or return to the dark zone for further affinity maturation (Fate 2). (11) The MZ B cells function as part of the adaptive immune system carrying antigens to the germinal centers for more efficient generation of memory B cells and glandular MZB cells are proliferative, activated, and produce autoantibodies. Lastly, (12) plasma cells exhibit hyperactivity and are responsible for the production of pathogenic autoantibodies. Created with BioRender.com.

Author Contributions: R.W. and S.G. conceptualized, prepared, and edited the manuscript. R.W. and S.G. created the table, and S.G. made the figure. C.Q.N. conceptualized, reviewed, and revised the manuscript and provided suggestions. All authors have read and agreed to the published version of the manuscript.

Funding: CQN was supported financially in part by Public Health Service (PHS) grants AI130561, DE026450, and DE028544 from the National Institutes of Health. RW is supported by the T90/R90 Comprehensive Training Program in Oral Biology (NIDCR, T90 DE21990). The content is solely the responsibility of the authors and does not necessarily represent the official views of the National Institutes of Health.

Conflicts of Interest: The authors declare no conflict of interest.

References

1. Helmick, C.G.; Felson, D.T.; Lawrence, R.C.; Gabriel, S.; Hirsch, R.; Kwoh, C.K.; Liang, M.H.; Kremers, H.M.; Mayes, M.D.; Merkel, P.A.; et al. Estimates of the prevalence of arthritis and other rheumatic conditions in the United States. Part I. *Arthritis Rheum.* **2008**, *58*, 15–25. [CrossRef]
2. Vivino, F.B.; Bunya, V.Y.; Massaro-Giordano, G.; Johr, C.R.; Giattino, S.L.; Schorpion, A.; Shafer, B.; Peck, A.; Sivils, K.; Rasmussen, A.; et al. Sjogren's syndrome: An update on disease pathogenesis, clinical manifestations and treatment. *Clin. Immunol.* **2019**, *203*, 81–121. [CrossRef]
3. Kassan, S.S.; Thomas, T.L.; Moutsopoulos, H.M.; Hoover, R.; Kimberly, R.P.; Budman, D.R.; Costa, J.; Decker, J.L.; Chused, T.M. Increased risk of lymphoma in sicca syndrome. *Ann. Intern. Med.* **1978**, *89*, 888–892. [CrossRef] [PubMed]
4. Risselada, A.P.; Looije, M.F.; Kruize, A.A.; Bijlsma, J.W.; van Roon, J.A. The role of ectopic germinal centers in the immunopathology of primary Sjögren's syndrome: A systematic review. *Semin. Arthritis Rheum.* **2013**, *42*, 368–376. [CrossRef] [PubMed]
5. Lee, K.E.; Kang, J.H.; Yim, Y.R.; Kim, J.E.; Lee, J.W.; Wen, L.; Park, D.J.; Kim, T.J.; Park, Y.W.; Yoon, K.C.; et al. The Significance of ectopic germinal centers in the minor salivary gland of patients with Sjögren's Syndrome. *J. Korean Med. Sci.* **2016**, *31*, 190–195. [CrossRef]
6. Reksten, T.R.; Jonsson, M.V. Sjögren's syndrome: An update on epidemiology and current insights on pathophysiology. *Oral Maxillofac. Surg. Clin. N. Am.* **2014**, *26*, 1–12. [CrossRef] [PubMed]
7. Ainola, M.; Porola, P.; Takakubo, Y.; Przybyla, B.; Kouri, V.P.; Tolvanen, T.A.; Hänninen, A.; Nordström, D.C. Activation of plasmacytoid dendritic cells by apoptotic particles - mechanism for the loss of immunological tolerance in Sjögren's syndrome. *Clin. Exp. Immunol.* **2018**, *191*, 301–310. [CrossRef] [PubMed]

8. Hillen, M.R.; Ververs, F.A.; Kruize, A.A.; Van Roon, J.A. Dendritic cells, T-cells and epithelial cells: A crucial interplay in immunopathology of primary Sjögren's syndrome. *Expert Rev. Clin. Immunol.* **2014**, *10*, 521–531. [CrossRef]
9. Jonsson, R.; Nginamau, E.; Szyszko, E.; Brokstad, K.A. Role of B cells in Sjögren's syndrome–from benign lymphoproliferation to overt malignancy. *Front. Biosci.* **2007**, *12*, 2159–2170. [CrossRef] [PubMed]
10. Pers, J.O.; Youinou, P. Are the B cells cast with the leading part in the Sjogren's syndrome scenario? *Oral Dis.* **2014**, *20*, 529–537. [CrossRef]
11. Singh, N.; Cohen, P.L. The T cell in Sjogren's syndrome:F majeure, not spectateur. *J. Autoimmun.* **2012**, *39*, 229–233. [CrossRef] [PubMed]
12. Kiripolsky, J.; McCabe, L.G.; Kramer, J.M. Innate immunity in Sjögren's syndrome. *Clin. Immunol.* **2017**, *182*, 4–13. [CrossRef] [PubMed]
13. Nakamura, H.; Shimizu, T.; Kawakami, A. Role of viral infections in the pathogenesis of Sjögren's syndrome: Different characteristics of Epstein-Barr virus and HTLV-1. *J. Clin. Med.* **2020**, *9*, 1459. [CrossRef] [PubMed]
14. Lessard, C.J.; Li, H.; Adrianto, I.; Ice, J.A.; Rasmussen, A.; Grundahl, K.M.; Kelly, J.A.; Dozmorov, M.G.; Miceli-Richard, C.; Bowman, S.; et al. Variants at multiple loci implicated in both innate and adaptive immune responses are associated with Sjögren's syndrome. *Nat. Genet.* **2013**, *45*, 1284–1292. [CrossRef]
15. Song, I.W.; Chen, H.C.; Lin, Y.F.; Yang, J.H.; Chang, C.C.; Chou, C.T.; Lee, M.M.; Chou, Y.C.; Chen, C.H.; Chen, Y.T.; et al. Identification of susceptibility gene associated with female primary Sjögren's syndrome in Han Chinese by genome-wide association study. *Hum. Genet.* **2016**, *135*, 1287–1294. [CrossRef]
16. Li, H.; Ice, J.A.; Lessard, C.J.; Sivils, K.L. Interferons in Sjögren's syndrome: Genes, mechanisms, and effects. *Front. Immunol.* **2013**, *4*, 290. [CrossRef]
17. Marketos, N.; Cinoku, I.; Rapti, A.; Mavragani, C.P. Type I interferon signature in Sjögren's syndrome: Pathophysiological and clinical implications. *Clin. Exp. Rheumatol.* **2019**, *37* (Suppl. S118), 185–191.
18. Brkic, Z.; Maria, N.I.; van Helden-Meeuwsen, C.G.; van de Merwe, J.P.; van Daele, P.L.; Dalm, V.A.; Wildenberg, M.E.; Beumer, W.; Drexhage, H.A.; Versnel, M.A. Prevalence of interferon type I signature in CD14 monocytes of patients with Sjogren's syndrome and association with disease activity and BAFF gene expression. *Ann. Rheum. Dis.* **2013**, *72*, 728–735. [CrossRef]
19. Min, H.K.; Moon, S.J.; Park, K.S.; Kim, K.J. Integrated systems analysis of salivary gland transcriptomics reveals key molecular networks in Sjögren's syndrome. *Arthritis Res. Ther.* **2019**, *21*, 294. [CrossRef]
20. Nezos, A.; Gravani, F.; Tassidou, A.; Kapsogeorgou, E.K.; Voulgarelis, M.; Koutsilieris, M.; Crow, M.K.; Mavragani, C.P. Type I and II interferon signatures in Sjogren's syndrome pathogenesis: Contributions in distinct clinical phenotypes and Sjogren's related lymphomagenesis. *J. Autoimmun.* **2015**, *63*, 47–58. [CrossRef]
21. Maria, N.I.; Vogelsang, P.; Versnel, M.A. The clinical relevance of animal models in Sjögren's syndrome: The interferon signature from mouse to man. *Arthritis Res. Ther.* **2015**, *17*, 172. [CrossRef] [PubMed]
22. Szczerba, B.M.; Rybakowska, P.D.; Dey, P.; Payerhin, K.M.; Peck, A.B.; Bagavant, H.; Deshmukh, U.S. Type I interferon receptor deficiency prevents murine Sjogren's syndrome. *J. Dent. Res.* **2013**, *92*, 444–449. [CrossRef] [PubMed]
23. Cha, S.; Brayer, J.; Gao, J.; Brown, V.; Killedar, S.; Yasunari, U.; Peck, A.B. A dual role for interferon-gamma in the pathogenesis of Sjogren's syndrome-like autoimmune exocrinopathy in the nonobese diabetic mouse. *Scand. J. Immunol.* **2004**, *60*, 552–565. [CrossRef] [PubMed]
24. Meyer, O. Interferons and autoimmune disorders. *Joint Bone Spine* **2009**, *76*, 464–473. [CrossRef] [PubMed]
25. Le Page, C.; Génin, P.; Baines, M.G.; Hiscott, J. Interferon activation and innate immunity. *Rev. Immunogenet.* **2000**, *2*, 374–386.
26. Mavragani, C.P.; Moutsopoulos, H.M. Sjögren's syndrome: Old and new therapeutic targets. *J. Autoimmun.* **2020**, *110*, 102364. [CrossRef]
27. Donate, A.; Voigt, A.; Nguyen, C.Q. The value of animal models to study immunopathology of primary human Sjögren's syndrome symptoms. *Expert Rev. Clin. Immunol.* **2014**, *10*, 469–481. [CrossRef]
28. Turpie, B.; Yoshimura, T.; Gulati, A.; Rios, J.D.; Dartt, D.A.; Masli, S. Sjogren's syndrome-like ocular surface disease in thrombospondin-1 deficient mice. *Am. J. Pathol.* **2009**, *175*, 1136–1147. [CrossRef]
29. Lavoie, T.N.; Lee, B.H.; Nguyen, C.Q. Current concepts: Mouse models of Sjögren's syndrome. *J. Biomed. Biotechnol.* **2011**, *2011*, 549107. [CrossRef]

30. Brayer, J.; Lowry, J.; Cha, S.; Robinson, C.P.; Yamachika, S.; Peck, A.B.; Humphreys-Beher, M.G. Alleles from chromosomes 1 and 3 of NOD mice combine to influence Sjogren's syndrome-like autoimmune exocrinopathy. *J. Rheumatol.* **2000**, *27*, 1896–1904.
31. Cha, S.; Nagashima, H.; Brown, V.B.; Peck, A.B.; Humphreys-Beher, M.G. Two NOD Idd-associated intervals contribute synergistically to the development of autoimmune exocrinopathy (Sjögren's syndrome) on a healthy murine background. *Arthritis Rheum.* **2002**, *46*, 1390–1398. [CrossRef] [PubMed]
32. Roescher, N.; Lodde, B.M.; Vosters, J.L.; Tak, P.P.; Catalan, M.A.; Illei, G.G.; Chiorini, J.A. Temporal changes in salivary glands of non-obese diabetic mice as a model for Sjögren's syndrome. *Oral Dis.* **2012**, *18*, 96–106. [CrossRef] [PubMed]
33. Vogelsang, P.; Jonsson, M.V.; Dalvin, S.T.; Appel, S. Role of dendritic cells in Sjögren's syndrome. *Scand. J. Immunol.* **2006**, *64*, 219–226. [CrossRef]
34. Cravens, P.D.; Lipsky, P.E. Dendritic cells, chemokine receptors and autoimmune inflammatory diseases. *Immunol. Cell Biol.* **2002**, *80*, 497–505. [CrossRef] [PubMed]
35. Park, C.S.; Choi, Y.S. How do follicular dendritic cells interact intimately with B cells in the germinal centre? *Immunology* **2005**, *114*, 2–10. [CrossRef]
36. van Blokland, S.C.; Wierenga-Wolf, A.F.; van Helden-Meeuwsen, C.G.; Drexhage, H.A.; Hooijkaas, H.; van de Merwe, J.P.; Versnel, M.A. Professional antigen presenting cells in minor salivary glands in Sjögren's syndrome: Potential contribution to the histopathological diagnosis? *Lab. Investig.* **2000**, *80*, 1935–1941. [CrossRef]
37. van Blokland, S.C.; van Helden-Meeuwsen, C.G.; Wierenga-Wolf, A.F.; Drexhage, H.A.; Hooijkaas, H.; van de Merwe, J.P.; Versnel, M.A. Two different types of sialoadenitis in the NOD- and MRL/lpr mouse models for Sjögren's syndrome: A differential role for dendritic cells in the initiation of sialoadenitis? *Lab. Investig.* **2000**, *80*, 575–585. [CrossRef]
38. Christodoulou, M.I.; Kapsogeorgou, E.K.; Moutsopoulos, H.M. Characteristics of the minor salivary gland infiltrates in Sjögren's syndrome. *J. Autoimmun.* **2010**, *34*, 400–407. [CrossRef]
39. Dieu, M.C.; Vanbervliet, B.; Vicari, A.; Bridon, J.M.; Oldham, E.; Aït-Yahia, S.; Brière, F.; Zlotnik, A.; Lebecque, S.; Caux, C. Selective recruitment of immature and mature dendritic cells by distinct chemokines expressed in different anatomic sites. *J. Exp. Med.* **1998**, *188*, 373–386. [CrossRef]
40. Steinman, R.M.; Hawiger, D.; Nussenzweig, M.C. Tolerogenic dendritic cells. *Annu. Rev. Immunol.* **2003**, *21*, 685–711. [CrossRef]
41. Ozaki, Y.; Amakawa, R.; Ito, T.; Iwai, H.; Tajima, K.; Uehira, K.; Kagawa, H.; Uemura, Y.; Yamashita, T.; Fukuhara, S. Alteration of peripheral blood dendritic cells in patients with primary Sjögren's syndrome. *Arthritis Rheum.* **2001**, *44*, 419–431. [CrossRef]
42. Ozaki, Y.; Ito, T.; Son, Y.; Amuro, H.; Shimamoto, K.; Sugimoto, H.; Katashiba, Y.; Ogata, M.; Miyamoto, R.; Murakami, N.; et al. Decrease of blood dendritic cells and increase of tissue-infiltrating dendritic cells are involved in the induction of Sjögren's syndrome but not in the maintenance. *Clin. Exp. Immunol.* **2010**, *159*, 315–326. [CrossRef] [PubMed]
43. Wildenberg, M.E.; van Helden-Meeuwsen, C.G.; van de Merwe, J.P.; Moreno, C.; Drexhage, H.A.; Versnel, M.A. Lack of CCR5 on dendritic cells promotes a proinflammatory environment in submandibular glands of the NOD mouse. *J. Leukoc. Biol.* **2008**, *83*, 1194–1200. [CrossRef] [PubMed]
44. Vogelsang, P.; Karlsen, M.; Brun, J.G.; Jonsson, R.; Appel, S. Altered phenotype and Stat1 expression in Toll-like receptor 7/8 stimulated monocyte-derived dendritic cells from patients with primary Sjögren's syndrome. *Arthritis Res. Ther.* **2014**, *16*, R166. [CrossRef]
45. Shi, B.; Qi, J.; Yao, G.; Feng, R.; Zhang, Z.; Wang, D.; Chen, C.; Tang, X.; Lu, L.; Chen, W.; et al. Mesenchymal stem cell transplantation ameliorates Sjögren's syndrome via suppressing IL-12 production by dendritic cells. *Stem. Cell Res. Ther.* **2018**, *9*, 308. [CrossRef] [PubMed]
46. Swiecki, M.; Colonna, M. The multifaceted biology of plasmacytoid dendritic cells. *Nat. Rev. Immunol.* **2015**, *15*, 471–485. [CrossRef]
47. Båve, U.; Nordmark, G.; Lövgren, T.; Rönnelid, J.; Cajander, S.; Eloranta, M.L.; Alm, G.V.; Rönnblom, L. Activation of the type I interferon system in primary Sjögren's syndrome: A possible etiopathogenic mechanism. *Arthritis Rheum.* **2005**, *52*, 1185–1195. [CrossRef]

48. Vogelsang, P.; Brun, J.G.; Oijordsbakken, G.; Skarstein, K.; Jonsson, R.; Appel, S. Levels of plasmacytoid dendritic cells and type-2 myeloid dendritic cells are reduced in peripheral blood of patients with primary Sjögren's syndrome. *Ann. Rheum. Dis.* **2010**, *69*, 1235–1238. [CrossRef] [PubMed]
49. Wildenberg, M.E.; van Helden-Meeuwsen, C.G.; van de Merwe, J.P.; Drexhage, H.A.; Versnel, M.A. Systemic increase in type I interferon activity in Sjögren's syndrome: A putative role for plasmacytoid dendritic cells. *Eur. J. Immunol.* **2008**, *38*, 2024–2033. [CrossRef]
50. Gottenberg, J.E.; Cagnard, N.; Lucchesi, C.; Letourneur, F.; Mistou, S.; Lazure, T.; Jacques, S.; Ba, N.; Ittah, M.; Lepajolec, C.; et al. Activation of IFN pathways and plasmacytoid dendritic cell recruitment in target organs of primary Sjögren's syndrome. *Proc. Natl. Acad. Sci. USA* **2006**, *103*, 2770–2775. [CrossRef]
51. Hillen, M.R.; Chouri, E.; Wang, M.; Blokland, S.L.M.; Hartgring, S.A.Y.; Concepcion, A.N.; Kruize, A.A.; Burgering, B.M.T.; Rossato, M.; van Roon, J.A.G.; et al. Dysregulated miRNome of plasmacytoid dendritic cells from patients with Sjögren's syndrome is associated with processes at the centre of their function. *Rheumatology (Oxford)* **2019**, *58*, 2305–2314. [CrossRef] [PubMed]
52. Hillen, M.R.; Pandit, A.; Blokland, S.L.M.; Hartgring, S.A.Y.; Bekker, C.P.J.; van der Heijden, E.H.M.; Servaas, N.H.; Rossato, M.; Kruize, A.A.; van Roon, J.A.G.; et al. Plasmacytoid DCs from patients with Sjögren's syndrome are transcriptionally primed for enhanced pro-inflammatory cytokine production. *Front. Immunol.* **2019**, *10*, 2096. [CrossRef] [PubMed]
53. Tew, J.G.; Wu, J.; Qin, D.; Helm, S.; Burton, G.F.; Szakal, A.K. Follicular dendritic cells and presentation of antigen and costimulatory signals to B cells. *Immunol. Rev.* **1997**, *156*, 39–52. [CrossRef] [PubMed]
54. Jonsson, M.V.; Skarstein, K. Follicular dendritic cells confirm lymphoid organization in the minor salivary glands of primary Sjögren's syndrome. *J. Oral Pathol. Med.* **2008**, *37*, 515–521. [CrossRef]
55. Bombardieri, M.; Barone, F.; Humby, F.; Kelly, S.; McGurk, M.; Morgan, P.; Challacombe, S.; De Vita, S.; Valesini, G.; Spencer, J.; et al. Activation-induced cytidine deaminase expression in follicular dendritic cell networks and interfollicular large B cells supports functionality of ectopic lymphoid neogenesis in autoimmune sialoadenitis and MALT lymphoma in Sjögren's syndrome. *J. Immunol.* **2007**, *179*, 4929–4938. [CrossRef]
56. Wynn, T.A.; Chawla, A.; Pollard, J.W. Macrophage biology in development, homeostasis and disease. *Nature* **2013**, *496*, 445–455. [CrossRef]
57. Cuello, C.; Palladinetti, P.; Tedla, N.; Di Girolamo, N.; Lloyd, A.R.; McCluskey, P.J.; Wakefield, D. Chemokine expression and leucocyte infiltration in Sjögren's syndrome. *Br. J. Rheumatol.* **1998**, *37*, 779–783. [CrossRef]
58. Hernández-Molina, G.; Michel-Peregrina, M.; Hernández-Ramírez, D.F.; Sánchez-Guerrero, J.; Llorente, L. Chemokine saliva levels in patients with primary Sjögren's syndrome, associated Sjögren's syndrome, pre-clinical Sjögren's syndrome and systemic autoimmune diseases. *Rheumatology (Oxford)* **2011**, *50*, 1288–1292. [CrossRef]
59. Manoussakis, M.N.; Boiu, S.; Korkolopoulou, P.; Kapsogeorgou, E.K.; Kavantzas, N.; Ziakas, P.; Patsouris, E.; Moutsopoulos, H.M. Rates of infiltration by macrophages and dendritic cells and expression of interleukin-18 and interleukin-12 in the chronic inflammatory lesions of Sjögren's syndrome: Correlation with certain features of immune hyperactivity and factors associated with high risk of lymphoma development. *Arthritis Rheum.* **2007**, *56*, 3977–3988. [CrossRef]
60. Ma, W.T.; Gao, F.; Gu, K.; Chen, D.K. The role of monocytes and macrophages in autoimmune diseases: A comprehensive review. *Front. Immunol.* **2019**, *10*, 1140. [CrossRef]
61. Greenwell-Wild, T.; Moutsopoulos, N.M.; Gliozzi, M.; Kapsogeorgou, E.; Rangel, Z.; Munson, P.J.; Moutsopoulos, H.M.; Wahl, S.M. Chitinases in the salivary glands and circulation of patients with Sjögren's syndrome: Macrophage harbingers of disease severity. *Arthritis Rheum.* **2011**, *63*, 3103–3115. [CrossRef]
62. Gliozzi, M.; Greenwell-Wild, T.; Jin, W.; Moutsopoulos, N.M.; Kapsogeorgou, E.; Moutsopoulos, H.M.; Wahl, S.M. A link between interferon and augmented plasmin generation in exocrine gland damage in Sjögren's syndrome. *J. Autoimmun.* **2013**, *40*, 122–133. [CrossRef] [PubMed]
63. Yarom, N.; Dayan, D.; Buchner, A.; Vered, M. Immunoprofile of focal lymphocytic infiltration in minor salivary glands of healthy individuals. *Oral Dis.* **2007**, *13*, 274–278. [CrossRef] [PubMed]
64. Baban, B.; Liu, J.Y.; Abdelsayed, R.; Mozaffari, M.S. Reciprocal relation between GADD153 and Del-1 in regulation of salivary gland inflammation in Sjögren syndrome. *Exp. Mol. Pathol.* **2013**, *95*, 288–297. [CrossRef] [PubMed]
65. Nagata, S. Apoptosis and clearance of apoptotic cells. *Annu. Rev. Immunol.* **2018**, *36*, 489–517. [CrossRef]

66. Ballantine, L.; Midgley, A.; Harris, D.; Richards, E.; Burgess, S.; Beresford, M.W. Increased soluble phagocytic receptors sMer, sTyro3 and sAxl and reduced phagocytosis in juvenile-onset systemic lupus erythematosus. *Pediatr. Rheumatol. Online J.* **2015**, *13*, 10. [CrossRef]
67. Kawano, M.; Nagata, S. Efferocytosis and autoimmune disease. *Int. Immunol.* **2018**, *30*, 551–558. [CrossRef]
68. Manganelli, P.; Fietta, P. Apoptosis and Sjögren syndrome. *Semin. Arthritis Rheum.* **2003**, *33*, 49–65. [CrossRef]
69. Kramer, J.M. Early events in Sjögren's syndrome pathogenesis: The importance of innate immunity in disease initiation. *Cytokine* **2014**, *67*, 92–101. [CrossRef]
70. Hauk, V.; Fraccaroli, L.; Grasso, E.; Eimon, A.; Ramhorst, R.; Hubscher, O.; Pérez Leirós, C. Monocytes from Sjögren's syndrome patients display increased vasoactive intestinal peptide receptor 2 expression and impaired apoptotic cell phagocytosis. *Clin. Exp. Immunol.* **2014**, *177*, 662–670. [CrossRef] [PubMed]
71. Manoussakis, M.N.; Fragoulis, G.E.; Vakrakou, A.G.; Moutsopoulos, H.M. Impaired clearance of early apoptotic cells mediated by inhibitory IgG antibodies in patients with primary Sjögren's syndrome. *PLoS ONE* **2014**, *9*, e112100. [CrossRef] [PubMed]
72. O'Brien, B.A.; Huang, Y.; Geng, X.; Dutz, J.P.; Finegood, D.T. Phagocytosis of apoptotic cells by macrophages from NOD mice is reduced. *Diabetes* **2002**, *51*, 2481–2488. [CrossRef] [PubMed]
73. Witas, R.; Peck, A.B.; Ambrus, J.L.; Nguyen, C.Q. Sjogren's syndrome and TAM receptors: A possible contribution to disease onset. *J. Immunol. Res.* **2019**, *2019*, 4813795. [CrossRef] [PubMed]
74. Ciccia, F.; Guggino, G.; Rizzo, A.; Ferrante, A.; Raimondo, S.; Giardina, A.; Dieli, F.; Campisi, G.; Alessandro, R.; Triolo, G. Potential involvement of IL-22 and IL-22-producing cells in the inflamed salivary glands of patients with Sjogren's syndrome. *Ann. Rheum. Dis.* **2012**, *71*, 295–301. [CrossRef]
75. Cortez, V.S.; Cervantes-Barragan, L.; Robinette, M.L.; Bando, J.K.; Wang, Y.; Geiger, T.L.; Gilfillan, S.; Fuchs, A.; Vivier, E.; Sun, J.C.; et al. Transforming growth factor-β signaling guides the differentiation of innate lymphoid cells in salivary glands. *Immunity* **2016**, *44*, 1127–1139. [CrossRef]
76. Robertson, M.J.; Ritz, J. Biology and clinical relevance of human natural killer cells. *Blood* **1990**, *76*, 2421–2438. [CrossRef]
77. Seaman, W.E. Natural killer cells and natural killer T cells. *Arthritis Rheum.* **2000**, *43*, 1204–1217. [CrossRef]
78. Szodoray, P.; Papp, G.; Horvath, I.F.; Barath, S.; Sipka, S.; Nakken, B.; Zeher, M. Cells with regulatory function of the innate and adaptive immune system in primary Sjögren's syndrome. *Clin. Exp. Immunol.* **2009**, *157*, 343–349. [CrossRef]
79. Sudzius, G.; Mieliauskaite, D.; Siaurys, A.; Viliene, R.; Butrimiene, I.; Characiejus, D.; Dumalakiene, I. Distribution of peripheral lymphocyte populations in primary Sjögren's syndrome patients. *J. Immunol. Res.* **2015**, *2015*, 854706. [CrossRef]
80. Struyf, N.J.; Snoeck, H.W.; Bridts, C.H.; De Clerck, L.S.; Stevens, W.J. Natural killer cell activity in Sjögren's syndrome and systemic lupus erythematosus: Stimulation with interferons and interleukin-2 and correlation with immune complexes. *Ann. Rheum. Dis.* **1990**, *49*, 690–693. [CrossRef]
81. Izumi, Y.; Ida, H.; Huang, M.; Iwanaga, N.; Tanaka, F.; Aratake, K.; Arima, K.; Tamai, M.; Kamachi, M.; Nakamura, H.; et al. Characterization of peripheral natural killer cells in primary Sjögren's syndrome: Impaired NK cell activity and low NK cell number. *J. Lab. Clin. Med.* **2006**, *147*, 242–249. [CrossRef] [PubMed]
82. Rusakiewicz, S.; Nocturne, G.; Lazure, T.; Semeraro, M.; Flament, C.; Caillat-Zucman, S.; Sène, D.; Delahaye, N.; Vivier, E.; Chaba, K.; et al. NCR3/NKp30 contributes to pathogenesis in primary Sjogren's syndrome. *Sci. Transl. Med.* **2013**, *5*, 195ra196. [CrossRef]
83. Deshmukh, U.S.; Bagavant, H. When killers become helpers. *Sci. Transl. Med.* **2013**, *5*, 195fs129. [CrossRef] [PubMed]
84. Manoussakis, M.N.; Kapsogeorgou, E.K. The role of intrinsic epithelial activation in the pathogenesis of Sjögren's syndrome. *J. Autoimmun.* **2010**, *35*, 219–224. [CrossRef]
85. Goules, A.V.; Kapsogeorgou, E.K.; Tzioufas, A.G. Insight into pathogenesis of Sjögren's syndrome: Dissection on autoimmune infiltrates and epithelial cells. *Clin. Immunol.* **2017**, *182*, 30–40. [CrossRef]
86. Tsunawaki, S.; Nakamura, S.; Ohyama, Y.; Sasaki, M.; Ikebe-Hiroki, A.; Hiraki, A.; Kadena, T.; Kawamura, E.; Kumamaru, W.; Shinohara, M.; et al. Possible function of salivary gland epithelial cells as nonprofessional antigen-presenting cells in the development of Sjögren's syndrome. *J. Rheumatol.* **2002**, *29*, 1884–1896. [PubMed]

87. Jin, J.O.; Shinohara, Y.; Yu, Q. Innate immune signaling induces interleukin-7 production from salivary gland cells and accelerates the development of primary Sjögren's syndrome in a mouse model. *PLoS ONE* **2013**, *8*, e77605. [CrossRef]
88. Amft, N.; Curnow, S.J.; Scheel-Toellner, D.; Devadas, A.; Oates, J.; Crocker, J.; Hamburger, J.; Ainsworth, J.; Mathews, J.; Salmon, M.; et al. Ectopic expression of the B cell-attracting chemokine BCA-1 (CXCL13) on endothelial cells and within lymphoid follicles contributes to the establishment of germinal center-like structures in Sjögren's syndrome. *Arthritis Rheum.* **2001**, *44*, 2633–2641. [CrossRef]
89. Barone, F.; Bombardieri, M.; Rosado, M.M.; Morgan, P.R.; Challacombe, S.J.; De Vita, S.; Carsetti, R.; Spencer, J.; Valesini, G.; Pitzalis, C. CXCL13, CCL21, and CXCL12 expression in salivary glands of patients with Sjögren's syndrome and MALT lymphoma: Association with reactive and malignant areas of lymphoid organization. *J. Immunol.* **2008**, *180*, 5130–5140. [CrossRef]
90. Salomonsson, S.; Larsson, P.; Tengnér, P.; Mellquist, E.; Hjelmström, P.; Wahren-Herlenius, M. Expression of the B cell-attracting chemokine CXCL13 in the target organ and autoantibody production in ectopic lymphoid tissue in the chronic inflammatory disease Sjögren's syndrome. *Scand. J. Immunol.* **2002**, *55*, 336–342. [CrossRef]
91. Gong, Y.Z.; Nititham, J.; Taylor, K.; Miceli-Richard, C.; Sordet, C.; Wachsmann, D.; Bahram, S.; Georgel, P.; Criswell, L.A.; Sibilia, J.; et al. Differentiation of follicular helper T cells by salivary gland epithelial cells in primary Sjögren's syndrome. *J. Autoimmun.* **2014**, *51*, 57–66. [CrossRef]
92. Ittah, M.; Miceli-Richard, C.; Gottenberg, J.E.; Sellam, J.; Eid, P.; Lebon, P.; Pallier, C.; Lepajolec, C.; Mariette, X. Viruses induce high expression of BAFF by salivary gland epithelial cells through TLR- and type-I IFN-dependent and -independent pathways. *Eur. J. Immunol.* **2008**, *38*, 1058–1064. [CrossRef] [PubMed]
93. Lavie, F.; Miceli-Richard, C.; Quillard, J.; Roux, S.; Leclerc, P.; Mariette, X. Expression of BAFF (BLyS) in T cells infiltrating labial salivary glands from patients with Sjögren's syndrome. *J. Pathol.* **2004**, *202*, 496–502. [CrossRef] [PubMed]
94. Aqrawi, L.A.; Kvarnström, M.; Brokstad, K.A.; Jonsson, R.; Skarstein, K.; Wahren-Herlenius, M. Ductal epithelial expression of Ro52 correlates with inflammation in salivary glands of patients with primary Sjögren's syndrome. *Clin. Exp. Immunol.* **2014**, *177*, 244–252. [CrossRef] [PubMed]
95. Katsiougiannis, S.; Tenta, R.; Skopouli, F.N. Autoimmune epithelitis (Sjögren's syndrome); the impact of metabolic status of glandular epithelial cells on auto-immunogenicity. *J. Autoimmun.* **2019**, *104*, 102335. [CrossRef]
96. Kawakami, A.; Nakashima, K.; Tamai, M.; Nakamura, H.; Iwanaga, N.; Fujikawa, K.; Aramaki, T.; Arima, K.; Iwamoto, N.; Ichinose, K.; et al. Toll-like receptor in salivary glands from patients with Sjögren's syndrome: Functional analysis by human salivary gland cell line. *J. Rheumatol.* **2007**, *34*, 1019–1026.
97. Spachidou, M.P.; Bourazopoulou, E.; Maratheftis, C.I.; Kapsogeorgou, E.K.; Moutsopoulos, H.M.; Tzioufas, A.G.; Manoussakis, M.N. Expression of functional Toll-like receptors by salivary gland epithelial cells: Increased mRNA expression in cells derived from patients with primary Sjögren's syndrome. *Clin. Exp. Immunol.* **2007**, *147*, 497–503. [CrossRef]
98. Shimizu, T.; Nakamura, H.; Takatani, A.; Umeda, M.; Horai, Y.; Kurushima, S.; Michitsuji, T.; Nakashima, Y.; Kawakami, A. Activation of Toll-like receptor 7 signaling in labial salivary glands of primary Sjögren's syndrome patients. *Clin. Exp. Immunol.* **2019**, *196*, 39–51. [CrossRef]
99. Deshmukh, U.S.; Nandula, S.R.; Thimmalapura, P.R.; Scindia, Y.M.; Bagavant, H. Activation of innate immune responses through Toll-like receptor 3 causes a rapid loss of salivary gland function. *J. Oral Pathol. Med.* **2009**, *38*, 42–47. [CrossRef]
100. Manoussakis, M.N.; Spachidou, M.P.; Maratheftis, C.I. Salivary epithelial cells from Sjogren's syndrome patients are highly sensitive to anoikis induced by TLR-3 ligation. *J. Autoimmun.* **2010**, *35*, 212–218. [CrossRef]
101. Nakamura, H.; Horai, Y.; Suzuki, T.; Okada, A.; Ichinose, K.; Yamasaki, S.; Koji, T.; Kawakami, A. TLR3-mediated apoptosis and activation of phosphorylated Akt in the salivary gland epithelial cells of primary Sjogren's syndrome patients. *Rheumatol. Int.* **2013**, *33*, 441–450. [CrossRef] [PubMed]
102. Li, P.; Yang, Y.; Jin, Y.; Zhao, R.; Dong, C.; Zheng, W.; Zhang, T.; Li, J.; Gu, Z. B7-H3 participates in human salivary gland epithelial cells apoptosis through NF-κB pathway in primary Sjögren's syndrome. *J. Transl. Med.* **2019**, *17*, 268. [CrossRef] [PubMed]

103. Vakrakou, A.G.; Polyzos, A.; Kapsogeorgou, E.K.; Thanos, D.; Manoussakis, M.N. Impaired anti-inflammatory activity of PPARγ in the salivary epithelia of Sjögren's syndrome patients imposed by intrinsic NF-κB activation. *J. Autoimmun.* **2018**, *86*, 62–74. [CrossRef] [PubMed]
104. Ambrosi, A.; Wahren-Herlenius, M. Update on the immunobiology of Sjögren's syndrome. *Curr. Opin. Rheumatol.* **2015**, *27*, 468–475. [CrossRef] [PubMed]
105. Rosloniec, E.F.; Latham, K.; Guedez, Y.B. Paradoxical roles of IFN-gamma in models of Th1-mediated autoimmunity. *Arthritis Res.* **2002**, *4*, 333–336. [CrossRef] [PubMed]
106. Mosmann, T.R.; Coffman, R.L. TH1 and TH2 cells: Different patterns of lymphokine secretion lead to different functional properties. *Annu. Rev. Immunol.* **1989**, *7*, 145–173. [CrossRef] [PubMed]
107. Batten, M.; Fletcher, C.; Ng, L.G.; Groom, J.; Wheway, J.; Laâbi, Y.; Xin, X.; Schneider, P.; Tschopp, J.; Mackay, C.R.; et al. TNF deficiency fails to protect BAFF transgenic mice against autoimmunity and reveals a predisposition to B cell lymphoma. *J. Immunol.* **2004**, *172*, 812–822. [CrossRef]
108. Karabiyik, A.; Peck, A.B.; Nguyen, C.Q. The important role of T cells and receptor expression in Sjogren's syndrome. *Scand. J. Immunol.* **2013**, *78*, 157–166. [CrossRef]
109. Nguyen, C.Q.; Sharma, A.; Lee, B.H.; She, J.X.; McIndoe, R.A.; Peck, A.B. Differential gene expression in the salivary gland during development and onset of xerostomia in Sjogren's syndrome-like disease of the C57BL/6.NOD-Aec1Aec2 mouse. *Arthritis Res. Ther.* **2009**, *11*, R56. [CrossRef]
110. Zheng, Y.; Yang, W.; Aldape, K.; He, J.; Lu, Z. Epidermal growth factor (EGF)-enhanced vascular cell adhesion molecule-1 (VCAM-1) expression promotes macrophage and glioblastoma cell interaction and tumor cell invasion. *J. Biol. Chem.* **2013**, *288*, 31488–31495. [CrossRef]
111. Walsh, S.V.; Hopkins, A.M.; Nusrat, A. Modulation of tight junction structure and function by cytokines. *Adv. Drug Deliv. Rev.* **2000**, *41*, 303–313. [CrossRef]
112. Ewert, P.; Aguilera, S.; Alliende, C.; Kwon, Y.J.; Albornoz, A.; Molina, C.; Urzúa, U.; Quest, A.F.; Olea, N.; Pérez, P.; et al. Disruption of tight junction structure in salivary glands from Sjögren's syndrome patients is linked to proinflammatory cytokine exposure. *Arthritis Rheum.* **2010**, *62*, 1280–1289. [CrossRef] [PubMed]
113. Abu-Helu, R.F.; Dimitriou, I.D.; Kapsogeorgou, E.K.; Moutsopoulos, H.M.; Manoussakis, M.N. Induction of salivary gland epithelial cell injury in Sjogren's syndrome: In vitro assessment of T cell-derived cytokines and Fas protein expression. *J. Autoimmun.* **2001**, *17*, 141–153. [CrossRef] [PubMed]
114. Chaly, Y.; Barr, J.Y.; Sullivan, D.A.; Thomas, H.E.; Brodnicki, T.C.; Lieberman, S.M. Type I interferon signaling is required for dacryoadenitis in the nonobese diabetic mouse model of Sjögren syndrome. *Int. J. Mol. Sci.* **2018**, *19*, 3259. [CrossRef] [PubMed]
115. Jin, J.O.; Kawai, T.; Cha, S.; Yu, Q. Interleukin-7 enhances the Th1 response to promote the development of Sjögren's syndrome-like autoimmune exocrinopathy in mice. *Arthritis Rheum.* **2013**, *65*, 2132–2142. [CrossRef] [PubMed]
116. Okamoto, K.; Iwai, Y.; Oh-Hora, M.; Yamamoto, M.; Morio, T.; Aoki, K.; Ohya, K.; Jetten, A.M.; Akira, S.; Muta, T.; et al. IkappaBzeta regulates T(H)17 development by cooperating with ROR nuclear receptors. *Nature* **2010**, *464*, 1381–1385. [CrossRef]
117. Okuma, A.; Hoshino, K.; Ohba, T.; Fukushi, S.; Aiba, S.; Akira, S.; Ono, M.; Kaisho, T.; Muta, T. Enhanced apoptosis by disruption of the STAT3-IκB-ζ signaling pathway in epithelial cells induces Sjögren's syndrome-like autoimmune disease. *Immunity* **2013**, *38*, 450–460. [CrossRef]
118. Forbes, L.R.; Milner, J.; Haddad, E. Signal transducer and activator of transcription 3: A year in review. *Curr. Opin. Hematol.* **2016**, *23*, 23–27. [CrossRef]
119. Ivanov, I.I.; Zhou, L.; Littman, D.R. Transcriptional regulation of Th17 cell differentiation. *Semin. Immunol.* **2007**, *19*, 409–417. [CrossRef]
120. Sakai, A.; Sugawara, Y.; Kuroishi, T.; Sasano, T.; Sugawara, S. Identification of IL-18 and Th17 cells in salivary glands of patients with Sjogren's syndrome, and amplification of IL-17-mediated secretion of inflammatory cytokines from salivary gland cells by IL-18. *J. Immunol.* **2008**, *181*, 2898–2906. [CrossRef]
121. Bombardieri, M.; Barone, F.; Pittoni, V.; Alessandri, C.; Conigliaro, P.; Blades, M.C.; Priori, R.; McInnes, I.B.; Valesini, G.; Pitzalis, C. Increased circulating levels and salivary gland expression of interleukin-18 in patients with Sjogren's syndrome: Relationship with autoantibody production and lymphoid organization of the periductal inflammatory infiltrate. *Arthritis Res. Ther.* **2004**, *6*, R447–R456. [CrossRef] [PubMed]

122. Delaleu, N.; Immervoll, H.; Cornelius, J.; Jonsson, R. Biomarker profiles in serum and saliva of experimental Sjogren's syndrome: Associations with specific autoimmune manifestations. *Arthritis Res. Ther.* **2008**, *10*, R22. [CrossRef] [PubMed]
123. Del Prete, G.; Maggi, E.; Romagnani, S. Human Th1 and Th2 cells: Functional properties, mechanisms of regulation, and role in disease. *Lab Investig.* **1994**, *70*, 299–306. [PubMed]
124. León, B.; Ballesteros-Tato, A.; Lund, F.E. Dendritic cells and B cells: Unexpected partners in Th2 development. *J. Immunol.* **2014**, *193*, 1531–1537. [CrossRef]
125. Hartenstein, B.; Teurich, S.; Hess, J.; Schenkel, J.; Schorpp-Kistner, M.; Angel, P. Th2 cell-specific cytokine expression and allergen-induced airway inflammation depend on JunB. *EMBO J.* **2002**, *21*, 6321–6329. [CrossRef]
126. Zheng, W.; Flavell, R.A. The transcription factor GATA-3 is necessary and sufficient for Th2 cytokine gene expression in CD4 T cells. *Cell* **1997**, *89*, 587–596. [CrossRef]
127. Brayer, J.B.; Cha, S.; Nagashima, H.; Yasunari, U.; Lindberg, A.; Diggs, S.; Martinez, J.; Goa, J.; Humphreys-Beher, M.G.; Peck, A.B. IL-4-dependent effector phase in autoimmune exocrinopathy as defined by the NOD.IL-4-gene knockout mouse model of Sjögren's syndrome. *Scand. J. Immunol.* **2001**, *54*, 133–140. [CrossRef]
128. Gao, J.; Killedar, S.; Cornelius, J.G.; Nguyen, C.; Cha, S.; Peck, A.B. Sjögren's syndrome in the NOD mouse model is an interleukin-4 time-dependent, antibody isotype-specific autoimmune disease. *J. Autoimmun.* **2006**, *26*, 90–103. [CrossRef]
129. Nguyen, C.Q.; Gao, J.H.; Kim, H.; Saban, D.R.; Cornelius, J.G.; Peck, A.B. IL-4-STAT6 signal transduction-dependent induction of the clinical phase of Sjogren's syndrome-like disease of the nonobese diabetic mouse. *J. Immunol.* **2007**, *179*, 382–390. [CrossRef]
130. Matsui, K.; Sano, H. T Helper 17 cells in primary Sjögren's syndrome. *J. Clin. Med.* **2017**, *6*, 65. [CrossRef]
131. Veldhoen, M.; Hocking, R.J.; Atkins, C.J.; Locksley, R.M.; Stockinger, B. TGFbeta in the context of an inflammatory cytokine milieu supports de novo differentiation of IL-17-producing T cells. *Immunity* **2006**, *24*, 179–189. [CrossRef] [PubMed]
132. Hunter, C.A. New IL-12-family members: IL-23 and IL-27, cytokines with divergent functions. *Nat. Rev. Immunol.* **2005**, *5*, 521–531. [CrossRef] [PubMed]
133. de Jong, E.; Suddason, T.; Lord, G.M. Translational mini-review series on Th17 cells: Development of mouse and human T helper 17 cells. *Clin. Exp. Immunol.* **2010**, *159*, 148–158. [CrossRef] [PubMed]
134. Katsifis, G.E.; Rekka, S.; Moutsopoulos, N.M.; Pillemer, S.; Wahl, S.M. Systemic and local interleukin-17 and linked cytokines associated with Sjögren's syndrome immunopathogenesis. *Am. J. Pathol.* **2009**, *175*, 1167–1177. [CrossRef] [PubMed]
135. Jetten, A.M.; Takeda, Y.; Slominski, A.; Kang, H.S. Retinoic acid-related Orphan Receptor γ (RORγ): Connecting sterol metabolism to regulation of the immune system and autoimmune disease. *Curr. Opin. Toxicol.* **2018**, *8*, 66–80. [CrossRef]
136. Schraml, B.U.; Hildner, K.; Ise, W.; Lee, W.L.; Smith, W.A.; Solomon, B.; Sahota, G.; Sim, J.; Mukasa, R.; Cemerski, S.; et al. The AP-1 transcription factor Batf controls T(H)17 differentiation. *Nature* **2009**, *460*, 405–409. [CrossRef]
137. Kang, K.Y.; Kim, H.O.; Kwok, S.K.; Ju, J.H.; Park, K.S.; Sun, D.I.; Jhun, J.Y.; Oh, H.J.; Park, S.H.; Kim, H.Y. Impact of interleukin-21 in the pathogenesis of primary Sjögren's syndrome: Increased serum levels of interleukin-21 and its expression in the labial salivary glands. *Arthritis Res. Ther.* **2011**, *13*, R179. [CrossRef]
138. Li, L.; He, J.; Zhu, L.; Yang, Y.; Jin, Y.; Jia, R.; Liu, X.; Liu, Y.; Sun, X.; Li, Z. The clinical relevance of IL-17-producing CD4+CD161+ cell and its subpopulations in primary Sjögren's syndrome. *J. Immunol. Res.* **2015**, *2015*, 307453. [CrossRef]
139. Alunno, A.; Carubbi, F.; Bistoni, O.; Caterbi, S.; Bartoloni, E.; Bigerna, B.; Pacini, R.; Beghelli, D.; Cipriani, P.; Giacomelli, R.; et al. CD4(-)CD8(-) T-cells in primary Sjögren's syndrome: Association with the extent of glandular involvement. *J. Autoimmun.* **2014**, *51*, 38–43. [CrossRef]
140. Nguyen, C.Q.; Hu, M.H.; Li, Y.; Stewart, C.; Peck, A.B. Salivary gland tissue expression of interleukin-23 and interleukin-17 in Sjogren's syndrome: Findings in humans and mice. *Arthritis Rheum.* **2008**, *58*, 734–743. [CrossRef]

141. Voigt, A.; Esfandiary, L.; Wanchoo, A.; Glenton, P.; Donate, A.; Craft, W.F.; Craft, S.L.; Nguyen, C.Q. Sexual dimorphic function of IL-17 in salivary gland dysfunction of the C57BL/6.NOD-Aec1Aec2 model of Sjogren's syndrome. *Sci. Rep.* **2016**, *6*, 38717. [CrossRef] [PubMed]
142. Wanchoo, A.; Voigt, A.; Sukumaran, S.; Stewart, C.M.; Bhattacharya, I.; Nguyen, C.Q. Single-cell analysis reveals sexually dimorphic repertoires of Interferon-gamma and IL-17A producing T cells in salivary glands of Sjogren's syndrome mice. *Sci. Rep.* **2017**, *7*, 12512. [CrossRef] [PubMed]
143. Lin, X.; Rui, K.; Deng, J.; Tian, J.; Wang, X.; Wang, S.; Ko, K.H.; Jiao, Z.; Chan, V.S.; Lau, C.S.; et al. Th17 cells play a critical role in the development of experimental Sjogren's syndrome. *Ann. Rheum. Dis.* **2015**, *74*, 1302–1310. [CrossRef] [PubMed]
144. Iizuka, M.; Tsuboi, H.; Matsuo, N.; Asashima, H.; Hirota, T.; Kondo, Y.; Iwakura, Y.; Takahashi, S.; Matsumoto, I.; Sumida, T. A crucial role of RORγt in the development of spontaneous Sialadenitis-like Sjögren's syndrome. *J. Immunol.* **2015**, *194*, 56–67. [CrossRef] [PubMed]
145. Lee, B.H.; Carcamo, W.C.; Chiorini, J.A.; Peck, A.B.; Nguyen, C.Q. Gene therapy using IL-27 ameliorates Sjögren's syndrome-like autoimmune exocrinopathy. *Arthritis Res. Ther.* **2012**, *14*, R172. [CrossRef] [PubMed]
146. Iizuka, M.; Wakamatsu, E.; Tsuboi, H.; Nakamura, Y.; Hayashi, T.; Matsui, M.; Goto, D.; Ito, S.; Matsumoto, I.; Sumida, T. Pathogenic role of immune response to M3 muscarinic acetylcholine receptor in Sjogren's syndrome-like sialoadenitis. *J. Autoimmun.* **2010**, *35*, 383–389. [CrossRef]
147. Iizuka, M.; Tsuboi, H.; Matsuo, N.; Kondo, Y.; Asashima, H.; Matsui, M.; Matsumoto, I.; Sumida, T. The crucial roles of IFN-γ in the development of M3 muscarinic acetylcholine receptor induced Sjögren's syndrome-like sialadenitis. *Mod. Rheumatol.* **2013**, *23*, 614–616. [CrossRef] [PubMed]
148. Liu, R.; Gao, C.; Chen, H.; Li, Y.; Jin, Y.; Qi, H. Analysis of Th17-associated cytokines and clinical correlations in patients with dry eye disease. *PLoS ONE* **2017**, *12*, e0173301. [CrossRef]
149. De Paiva, C.S.; Hwang, C.S.; Pitcher, J.D.; Pangelinan, S.B.; Rahimy, E.; Chen, W.; Yoon, K.C.; Farley, W.J.; Niederkorn, J.Y.; Stern, M.E.; et al. Age-related T-cell cytokine profile parallels corneal disease severity in Sjogren's syndrome-like keratoconjunctivitis sicca in CD25KO mice. *Rheumatology (Oxford)* **2010**, *49*, 246–258. [CrossRef]
150. Grosskreutz, C.L.; Hockey, H.U.; Serra, D.; Dryja, T.P. Dry eye signs and symptoms persist during systemic neutralization of IL-1β by canakinumab or IL-17A by secukinumab. *Cornea* **2015**, *34*, 1551–1556. [CrossRef]
151. Ramsdell, F.; Ziegler, S.F. FOXP3 and scurfy: How it all began. *Nat. Rev. Immunol.* **2014**, *14*, 343–349. [CrossRef] [PubMed]
152. Sarigul, M.; Yazisiz, V.; Bassorgun, C.I.; Ulker, M.; Avci, A.B.; Erbasan, F.; Gelen, T.; Gorczynski, R.M.; Terzioglu, E. The numbers of Foxp3 + Treg cells are positively correlated with higher grade of infiltration at the salivary glands in primary Sjogren's syndrome. *Lupus* **2010**, *19*, 138–145. [CrossRef] [PubMed]
153. Christodoulou, M.I.; Kapsogeorgou, E.K.; Moutsopoulos, N.M.; Moutsopoulos, H.M. Foxp3+ T-regulatory cells in Sjogren's syndrome: Correlation with the grade of the autoimmune lesion and certain adverse prognostic factors. *Am. J. Pathol.* **2008**, *173*, 1389–1396. [CrossRef]
154. Li, X.; Qian, L.; Wang, G.; Zhang, H.; Wang, X.; Chen, K.; Zhai, Z.; Li, Q.; Wang, Y.; Harris, D.C. T regulatory cells are markedly diminished in diseased salivary glands of patients with primary Sjögren's syndrome. *J. Rheumatol.* **2007**, *34*, 2438–2445. [PubMed]
155. Liu, M.F.; Lin, L.H.; Weng, C.T.; Weng, M.Y. Decreased CD4+CD25+bright T cells in peripheral blood of patients with primary Sjogren's syndrome. *Lupus* **2008**, *17*, 34–39. [CrossRef] [PubMed]
156. Banica, L.; Besliu, A.; Pistol, G.; Stavaru, C.; Ionescu, R.; Forsea, A.M.; Tanaseanu, C.; Dumitrache, S.; Otelea, D.; Tamsulea, I.; et al. Quantification and molecular characterization of regulatory T cells in connective tissue diseases. *Autoimmunity* **2009**, *42*, 41–49. [CrossRef]
157. Alunno, A.; Petrillo, M.G.; Nocentini, G.; Bistoni, O.; Bartoloni, E.; Caterbi, S.; Bianchini, R.; Baldini, C.; Nicoletti, I.; Riccardi, C.; et al. Characterization of a new regulatory CD4+ T cell subset in primary Sjögren's syndrome. *Rheumatology (Oxford)* **2013**, *52*, 1387–1396. [CrossRef]
158. Gottenberg, J.E.; Lavie, F.; Abbed, K.; Gasnault, J.; Le Nevot, E.; Delfraissy, J.F.; Taoufik, Y.; Mariette, X. CD4 CD25high regulatory T cells are not impaired in patients with primary Sjögren's syndrome. *J. Autoimmun.* **2005**, *24*, 235–242. [CrossRef]
159. Miyara, M.; Amoura, Z.; Parizot, C.; Badoual, C.; Dorgham, K.; Trad, S.; Nochy, D.; Debré, P.; Piette, J.C.; Gorochov, G. Global natural regulatory T cell depletion in active systemic lupus erythematosus. *J. Immunol.* **2005**, *175*, 8392–8400. [CrossRef]

160. Furuzawa-Carballeda, J.; Hernández-Molina, G.; Lima, G.; Rivera-Vicencio, Y.; Férez-Blando, K.; Llorente, L. Peripheral regulatory cells immunophenotyping in primary Sjögren's syndrome: A cross-sectional study. *Arthritis Res. Ther.* **2013**, *15*, R68. [CrossRef]
161. Coursey, T.G.; Bian, F.; Zaheer, M.; Pflugfelder, S.C.; Volpe, E.A.; de Paiva, C.S. Age-related spontaneous lacrimal keratoconjunctivitis is accompanied by dysfunctional T regulatory cells. *Mucosal Immunol.* **2017**, *10*, 743–756. [CrossRef] [PubMed]
162. Maria, N.I.; van Helden-Meeuwsen, C.G.; Brkic, Z.; Paulissen, S.M.; Steenwijk, E.C.; Dalm, V.A.; van Daele, P.L.; Martin van Hagen, P.; Kroese, F.G.; van Roon, J.A.; et al. Association of increased Treg cell levels with elevated Indoleamine 2,3-Dioxygenase activity and an imbalanced Kynurenine pathway in interferon-positive primary Sjögren's syndrome. *Arthritis Rheumatol.* **2016**, *68*, 1688–1699. [CrossRef]
163. Noack, M.; Miossec, P. Th17 and regulatory T cell balance in autoimmune and inflammatory diseases. *Autoimmun. Rev.* **2014**, *13*, 668–677. [CrossRef] [PubMed]
164. Yao, Y.; Ma, J.F.; Chang, C.; Xu, T.; Gao, C.Y.; Gershwin, M.E.; Lian, Z.X. Immunobiology of T Cells in Sjögren's syndrome. *Clin. Rev. Allergy Immunol.* **2020**. [CrossRef] [PubMed]
165. Nurieva, R.I.; Chung, Y.; Martinez, G.J.; Yang, X.O.; Tanaka, S.; Matskevitch, T.D.; Wang, Y.H.; Dong, C. Bcl6 mediates the development of T follicular helper cells. *Science* **2009**, *325*, 1001–1005. [CrossRef] [PubMed]
166. Verstappen, G.M.; Kroese, F.G.; Meiners, P.M.; Corneth, O.B.; Huitema, M.G.; Haacke, E.A.; van der Vegt, B.; Arends, S.; Vissink, A.; Bootsma, H.; et al. B cell depletion therapy normalizes circulating follicular Th cells in primary Sjögren syndrome. *J. Rheumatol.* **2017**, *44*, 49–58. [CrossRef]
167. Vinuesa, C.G.; Linterman, M.A.; Yu, D.; MacLennan, I.C. Follicular helper T cells. *Annu. Rev. Immunol.* **2016**, *34*, 335–368. [CrossRef]
168. Szabo, K.; Papp, G.; Dezso, B.; Zeher, M. The histopathology of labial salivary glands in primary Sjögren's syndrome: Focusing on follicular helper T cells in the inflammatory infiltrates. *Mediat. Inflamm.* **2014**, *2014*, 631787. [CrossRef]
169. Moens, L.; Tangye, S.G. Cytokine-Mediated Regulation of Plasma Cell Generation: IL-21 Takes Center Stage. *Front. Immunol.* **2014**, *5*, 65. [CrossRef]
170. Crotty, S. T follicular helper cell differentiation, function, and roles in disease. *Immunity* **2014**, *41*, 529–542. [CrossRef]
171. Deenick, E.K.; Ma, C.S. The regulation and role of T follicular helper cells in immunity. *Immunology* **2011**, *134*, 361–367. [CrossRef]
172. Santamaria, P. Effector lymphocytes in autoimmunity. *Curr. Opin. Immunol.* **2001**, *13*, 663–669. [CrossRef]
173. Gao, C.Y.; Yao, Y.; Li, L.; Yang, S.H.; Chu, H.; Tsuneyama, K.; Li, X.M.; Gershwin, M.E.; Lian, Z.X. Tissue-resident memory CD8+ T cells acting as mediators of salivary gland damage in a murine model of Sjögren's syndrome. *Arthritis Rheumatol.* **2019**, *71*, 121–132. [CrossRef] [PubMed]
174. Mingueneau, M.; Boudaoud, S.; Haskett, S.; Reynolds, T.L.; Nocturne, G.; Norton, E.; Zhang, X.; Constant, M.; Park, D.; Wang, W.; et al. Cytometry by time-of-flight immunophenotyping identifies a blood Sjögren's signature correlating with disease activity and glandular inflammation. *J. Allergy Clin. Immunol.* **2016**, *137*, 1809–1821.e1812. [CrossRef] [PubMed]
175. Tasaki, S.; Suzuki, K.; Nishikawa, A.; Kassai, Y.; Takiguchi, M.; Kurisu, R.; Okuzono, Y.; Miyazaki, T.; Takeshita, M.; Yoshimoto, K.; et al. Multiomic disease signatures converge to cytotoxic CD8 T cells in primary Sjögren's syndrome. *Ann. Rheum. Dis.* **2017**, *76*, 1458–1466. [CrossRef]
176. Caldeira-Dantas, S.; Furmanak, T.; Smith, C.; Quinn, M.; Teos, L.Y.; Ertel, A.; Kurup, D.; Tandon, M.; Alevizos, I.; Snyder, C.M. The chemokine receptor CXCR3 promotes CD8. *J. Immunol.* **2018**, *200*, 1133–1145. [CrossRef]
177. Barr, J.Y.; Wang, X.; Meyerholz, D.K.; Lieberman, S.M. CD8 T cells contribute to lacrimal gland pathology in the nonobese diabetic mouse model of Sjögren syndrome. *Immunol. Cell Biol.* **2017**, *95*, 684–694. [CrossRef]
178. Cerutti, A.; Cols, M.; Puga, I. Marginal zone B cells: Virtues of innate-like antibody-producing lymphocytes. *Nat. Rev. Immunol.* **2013**, *13*, 118–132. [CrossRef]
179. Martin, F.; Kearney, J.F. Marginal-zone B cells. *Nat. Rev. Immunol.* **2002**, *2*, 323–335. [CrossRef]
180. Grasseau, A.; Boudigou, M.; Le Pottier, L.; Chriti, N.; Cornec, D.; Pers, J.O.; Renaudineau, Y.; Hillion, S. Innate B cells: The archetype of protective immune cells. *Clin. Rev. Allergy Immunol.* **2020**, *58*, 92–106. [CrossRef]
181. Weill, J.C.; Weller, S.; Reynaud, C.A. Human marginal zone B cells. *Annu. Rev. Immunol.* **2009**, *27*, 267–285. [CrossRef] [PubMed]

182. Chen, X.; Martin, F.; Forbush, K.A.; Perlmutter, R.M.; Kearney, J.F. Evidence for selection of a population of multi-reactive B cells into the splenic marginal zone. *Int. Immunol.* **1997**, *9*, 27–41. [CrossRef] [PubMed]
183. Peeva, E.; Michael, D.; Cleary, J.; Rice, J.; Chen, X.; Diamond, B. Prolactin modulates the naive B cell repertoire. *J. Clin. Investig.* **2003**, *111*, 275–283. [CrossRef] [PubMed]
184. Grimaldi, C.M.; Michael, D.J.; Diamond, B. Cutting edge: Expansion and activation of a population of autoreactive marginal zone B cells in a model of estrogen-induced lupus. *J. Immunol.* **2001**, *167*, 1886–1890. [CrossRef] [PubMed]
185. Li, Y.; Li, H.; Ni, D.; Weigert, M. Anti-DNA B cells in MRL/lpr mice show altered differentiation and editing pattern. *J. Exp. Med.* **2002**, *196*, 1543–1552. [CrossRef] [PubMed]
186. Voulgarelis, M.; Ziakas, P.D.; Papageorgiou, A.; Baimpa, E.; Tzioufas, A.G.; Moutsopoulos, H.M. Prognosis and outcome of non-Hodgkin lymphoma in primary Sjögren syndrome. *Medicine (Baltimore)* **2012**, *91*, 1–9. [CrossRef]
187. Daridon, C.; Pers, J.O.; Devauchelle, V.; Martins-Carvalho, C.; Hutin, P.; Pennec, Y.L.; Saraux, A.; Youinou, P. Identification of transitional type II B cells in the salivary glands of patients with Sjögren's syndrome. *Arthritis Rheum.* **2006**, *54*, 2280–2288. [CrossRef]
188. Groom, J.; Kalled, S.L.; Cutler, A.H.; Olson, C.; Woodcock, S.A.; Schneider, P.; Tschopp, J.; Cachero, T.G.; Batten, M.; Wheway, J.; et al. Association of BAFF/BLyS overexpression and altered B cell differentiation with Sjögren's syndrome. *J. Clin. Investig.* **2002**, *109*, 59–68. [CrossRef]
189. Mackay, F.; Woodcock, S.A.; Lawton, P.; Ambrose, C.; Baetscher, M.; Schneider, P.; Tschopp, J.; Browning, J.L. Mice transgenic for BAFF develop lymphocytic disorders along with autoimmune manifestations. *J. Exp. Med.* **1999**, *190*, 1697–1710. [CrossRef]
190. Fletcher, C.A.; Sutherland, A.P.; Groom, J.R.; Batten, M.L.; Ng, L.G.; Gommerman, J.; Mackay, F. Development of nephritis but not sialadenitis in autoimmune-prone BAFF transgenic mice lacking marginal zone B cells. *Eur. J. Immunol.* **2006**, *36*, 2504–2514. [CrossRef]
191. Shen, L.; Gao, C.; Suresh, L.; Xian, Z.; Song, N.; Chaves, L.D.; Yu, M.; Ambrus, J.L., Jr. Central role for marginal zone B cells in an animal model of Sjogren's syndrome. *Clin. Immunol.* **2016**, *168*, 30–36. [CrossRef] [PubMed]
192. Cuenca, M.; Romero, X.; Sintes, J.; Terhorst, C.; Engel, P. Targeting of Ly9 (CD229) disrupts marginal zone and B1 B cell homeostasis and antibody responses. *J. Immunol.* **2016**, *196*, 726–737. [CrossRef] [PubMed]
193. Puñet-Ortiz, J.; Sáez Moya, M.; Cuenca, M.; Caleiras, E.; Lazaro, A.; Engel, P. Ly9 (CD229) antibody targeting depletes marginal zone and germinal center B cells in lymphoid tissues and reduces salivary gland inflammation in a mouse model of Sjögren's Syndrome. *Front. Immunol.* **2018**, *9*, 2661. [CrossRef] [PubMed]
194. Maruyama, M.; Lam, K.P.; Rajewsky, K. Memory B-cell persistence is independent of persisting immunizing antigen. *Nature* **2000**, *407*, 636–642. [CrossRef]
195. Schittek, B.; Rajewsky, K. Maintenance of B-cell memory by long-lived cells generated from proliferating precursors. *Nature* **1990**, *346*, 749–751. [CrossRef]
196. Giesecke, C.; Frölich, D.; Reiter, K.; Mei, H.E.; Wirries, I.; Kuhly, R.; Killig, M.; Glatzer, T.; Stölzel, K.; Perka, C.; et al. Tissue distribution and dependence of responsiveness of human antigen-specific memory B cells. *J. Immunol.* **2014**, *192*, 3091–3100. [CrossRef]
197. Steiniger, B.; Timphus, E.M.; Jacob, R.; Barth, P.J. CD27+ B cells in human lymphatic organs: Re-evaluating the splenic marginal zone. *Immunology* **2005**, *116*, 429–442. [CrossRef]
198. Manzo, A.; Vitolo, B.; Humby, F.; Caporali, R.; Jarrossay, D.; Dell'accio, F.; Ciardelli, L.; Uguccioni, M.; Montecucco, C.; Pitzalis, C. Mature antigen-experienced T helper cells synthesize and secrete the B cell chemoattractant CXCL13 in the inflammatory environment of the rheumatoid joint. *Arthritis Rheum.* **2008**, *58*, 3377–3387. [CrossRef]
199. Rupprecht, T.A.; Plate, A.; Adam, M.; Wick, M.; Kastenbauer, S.; Schmidt, C.; Klein, M.; Pfister, H.W.; Koedel, U. The chemokine CXCL13 is a key regulator of B cell recruitment to the cerebrospinal fluid in acute Lyme neuroborreliosis. *J. Neuroinflamm.* **2009**, *6*, 42. [CrossRef]
200. Sáez de Guinoa, J.; Barrio, L.; Mellado, M.; Carrasco, Y.R. CXCL13/CXCR5 signaling enhances BCR-triggered B-cell activation by shaping cell dynamics. *Blood* **2011**, *118*, 1560–1569. [CrossRef]
201. Hoffman, W.; Lakkis, F.G.; Chalasani, G. B Cells, antibodies, and more. *Clin. J. Am. Soc. Nephrol.* **2016**, *11*, 137–154. [CrossRef] [PubMed]

202. Fazilleau, N.; McHeyzer-Williams, L.J.; Rosen, H.; McHeyzer-Williams, M.G. The function of follicular helper T cells is regulated by the strength of T cell antigen receptor binding. *Nat. Immunol.* **2009**, *10*, 375–384. [CrossRef] [PubMed]
203. Moisini, I.; Davidson, A. BAFF: A local and systemic target in autoimmune diseases. *Clin. Exp. Immunol.* **2009**, *158*, 155–163. [CrossRef] [PubMed]
204. Ittah, M.; Miceli-Richard, C.; Eric Gottenberg, J.; Lavie, F.; Lazure, T.; Ba, N.; Sellam, J.; Lepajolec, C.; Mariette, X. B cell-activating factor of the tumor necrosis factor family (BAFF) is expressed under stimulation by interferon in salivary gland epithelial cells in primary Sjögren's syndrome. *Arthritis Res. Ther.* **2006**, *8*, R51. [CrossRef]
205. Brito-Zerón, P.; Ramos-Casals, M.; Nardi, N.; Cervera, R.; Yagüe, J.; Ingelmo, M.; Font, J. Circulating monoclonal immunoglobulins in Sjögren syndrome: Prevalence and clinical significance in 237 patients. *Medicine (Baltimore)* **2005**, *84*, 90–97. [CrossRef]
206. Szyszko, E.A.; Brokstad, K.A.; Oijordsbakken, G.; Jonsson, M.V.; Jonsson, R.; Skarstein, K. Salivary glands of primary Sjogren's syndrome patients express factors vital for plasma cell survival. *Arthritis Res. Ther.* **2011**, *13*, R2. [CrossRef]
207. Tengnér, P.; Halse, A.K.; Haga, H.J.; Jonsson, R.; Wahren-Herlenius, M. Detection of anti-Ro/SSA and anti-La/SSB autoantibody-producing cells in salivary glands from patients with Sjögren's syndrome. *Arthritis Rheum.* **1998**, *41*, 2238–2248. [CrossRef]
208. Halse, A.; Harley, J.B.; Kroneld, U.; Jonsson, R. Ro/SS-A-reactive B lymphocytes in salivary glands and peripheral blood of patients with Sjögren's syndrome. *Clin. Exp. Immunol.* **1999**, *115*, 203–207. [CrossRef]
209. Aqrawi, L.A.; Skarstein, K.; Øijordsbakken, G.; Brokstad, K.A. Ro52- and Ro60-specific B cell pattern in the salivary glands of patients with primary Sjögren's syndrome. *Clin. Exp. Immunol.* **2013**, *172*, 228–237. [CrossRef]
210. Aqrawi, L.A.; Brokstad, K.A.; Jakobsen, K.; Jonsson, R.; Skarstein, K. Low number of memory B cells in the salivary glands of patients with primary Sjögren's syndrome. *Autoimmunity* **2012**, *45*, 547–555. [CrossRef]
211. Szabó, K.; Papp, G.; Szántó, A.; Tarr, T.; Zeher, M. A comprehensive investigation on the distribution of circulating follicular T helper cells and B cell subsets in primary Sjögren's syndrome and systemic lupus erythematosus. *Clin. Exp. Immunol.* **2016**, *183*, 76–89. [CrossRef] [PubMed]
212. Nimmerjahn, F.; Ravetch, J.V. Fcgamma receptors as regulators of immune responses. *Nat. Rev. Immunol.* **2008**, *8*, 34–47. [CrossRef]
213. Pierpont, T.M.; Limper, C.B.; Richards, K.L. Past, present, and future of rituximab-the world's first oncology monoclonal antibody therapy. *Front. Oncol.* **2018**, *8*, 163. [CrossRef] [PubMed]
214. McGinley, M.P.; Moss, B.P.; Cohen, J.A. Safety of monoclonal antibodies for the treatment of multiple sclerosis. *Expert. Opin. Drug. Saf.* **2017**, *16*, 89–100. [CrossRef] [PubMed]
215. Blüml, S.; McKeever, K.; Ettinger, R.; Smolen, J.; Herbst, R. B-cell targeted therapeutics in clinical development. *Arthritis Res. Ther.* **2013**, *15* (Suppl. S1), S4. [CrossRef]
216. Pertovaara, M.; Antonen, J.; Hurme, M. Th2 cytokine genotypes are associated with a milder form of primary Sjogren's syndrome. *Ann. Rheum. Dis.* **2006**, *65*, 666–670. [CrossRef]
217. Fernández-Fernández, F.J. Comment on: Th17 cells and IL-17A–focus on immunopathogenesis and immunotherapeutics. *Semin. Arthritis Rheum.* **2014**, *44*, e3. [CrossRef]
218. Kleinewietfeld, M.; Hafler, D.A. The plasticity of human Treg and Th17 cells and its role in autoimmunity. *Semin. Immunol.* **2013**, *25*, 305–312. [CrossRef]
219. Sakaguchi, S.; Sakaguchi, N.; Asano, M.; Itoh, M.; Toda, M. Immunologic self-tolerance maintained by activated T cells expressing IL-2 receptor alpha-chains (CD25). Breakdown of a single mechanism of self-tolerance causes various autoimmune diseases. *J. Immunol.* **1995**, *155*, 1151–1164.
220. MacLennan, I.C. Germinal centers. *Annu. Rev. Immunol.* **1994**, *12*, 117–139. [CrossRef]
221. Nocturne, G.; Mariette, X. B cells in the pathogenesis of primary Sjögren syndrome. *Nat. Rev. Rheumatol.* **2018**, *14*, 133–145. [CrossRef] [PubMed]

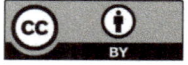

© 2020 by the authors. Licensee MDPI, Basel, Switzerland. This article is an open access article distributed under the terms and conditions of the Creative Commons Attribution (CC BY) license (http://creativecommons.org/licenses/by/4.0/).

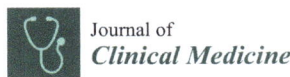

Review

Imaging in Primary Sjögren's Syndrome

Martha S. van Ginkel [1,*], Andor W.J.M. Glaudemans [2], Bert van der Vegt [3], Esther Mossel [1], Frans G.M. Kroese [1], Hendrika Bootsma [1] and Arjan Vissink [4,*]

1. Department of Rheumatology and Clinical Immunology, University of Groningen, University Medical Center Groningen, 9713 GZ Groningen, The Netherlands; e.mossel@umcg.nl (E.M.); f.g.m.kroese@umcg.nl (F.G.M.K.); h.bootsma@umcg.nl (H.B.)
2. Department of Nuclear Medicine and Molecular Imaging, University of Groningen, University Medical Center Groningen, 9713 GZ Groningen, The Netherlands; a.w.j.m.glaudemans@umcg.nl
3. Department of Pathology and Medical Biology, University of Groningen, University Medical Center Groningen, 9713 GZ Groningen, The Netherlands; b.van.der.vegt@umcg.nl
4. Department of Oral and Maxillofacial Surgery, University of Groningen, University Medical Center Groningen, 9713 GZ Groningen, The Netherlands
* Correspondence: m.s.van.ginkel@umcg.nl (M.S.v.G.); a.vissink@umcg.nl (A.V.); Tel.: +316-50-36-16-604 (M.S.v.G.); +316-50-36-13-841 (A.V.)

Received: 10 July 2020; Accepted: 30 July 2020; Published: 3 August 2020

Abstract: Primary Sjögren's syndrome (pSS) is a systemic autoimmune disease characterized by dysfunction and lymphocytic infiltration of the salivary and lacrimal glands. Besides the characteristic sicca complaints, pSS patients can present a spectrum of signs and symptoms, which challenges the diagnostic process. Various imaging techniques can be used to assist in the diagnostic work-up and follow-up of pSS patients. Developments in imaging techniques provide new opportunities and perspectives. In this descriptive review, we discuss imaging techniques that are used in pSS with a focus on the salivary glands. The emphasis is on the contribution of these techniques to the diagnosis of pSS, their potential in assessing disease activity and disease progression in pSS, and their contribution to diagnosing and staging of pSS-associated lymphomas. Imaging findings of the salivary glands will be linked to histopathological changes in the salivary glands of pSS patients.

Keywords: primary Sjögren's syndrome; imaging; salivary gland; sialography; salivary gland ultrasonography; magnetic resonance imaging; sialendoscopy; salivary gland scintigraphy; positron emission tomography

1. Introduction

Primary Sjögren's syndrome (pSS) is a chronic, systemic, autoimmune disease characterized by dry mouth and dry eyes. As a heterogeneous systemic disease, many patients suffer from extraglandular symptoms, and almost all organs can be involved [1]. Because of the heterogeneity of the disease, pSS patients can present a broad spectrum of signs and symptoms, thereby making the diagnostic process challenging. The characteristic sicca symptoms of mouth and eyes, however, remain the most common manifestation of pSS. The dysfunction of the salivary glands and lacrimal glands is usually associated with chronic inflammation. For this reason, salivary gland biopsies are part of the standard diagnostic work-up, and the typical periductal lymphocytic infiltrates are an important criterion for pSS [2]. However, taking biopsies is an invasive surgical procedure and cannot be performed in all diagnostic centers. Imaging techniques, on the other hand, are noninvasive. It has been shown that imaging techniques can assist in the diagnostic process of pSS [3]. Imaging techniques could also be of value in assessing disease activity and detecting disease progression in pSS, which has already been shown in other systemic autoimmune diseases [4].

PSS patients have an increased risk of developing a non-Hodgkin's lymphoma, mostly of the mucosa-associated lymphoid tissue (MALT) type. The prevalence of lymphoma development in pSS patients varies in different studies from 2.7% to 9.8% [5]. In pSS patients, MALT lymphomas most commonly arise within the parotid glands, but they can also develop at other extranodal locations, such as the lungs, lacrimal glands, or stomach [6–8]. Although the usefulness of imaging techniques in the diagnosis, staging, and treatment response evaluation in lymphomas in general is widely known [9,10], the value of imaging techniques in pSS-associated lymphomas is not yet clear.

In this descriptive review, we discuss the various imaging techniques used in pSS and link imaging findings to histopathological changes that occur in the salivary glands. We review the potential contribution of radiological and nuclear imaging techniques to the diagnostic work-up of pSS, and their role in assessing disease activity and disease progression. We also discuss imaging techniques that are currently used for the diagnosis and staging of pSS-associated lymphomas.

2. Diagnosis and Classification of pSS

Currently, there is no "gold standard" test or diagnostic criteria set to support diagnosis of this heterogenous and multisystemic autoimmune disease [11,12]. Therefore, diagnosis of pSS is still based on expert opinion, which relies on interpretation of a combination of several assessments. Although there is no consensus yet which assessments are necessary for diagnosing pSS, the diagnostic work-up can consist of different items, such as clinical examination, serological tests, oral and ocular tests, imaging techniques, and histopathology of the salivary gland. In the past years, multiple classification criteria sets were developed for pSS. These classification criteria were developed for research purposes, to allow selection of well-defined and homogenous populations of pSS patients for clinical studies. However, the terms diagnosis and classification in pSS are often used interchangeably since diagnosis and classification depend on similar items/tests. Table 1 shows the items that are included in the various classification criteria sets. In this review, we focus on the value of imaging techniques in the diagnostic work-up of pSS. When we specifically discuss imaging techniques as items of classification criteria sets, we add the term classification.

Table 1. Comparison of classification criteria sets for pSS [13].

	2016-ACR-EULAR [14]	2012-ACR [15]	2002-AECG [16]
ESSDAI ≥ 1	+ (Entry Criterion)	−	−
Sicca Symptoms	+ (Entry Criterion)	−	+
Salivary Gland Biopsy	+	+	+
Serology			
Anti-Ro/SSA	+	+	+
Anti-La/SSB	−	+	+
Antinuclear Antibodies	−	+	−
Rheumatoid Factor	−	+	−
Oral Signs			
UWS ≤ 0.1mL/Min	+	−	+
Sialography	−	−	+
Scintigraphy	−	−	+
Ocular Signs			
Schirmer's Test ≤ 5	+	−	+
Ocular Staining (OSS or vBv)	+	+	+

ACR-EULAR: American College of Rheumatology-European League Against Rheumatism; ACR: American College of Rheumatology; AECG: American European Consensus Group; ESSDAI: EULAR Sjögren's Syndrome Disease Activity Index; UWS: unstimulated whole saliva; OSS: ocular staining score; vBv: van Bijsterveld score.

3. Histopathology of the Salivary Gland

For decades, salivary gland histopathology has played a major role in diagnosing pSS. The characteristic finding within labial and parotid gland biopsies is the presence of infiltrates around striated ducts, mainly consisting of B- and T-lymphocytes. From the number of periductal foci (clusters of >50 lymphocytes) per 4 mm^2, the focus score can be calculated, which is used in classification criteria sets for pSS [2,14]. Another scoring system is the grading system by Chisholm and Mason. In this grading system, stage 0, 1, and 2 indicate no, slight, or moderate infiltration with less than one focus per 4 mm^2, respectively. Stage 3 and 4 correspond with a positive focus score (≥1 focus per 4 mm^2) [17]. Besides the presence of periductal foci, other characteristic features can be found within the salivary glands of pSS patients, such as influx of IgG plasma cells and the presence of lymphoepithelial lesions (LELs) and germinal centers [18–20]. LELs are defined as hyperplastic ductal epithelial cells with infiltrating lymphocytes. LELs can eventually lead to complete obstruction of ducts (Figure 1). In addition to these characteristic features, proportions of fibrosis and acinar atrophy within salivary gland tissue are higher in pSS patients compared to controls [21,22]. There is no agreement yet whether fatty infiltration is age-associated or specific for pSS [23,24]. Besides their role in the diagnostic work-up of pSS, biopsies may also be used to assess prognosis (Table 2). Higher focus score is associated with higher European League Against Rheumatism (EULAR) Sjögren's syndrome disease activity index (ESSDAI) scores, severe serological profiles, and an increased risk of lymphoma development [25,26]. PSS-associated salivary gland MALT lymphomas are diagnosed on histomorphological appearance (Figure 1) in combination with clonal analysis of immunoglobulin heavy chain (IGH) variable(V)-diversity(D)-joining(J) (VDJ) gene segments [27]. The following sections will discuss whether the characteristic histopathological findings correspond with imaging findings found in pSS patients.

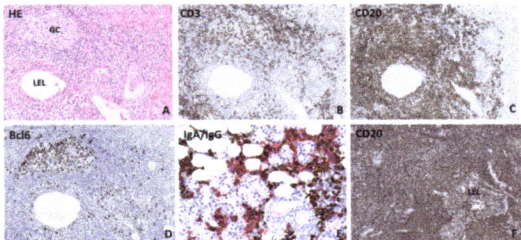

Figure 1. Histopathological features in parotid salivary glands of primary Sjögren's syndrome patients (**A**) Lymphocytic infiltrate located around a hyperplastic striated duct (lymphoepithelial lesion: LEL) without obstructed lumen. Both (**B**) CD3+ T-lymphocytes and (**C**) CD20+ B-lymphocytes are present in the periductal infiltrate and within the ductal epithelium. (**D**) Presence of a germinal center, which was revealed by the presence of a cluster of ≥5 adjacent Bcl6-positive cells within a focus [28]. (**E**) Immunoglobulin A (IgA) (red) and immunoglobulin G (IgG) (brown) staining shows a plasma cell shift towards IgG plasma cells. (**F**) Salivary gland mucosa associated lymphoid tissue (MALT) lymphoma biopsy, which shows a diffuse CD20+ B-lymphocytic infiltrate around lymphoepithelial lesions in the absence of normal salivary gland parenchyma.

Table 2. Contribution of imaging techniques to the diagnostic work-up and follow-up of pSS patients.

	Contribution To:				Advantages	Disadvantages
	Diagnosing pSS	Assessing Disease Activity/Disease Progression	Diagnosing pSS-Associated Lymphoma	Staging pSS-Associated Lymphoma		
Salivary Gland Biopsy	+++	+	+++	−	-Gold Standard of Salivary and Lacrimal Gland MALT Lymphoma Diagnosis	-Invasive -Risk of Sampling Error
Sialography	+	+	−	−	-Moderate to High Sensitivity and Specificity	-Invasive -Contrast Medium
MRI	+	+	+	+	-High Spatial Resolution -Useful in Local Staging of PSS-Associated Lymphomas of Salivary and Lacrimal Glands	-Expensive -Moderate Differentiation Between Benign and Malignant Lesions of Salivary and Lacrimal Glands
Ultrasound	++	+	−	−	-Noninvasive -Widely Available	-No Consensus Scoring System
Sialendoscopy	−	−	−	−	-Possible Therapeutic Effect of Rinsing the Ductal System	-Invasive -No Added Value in Diagnostic Work-Up
Scintigraphy with ^{99m}Tc-Pertechnetate	+	+	−	−	-Possibility of Whole-Body Imaging	-Low Specificity -Low Spatial Resolution
^{18}F-FDG-PET/CT	+	++	+	+++	-Whole-Body Imaging -Useful in Assessing Treatment Response -Objective Quantification Possible	-Expensive -No Exact Interpretation Criteria for pSS Available

MRI: magnetic resonance imaging; PET/CT: positron emission tomography/computed tomography; MALT: mucosa-associated lymphoid tissue. Plus and minus signs are entered as follows: (+++) in case the imaging technique has an excellent contribution to the specific item, (++) for a good contribution, (+) in case the contribution is not yet clear or there is contradictive data, and (−) in case there is no evidence for contribution of the imaging technique to the specific item.

4. Radiology Techniques

4.1. Sialography

Sialography is a radiographic technique that visualizes the architecture of the ductal system by using X-ray projections after injection of contrast medium. In pSS patients, sialography shows sialectasis, which are collections of contrast material. The degree of sialectasis can be classified according to the scoring system developed by Rubin and Holt [29] (Figure 2). Sialectasis may be found at the location of cystic ductal dilatations in pSS patients. Another explanation could be that sialectasis represents extravasation of contrast material into the glandular parenchyma. A possible explanation for the leakage of contrast medium in pSS patients is dysfunction of tight junctions between striated ductal cells, due to the presence of proinflammatory cytokines [30]. In addition to sialectasis, sparsity of the ductal branching pattern can be found during sialography [3,31,32]. This could be due to obstruction of the ductal system, as a result of lymphocytic infiltration and proliferation of the ductal epithelium. However, direct associations with histopathological findings, such as the area of lymphocytic infiltrate or presence of LELs, have thus far not been reported.

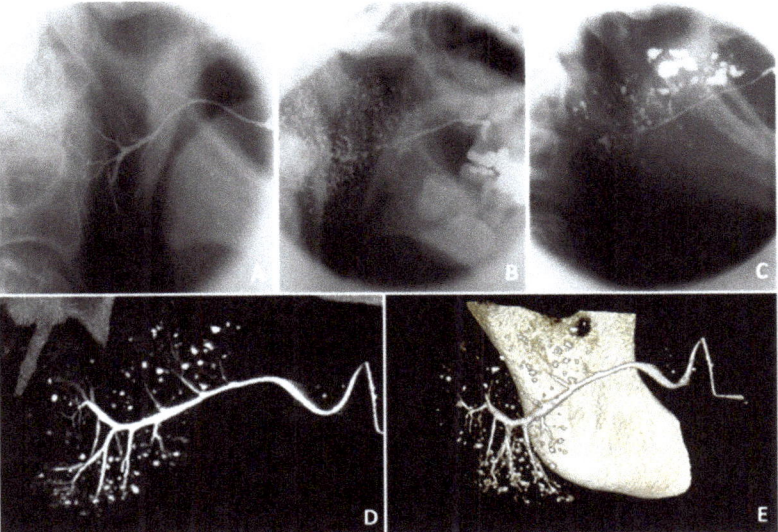

Figure 2. Findings on sialography. Sialographies of the parotid gland showing (**A**) no abnormalities in a healthy subject, (**B**) punctate/globular sialectasis in a pSS patient, and (**C**) globular/cavitary sialectasis in a pSS patient [29]. (**D**) Two-dimensional sialo-CBCT image and (**E**) three-dimensional sialo-CBCT image of the parotid gland of a pSS patient, showing normal width of the primary duct, moderate scarcity of ductal branches, and numerous diverse sialectasis. Thanks to Prof. D.J. Aframian and Dr. C. Nadler and colleagues who provided the sialo-CBCT images.

Sialography has been used for diagnosing pSS for decades and shows moderate to high sensitivity and specificity [3]. This technique was excluded from the 2016 American College of Rheumatology/European League Against Rheumatism (ACR-EULAR) classification criteria (Table 1) because of multiple drawbacks. It is an invasive technique with risk of complications and radiation exposure. Furthermore, there are multiple contraindications like acute infection, acute inflammation, and contrast allergy [3,31].

Alternative sialographic techniques have been developed, such as sialo-cone-beam computerized tomography (sialo-CBCT) and magnetic resonance (MR) sialography. These techniques have an increased spatial resolution and provide three-dimensional, instead of two-dimensional, images of the ductal system. Keshet et al. [33] described correlations between sialo-CBCT findings and clinical data, such as xerostomia and serological parameters. However, since only 6 out of 67 sicca patients fulfilled the American European Consensus Group (AECG) classification criteria for pSS in this cohort, the usefulness of sialo-CBCT in pSS should be further investigated. MR sialography can identify changes within the salivary glands without the injection of contrast medium. The typical finding in pSS is the presence of multiple high-signal-intensity spots, which are thought to arise after leakage of saliva from peripheral ducts. Kojima et al. [34] did not find correlations between MR sialography findings and salivary flow rate, which can be explained by the fact that MR sialography visualizes the ductal system instead of saliva-producing acinar cells. Although MR sialography seems to be more sensitive to detect early disease, magnetic resonance imaging (MRI) provides more information on pathological changes in the glandular parenchyma, as we describe below [35].

In conclusion, sialography is not commonly used in the diagnostic work-up and follow-up of pSS anymore. Although alternative sialographic techniques such as sialo-CBCT and MR sialography have been evaluated, their current role in the diagnostic work-up of pSS is limited.

4.2. Magnetic Resonance Imaging

The role of MRI of the salivary glands in pSS has been investigated during the past decades. The characteristic finding in salivary glands of pSS patients is a heterogeneous signal-intensity distribution on T1- and T2-weighted images. The multiple hypointense and hyperintense areas cause a so-called salt and pepper appearance [34]. In the advanced stages of pSS, cystic changes can be found with MRI, which are thought to arise from destruction of the salivary gland parenchyma and the presence of fibrosis and fatty infiltration [3,31,36]. Although fat fractions in salivary glands seem to increase with higher age and body mass index [37] and can account for 60% of the histological section of the parotid gland in healthy individuals [38], imaging studies found that premature fat deposition found on MRI images is associated with SS [39,40]. Histopathological studies, however, did not make clear whether fatty infiltration is a specific feature of pSS or age-associated. Since biopsies do not represent the entire gland, it remains difficult to correlate MRI findings to histopathological findings. Although correlations between the focus score of the labial gland and MRI findings of the parotid gland were found [41,42], further associations between MRI findings and histopathological findings, such as the area of lymphocytic infiltration, fibrosis, and fatty infiltration, have not been investigated yet.

Although MRI showed added value in the diagnostic work-up of pSS by detecting pSS-specific abnormalities of the salivary glands, this technique is not routinely applied in pSS. Findings on MRI showed good agreement with salivary gland ultrasonography (SGUS). Since SGUS has several advantages over MRI, such as its high spatial resolution in superficial organs and the fact that SGUS is more easily accessible, SGUS is a better alternative for the diagnostic work-up of pSS [3,43].

Kojima et al. [34] demonstrated, in a group of pSS patients, that a higher degree of glandular heterogeneity and a smaller volume of the parotid and submandibular glands on MRI images were associated with lower stimulated and unstimulated salivary flow rates. These associations were even more pronounced for the submandibular glands, compared to the parotid glands, indicating that MRI findings of the submandibular glands can reflect hyposalivation. A possible explanation for the differences in associations between both glands is that the function of the submandibular gland is impaired earlier in the disease process than the function of the parotid gland [34,44,45]. Collection of saliva from the individual glands would be a more direct approach to relate MRI findings with salivary gland functioning in pSS. Similar to the MRI findings of Kojima et al. [34], lacrimal flow rates were associated with lacrimal gland volumes of pSS patients. Lacrimal flow rates were lower in pSS patients with atrophic lacrimal glands compared to patients with hypertrophic and normal-sized glands [46]. No studies have been performed to evaluate associations between MRI findings of the salivary glands and systemic disease activity, but MRI is the most appropriate imaging technique to evaluate central or peripheral nervous system involvement in pSS [47,48].

MRI is also used for the evaluation of pSS-associated lymphomas in the head and neck region (Figure 3). MRI findings of salivary and lacrimal gland MALT lymphomas vary. Findings that have been described are glandular enlargement, (micro)cystic changes, and calcifications [49–51]. Zhu et al. [51] found that solid cystic appearances of MALT lymphomas can help to differentiate MALT from non-MALT lymphomas. However, benign and malignant lesions of salivary and lacrimal gland show overlap, which makes MRI a less reliable technique to differentiate between benign and malignant disorders of the exocrine glands [3,52,53]. Despite the indolent nature of pSS-associated lymphomas, these malignancies are able to disseminate to other mucosal sites or organs. MRI is used in local staging of the disease, by assessing the ingrowth in adjacent structures and spread to lymph nodes or other organs [50,54] (Table 2).

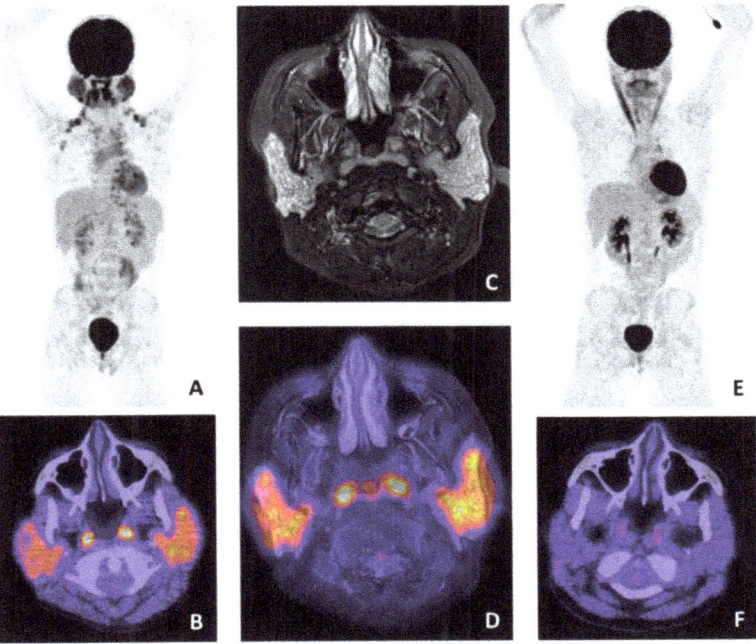

Figure 3. ^{18}F-fluorodeoxyglucose (FDG) positron emmison tomography/computed tomography (PET/CT) and magnetic resonance imaging (MRI) findings in a pSS patient with salivary gland mucosa associated lymphoid tissue (MALT) lymphoma. (**A**) Whole-body FDG-PET showing high heterogeneous FDG uptake in both parotid and submandibular glands. No other pathological lesions were found (axillary and clavicular regions with increased uptake represent brown fat). (**B**) FDG-PET/CT image showing pathological uptake in the parotid glands and physiological uptake in the tonsils. (**C**) MRI stir sequence showing a pathological, heterogeneous aspect of both parotid glands. (**D**) Manually fused FDG-PET/MRI image, showing pathological uptake in the parotid glands and physiological uptake in the tonsils. (**E**) Whole-body FDG-PET and (**F**) FDG-PET/CT image after treatment, showing no pathological uptake in the parotid glands, indicating complete remission.

Together, MRI is not often used in the standard diagnostic work-up of pSS. However, due to its high spatial resolution, MRI is the most useful imaging technique for local staging of pSS-associated salivary and lacrimal gland lymphomas.

4.3. Salivary Gland Ultrasonography

Within the past decade, salivary gland ultrasonography (SGUS) has gained more and more attention, and was proven to be effective for the detection of typical structural abnormalities in pSS [55,56]. Furthermore, various studies demonstrated that addition of SGUS improves the performance and feasibility of the 2016 ACR-EULAR classification criteria [57–60]. However, many different SGUS-based scoring systems are available, and international consensus on which scoring system should be used is lacking. This hampers addition of SGUS to the classification criteria [55,56]. Therefore, the Outcome Measures in Rheumatology Clinical Trials (OMERACT) SGUS task force group has recently developed ultrasound definitions and a novel SGUS scoring system with good and excellent inter and intraobserver reliabilities, respectively [61]. Further studies should validate this scoring system before SGUS can be added to the 2016 ACR-EULAR classification criteria.

Typical ultrasonographic abnormalities in pSS are hypoechogenic areas, hyperechogenic reflections, and poorly defined salivary gland borders [55] (Figure 4). Mossel et al. [62] demonstrated that the presence of hypoechogenic areas is the most important SGUS feature. However, it is still unknown what these hypoechogenic areas reflect at a histological level. It has been suggested that hypoechogenic areas consist of foci containing inflammatory cells. Histopathological foci, however, are smaller in size compared to the hypoechogenic areas. Preliminary results of Mossel et al. [63] show a good correlation between hypoechogenic areas and percentages of CD45+ leukocytic infiltrate. These results indicate that, despite the differences in size, hypoechogenic areas are somehow associated with foci of inflammatory cells. One explanation for this association could be that hypoechogenic areas originate from leakage of saliva that is transported through the ductal system into the periductal infiltrate, and eventually into the salivary gland parenchyma. Leakage of saliva from the ductal system can be a comparable phenomenon to leakage of contrast medium during sialography, due to dysfunction of tight junctions between striated ductal cells [30]. However, collections of saliva in the periductal infiltrates or parenchyma are not commonly seen in salivary gland biopsies of pSS patients. Another hypothesis is that the hypoechogenic areas represent fatty infiltration. However, fat tissue is most often visible as a hyperechogenic instead of hypoechogenic area [64]. Furthermore, preliminary results of Mossel et al. [63] show poor associations between hypoechogenic areas and the percentage of fat cells in the total salivary gland parenchyma, which contradicts the latter hypothesis.

As described before, the area from which the parotid biopsies are taken may not be representative for the ultrasonographic images. The biopsy is taken from the periphery of the gland, which does not contain larger excretory ducts. Therefore, correlating histopathology to SGUS findings remains difficult. A possibility to get a better understanding of what SGUS features in salivary glands of pSS patients represent is taking ultrasound-guided core needle biopsies. A recent study by Baer et al. [65] showed that taking core needle biopsies in pSS patients suspected of salivary gland lymphoma is a safe and useful procedure. Although the morphology of core needle biopsies is inferior compared to that of open biopsies, the core needle method allows biopsies to be taken from the exact location of hypoechogenic areas or hyperechogenic reflections.

Another unresolved question is whether current SGUS scoring systems are sensitive enough to assess (treatment-induced) differences that are seen histopathologically. Current SGUS scoring systems use subjective categorical scales. Hypoechogenic areas, for instance, are scored on a 0–3 scale. Therefore, major changes need to occur in order to change from one category to another. This could be an important drawback when using SGUS as an objective tool to assess disease progression as well as to assess changes in salivary gland involvement in clinical trials [56,66]. Scoring SGUS findings on a continuous scale and in a more objective way could increase the sensitivity to change. A possible way to do this is by using image segmentation and artificial intelligence. HarmonicSS, a multicenter and EU-supported project, is applying artificial intelligence to SGUS images in pSS. Preliminary results show that, among the tested algorithms, the multilayer perceptron classifier is the best performing algorithm. Since the HarmonicSS cohort will increase in size over time, further validation will follow [56,67].

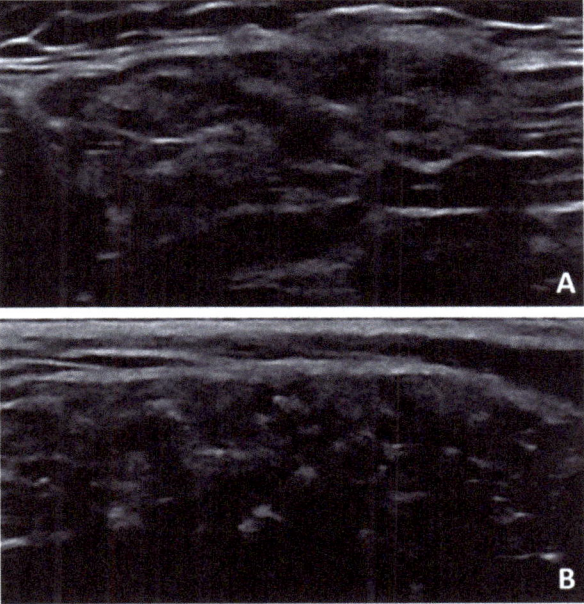

Figure 4. Salivary gland ultrasonography findings in pSS. Presence of hypoechogenic areas and hyperechogenic reflections in the (**A**) submandibular gland and (**B**) parotid gland of a pSS patient.

Despite the potential usefulness of SGUS in diagnosis and classification of pSS, the value of SGUS to assess disease activity and disease progression and to detect salivary gland MALT lymphoma needs to be established. SGUS scores seem to correlate with objective salivary gland function, as unstimulated salivary flow rates were found to be lower in SGUS-positive patients, compared to SGUS-negative patients [68–70]. Zabotti et al. [71] described that of all SGUS findings, the presence of hyperechogenic bands was independently associated with salivary flow rates. Although they suggested that damage of the glands is reflected by hyperechogenic bands, it is still unclear what these hyperechogenic bands reflect at a histological level. Several studies showed associations between SGUS scores and clinical parameters of disease activity, such as ESSDAI scores, IgG levels, and rheumatoid factor (RF) levels [68,72–75]. In contrast, other studies did not find correlations between SGUS scores and ESSDAI [69,76]. These discrepancies can be explained by differences in patient characteristics between cohorts, and by the fact that severe salivary gland involvement might not reflect systemic disease activity in all pSS patients.

Since previous studies found associations between SGUS findings and risk markers of lymphoma, such as cryoglobulinemia, lymphopenia, and persistent salivary gland swelling, Theander et al. [72] and Coiffier et al. [77] stated that SGUS can identify patients at risk of developing lymphoma. However, these results were found in retrospective cohorts, and longitudinal studies should be performed to assess whether SGUS findings are predictive of lymphoma [78]. Furthermore, the capability of SGUS to detect lymphoma compared to histopathology and MRI should be clarified.

The studies presented thus far provide evidence that SGUS has added value in the diagnostic work-up of pSS (Table 2). Further research should be performed on the development of a consensus scoring system. Furthermore, to assess the usefulness of SGUS in follow-up and lymphoma detection in pSS, longitudinal studies are needed. Several initiatives have started already, such as OMERACT and HarmonicSS projects, which will give us more insight into the potential of this imaging tool in pSS.

5. Sialendoscopy

Sialendoscopy is a minimally invasive technique used for both diagnosis and management of obstructive salivary gland disorders, such as sialolithiasis, anatomic ductal abnormalities and mucus plugs. With this gland-sparing technique, a sialendoscope is entered through the ductal orifice of major salivary glands for inspection and irrigation of the ductal system, after local or general anesthesia.

In pSS patients, sialendoscopic examination mainly shows strictures, but mucous plugs and a pale, minimally vascularized ductal wall of the larger excretory ducts can also be observed [79–81]. Ductal strictures can cause ductal obstruction and could therewith account for glandular swelling and pain in pSS. It is still unclear what these strictures reflect at a histological level. One hypothesis is that strictures are caused by large LELs that obstruct the ductal system, but no histological studies have been performed yet to prove this hypothesis. Since the sialendoscopic findings in pSS are not specific for the disease, the diagnostic value of this technique in pSS is limited. However, various studies show that dilatation of strictures in combination with irrigation of the ductal system with saline and/or corticosteroids by using sialendoscopy is a safe and effective treatment option for salivary gland dysfunction in pSS patients. Studies showed that both subjective and objective oral dryness improved after sialendoscopy [80,82,83]. Furthermore, visual analogue scale pain scores decreased after the procedure [79,84], and the number of episodes of glandular swelling declined after treatment [85]. However, the above mentioned (pilot) studies included relatively small numbers of patients. The clinical benefits for pSS patients after sialendoscopy should be further explored in larger cohorts.

Although complications, such as infections and postoperative pain, seem to be limited [86], multiple studies reported that the sialendoscopic procedure was not successful in all pSS patients because of technical issues [79,80]. The most common difficulties reported were problems with identification or dilatation of the papilla before introducing the sialendoscope, which occurred more often during sialendoscopy of the submandibular gland compared to the parotid gland. These problems might be associated with characteristic features of severe stages of pSS, such as the presence of extreme hyposalivation and atrophic changes. Using salivary gland ultrasonography to assess the stage of the disease was suggested to predict whether patients would benefit from sialendoscopic treatment [80]. It would be of value to study this suggestion.

In summary, although sialendoscopy has no added value in the diagnostic work-up of pSS, recent studies have drawn attention to the fact that rinsing the ductal system, a procedure that accompanies sialendoscopy, might be useful in the management of oral symptoms.

6. Nuclear Medicine Techniques

6.1. Conventional Nuclear Medicine

Nuclear medicine imaging uses specific radiopharmaceuticals to visualize (patho)physiological processes in the body. Imaging with a a gamma camera system that provides two-dimensional planar images forms the basis of conventional nuclear medicine. However, it is often difficult to determine the exact location of increased tracer uptake by using these two-dimensional images. Three-dimensional images can be created by collecting images from different angles around the patient. This technique, called single photon emission computed tomography (SPECT), leads to a higher contrast and improves sensitivity, compared to two-dimensional nuclear medicine. Combining SPECT with a low dose or contrast-enhanced CT scan enables determination of the exact location of the area with increased uptake.

6.1.1. ^{99m}Tc-Pertechnetate Scintigraphy

Scintigraphy of the major salivary glands is a nuclear imaging technique that evaluates salivary gland function by uptake and secretion patterns of the radioactive tracer Technetium-99m pertechnetate (^{99m}Tc-pertechnetate). ^{99m}Tc-pertechnetate is actively taken up by salivary gland epithelial cells, probably by using Na+/I− symporters, and secreted into the ductal lumen along with saliva [87]. The technique was included in previous classification criteria of pSS, in which a positive scintigraphy was defined as delayed uptake, reduced concentration, and/or delayed excretion of the tracer [16]. However, due to the low specificity and the inability to differentiate uptake failure from secretory failure, scintigraphy was omitted from the ACR-EULAR classification criteria [14,88]. Various studies stated that scintigraphic examination should focus on the degree of salivary gland dysfunction in pSS, instead of the differentiation between pSS and non-SS [31,89].

Several studies found a relationship between scintigraphic findings and severity of the disease. Brito-Zéron et al. [90] concluded that severe scintigraphic patterns were a prognostic factor for developing extraglandular manifestations. In a large retrospective study by Ramos-Casals et al. [89], patients presenting with severe involvement of the salivary glands according to the scintigraphic examination not only showed increased risk of developing serious extraglandular manifestations, but also a higher risk of developing lymphoma and a lower survival rate. The latter authors also reported that scintigraphic findings worsened during follow-up in 32% of patients. This subgroup of patients also had higher prevalence of high ANA titers, compared to patients with stabilization or improvement of scintigraphy [89]. Furthermore, scintigraphy was associated with histopathological findings within labial salivary glands of pSS patients, as scintigraphic parameters decreased significantly with higher stages of lymphocytic infiltrates graded by Chisholm and Mason's grading system [91–93].

6.1.2. Future Promising Scintigraphic Tracers

Another scintigraphic tracer studied in pSS patients is ^{99m}Tc-EDDA/Tricine-HYNIC-Tyr(3)-Octreotide (^{99m}Tc-HYNIC-TOC). This tracer binds to somatostatin receptors on cell membranes. These receptors were shown to be overexpressed in various inflammatory and autoimmune diseases, and were found on, among others, activated lymphocytes, endothelial cells, and the monocyte lineage in synovium of rheumatoid arthritis (RA) patients [94–96]. Anzola et al. [97] showed increased ^{99m}Tc-HYNIC-TOC uptake within salivary glands of pSS patients compared to controls, as well as a considerably higher sensitivity of ^{99m}Tc-HYNIC-TOC scintigraphy compared to conventional scintigraphy. Furthermore, they demonstrated that ^{99m}Tc-HYNIC-TOC scintigraphy was able to identify joint involvement in a cohort of 62 pSS patients, of which many patients (87%) reported joint pain. Another tracer with potential applicability for pSS is ^{99m}Tc labeled with rituximab, which is an anti-CD20 tracer that images B-lymphocytes. In a small experimental setting, this tracer showed variable uptake in salivary glands and moderate uptake in lacrimal glands in two pSS patients [98].

Together, ^{99m}Tc-pertechnetate scintigraphy is in many institutes no longer used as an imaging technique in the diagnostic work-up and follow-up of pSS. Although promising new scintigraphic tracers have been developed, conventional nuclear medicine has disadvantages, such as the limited resolution of 8-10 mm and the inability to quantify the exact uptake. Positron emission tomography (PET), combined with low dose or contrast-enhanced CT, has multiple advantages over conventional scintigraphy, such as better spatial resolution, faster imaging tracts, and the possibility to quantify tracer uptake. It would be of value to couple the promising tracers that are mentioned above to a PET radionuclide in order to study the added value of these PET tracers in pSS patients.

6.2. Positron Emission Tomography/Computed Tomography

PET is an imaging tool developed in the 1990s to visualize specific (patho)physiological processes of a particular area or of the whole body. The technique is based on injection of radioactive tracers, which are tracers attached to radionuclides that emit positrons (positively charged electrons) to become stable. Emitting positrons cannot exist freely and annihilate with antimatter (negatively charged electrons) by emitting two gamma-ray photons, each with the same energy (511 keV) in direct opposite directions. The PET camera system consists of a ring-shaped detector system which can detect the two photons when they arrive within a certain time frame. Recent developments in software of PET cameras have led to a correction method for the time these photons need to travel to the detector, the so-called Time-of-Flight technique. This improvement (since 2005) caused a higher efficacy in detecting photons. Since then, the use of PET imaging for clinical and research purposes increased considerably. Although PET was originally used in oncological diseases to detect malignancies, the usefulness of PET to image infection and inflammation has markedly increased during the last decade, and PET techniques evolved rapidly. Hybrid camera systems were developed to combine PET findings with CT or MRI to add anatomical information. These new camera systems provide better spatial resolution images (around 3–4 mm), decrease scan duration and radiation dose, and lead to increased diagnostic accuracy. Furthermore, the development of guidelines to standardize PET/CT techniques between centers by the European Association of Nuclear Medicine (EANM) enhances comparability of data and promotes multicenter research [99,100]. In addition, new and specific tracers to image infectious and inflammatory diseases are constantly being developed.

6.2.1. ^{18}F-FDG-PET/CT

The most commonly used PET tracer is ^{18}F-fluorodeoxyglucose (FDG). Uptake of this tracer is relatively higher in cells that are metabolically active, such as inflammatory cells. FDG is indicated in several infectious and inflammatory diseases and is useful for the diagnosis and follow-up of various autoimmune diseases [4,101,102]. In pSS patients, several case reports showed abnormal FDG uptake in salivary glands [103–105] (Figure 5). However, physiological FDG accumulation in salivary glands is highly variable, and subjects without known head and neck pathology frequently show increased FDG uptake in the salivary glands [106,107]. A possible explanation for the wide range in physiological uptake is that salivary glands of different subjects utilize different amounts of glucose for metabolism [108,109]. Which human salivary gland cells have the highest glucose uptake is not known, but in rodent salivary glands, both acinar and ductal cells seem to play a role in glucose uptake [110,111].

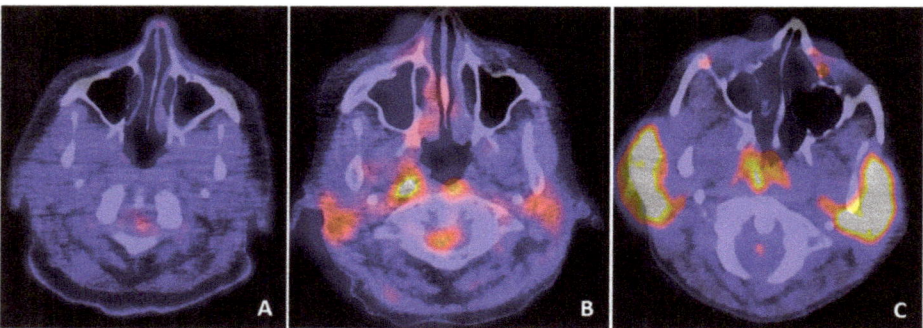

Figure 5. FDG-PET uptake patterns within the parotid glands. FDG-PET/CT showing (**A**) no increased uptake in the parotid glands of a subject without pathology in the head/neck region, (**B**) increased uptake in both parotid glands in a pSS patient, and (**C**) intense uptake in both parotid glands of a pSS patients with histologically confirmed parotid salivary gland MALT lymphoma.

Whether pSS patients show increased FDG uptake in inflamed salivary and lacrimal glands is not yet clear. Although Cohen et al. [112] reported increased FDG uptake in salivary glands of pSS patients compared to a control group of patients who underwent PET for an isolated pulmonary nodule, another study could not confirm this finding [36]. However, both studies used different scoring methods and camera settings, and standardized guidelines and EANM Research Ltd. (EARL) reconstructions were not applied in these studies.

Besides visualizing salivary gland inflammation, several authors reported the ability of FDG-PET/CT to detect systemic disease activity in pSS [104,105,112–115]. Abnormal FDG uptake was observed in 75–85% of pSS patients, mainly within salivary glands, lymph nodes, and lungs [112,113].

However, not all organ involvement in pSS can be visualized by FDG-PET/CT, such as neuropathies, cutaneous vasculitis, and other skin abnormalities, which is mainly due to limited spatial resolution of PET cameras. Since the optimal spatial resolution is around 3-4 mm in newer PET/CT systems, it would be of interest to use these newer systems to study the effectiveness of FDG-PET/CT in assessing systemic disease activity in representative pSS cohorts.

The applicability of FDG-PET/CT in MALT lymphomas is still controversial due to variable FDG avidity at different MALT locations. Pulmonary and head/neck MALT lymphomas seem to be most FDG avid, and FDG-PET/CT shows higher sensitivities at these regions [116,117]. Since pSS-associated MALT lymphomas frequently develop in the salivary glands and/or lungs, there may be a role for this technique in the detection of lymphomas associated with pSS [113,118,119] (Figure 3). Cohen et al. [112] reported a higher maximum standardized uptake value (SUVmax) in lymphoma patients compared to pSS patients without lymphoma. Since only four lymphoma patients were included in this retrospective cohort, the study was not powered to affirm the usefulness of FDG-PET/CT in the diagnosis of pSS-associated MALT lymphoma. In another retrospective study by Kerean et al. [113], 8 out of 15 pSS patients had confirmed salivary gland or pulmonary MALT lymphoma. They found that a SUVmax of ≥4.7 in the parotid glands and presence of focal lung lesions were associated with lymphoma. An important advantage of FDG-PET/CT is the possibility to detect extraglandular lymphoma locations by using whole-body imaging. In addition, Kerean et al. [113] showed that FDG-PET/CT is useful for biopsy guiding and for treatment response monitoring [113]. However, the mentioned SUVmax threshold found in this study cannot directly be used by others, as different nonstandardized camera systems were used in this multicenter study. Importantly, both retrospective studies state that the frequent presence of benign lymph node uptake in pSS patients can be misleading and should be taken into account when using FDG-PET/CT for the diagnosis of lymphoma in pSS patients [112,113].

6.2.2. Future Promising PET Tracers

Similar to conventional scintigraphy, specific PET tracers can be used to visualize inflammation in pSS. A case report showed intense uptake of ^{68}Ga-pentixafor, a radioligand of the chemokine receptor CXCR4. This receptor is involved in, among others, migration of leukocytes toward sites of inflammation. In this pSS patient, the increased uptake in salivary glands and lymph nodes was histologically proven to be attributed to inflammatory cell infiltration [120]. To further investigate the overexpression of somatostatin receptors in salivary glands and joints of pSS patients, as shown by ^{99m}Tc-HYNIC-TOC scintigraphy, the specific PET tracer ^{68}Ga-DOTATOC can be used [121]. Another pathological feature in pSS that could be visualized is the increased number of B-lymphocytes within salivary glands. Furthermore, by using whole-body B-lymphocyte imaging, not only B-lymphocytes within the salivary glands can be visualized, but also B-lymphocytes that are present in other organs associated with pSS. We previously showed that high numbers of B-lymphocytes within salivary glands of pSS patients predict response to rituximab (anti-CD20) therapy [122]. Whole-body imaging of B-lymphocytes could be an improved and noninvasive method to select pSS patients who are likely to respond to rituximab treatment. In rheumatoid arthritis and orbital inflammatory diseases, imaging of B-lymphocytes by using ^{89}Zr-rituximab has shown potential in the detection of B-lymphocyte-mediated diseases, in the evaluation of rituximab treatment, and also in the selection of rituximab responders [123,124]. Therefore, it is of interest to study whole-body B-lymphocyte imaging by using PET/CT in pSS patients, and to assess whether this specific PET tracer can detect treatment response and can identify rituximab responders at baseline. Since T-lymphocytes are thought to be predominant in salivary glands in early stages of pSS [125], imaging of these lymphocytes could also be of added value. Radiolabeled interleukin-2 (IL-2) can detect activated T-lymphocytes within affected organs in pSS since IL-2 receptors are overexpressed on activated T-lymphocytes [126].

Overall, PET seems to be a promising imaging technique in pSS. Although the added value of PET in the diagnostic process of pSS remains to be shown, FDG-PET/CT was found to be useful in the assessment of disease activity, the systemic staging of pSS-associated lymphomas, and the evaluation of treatment response.

7. Conclusions

Currently, various imaging techniques are used in the diagnostic work-up and follow-up of pSS patients, but none of them are included in the current 2016 ACR-EULAR classification criteria. Although sialography and scintigraphy have been part of previous classification criteria sets, both techniques are not commonly used in the diagnostic work-up of pSS anymore. An imaging technique that has proven to be of added value in diagnosing and classifying pSS is SGUS. The next step is to incorporate a consensus SGUS scoring system into the 2016 ACR-EULAR criteria, after its validation in independent cohorts. In addition, longitudinal observational studies and clinical trials are needed to understand the usefulness of SGUS in assessing disease activity and disease progression in pSS. Several initiatives were started already, such as OMERACT and HarmonicSS, which will give us more insight into the potential of this promising imaging tool in pSS. Another emerging technique in the evaluation of salivary gland and systemic involvement in pSS is PET, combined with CT or MRI. Additional studies are needed to further elucidate the presumed role of FDG-PET/CT in pSS, by using larger and representative cohorts, standardized scanning procedures, and harmonization between centers. Besides, new pSS-specific PET tracers should be further explored since they may provide promising insights into pathological processes. Regarding imaging of pSS-associated lymphomas, findings on MRI, SGUS, and FDG-PET/CT should be compared to histopathological findings in order to investigate which imaging technique is most appropriate for the detection and staging of pSS-associated lymphomas. Furthermore, it is still not known what the various imaging findings in salivary glands of pSS patients represent at a histological level. Further research, for example, by performing ultrasound-guided biopsies, is needed to answer this question.

Author Contributions: M.S.v.G., A.V. and A.W.G. were involved in writing and preparing the original draft. B.v.d.V., E.M., F.G.K. and H.B. critically revised the manuscript. All authors have read and agreed to the final version of the review. All authors have read and agreed to the published version of the manuscript.

Funding: This work was supported by Horizon 2020, a research project supported by the European Commission [H2020-SC1-2016-RTD, proposal 731944].

Conflicts of Interest: The authors declare no conflict of interest.

References

1. Ramos-Casals, M.; Brito-Zerón, P.; Solans, R.; Camps, M.T.; Casanovas, A.; Sopeña, B.; Díaz-López, B.; Rascón, F.-J.; Qanneta, R.; Fraile, G.; et al. Systemic involvement in primary Sjogren's syndrome evaluated by the EULAR-SS disease activity index: Analysis of 921 Spanish patients (GEAS-SS Registry). *Rheumatology* **2014**, *53*, 321–331. [CrossRef]
2. Greenspan, J.S.; Daniels, T.E.; Talal, N.; Sylvester, R.A. The histopathology of Sjögren's syndrome in labial salivary gland biopsies. *Oral Surg. Oral Med. Oral Pathol.* **1974**, *37*, 217–229. [CrossRef]
3. Baldini, C.; Zabotti, A.; Filipovic, N.; Vukicevic, A.; Luciano, N.; Ferro, F.; Lorenzon, M.; De Vita, S. Imaging in primary Sjögren's syndrome: The "obsolete and the new.". *Clin. Exp. Rheumatol.* **2018**, *36*, S215–S221.
4. Signore, A.; Anzola, K.L.; Auletta, S.; Varani, M.; Petitti, A.; Pacilio, M.; Galli, F.; Lauri, C. Current status of molecular imaging in inflammatory and autoimmune disorders. *Curr. Pharm. Des.* **2018**, *24*, 743–753. [CrossRef] [PubMed]
5. Goules, A.V.; Tzioufas, A.G. Lymphomagenesis in Sjögren's syndrome: Predictive biomarkers towards precision medicine. *Autoimmun. Rev.* **2019**, *18*, 137–143. [CrossRef] [PubMed]
6. Routsias, J.G.; Goules, J.D.; Charalampakis, G.; Tzima, S.; Papageorgiou, A.; Voulgarelis, M. Malignant lymphoma in primary Sjögren's syndrome: An update on the pathogenesis and treatment. *Semin. Arthritis Rheum.* **2013**, *43*, 178–186. [CrossRef]

7. Royer, B.; Cazals-Hatem, D.; Sibilia, J.; Agbalika, F.; Cayuela, J.M.; Soussi, T.; Maloisel, F.; Clauvel, J.P.; Brouet, J.C.; Mariette, X. Lymphomas in patients with Sjogren's syndrome are marginal zone B-cell neoplasms, arise in diverse extranodal and nodal sites, and are not associated with viruses. *Blood* **1997**, *90*, 766–775. [CrossRef]
8. Voulgarelis, M.; Dafni, U.G.; Isenberg, D.A.; Moutsopoulos, H.M. Malignant lymphoma in primary Sjögren's syndrome: A multicenter, retrospective, clinical study by the European concerted action on Sjögren's syndrome. *Arthritis Rheum.* **1999**, *42*, 1765–1772. [CrossRef]
9. Johnson, S.A.; Kumar, A.; Matasar, M.J.; Schöder, H.; Rademaker, J. Imaging for staging and response assessment in lymphoma. *Radiology* **2015**, *276*, 323–338. [CrossRef]
10. Barrington, S.F.; Mikhaeel, N.G.; Kostakoglu, L.; Meignan, M.; Hutchings, M.; Müeller, S.P.; Schwartz, L.H.; Zucca, E.; Fisher, R.I.; Trotman, J.; et al. Role of imaging in the staging and response assessment of lymphoma: Consensus of the international conference on malignant lymphomas imaging working group. *J. Clin. Oncol.* **2014**, *32*, 3048–3058. [CrossRef]
11. Vitali, C.; Del Papa, N. Classification and diagnostic criteria in Sjögren's syndrome: A long-standing and still open controversy. *Ann. Rheum. Dis.* **2017**, *76*, 1953–1954. [CrossRef] [PubMed]
12. Bootsma, H.; Spijkervet, F.K.L.; Kroese, F.G.M.; Vissink, A. Toward new classification criteria for Sjögren's syndrome? *Arthritis Rheum.* **2013**, *65*, 21–23. [CrossRef] [PubMed]
13. Van Nimwegen, J.F.; Van Ginkel, M.S.; Arends, S.; Haacke, E.A.; van der Vegt, B.; Sillevis Smitt-Kamminga, N.; Spijkervet, F.K.L.; Kroese, F.G.M.; Stel, A.J.; Brouwer, E.; et al. Validation of the ACR-EULAR criteria for primary Sjögren's syndrome in a Dutch prospective diagnostic cohort. *Rheumatology* **2018**, *57*, 818–825. [CrossRef] [PubMed]
14. Shiboski, C.H.; Shiboski, S.C.; Seror, R.; Criswell, L.A.; Labetoulle, M.; Lietman, T.M.; Rasmussen, A.; Scofield, H.; Vitali, C.; Bowman, S.J.; et al. 2016 American College of Rheumatology/European League Against Rheumatism classification criteria for primary Sjögren's syndrome: A consensus and data-driven methodology involving three international patient cohorts. *Ann. Rheum. Dis.* **2017**, *76*, 9–16. [CrossRef]
15. Shiboski, S.C.; Shiboski, C.H.; Criswell, L.A.; Baer, A.N.; Challacombe, S.; Lanfranchi, H.; Schiødt, M.; Umehara, H.; Vivino, F.; Zhao, Y.; et al. American College of rheumatology classification criteria for Sjögren's syndrome: A data-driven, expert consensus approach in the Sjögren's International Collaborative Clinical Alliance cohort. *Arthritis Care Res.* **2012**, *64*, 475–487. [CrossRef]
16. Vitali, C.; Bombardieri, S.; Jonsson, R.; Moutsopoulos, H.M.; Alexander, E.L.; Carsons, S.E.; Daniels, T.E.; Fox, P.C.; Fox, R.I.; Kassan, S.S.; et al. Classification criteria for Sjogren's syndrome: A revised version of the European criteria proposed by the American-European Consensus Group. *Ann. Rheum. Dis.* **2002**, *61*, 554–558. [CrossRef]
17. Chisholm, D.M.; Mason, D.K. Labial salivary gland biopsy in Sjögren's disease. *J. Clin. Pathol.* **1968**, *21*, 656–660. [CrossRef]
18. Bodeutsch, C.; De Wilde, P.C.M.; Kater, L.; Van Houwelingen, J.C.; Van Den Hoogen, F.H.J.; Kruize, A.A.; Hené, R.J.; Van De Putte, L.B.A.; Vooijs, G.P. Quantitative immunohistologic criteria are superior to the lymphocytic focus score criterion for the diagnosis of Sjögren's syndrome. *Arthritis Rheum.* **1992**, *35*, 1075–1087. [CrossRef]
19. Leroy, J.P.; Pennec, Y.L.; Letoux, G.; Youinou, P. Lymphocytic infiltration of salivary ducts: A histopathologic lesion specific for primary Sjögren's syndrome? *Arthritis Rheum.* **1992**, *35*, 481–482. [CrossRef]
20. Ihrler, S.; Zietz, C.; Sendelhofert, A.; Riederer, A.; Löhrs, U. Lymphoepithelial duct lesions in Sjogren-type sialadenitis. *Virchows Arch.* **1999**, *434*, 315–323. [CrossRef]
21. Llamas-Gutierrez, F.J.; Reyes, E.; Martínez, B.; Hernández-Molina, G. Histopathological environment besides the focus score in Sjögren's syndrome. *Int. J. Rheum. Dis.* **2014**, *17*, 898–903. [CrossRef] [PubMed]
22. Leehan, K.M.; Pezant, N.P.; Rasmussen, A.; Grundahl, K.; Moore, J.S.; Radfar, L.; Lewis, D.M.; Stone, D.U.; Lessard, C.J.; Rhodus, N.L.; et al. Minor salivary gland fibrosis in Sjögren's syndrome is elevated, associated with focus score and not solely a consequence of aging. *Clin. Exp. Rheumatol.* **2018**, *36*, S80–S88.
23. Leehan, K.M.; Pezant, N.P.; Rasmussen, A.; Grundahl, K.; Moore, J.S.; Radfar, L.; Lewis, D.M.; Stone, D.U.; Lessard, C.J.; Rhodus, N.L.; et al. Fatty infiltration of the minor salivary glands is a selective feature of aging but not Sjögren's syndrome. *Autoimmunity* **2017**, *50*, 451–457. [CrossRef] [PubMed]

24. Skarstein, K.; Aqrawi, L.A.; Øijordsbakken, G.; Jonsson, R.; Jensen, J.L. Adipose tissue is prominent in salivary glands of Sjögren's syndrome patients and appears to influence the microenvironment in these organs. *Autoimmunity* **2016**, *49*, 338–346. [CrossRef] [PubMed]
25. Risselada, A.P.; Kruize, A.A.; Goldschmeding, R.; Lafeber, F.P.J.G.; Bijlsma, J.W.J.; Van Roon, J.A.G. The prognostic value of routinely performed minor salivary gland assessments in primary Sjögren's syndrome. *Ann. Rheum. Dis.* **2014**, *73*, 1537–1540. [CrossRef] [PubMed]
26. Carubbi, F.; Alunno, A.; Cipriani, P.; Bartoloni, E.; Baldini, C.; Quartuccio, L.; Priori, R.; Valesini, G.; De Vita, S.; Bombardieri, S.; et al. A retrospective, multicenter study evaluating the prognostic value of minor salivary gland histology in a large cohort of patients with primary Sjögren's syndrome. *Lupus* **2015**, *24*, 315–320. [CrossRef]
27. De Re, V.; De Vita, S.; Carbone, A.; Ferraccioli, G.; Gloghini, A.; Marzotto, A.; Pivetta, B.; Dolcetti, R.; Boiocchi, M. The relevance of VDJ PCR protocols in detecting B-cell clonal expansion in lymphomas and other lymphoproliferative disorders. *Tumori* **1995**, *81*, 405–409. [CrossRef]
28. Nakshbandi, U.; Haacke, E.A.; Bootsma, H.; Vissink, A.; Spijkervet, F.K.L.; Van Der Vegt, B.; Kroese, F.G.M. Bcl6 for identification of germinal centres in salivary gland biopsies in primary Sjögren's syndrome. *Oral Dis.* **2020**, *26*, 707–710. [CrossRef]
29. Rubin, P.; Holt, J. Secretory sialography in diseases of the major salivary glands. *Am. J. Roentgenol. Radium Ther. Nucl. Med.* **1957**, *77*, 575–598.
30. Wang, X.; Bootsma, H.; Terpstra, J.; Vissink, A.; Van Der Vegt, B.; Spijkervet, F.K.L.; Kroese, F.G.M.; Pringle, S. Progenitor cell niche senescence reflects pathology of the parotid salivary gland in primary Sjögren's syndrome. *Rheumatology* **2020**, in press. [CrossRef]
31. Swiecka, M.; Maślińska, M.; Paluch, L.; Zakrzewski, J.; Kwiatkowska, B. Imaging methods in primary Sjögren's syndrome as potential tools of disease diagnostics and monitoring. *Reumatologia* **2019**, *57*, 336–342. [CrossRef] [PubMed]
32. Golder, W.; Stiller, M. Verteilungsmuster des Sjögren-Syndroms: Eine sialographische Studie. *Z. Rheumatol.* **2014**, *73*, 928–933. [CrossRef] [PubMed]
33. Keshet, N.; Aricha, A.; Friedlander-Barenboim, S.; Aframian, D.J.; Nadler, C. Novel parotid sialo-cone-beam computerized tomography features in patients with suspected Sjogren's syndrome. *Oral Dis.* **2019**, *25*, 126–132. [CrossRef] [PubMed]
34. Kojima, I.; Sakamoto, M.; Iikubo, M.; Shimada, Y.; Nishioka, T.; Sasano, T. Relationship of MR imaging of submandibular glands to hyposalivation in Sjögren's syndrome. *Oral Dis.* **2019**, *25*, 117–125. [CrossRef] [PubMed]
35. Niemelä, R.K.; Pääkkö, E.; Suramo, I.; Takalo, R.; Hakala, M. Magnetic Resonance Imaging and Magnetic Resonance Sialography of Parotid Glands in Primary Sjogren's Syndrome. *Arthritis Rheum.* **2001**, *45*, 512–518. [CrossRef]
36. Shimizu, M.; Okamura, K.; Kise, Y.; Takeshita, Y.; Furuhashi, H.; Weerawanich, W.; Moriyama, M.; Ohyama, Y.; Furukawa, S.; Nakamura, S.; et al. Effectiveness of imaging modalities for screening IgG4-related dacryoadenitis and sialadenitis (Mikulicz's disease) and for differentiating it from Sjögren's syndrome (SS), with an emphasis on sonography. *Arthritis Res.* **2015**, *17*, 223. [CrossRef]
37. Su, G.Y.; Wang, C.B.; Hu, H.; Liu, J.; Ding, H.Y.; Xu, X.Q.; Wu, F.Y. Effect of laterality, gender, age and body mass index on the fat fraction of salivary glands in healthy volunteers: Assessed using iterative decomposition of water and fat with echo asymmetry and least-squares estimation method. *Dentomaxillofac. Radiol.* **2019**, *48*, 20180263. [CrossRef]
38. Scott, J.; Flower, E.A.; Burns, J. A quantitative study of histological changes in the human parotid gland occurring with adult age. *J. Oral Pathol. Med.* **1987**, *16*, 505–510. [CrossRef]
39. Izumi, M.; Eguchi, K.; Nakamura, H.; Nagataki, S.; Nakamura, T. Premature fat deposition in the salivary glands associated with Sjogren syndrome: MR and CT evidence. *Am. J. Neuroradiol.* **1997**, *18*, 951–958.
40. Ren, Y.D.; Li, X.R.; Zhang, J.; Long, L.L.; Li, W.X.; Han, Y.Q. Conventional MRI techniques combined with MR sialography on T2-3D-DRIVE in Sjögren syndrome. *Int. J. Clin. Exp. Med.* **2015**, *8*, 3974–3982.
41. Niemelä, R.K.; Takalo, R.; Pääkkö, E.; Suramo, I.; Päivänsalo, M.; Salo, T.; Hakala, M. Ultrasonography of salivary glands in primary Sjögren's syndrome. A comparison with magnetic resonance imaging and magnetic resonance sialography of parotid glands. *Rheumatology* **2004**, *43*, 875–879. [CrossRef] [PubMed]

42. Izumi, M.; Eguchi, K.; Ohki, M.; Uetani, M.; Hayashi, K.; Kita, M.; Nagataki, S.; Nakamura, T. MR imaging of the parotid gland in Sjögren's syndrome: A proposal for new diagnostic criteria. *Am. J. Roentgenol.* **1996**, *166*, 1483–1487. [CrossRef] [PubMed]
43. El Miedany, Y.M.; Ahmed, I.; Mourad, H.G.; Mehanna, A.N.; Aty, S.A.; Gamal, H.M.; El Baddini, M.; Smith, P.; El Gafaary, M. Quantitative ultrasonography and magnetic resonance imaging of the parotid gland: Can they replace the histopathologic studies in patients with Sjogren's syndrome? *Jt. Bone Spine* **2004**, *71*, 29–38. [CrossRef] [PubMed]
44. Pijpe, J.; Kalk, W.W.I.; Bootsma, H.; Spijkervet, F.K.L.; Kallenberg, C.G.M.; Vissink, A. Progression of salivary gland dysfunction in patients with Sjögren's syndrome. *Ann. Rheum. Dis.* **2007**, *66*, 107–112. [CrossRef]
45. Atkinson, J.; Travis, W.; Pillemer, S.; Bermudez, D.; Wolff, A.; Fox, P. Major salivary gland function in primary Sjögren's syndrome and its relationship to clinical features. *J. Rheumatol.* **1990**, *17*, 318–322.
46. Izumi, M.; Eguchi, K.; Uetani, M.; Nakamura, H.; Takagi, Y.; Hayashi, K.; Nakamura, T. MR features of the lacrimal gland in Sjogren's syndrome. *Am. J. Roentgenol.* **1998**, *170*, 1661–1666. [CrossRef]
47. Morgen, K.; McFarland, H.F.; Pillemer, S.R. Central nervous system disease in primary Sjögren's syndrome: The role of magnetic resonance imaging. *Semin. Arthritis Rheum.* **2004**, *34*, 623–630. [CrossRef]
48. McCoy, S.S.; Baer, A.N. Neurological complications of Sjögren's syndrome: Diagnosis and Management. *Curr. Treat. Options Rheumatol.* **2017**, *3*, 275–288. [CrossRef]
49. Cassidy, D.T.; McKelvie, P.; Harris, G.J.; Rose, G.E.; McNab, A.A. Lacrimal gland orbital lobe cysts associated with MALT lymphoma and primary Sjögren's syndrome. *Orbit* **2005**, *24*, 257–263. [CrossRef]
50. Tonami, H.; Matoba, M.; Kuginuki, Y.; Yokota, H.; Higashi, K.; Yamamoto, I.; Sugai, S. Clinical and imaging findings of lymphoma in patients with Sjögren syndrome. *J. Comput. Assist. Tomogr.* **2003**, *27*, 517–524. [CrossRef]
51. Zhu, L.; Wang, P.; Yang, J.; Yu, Q. Non-Hodgkin lymphoma involving the parotid gland: CT and MR imaging findings. *Dentomaxillofac. Radiol.* **2013**, *42*, 20130046. [CrossRef] [PubMed]
52. Tonami, H.; Matoba, M.; Yokota, H.; Higashi, K.; Yamamoto, I.; Sugai, S. CT and MR findings of bilateral lacrimal gland enlargement in Sjögren syndrome. *Clin. Imaging* **2002**, *26*, 392–396. [CrossRef]
53. Grevers, G.; Ihrler, S.; Vogl, T.J.; Weiss, M. A comparison of clinical, pathological and radiological findings with magnetic resonance imaging studies of lymphomas in patients with Sjögren's syndrome. *Eur. Arch. Oto-Rhino-Laryngol.* **1994**, *251*, 214–217. [CrossRef] [PubMed]
54. Tonami, H.; Matoba, M.; Yokota, H.; Higashi, K.; Yamamoto, I.; Sugai, S. Mucosa-associated lymphoid tissue lymphoma in Sjögren's syndrome: Initial and follow-up imaging features. *Am. J. Roentgenol.* **2002**, *179*, 485–489. [CrossRef] [PubMed]
55. Carotti, M.; Salaffi, F.; Di Carlo, M.; Barile, A.; Giovagnoni, A. Diagnostic value of major salivary gland ultrasonography in primary Sjögren's syndrome: The role of grey-scale and colour/power Doppler sonography. *Gland Surg.* **2019**, *8*, S159–S167. [CrossRef]
56. Devauchelle-Pensec, V.; Zabotti, A.; Carvajal-Alegria, G.; Filipovic, N.; Jousse-Joulin, S.; De Vita, S. Salivary gland ultrasonography in primary Sjögren's syndrome: Opportunities and challenges. *Rheumatology* **2019**, in press. [CrossRef]
57. Le Goff, M.; Cornec, D.; Jousse-Joulin, S.; Guellec, D.; Costa, S.; Marhadour, T.; Le Berre, R.; Genestet, S.; Cochener, B.; Boisrame-Gastrin, S.; et al. Comparison of 2002 AECG and 2016 ACR/EULAR classification criteria and added value of salivary gland ultrasonography in a patient cohort with suspected primary Sjögren's syndrome. *Arthritis Res.* **2017**, *19*, 269. [CrossRef]
58. Jousse-Joulin, S.; Gatineau, F.; Baldini, C.; Baer, A.; Barone, F.; Bootsma, H.; Bowman, S.; Brito-Zerón, P.; Cornec, D.; Dorner, T.; et al. Weight of salivary gland ultrasonography compared to other items of the 2016 ACR/EULAR classification criteria for Primary Sjögren's syndrome. *J. Intern. Med.* **2020**, *287*, 180–188. [CrossRef]
59. Takagi, Y.; Nakamura, H.; Sumi, M.; Shimizu, T.; Hirai, Y.; Horai, Y.; Takatani, A.; Kawakami, A.; Eida, S.; Sasaki, M.; et al. Combined classification system based on ACR/EULAR and ultrasonographic scores for improving the diagnosis of Sjögren's syndrome. *PLoS ONE* **2018**, *13*, e0195113. [CrossRef]
60. Van Nimwegen, J.F.; Mossel, E.; Delli, K.; van Ginkel, M.S.; Stel, A.J.; Kroese, F.G.M.; Spijkervet, F.K.L.; Vissink, A.; Arends, S.; Bootsma, H. Incorporation of Salivary Gland Ultrasonography into the American College of Rheumatology/European League Against Rheumatism Criteria for Primary Sjögren's Syndrome. *Arthritis Care Res.* **2020**, *72*, 583–590. [CrossRef]

61. Jousse-Joulin, S.; D'Agostino, M.A.; Nicolas, C.; Naredo, E.; Ohrndorf, S.; Backhaus, M.; Tamborrini, G.; Chary-Valckenaere, I.; Terslev, L.; Iagnocco, A.; et al. Video clip assessment of a salivary gland ultrasound scoring system in Sjögren's syndrome using consensual definitions: An OMERACT ultrasound working group reliability exercise. *Ann. Rheum. Dis.* **2019**, *78*, 967–973. [CrossRef] [PubMed]
62. Mossel, E.; Arends, S.; Van Nimwegen, J.F.; Delli, K.; Stel, A.J.; Kroese, F.G.M.; Spijkervet, F.K.L.; Vissink, A.; Bootsma, H. Scoring hypoechogenic areas in one parotid and one submandibular gland increases feasibility of ultrasound in primary Sjögren's syndrome. *Ann. Rheum. Dis.* **2018**, *77*, 556–562. [CrossRef] [PubMed]
63. Mossel, E. Comparing ultrasound, histopathology and saliva production of the parotid gland in patients with primary Sjögren's syndrome. Unpublished work.
64. Rahmani, G.; McCarthy, P.; Bergin, D. The diagnostic accuracy of ultrasonography for soft tissue lipomas: A systematic review. *Acta Radiol. Open* **2017**, *6*. [CrossRef] [PubMed]
65. Baer, A.N.; Grader-Beck, T.; Antiochos, B.; Birnbaum, J.; Fradin, J.M. Ultrasound-guided biopsy of suspected salivary gland lymphoma in Sjögren's syndrome. *Arthritis Care Res.* **2020**, in press. [CrossRef] [PubMed]
66. Mossel, E.; Delli, K.; Arends, S.; Haacke, E.A.; Van Der Vegt, B.; Van Nimwegen, J.F.; Stel, A.J.; Spijkervet, F.K.L.; Vissink, A.; Kroese, F.G.M.; et al. Can ultrasound of the major salivary glands assess histopathological changes induced by treatment with rituximab in primary Sjögren's syndrome? *Ann. Rheum. Dis.* **2019**, *78*, e27. [CrossRef]
67. Radovic, M.; Vukicevic, A.; Zabotti, A.; Milic, V.; De Vita, S.; Filipovic, N. Deep learning based approach for assessment of primary Sjögren's syndrome from salivary gland ultrasonography images. In *Computational Bioengineering and Bioinformatics. Learning and Analytics in Intelligent Systems. Proceedings of the ICCB 2019 8th International Conference on Computational Bioengineering, Belgrade, Serbia, 4–6 September 2019*; Filipovic, N., Ed.; Springer: Cham, Switzerland, 2020; Volume 11.
68. Fidelix, T.; Czapkowski, A.; Azjen, S.; Andriolo, A.; Trevisani, V.F.M. Salivary gland ultrasonography as a predictor of clinical activity in Sjögren's syndrome. *PLoS ONE* **2017**, *12*, e0182287. [CrossRef]
69. Inanc, N.; Sahinkaya, Y.; Mumcu, G.; Özdemir, F.T.; Paksoy, A.; Ertürk, Z.; Direskeneli, H.; Bruyn, G.A. Evaluation of salivary gland ultrasonography in primary Sjögren's syndrome: Does it reflect clinical activity and outcome of the disease? *Clin. Exp. Rheumatol.* **2019**, *37*, S140–S145.
70. Cornec, D.; Jousse-Joulin, S.; Costa, S.; Marhadour, T.; Marcorelles, P.; Berthelot, J.M.; Hachulla, E.; Hatron, P.Y.; Goeb, V.; Vittecoq, O.; et al. High-grade salivary-gland involvement, assessed by histology or ultrasonography, is associated with a poor response to a single rituximab course in primary Sjögren's syndrome: Data from the TEARS randomized trial. *PLoS ONE* **2016**, *11*, e0162787. [CrossRef]
71. Zabotti, A.; Callegher, S.Z.; Gandolfo, S.; Valent, F.; Giovannini, I.; Cavallaro, E.; Lorenzon, M.; De Vita, S. Hyperechoic bands detected by salivary gland ultrasonography are related to salivary impairment in established Sjögren's syndrome. *Clin. Exp. Rheumatol.* **2019**, *37*, S146–S152.
72. Theander, E.; Mandl, T. Primary Sjögren's syndrome: Diagnostic and prognostic value of salivary gland ultrasonography using a simplified scoring system. *Arthritis Care Res.* **2014**, *66*, 1102–1107. [CrossRef]
73. Milic, V.; Colic, J.; Cirkovic, A.; Stanojlovic, S.; Damjanov, N. Disease activity and damage in patients with primary Sjogren's syndrome: Prognostic value of salivary gland ultrasonography. *PLoS ONE* **2019**, *14*, e0226498. [CrossRef] [PubMed]
74. Mossel, E.; van Nimwegen, J.F.; Stel, A.J.; Wijnsma, R.; Delli, K.; van Zuiden, G.S.; Olie, L.; Vehof, J.; Los, L.; Vissink, A.; et al. Clinical phenotyping of primary Sjögren's patients using salivary gland ultrasonography—Data from the REgistry of Sjögren syndrome in Umcg LongiTudinal (RESULT) cohort. Unpublished work.
75. Kim, J.W.; Lee, H.; Park, S.H.; Kim, S.K.; Choe, J.Y.; Kim, J.K. Salivary gland ultrasonography findings are associated with clinical, histological, and serologic features of Sjögren's syndrome. *Scand. J. Rheumatol.* **2018**, *47*, 303–310. [CrossRef] [PubMed]
76. Lee, K.A.; Lee, S.H.; Kim, H.R. Diagnostic and predictive evaluation using salivary gland ultrasonography in primary Sjögren's syndrome. *Clin. Exp. Rheumatol.* **2018**, *36*, S165–S172.
77. Coiffier, G.; Martel, A.; Albert, J.D.; Lescoat, A.; Bleuzen, A.; Perdriger, A.; De Bandt, M.; Maillot, F. Ultrasonographic damages of major salivary glands are associated with cryoglobulinemic vasculitis and lymphoma in primary Sjogren's syndrome: Are the ultrasonographic features of the salivary glands new prognostic markers in Sjögren's syndrome? *Ann. Rheum. Dis* **2019**, in press. [CrossRef]

78. Jousse-Joulin, S.; D'agostino, M.A.; Hočevar, A.; Naredo, E.; Terslev, L.; Ohrndorf, S.; Iagnocco, A.; Schmidt, W.A.; Finzel, S.; Alavi, Z.; et al. Could we use salivary gland ultrasonography as a prognostic marker in Sjogren's syndrome? Response to: Ultrasonographic damages of major salivary glands are associated with cryoglobulinemic vasculitis and lymphoma in primary Sjögren's syndrome: Are the ultrasonographic features of the salivary glands new prognostic markers in Sjögren's syndrome? *Ann. Rheum. Dis* **2019**, in press.
79. De Luca, R.; Trodella, M.; Vicidomini, A.; Colella, G.; Tartaro, G. Endoscopic management of salivary gland obstructive diseases in patients with Sjögren's syndrome. *J. Cranio-Maxillofac. Surg.* **2015**, *43*, 1643–1649. [CrossRef]
80. Hakki Karagozoglu, K.; Vissink, A.; Forouzanfar, T.; Brand, H.S.; Maarse, F.; Jan Jager, D.H. Sialendoscopy enhances salivary gland function in Sjögren's syndrome: A 6-month follow-up, randomised and controlled, single blind study. *Ann. Rheum. Dis.* **2018**, *77*, 1025–1031. [CrossRef]
81. Gallo, A.; Martellucci, S.; Fusconi, M.; Pagliuca, G.; Greco, A.; De Virgilio, A.; De Vincentiis, M. Sialendoscopic management of autoimmune sialadenitis: A review of literature. *Acta Otorhinolaryngol. Ital.* **2017**, *37*, 148–154.
82. Jager, D.J.; Karagozoglu, K.H.; Maarse, F.; Brand, H.S.; Forouzanfar, T. Sialendoscopy of salivary glands affected by Sjögren syndrome: A randomized controlled pilot study. *J. Oral Maxillofac. Surg.* **2016**, *74*, 1167–1174. [CrossRef]
83. Shacham, R.; Puterman, M.B.; Ohana, N.; Nahlieli, O. Endoscopic treatment of salivary glands affected by autoimmune diseases. *J. Oral Maxillofac. Surg.* **2011**, *69*, 476–481. [CrossRef]
84. Guo, Y.; Sun, N.; Wu, C.; Xue, L.; Zhou, Q. Sialendoscopy-assisted treatment for chronic obstructive parotitis related to Sjogren syndrome. *Oral Surg. Oral Med. Oral Pathol. Oral Radiol.* **2017**, *123*, 305–309. [CrossRef] [PubMed]
85. Capaccio, P.; Canzi, P.; Torretta, S.; Rossi, V.; Benazzo, M.; Bossi, A.; Vitali, C.; Cavagna, L.; Pignataro, L. Combined interventional sialendoscopy and intraductal steroid therapy for recurrent sialadenitis in Sjögren's syndrome: Results of a pilot monocentric trial. *Clin. Otolaryngol.* **2018**, *43*, 96–102. [CrossRef] [PubMed]
86. Karagozoglu, K.H.; De Visscher, J.G.; Forouzanfar, T.; van der Meij, E.H.; Jager, D.J. Complications of Sialendoscopy in Patients with Sjögren Syndrome. *J. Oral Maxillofac. Surg.* **2017**, *75*, 978–983. [CrossRef]
87. Nakayama, M.; Okizaki, A.; Nakajima, K.; Takahashi, K. Approach to Diagnosis of Salivary Gland Disease from Nuclear Medicine Images, Salivary Glands—New Approaches in Diagnostics and Treatment, Işıl Adadan Güvenç, IntechOpen. Available online: https://www.intechopen.com/books/salivary-glands-new-approaches-in-diagnostics-and-treatment/approach-to-diagnosis-of-salivary-gland-disease-from-nuclear-medicine-images (accessed on 3 July 2020).
88. Soto-Rojas, A.E.; Kraus, A. The oral side of Sjögren syndrome. Diagnosis and treatment. A review. *Arch. Med. Res.* **2002**, *33*, 95–106. [CrossRef]
89. Ramos-Casals, M.; Brito-Zerón, P.; Perez-De-Lis, M.; Diaz-Lagares, C.; Bove, A.; Soto, M.J.; Jimenez, I.; Belenguer, R.; Siso, A.; Muxí, A.; et al. Clinical and prognostic significance of parotid scintigraphy in 405 patients with primary Sjögren's syndrome. *J. Rheumatol.* **2010**, *37*, 585–590. [CrossRef] [PubMed]
90. Brito-Zero, P.; Ramos-Casals, M.; Bove, A.; Sentis, J.; Font, J. Predicting adverse outcomes in primary Sjögren's syndrome: Identification of prognostic factors. *Rheumatology* **2007**, *46*, 1359–1362. [CrossRef]
91. Huang, J.; Wu, J.; Zhao, L.; Liu, W.; Wei, J.; Hu, Z.; Hao, B.; Wu, H.; Sun, L.; Chen, H. Quantitative evaluation of salivary gland scintigraphy in Sjögren's syndrome: Comparison of diagnostic efficacy and relationship with pathological features of the salivary glands. *Ann. Nucl. Med.* **2020**, *34*, 289–298. [CrossRef]
92. Aung, W.; Murata, Y.; Ishida, R.; Takahashi, Y.; Okada, N.; Shibuya, H. Study of Quantitative Oral Radioactivity in Salivary Gland Scintigraphy and Determination of the Clinical Stage of Sjögren's Syndrome. *J. Nucl. Med.* **2001**, *42*, 38–43.
93. Aksoy, T.; Kiratli, P.O.; Erbas, B. Correlations between histopathologic and scintigraphic parameters of salivary glands in patients with Sjögren's syndrome. *Clin. Rheumatol.* **2012**, *31*, 1365–1370. [CrossRef]
94. Ferone, D.; Lombardi, G.; Colao, A. Somatostatin Receptors in Immune System Cells. *Minerva Endocrinol.* **2001**, *26*, 165–173.
95. Duet, M.; Lioté, F. Somatostatin and somatostatin analog scintigraphy: Any benefits for rheumatology patients? *Jt. Bone Spine* **2004**, *71*, 530–535. [CrossRef] [PubMed]

96. Ferone, D.; Van Hagen, P.M.; Semino, C.; Dalm, V.A.; Barreca, A.; Colao, A.; Lamberts, S.W.J.; Minuto, F.; Hofland, L.J. Somatostatin receptor distribution and function in immune system. *Dig. Liver Dis.* **2004**, *36*, S68–S77. [CrossRef] [PubMed]
97. Anzola, L.K.; Rivera, J.N.; Dierckx, R.A.; Lauri, C.; Valabrega, S.; Galli, F.; Moreno Lopez, S.; Glaudemans, A.W.J.M.; Signore, A. Value of Somatostatin Receptor Scintigraphy with 99mTc-HYNIC-TOC in Patients with Primary Sjögren Syndrome. *J. Clin. Med.* **2019**, *8*, 763. [CrossRef] [PubMed]
98. Malviya, G.; Anzola, K.L.; Podestà, E.; Laganà, B.; Del Mastro, C.; Dierckx, R.A.; Scopinaro, F.; Signore, A. 99mTc-labeled rituximab for imaging B lymphocyte infiltration in inflammatory autoimmune disease patients. *Mol. Imaging Biol.* **2012**, *14*, 637–646. [CrossRef] [PubMed]
99. Jamar, F.; Buscombe, J.; Chiti, A.; Christian, P.E.; Delbeke, D.; Donohoe, K.J.; Israel, O.; Martin-Comin, J.; Signore, A. EANM/SNMMI guideline for 18F-FDG use in inflammation and infection. *J. Nucl. Med.* **2013**, *54*, 647–658. [CrossRef]
100. EARL. An EANM Initiative. Available online: http://earl.eanm.org/cms/website.php (accessed on 29 June 2020).
101. Pelletier-Galarneau, M.; Ruddy, T.D. PET/CT for Diagnosis and Management of Large-Vessel Vasculitis. *Curr. Cardiol. Rep.* **2019**, *21*, 34. [CrossRef]
102. Zhang, J.; Chen, H.; Ma, Y.; Xiao, Y.; Niu, N.; Lin, W.; Wang, X.; Liang, Z.; Zhang, F.; Li, F.; et al. Characterizing IgG4-related disease with 18F-FDG PET/CT: A prospective cohort study. *Eur. J. Nucl. Med. Mol. Imaging* **2014**, *41*, 1624–1634. [CrossRef]
103. Jadvar, H.; Bonyadlou, S.; Iagaru, A.; Colletti, P.M. FDG PET-CT demonstration of Sjogren's sialoadenitis. *Clin. Nucl. Med.* **2005**, *30*, 698–699. [CrossRef]
104. Kumar, P.; Jaco, M.J.; Pandit, A.G.; Shanmughanandan, K.; Jain, A.; Rajeev; Ravina, M. Miliary sarcoidosis with secondary sjogren's syndrome. *J. Assoc. Physicians India* **2013**, *61*, 505–507.
105. Sharma, P.; Chatterjee, P. 18F-FDG PET/CT in multisystem Sjögren Syndrome. *Clin. Nucl. Med.* **2015**, *40*, e293-4. [CrossRef]
106. Nakamoto, Y.; Tatsumi, M.; Hammoud, D.; Cohade, C.; Osman, M.M.; Wahl, R.L. Normal FDG distribution patterns in the head and neck: PET/CT evaluation. *Radiology* **2005**, *234*, 879–885. [CrossRef] [PubMed]
107. Zincirkeser, S.; Sahin, E.; Halac, M.; Sager, S. Standardized uptake values of normal organs on 18F-fluorodeoxyglucose positron emission tomography and computed tomography imaging. *J. Int. Med. Res.* **2007**, *35*, 231–236. [CrossRef] [PubMed]
108. Carter, K.R.; Kotlyarov, E. Common causes of false positive F18 FDG PET/CT scans in oncology. *Braz. Arch. Biol. Technol.* **2007**, *50*, 29–35. [CrossRef]
109. Nicolau, J.; Sassaki, K.T. Metabolism of carbohydrate in the major salivary glands of rats. *Arch. Oral Biol.* **1976**, *21*, 659–661. [CrossRef]
110. Jurysta, C.; Nicaise, C.; Cetik, S.; Louchami, K.; Malaisse, W.J.; Sener, A. Glucose Transport by Acinar Cells in Rat Parotid Glands. *Cell. Physiol. Biochem.* **2012**, *29*, 325–330. [CrossRef]
111. Cetik, S.; Hupkens, E.; Malaisse, W.J.; Sener, A.; Popescu, I.R. Expression and Localization of Glucose Transporters in Rodent Submandibular Salivary Glands. *Cell. Physiol. Biochem.* **2014**, *33*, 1149–1161. [CrossRef]
112. Cohen, C.; Mekinian, A.; Uzunhan, Y.; Fauchais, A.L.; Dhote, R.; Pop, G.; Eder, V.; Nunes, H.; Brillet, P.Y.; Valeyre, D.; et al. 18F-fluorodeoxyglucose positron emission tomography/computer tomography as an objective tool for assessing disease activity in Sjögren's syndrome. *Autoimmun. Rev.* **2013**, *12*, 1109–1114. [CrossRef]
113. Keraen, J.; Blanc, E.; Besson, F.L.; Leguern, V.; Meyer, C.; Henry, J.; Belkhir, R.; Nocturne, G.; Mariette, X.; Seror, R. Usefulness of 18F-Labeled Fluorodeoxyglucose–Positron Emission Tomography for the Diagnosis of Lymphoma in Primary Sjögren's Syndrome. *Arthritis Rheumatol.* **2019**, *71*, 1147–1157. [CrossRef]
114. Serizawa, I.; Inubushi, M.; Kanegae, K.; Morita, K.; Inoue, T.; Shiga, T.; Itoh, T.; Fukae, J.; Koike, T.; Tamaki, N. Lymphadenopathy due to amyloidosis secondary to Sjögren syndrome and systemic lupus erythematosus detected by F-18 FDG PET. *Clin. Nucl. Med.* **2007**, *32*, 881–882. [CrossRef]
115. Ma, D.; Lu, H.; Qu, Y.; Wang, S.; Ying, Y.; Xiao, W. Primary Sjögren's syndrome accompanied by pleural effusion: A case report and literature review. *Int. J. Clin. Exp. Pathol.* **2015**, *8*, 15322–15327.

116. Perry, C.; Herishanu, Y.; Metzer, U.; Bairey, O.; Ruchlemer, R.; Trejo, L.; Naparstek, E.; Sapir, E.E.; Polliack, A. Diagnostic accuracy of PET/CT in patients with extranodal marginal zone MALT lymphoma. *Eur. J. Haematol.* **2007**, *79*, 205–209. [CrossRef] [PubMed]
117. Albano, D.; Durmo, R.; Treglia, G.; Giubbini, R.; Bertagna, F. 18F-FDG PET/CT or PET Role in MALT Lymphoma: An Open Issue not Yet Solved—A Critical Review. *Clin. Lymphoma Myeloma Leuk.* **2020**, *20*, 137–146. [CrossRef] [PubMed]
118. Bural, G. Rare case of Primary Pulmonary Extranodal Non-Hodgkin's Lymphoma in a Patient with Sjogrens Syndrome: Role of FDG-PET/CT in the Initial Staging and Evaluating Response to Treatment. *Mol. Imaging Radionucl. Ther.* **2012**, *21*, 117–120. [PubMed]
119. Shih, W.J.; Ghesani, N.; Hongming, Z.; Alavi, A.; Schusper, S.; Mozley, D. F-18 FDG positron emission tomography demonstrates resolution of non-Hodgkin's lymphoma of the parotid gland in a patient with Sjogren's syndrome before and after anti-CD20 antibody rituximab therapy. *Clin. Nucl. Med.* **2002**, *27*, 142–143. [CrossRef]
120. Cytawa, W.; Kircher, S.; Schirbel, A.; Shirai, T.; Fukushima, K.; Buck, A.K.; Wester, H.J.; Lapa, C. Chemokine Receptor 4 Expression in Primary Sjögren's Syndrome. *Clin. Nucl. Med.* **2018**, *43*, 835–836. [CrossRef]
121. Ambrosini, V.; Nanni, C.; Fanti, S. The use of gallium-68 labeled somatostatin receptors in PET/CT imaging. *PET Clin.* **2014**, *9*, 323–329. [CrossRef]
122. Delli, K.; Haacke, E.A.; Kroese, F.G.M.; Pollard, R.P.; Ihrler, S.; van der Vegt, B.; Vissink, A.; Bootsma, H.; Spijkervet, F.K.L. Towards personalised treatment in primary Sjögren's syndrome: Baseline parotid histopathology predicts responsiveness to rituximab treatment. *Ann. Rheum. Dis.* **2016**, *75*, 1933–1938. [CrossRef]
123. Laban, K.G.; Kalmann, R.; Leguit, R.J.; De Keizer, B. Zirconium-89-labelled rituximab PET-CT in orbital inflammatory disease. *EJNMMI Res.* **2019**, *9*, 69. [CrossRef]
124. Bruijnen, S.; Tsang-A-Sjoe, M.; Raterman, H.; Ramwadhdoebe, T.; Vugts, D.; van Dongen, G.; Huisman, M.; Hoekstra, O.; Tak, P.P.; Voskuyl, A.; et al. B-cell imaging with zirconium-89 labelled rituximab PET-CT at baseline is associated with therapeutic response 24weeks after initiation of rituximab treatment in rheumatoid arthritis patients. *Arthritis Res. Ther.* **2016**, *18*, 266. [CrossRef]
125. Voulgarelis, M.; Tzioufas, A.G. Pathogenetic mechanisms in the initiation and perpetuation of Sjogren's syndrome. *Nat. Rev.* **2010**, *6*, 529–537. [CrossRef]
126. Di Gialleonardo, V.; Signore, A.; Glaudemans, A.W.J.M.; Dierckx, R.A.J.O.; De Vries, E.F.J. N-(4-18F-fluorobenzoyl)interleukin-2 for PET of human-activated T lymphocytes. *J. Nucl. Med.* **2012**, *53*, 679–686. [CrossRef] [PubMed]

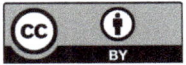

© 2020 by the authors. Licensee MDPI, Basel, Switzerland. This article is an open access article distributed under the terms and conditions of the Creative Commons Attribution (CC BY) license (http://creativecommons.org/licenses/by/4.0/).

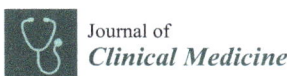
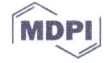

Review

Radiation-Induced Salivary Gland Dysfunction: Mechanisms, Therapeutics and Future Directions

Kimberly J. Jasmer [1,*], Kristy E. Gilman [2], Kevin Muñoz Forti [1], Gary A. Weisman [1] and Kirsten H. Limesand [2]

1. Christopher S. Bond Life Sciences Center, Department of Biochemistry, The University of Missouri, Columbia, MO 65211-7310, USA; kmunoz@mail.missouri.edu (K.M.F.); WeismanG@missouri.edu (G.A.W.)
2. Department of Nutritional Sciences, The University of Arizona, Tucson, AZ 85721, USA; gilmankr@email.arizona.edu (K.E.G.); limesank@arizona.edu (K.H.L.)
* Correspondence: JasmerK@missouri.edu

Received: 30 November 2020; Accepted: 17 December 2020; Published: 18 December 2020

Abstract: Salivary glands sustain collateral damage following radiotherapy (RT) to treat cancers of the head and neck, leading to complications, including mucositis, xerostomia and hyposalivation. Despite salivary gland-sparing techniques and modified dosing strategies, long-term hypofunction remains a significant problem. Current therapeutic interventions provide temporary symptom relief, but do not address irreversible glandular damage. In this review, we summarize the current understanding of mechanisms involved in RT-induced hyposalivation and provide a framework for future mechanistic studies. One glaring gap in published studies investigating RT-induced mechanisms of salivary gland dysfunction concerns the effect of irradiation on adjacent non-irradiated tissue via paracrine, autocrine and direct cell–cell interactions, coined the bystander effect in other models of RT-induced damage. We hypothesize that purinergic receptor signaling involving P2 nucleotide receptors may play a key role in mediating the bystander effect. We also discuss promising new therapeutic approaches to prevent salivary gland damage due to RT.

Keywords: radiation; hyposalivation; xerostomia; purinergic signaling; bystander effect; saliva; salivary gland; P2 receptors; radioprotection; head and neck cancer

1. Introduction

Advances in radiotherapy (RT) for cancer have aimed at minimizing damage to surrounding tissues through modified treatment regimens, technological improvements affording more precise RT delivery and novel radiation sources. These efforts notwithstanding, damage to surrounding tissues such as salivary glands following RT for head and neck cancer (HNC) remains a significant problem. Despite being a highly differentiated, slowly proliferating tissue, salivary glands are surprisingly sensitive to RT [1], a phenomenon attributed to disruption of the plasma membrane on secretory salivary acinar cells and apoptosis [2–9]. RT-induced salivary gland dysfunction results in hyposalivation (i.e., measured reduction in saliva production), xerostomia (i.e., the sensation of oral dryness), mucositis, nutritional deficiencies, oral infections and functional changes, such as difficulties with mastication, dysphagia (i.e., problems with swallowing) and loss of taste, which can significantly reduce the quality of life for afflicted patients [10,11]. It is estimated that >80% of HNC patients exhibit xerostomia and salivary gland hypofunction following RT [12]. Depending on the RT dose, delivery method and salivary gland-sparing techniques employed, chronic xerostomia affects 64–91% of RT patients with HNC [12–14]. There are limited treatment options for RT-induced hyposalivation. The muscarinic receptor agonists pilocarpine and cevimeline that induce saliva secretion from residual acinar cells [15] and artificial saliva provide only temporary symptom relief, which comes at a substantial long-term financial cost [12]. Amifostine is the only FDA-approved radioprotective therapeutic aimed at preventing damage to normal tissues, including salivary glands [16]. However, due to toxicity and potential tumor-protective effects, amifostine is not widely used [17]. Thus, development of innovative approaches to restore or retain salivary function in HNC patients receiving RT is essential [9]. The lack of treatment options to prevent dysfunction or recover function in irradiated salivary glands is compounded by a limited understanding of the underlying mechanisms and the range of variable responses to different RT regimens. In the present review, we explore the mechanisms underlying short- and long-term RT-induced salivary gland dysfunction as well as current and promising future therapeutics.

2. Clinical Presentation

Fractionated radiotherapy is the most common treatment regimen for head and neck squamous cell carcinoma (HNSCC), which consists of daily radiotherapy, usually 2 gray (Gy) per fraction, five days per week, to a total dose of 70 Gy to the tumor [18]. For HNC patients receiving radiotherapy, acute hyposalivation occurs within the first week after RT with a 50–60% loss of saliva flow [19]. In addition to patient-reported xerostomia, which is scored using quality of life (QoL) questionnaires, RT-induced salivary gland dysfunction is verified by an objective measure of salivary gland flow rates or scintigraphic assessment of gland function [20–22]. Rapid RT dose-dependent loss of secretory function seems to result from a marked loss of salivary acinar epithelial cells [23,24], a finding that has been supported in animal studies [3–7]. During the first three weeks after RT, nearly all patients present with mucositis due to significant inflammatory damage to the mucosal surfaces [25]. Interestingly, the incidence of mucositis is highest following fractionated radiation treatment regimens [26]. While these lesions usually resolve within a few weeks, they are reportedly painful and can be so severe as to disrupt HNC treatment regimens [11]. In addition to decreased volume, changes in saliva quality (e.g., pH, protein composition, consistency) affect the buffering capacity and digestive functions of saliva, as well as the composition of oral microbiota [27–30].

Chronic hyposalivation, usually lasting at least 6 months, is commonly experienced by HNC patients undergoing RT [12–14,19,31]. Chronic salivary gland dysfunction is attributed in part due to failure to regenerate functional acini and the development of glandular fibrosis [32–36], although the degree of acute dysfunction is predictive of long-term complications [37,38]. Chronic xerostomia is responsible for a host of complications, including functional impairments in speaking, swallowing and eating [37], poor oral clearance and altered saliva quality that lead to increased incidence of oral bacterial, yeast and fungal infections, dental caries, periodontitis [39,40], digestive disorders and nutritional deficiencies [19], which significantly reduce the quality of life of afflicted patients [20]. Thus management of chronic xerostomia is critical. Unfortunately, current management strategies are inadequate, relying on transient symptom relief afforded by artificial saliva products [41,42] or sialagogues that promote saliva production from residual acinar cells, as discussed in the therapeutics section of the present review [15]. However, there are some promising strategies for RT-induced salivary gland dysfunction, such as recently evaluated oral probiotic lozenges [30]. We will discuss novel therapies being investigated for radioprotection or salivary gland regeneration at the end of this review.

3. Animal Models Provide Mechanistic Insight into Radiation-Induced Salivary Gland Dysfunction

Preclinical animal models have provided many clues to the underlying mechanisms of radiation-induced salivary gland damage. Previous studies from our labs and others have utilized mouse models of ionizing radiation (IR)-induced salivary gland damage to show that acute hyposalivation detected immediately after IR and before onset of obvious gland damage is associated with aberrant calcium signaling, rapid apoptosis of acinar cells, DNA damage and enhanced reactive oxygen species (ROS) production [1,2,4,8,9,43–48]. Sustained IR-induced salivary dysfunction is additionally impacted by inflammation, neuronal and vascular changes, senescence or dysfunction of adult progenitor cell populations, cytoskeletal rearrangements and replacement of normal parenchyma with fibrotic tissue [1,44,45,49–55] (Figure 1). In mouse and rat models, the events giving rise to early loss of salivary gland function occur within the first 3 days following IR. Thus, we have defined acute time points for animal models as the first 3 days and chronic time points as ≥30 days post-IR. Acute IR-induced hyposalivation in mice is observed within the first few hours following IR with a marked loss of acinar cells, a decrease in saliva flow and altered saliva composition [1,4,56]. Available research investigates chronic hyposalivation anywhere from 30 to 300 days post-IR with fibrosis developing between 4 and 6 months [1,44] and as early as 30 days post-fractionated IR in minipigs [57]. Here, we summarize and discuss the signaling processes involved in IR-induced hyposalivation during both acute and chronic time points post-IR.

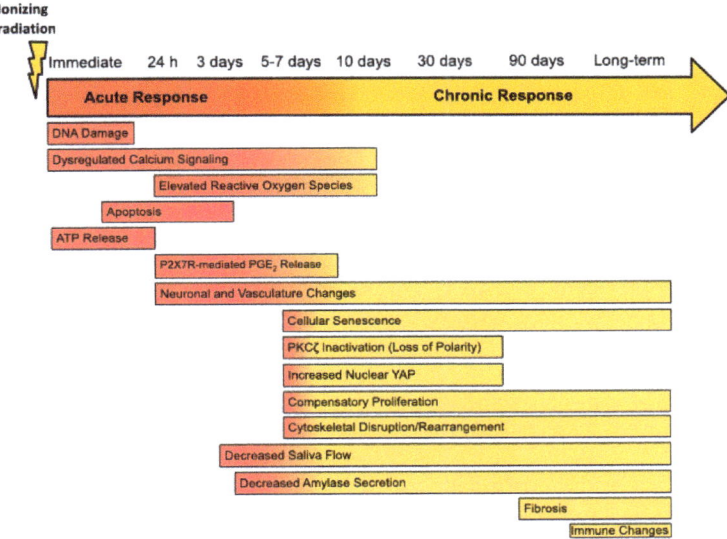

Figure 1. Timeline of Radiation-Induced Changes in the Rodent Salivary Gland. Following irradiation, rodent models show decreased saliva flow at approximately 3 days and a loss of amylase secretion reported as early as 4 days in rats post-IR [2,56,58]. In the acute phase, immediate DNA damage [6,59], rapid apoptosis of acinar cells [4,6,58], and elevated levels of intracellular calcium [45,46] and reactive oxygen species [45,46,60,61] contribute to acute loss of glandular function following irradiation. This period is also marked by release of ATP, which activates the P2X7 receptor (P2X7R), and P2X7R-dependent release of prostaglandin E_2 (PGE$_2$) in murine parotid cells [48]. During the transition phase, loss of apical/basolateral polarity as a result of PKCζ inactivation [55,62,63], increases nuclear Yes-associated protein (Yap) levels [55,64], compensatory proliferation [62,65,66], cellular senescence [60,67,68], and cytoskeletal rearrangements [50,69], which contribute to long-term dysfunction. Changes in innervation and vasculature have been reported as early as 24 h post-IR [53], as well as at chronic time points [54,70]. Though inconsistently reported, fibrosis generally appears between 4 and 6 months following irradiation [1,44,71]. There is little information regarding the effect of irradiation on the immune landscape of the salivary glands in rodent models, although one study indicates changes at 300 days post-IR in mice [54].

3.1. DNA Damage, Insufficient DNA Repair and Cell Cycle Arrest

Administration of IR to salivary glands activates an array of signaling pathways that influence the development of acute hyposalivation. Within minutes of IR exposure, DNA double-strand breaks were detected in mouse parotid glands using a neutral comet assay and were associated with increased phosphorylation of the H2A histone family member X (referred to as γH2AX) [59]. Furthermore,

DNA strand breaks were insufficiently repaired in parotid glands due to reduced activity of the stress-induced deacetylase, sirtuin-1, that results in reduced phosphorylation of the DNA repair protein, NBS1, likely due to inadequate deacetylation that is necessary for optimum kinase function and initiation of the DNA damage response [59]. Insulin-like growth factor (IGF)-1 pretreatment in mice preserved salivary gland function following IR exposure [5]. Mice pretreated with IGF-1 had reduced γH2AX levels, increased NBS1 phosphorylation and improved DNA repair capabilities. Blocking sirtuin-1 activity using a pharmacological inhibitor in combination with IGF-1 therapy decreased DNA repair efficiency, confirming the importance of sirtuin-1-mediated DNA repair in conserving parotid gland function post-IR, especially in the context of IGF-1-mediated preservation of glandular function [59].

Following IR-induced damage, salivary glands insufficiently undergo cell cycle arrest that would allow for complete DNA repair. Following 5 Gy IR, parotid glands exhibit reduced cell cycle arrest, with a low percentage of cells in the G2/M phase at 8 h post-IR, as well as reduced levels of the cell cycle arrest gene, *p21*, at 24 h post-IR [47]. At 8 and 24 h post-IR, there were elevated levels of total and phosphorylated p53 tumor suppressor protein and increases in the truncated, inhibitory isoform of the p53 homolog, p63, (ΔNp63) which is known to block transcription of genes, including *p21*. In the IR-induced salivary gland damage model, IGF-1 pretreatment reduced salivary dysfunction in mice through induction of cell cycle arrest by increasing *p21* transcription due to reduced ΔNp63 binding and increased p53 binding to the *p21* promoter 8 h post-IR [47]. Interestingly, pretreatment of mice with roscovitine, a cell cycle inhibitor, 2 h prior to IR, increased G2/M phase cell cycle arrest and p21 protein content within 6 h post-IR [72]. Compared to vehicle treatment, roscovitine increased phosphorylation of protein kinase B (Akt), a master regulator of cell survival, and mouse double minute 2 homolog (MDM2), an E3 ubiquitin ligase that negatively regulates p53, at 6 h post-IR, which correlates with reduced apoptosis at 24 h post-IR and improved salivary output at days 3 and 30 post-IR [72]. These results confirm the importance of cell cycle inhibition immediately following IR-induced damage to enhance DNA repair and reduce apoptosis in salivary glands.

3.2. Reactive Oxygen Species Generation

Reactive oxygen species (ROS) production is a known consequence of IR treatment and typically induces cellular damage immediately following IR exposure. In rats receiving 5 Gy IR, there was a significant reduction in the activity of the free radical scavenging enzymes superoxide dismutase, glutathione peroxidase and glutathione S-transferase that correlates with elevated levels of the oxidative stress markers, malondialdehyde and xanthine oxidase, as well as increased levels of peroxynitrite, nitric oxide synthase and nitric oxide in salivary glands at day 10 post-IR [61]. In mouse primary submandibular gland (SMG) cells, mitochondrial ROS levels were increased by days 1–3 post-IR with a reduction in ROS levels observed in cells deficient in transient receptor potential melastatin-related 2 (TRPM2), a calcium-permeable cation channel that is activated by oxidative stress and the DNA damage responsive protein, poly (ADP-ribose) polymerase 1 (PARP1), which correlates with improved salivary secretory function post-IR [45]. Furthermore, pharmacologically quenching ROS levels with Tempol improved salivary gland function in mice post-IR [46]. Another group showed that ROS and malondialdehyde levels remained elevated at day 7 post-5 Gy IR in SMGs, but were reduced by adenoviral induction of Sonic Hedgehog signaling at day 3 post-IR, which promoted DNA damage repair [60]. In rats receiving 18 Gy IR, there were elevated levels of the ROS-generating enzyme, NADPH oxidase at days 4–7 post-IR and increased DNA oxidation, measured as enhanced oxidized deoxyguanosine production by 4 days post-IR [58]. This phenotype was reversed following treatment with the antioxidant, α-lipoic acid, that correlated with increased amylase content and salivary function in SMGs [58]. Taken together, these results indicate that IR-induced ROS generation is detrimental to salivary gland function.

3.3. Dysregulated Calcium Signaling

Intracellular calcium levels are tightly regulated and impact a multitude of signaling pathways, including induction of saliva secretion, and have been shown to be dysregulated following irradiation of SMGs [45,46]. Blocking activation of the calcium-permeable cation channel, TRPM2, by pharmacologically scavenging free radicals with Tempol or inhibiting PARP1 activity, attenuates ROS production and preserves salivary gland function at days 10–30 following administration of 15 Gy IR, which was also seen in TRPM2$^{-/-}$ mice [46]. Further evaluation of this pathway illustrated that TRPM2 activation and mitochondrial calcium uniporter (MCU) activity induced cleavage of the stromal interaction molecule 1 (STIM1) via caspase-3 activation within 48 h of IR exposure [45]. STIM1 function is necessary for regulating calcium stores in the endoplasmic reticulum and mediates store-operated calcium entry into acinar cells, with alterations in this pathway leading to reduced saliva secretion at day 30 post-IR. Blocking TRPM2, MCU or caspase-3 function with siRNA or pharmacological inhibitors reversed the hyposalivation phenotype. Likewise, adenovirus-induced expression of STIM1 at day 15 post-IR improved salivary gland function by day 30 following IR-induced damage [45]. These results suggest a key role for the regulation of intracellular calcium signaling in preserving salivary gland function post-IR.

3.4. Generation of Inflammatory Responses

Inflammatory responses may also contribute to IR-induced salivary gland dysfunction. Extracellular ATP (eATP), a damage-associated molecular pattern (DAMP) that commonly activates neighboring cells due to ATP release from adjacent damaged cells, is released from primary parotid gland cells immediately following 2–10 Gy IR exposure [48]. Additionally, levels of the inflammation-associated lipid, prostaglandin E_2 (PGE_2), are increased in parotid acinar cell culture supernatant 24–72 h following 5 Gy IR, with reduced levels of eATP and PGE_2 release shown in mice deficient in the ATP-activated, P2X7 purinergic receptor (P2X7R), which correlates with improved saliva flow by days 3–30 post-IR [48]. Surprisingly, these pathways do not impact cell death induction in parotid glands post-IR [48], but may play a role in the inflammatory response to IR-induced salivary gland damage. It also has been observed that mRNA levels of the inflammatory cytokine interleukin (IL)-6 in irradiated salivary glands increased at 3 h post-13 Gy IR exposure and were reduced by 6 h post-IR, but increased again by day 14 post-IR. Interestingly, this increase correlated with elevated serum IL-6 levels at 6–12 h post-IR and again by day 14 [67]. IL-6 is a pro-inflammatory cytokine with diverse functions. However, the exact role that IL-6 plays in salivary glands post-IR has not been well defined. These data suggest that IR-induced damage to salivary glands leads to diverse inflammatory responses that should be further investigated.

3.5. Apoptosis, Autophagy and Cellular Senescence

Apoptosis of salivary acinar cells occurs at 8–72 h post-IR in mice, with the peak commonly occurring at 24 h post-IR in both parotid glands and SMGs [3–6,48,53]. Apoptosis levels have been quantitated in a multitude of ways to characterize this acute mechanistic phenotype, including via elevated mRNA expression of the apoptosis regulators Bax and Puma [4,6,73], increased caspase-3 protein cleavage [3,6,48,73,74] or enhanced caspase-3 activity [6] or via the terminal deoxynucleotidyl transferase dUTP nick end labelling (TUNEL) assay [3,48,58,73,75,76].

In rats treated by total body irradiation with 5 Gy Cesium-137, there were elevated apoptosis levels, reduced aquaporin-5 content, histological scores in SMGs indicative of tissue degeneration and a concomitant reduction in gland size and saliva secretion by days 10–30 post-IR [76]. Furthermore, in rats receiving 18 Gy IR, there were elevated levels of TUNEL-positive cells and increased cleavage of caspase-9, the upstream regulatory caspase that promotes caspase-3 activation [58]. Importantly, rats receiving α-lipoic acid treatment 1 h post-IR exhibit reduced apoptosis markers and improved saliva secretion at days 4–56 post-IR [58].

Mice lacking the tumor suppressor protein, p53, show improved salivary flow rates at days 3 and 30 following 2 or 5 Gy IR, which correlates with reduced expression of the apoptosis regulators Puma and Bax and a reduction in cleaved caspase-3 levels in histological salivary gland sections [4]. Similarly, mice with constitutive activation of Akt show reduced apoptosis of salivary acinar cells due to inhibition of p53-mediated apoptosis, which was shown to be dependent on Akt-induced phosphorylation and activation of MDM2, leading to p53 ubiquitination and degradation, reduced mRNA and protein levels of the cell cycle regulator p21 and reduced expression of the p53 homologs, p63 and p73 at 24 h post-IR [6]. Constitutive Akt activity reduced apoptosis levels 8–24 h following various doses of IR [5,6] that correlated with reduced p21 and Bax mRNA levels at 12 h post-IR, which improved salivary flow rates at days 3 and 30 post-IR [5]. Another group reiterated the importance of this pathway in mouse and human salivary gland cell cultures, with p53-mediated apoptosis being reduced in mice treated with keratinocyte growth factor-1 (KGF-1) 1 h prior to and immediately following 15 Gy IR, which correlated with improved salivary gland function and increased amylase content of saliva at 16 weeks post-IR [75].

Another study evaluated the potential use of human adipose mesenchymal stem cells (hAMSCs) to preserve salivary gland architecture and function and found that treatment of human parotid gland organoid cultures with hAMSCs increased the release of fibroblast growth factor 10 (FGF10), which reduced IR-induced (10 Gy) apoptosis measured by the TUNEL assay, decreased DNA damage as measured by γH2AX staining, and reduced levels of p53 phosphorylation, Puma and Bax protein and caspase-3 cleavage [73]. Further evaluation of FGF10 signaling showed that activation of the FGFR2-PI3K-Akt pathway increased phosphorylation of BAD and MDM2 and reduced p53-mediated apoptosis, which could be inhibited by pharmacological blockade of FGF10, FGFR2 or phosphatidylinositol-3-kinase (PI3K) activity. Injection of hAMSCs into SMGs of mice 4 weeks post-IR (15 Gy) increased amylase levels, glycoprotein content, gland weight and salivary flow rates and reduced levels of fibrosis at 12 weeks post-injection [73]. These results further support the importance of targeting p53-mediated cell death to improve salivary function post-IR.

Interestingly, knocking down expression of the apoptosis mediator, protein kinase C delta (PKCδ), in mice led to a reduction in 1 or 5 Gy IR-induced apoptosis in parotid glands 24 h post-IR [63]. Additionally, blocking the activity of PKCδ with nanoparticles containing PKCδ siRNA reduced apoptosis levels in mouse SMGs 48 h following 10 Gy IR [3]. The use of siRNA or the tyrosine kinase inhibitors, dasatinib or imatinib, to block the non-receptor tyrosine kinases c-Abl and c-Src, known upstream regulators of PKCδ, caused a similar reduction in apoptosis levels and improved saliva secretion post-IR [77,78]. Importantly, tyrosine kinase inhibition did not enhance survival or growth of HNC cell lines or tumors in mice following radiotherapy [78]. These results suggest apoptosis of salivary acinar cells is a major mechanistic component of the acute response to radiation and can occur via p53- and PKCδ-mediated apoptosis.

Autophagy is the process of "self-eating" damaged cellular components (e.g., organelles or cytoplasmic molecules) to support cell survival and healthy cell regeneration. While 5 Gy irradiation of FVB mouse salivary glands only modestly induced autophagy, pretreatment with IGF-1 followed by IR promoted autophagy activation in salivary glands as measured by conversion of microtubule-associated protein light chain 3 (LC3)-1 to LC3-II, concomitant with decreased levels of the autophagy substrate, p62, and increased interaction of the autophagy regulator Ambra-1 with Beclin-1 [56]. Notably, mice that do not exhibit autophagy in parotid acinar cells 24–48 h post-IR have increased salivary gland apoptosis levels, as well as reduced saliva flow rates that cannot be rescued with IGF-1 therapy [56]. Additionally, inhibition of autophagy leads to increased compensatory cell proliferation at 1–30 days post-IR [56]. Despite the fact that autophagosome formation was only minimally observed in irradiated salivary glands, the combined data suggest a critical role of autophagy in the damage response to irradiation, especially in the context of damage prevention using IGF-1 therapy. In a translational model utilizing miniature pigs, there is reduced levels of microtubule-associated protein light chain 3B (LC3B) and increased p62 levels in parotid glands post-IR (20 Gy) that correlates with a reduction in gland weight, acinar area, aquaporin-5 expression and saliva secretion [52]. Remarkably, activation of the Sonic Hedgehog (Shh) pathway by intraglandular delivery of adenoviral vectors expressing Shh at 4 weeks post-IR reversed this phenotype and improved saliva output in minipigs [52]. These studies suggest that further understanding of the role played by autophagy in post-IR damage may provide alternative strategies for drug development to preserve salivary gland function in HNC patients receiving RT.

Cellular senescence may play a role in IR-induced hyposalivation. Senescence has been suggested to occur in a subset of SMG cells that exhibit elevated DNA damage, measured by an increase in γH2AX+ cells and p21 mRNA by day 7 following 15 Gy IR in mice [60] and by 5 weeks following 20 Gy IR in minipigs [52]. Another study utilizing a 13 Gy dose of IR found increased levels of γH2AX+ cells, p53 binding protein-1 and mRNAs for senescence-associated markers p21, p19, decoy receptor 2, plasminogen activator-1 and IL-6 in SMGs, which were maintained above baseline 6 weeks later [67]. Interestingly, both IL-6-deficient mice and mice receiving IL-6 treatment prior to irradiation showed a reduction in these markers of senescence and improved saliva flow rates 8 weeks post-IR [67], suggesting a key role for senescence in the IR-induced damage response of salivary glands.

3.6. Neuronal and Vascular Changes

Alternative pathways that may be influencing IR-induced hyposalivation include damage to non-epithelial tissue within the salivary gland, such as neurons or vasculature. Importantly, parasympathetic neurons have been suggested to play a role in salivary gland regeneration post-IR damage. During embryonal development, SMGs that receive IR exposure exhibit increased epithelial and neuronal cell apoptosis at 24 and 72 h post-IR, respectively [53]. Neurturin (NRTN) is essential for parasympathetic neuronal development and survival, including in murine salivary glands [53,79,80]. Delivery of human NRTN by adenovirus serotype 5 vector (AdNRTN) to murine SMGs 24 h prior to IR (5 Gy) preserved function at 60 days post-IR [81]. Additionally, NRTN delivery by adeno-associated virus serotype 2 (AAV2) in CH3 mice and minipigs prior to IR improved saliva flow rate at 300 days and 16 weeks, respectively [54]. Treatment with NRTN has been shown to enhance parasympathetic innervation and reduce epithelial apoptosis post-IR, consistent with increased end bud formation within SMGs, supporting a potential regenerative role for neurotrophic signaling in the repair of IR-induced salivary gland damage [53]. Rats administered 18 Gy IR exhibit reduced levels of the neurotrophic factors brain-derived neurotrophic factor (BDNF) and NTRN as well as decreased levels of the neurotrophic factor receptor, GRFα2, acetylcholinesterase and neurofilament staining in SMGs, which could be reversed with α-lipoic acid treatment [70]. In minipigs following 20 Gy IR, there is a reduction in levels of BDNF, NTRN, acetylcholinesterase and the acetylcholine receptor, Chrm1, indicative of decreased parasympathetic innervation, responses that can be reversed with intraglandular adenoviral delivery of Shh at 4 weeks post-IR [52].

As for the vasculature in salivary glands, endothelial cell death occurs 4 h after 15 Gy IR, measured as an increase in caspase-3 cleavage in platelet endothelial cell adhesion molecule (CD31) positive cells, which correlates with an overall reduction in microvessel content in salivary gland tissue sections, responses modulated by treatment with the ROS scavenger Tempol for 10 min prior to IR in mice [82]. Minipigs receiving 20 Gy IR exhibit reduced blood flow and CD31 and vascular endothelial growth factor (VEGF) levels in parotid glands 20 weeks post-IR, indicative of the microvascular damage induced by IR [52]. At 90 days following 15 Gy IR, mice show an increase in blood vessel dilation in SMGs that coincides with a reduction in total capillary volume and diminished salivary function. Interestingly, co-treatment of mice with FMS-like tyrosine kinase-3 ligand (Flt-3L), stem cell factor (SCF) and granulocyte colony-stimulating factor (G-CSF) (i.e., F/S/G treatment) one month following IR promoted increased endothelial cell division, capillary content and endothelial nitric oxide synthase and endoglin expression due to bone-marrow-derived immune cell recruitment and activation of endothelial cells by F/S/G, which correlated with increased acinar cell number and saliva flow at day

90 [83]. Overall, these data suggest that repair of acute and chronic IR-induced damage to salivary glands likely requires contributions from neuronal and vascular cells.

3.7. Stem/Progenitor Cell Dysfunction

In addition to restoring proper innervation and vascularization, the ability of salivary glands to regain function following irradiation relies on the presence of stem and/or progenitor cells to regenerate depleted acinar cells [2]. One group reported that stem/progenitor cells are not evenly distributed within the salivary glands, but rather are localized to salivary ducts in rat and human parotid glands [84]. This suggests that preventing IR from damaging these stem/progenitor cell populations may improve salivary gland function following IR. Indeed, the same group found that irradiation of the cranial 50% of the rat parotid gland—where the authors speculate that the preponderance of progenitor cells reside—had considerably more devastating effects on saliva production at 1 year post-IR than irradiating the caudal region [84]. However, other groups have reported that progenitor cells localized to the acinar compartment of mouse parotid glands and SMGs are capable of self-renewal [55,85]. This discrepancy may be due to the markers used to identify various salivary gland progenitor cell populations. Isolation of Sca-1-, c-Kit- and Musashi-1-expressing mouse salivary gland stem cells has been achieved by in vitro culture of salispheres followed by fluorescence-activated cell sorting (FACS) enrichment using c-Kit as a marker [86]. These cells were capable of differentiating into functional amylase-producing acinar cells. This same group investigated the effect of transplanting salisphere cultures in 15 Gy irradiated female mouse salivary gland. Ninety days after salisphere transplantation, irradiated salivary glands in mice had similar morphology to non-irradiated glands and exhibited restoration of acinar cell populations and improved saliva production compared to irradiated, untreated glands [86].

Senescence as a result of IR can similarly inhibit regenerative potential. In a recent study, C57BL/6 mice receiving 15 Gy X-ray IR were treated with the senolytic drug, ABT263, by oral gavage at 8 or 11 weeks post-IR [68]. ABT263, which inhibits BCL-2 and BCL-xL, selectively eliminates senescent cells. Pilocarpine-stimulated saliva secretion demonstrated a restoration of salivary gland function in irradiated mice receiving ABT263, compared to those receiving IR and vehicle [68]. Additionally, these mice had reduced expression of senescence markers and an increase in aquaporin 5-expressing acinar cells in the SMGs [68]. The authors conclude that clearance of senescent cells promotes self-renewal of the stem/progenitor niche and restoration of salivary gland function [68]. Together, these data underscore the importance of salivary progenitor/stem cells in the regeneration of salivary gland function post-IR. These preclinical studies suggest that stem cell therapies may be a promising approach for the treatment of RT-induced hyposalivation in HNC patients.

Importantly, another group reported that regeneration following salivary gland damage due to duct ligation or under normal homeostatic conditions could occur through self-duplication of acinar cells [85]. More recently, this same group showed that while regeneration following glandular damage in mice under homeostatic conditions or following duct ligation was limited to lineage-restricted progenitors, both differentiated acinar and ductal cells in the adult mouse salivary gland were capable of contributing to acinar regeneration following irradiation [87]. Because permanent acinar cell depletion following irradiation has been reported [2], the ability of ductal cells to regenerate acinar cells is significant. If this cellular plasticity and self-duplication are also observed in human adult salivary acinar and ductal cells following radiotherapy, treatment options involving expansion or stimulation of endogenous populations without the need for isolating salivary gland stem cells may prove promising.

3.8. Compensatory Proliferation

Compensatory proliferation is a common reparative response to tissue damage that typically leads to replacement of dead cells following an injury. In irradiated murine salivary glands, induction of proliferation, as measured by increased expression of proliferating cell nuclear antigen (PCNA) or pKi67, is observed as early as 48 h post-IR [47,72] and continues through chronic time points (i.e.,

30–90 days) [62,65,66,74]. Despite the increase in cell number, salivary glands remain non-functional post-IR, which correlates with reduced levels of salivary amylase, a marker of differentiated acinar cells, suggesting that the newly generated cells are maintained in an undifferentiated state [56,65,66]. Ectodysplasin A-1 receptor (EDAR) signaling typically occurs during embryogenesis to allow for fetal development of ectodermal tissues, such as skin, hair and exocrine glands, including salivary glands. Interestingly, activating this pathway with an EDAR-agonist monoclonal antibody restores salivary gland function post-IR, which correlates with a reduction in compensatory proliferation and increased levels of salivary amylase at days 30–90 [65]. The mammalian target of rapamycin (mTOR) is a critical signaling mediator that controls cell metabolism, growth, proliferation and survival, which is inhibited by rapamycin. Treating mice with the rapamycin analog, CCI-779, reduces proliferation rates while increasing levels of amylase and saliva flow rates at day 30 post-IR [88]. Likewise, post-IR IGF-1 treatment reduces the number of proliferating cells and enhances amylase levels and saliva secretion from days 9–90 post-IR [66].

Compensatory proliferation has been shown to be mediated by reduced activation of the apical polarity regulator, PKCζ, which leads to increased Jun kinase (JNK) signaling in parotid glands following IR [62]. The reduction in PKCζ activity is observed in a subset of stem and progenitor cells, as well as the entire acinar compartment at 5–30 days post-IR, which correlates with increased Ki67 levels [55,62]. Notably, mice lacking PKCζ have increased baseline proliferation rates that are unchanged post-IR and cannot be modulated by IGF-1 treatment [55,62]. Additionally, mice deficient in PKCζ and treated with IGF-1 do not show improvements in salivary gland function post-IR [55]. Together, these data illustrate the importance of the regulation of cell polarity and proliferation by PKCζ and its alteration due to the IR-induced damage response in parotid glands. Modulating proliferation downstream of PKCζ signaling may provide novel drug targets to preserve salivary gland function post-IR.

3.9. Alterations in Cell Structure

Modifications to cell junction protein interactions and actin cytoskeletal rearrangements are also observed in salivary glands following IR in mice [50] and rats [69]. Junctional regulators play a critical role in cell–cell contact and their interactions influence cell proliferation and differentiation, essential components of tissue repair. Claudins are tight junction proteins that comprise the paracellular barrier between neighboring cells and mediate intercellular permeability. In rat parotid glands, there is a transient increase in claudin-4 expression 2–3 days following 15 or 20 Gy irradiation and a reduction in levels of claudin-3 at days 7 and 30, responses that could be modulated in non-injured cells via Src kinase inhibition [69]. Epithelial (E)-cadherin is another junctional protein that is typically associated with the protein catenin, including α, β, γ or p120 isoforms that are known to play a critical role in cytoskeletal assembly and the regulation of cell adhesion, contraction and motility. A reduction in the interaction between E-cadherin and β-catenin leads to actin filament fragmentation in mouse parotid glands 7–30 days post-IR due to increased rho-associated kinase (ROCK) signaling that can be reversed by post-IR IGF-1 treatment [50]. Further evaluation of this pathway showed that ROCK signaling leads to activation and nuclear translocation of the transcriptional regulator Yes-associated protein (Yap) that is modulated by ROCK inhibition or IGF-1 treatment [64]. Yap activity is typically beneficial in injury models, although in salivary glands increased activation of Yap is seen in subsets of stem and progenitor cells, as well as the entire acinar compartment in parotid glands at days 5–30 post-IR in models that do not restore salivary function [55,64]. In contrast, post-IR IGF-1 treatment reduces Yap activity and improves salivary gland function in a PKCζ-dependent manner [55,64]. Together, these data support the mechanism whereby IR induces dissociation of tight junction proteins to promote loss of PKCζ-mediated apical/basolateral polarity, ROCK-dependent actin cytoskeletal rearrangements and loss of salivary gland function, responses that can be reversed by IGF-1 to restore salivary function of irradiated parotid glands.

3.10. Fibrosis

SMG biopsies from patients with advanced stage oropharyngeal cancer who received fractionated radiotherapy (1.8–2 Gy per fraction, ~35 fractions) showed glandular atrophy and periductal and parenchymal fibrosis that correlates with the degree of sialadenitis (i.e., lymphocytic infiltration of the gland). Destruction of salivary gland parenchyma with progressive replacement of functional tissue by extracellular matrix proteins impairs saliva production [33]. In rodent models, the development of fibrosis following irradiation is inconsistent, but has been reported to develop between 4 and 6 months post-IR [1,44,71]. In minipigs, IR-induced fibrosis has been reported at 30 days post-fractionated IR (200 cGy per fraction, 70 Gy total dose) [57]. Extensive fibrosis, measured by collagen deposition, was reported in CH3 mice and minipigs after 300 days and 16 weeks post-IR, respectively. In this study, CH3 mice received fractionated IR (5 × 6 Gy doses), whereas minipigs were exposed to a single 15 Gy dose of IR [54]. RNA-seq analysis of mouse SMGs 300 days post-IR revealed upregulation of genes involved in extracellular matrix remodeling and fibrosis (i.e., *Col23a1*, *Mmp2*, *Mmp3*, *Serping1*), whereas *Serping1* and *Mmp2* were also upregulated in minipigs at 16 weeks post-IR [54]. In a partial gland resection model utilized to investigate the mechanisms of salivary gland regeneration in the absence of confounding external stimuli, such as irradiation, genes involved in fibrotic development, ECM remodeling and the innate and adaptive immune system were similarly upregulated at days 3 and 14 post-resection in the murine SMG [89].

While humans [33,36,90] as well as mice and minipigs [1,44,54,57] show significant fibrotic damage to the salivary glands following irradiation, there is insufficient evidence to determine whether fibrosis is a cause or consequence of gland dysfunction. TGF-β, a known mediator of fibrogenesis in several tissues [91–94] is elevated in HNC patients following radiotherapy [95] and in murine models of IR-induced hyposalivation [96]. We have previously shown that TGF-β is upregulated in a mouse model of fibrosis caused by SMG excretory duct ligation and that in vivo administration of TGF-β inhibitors reduces duct ligation-induced salivary gland fibrosis [97]. TGF-β inhibition also efficiently reduces IR-induced lung [98,99] and rectal [100] fibrosis in mouse models. Further investigation is needed on the relationship of TGF-β and fibrosis to IR-induced hyposalivation and whether this pathway plays a significant role in chronic salivary gland dysfunction in RT.

3.11. Immunomodulation

The immunomodulatory effect of radiation on immune cells within tumors and normal tissue is a well-documented phenomenon in other models of IR-induced damage involving infiltration of immune cells of both the innate and adaptive immune system, as well as differentiation and gene expression changes within irradiated immune cell populations [101–103]. Lombaert et al. recently reported that female CH3 mice receiving fractionated IR (5 × 6 Gy) showed increased fibrosis, inflammation and expression of innate and adaptive immune markers (i.e., *Clec12a*, *Cma1*, *Pld4*, and *Lyz2*) in irradiated SMGs 300 days post-IR [54]. This is the first published evidence of IR-induced immunomodulation in mouse salivary glands, despite being an important area of research for other tissues and models of IR-induced damage, such as pneumonitis and pulmonary fibrosis following thoracic irradiation [102]. Similar changes in the expression patterns of these markers of immunomodulation have been shown in 15 Gy irradiated parotid glands of minipigs at 16 weeks post-IR [54].

In humans, there also is limited research on the effect of RT on salivary gland immune responses. SMG biopsies from patients receiving fractionated radiotherapy (1.8–2 Gy per fraction, 5 days per week, for a total dose of 60–70.6 Gy) revealed lymphocytic infiltration (i.e., sialadenitis), where the majority of lymphocytic infiltrates were $CD3^+$ T cells with a 1:1.8 ratio of $CD4^+$ to $CD8^+$ T cells and significant numbers of granzyme B-stained cytotoxic T cells [33]. Macrophages and monocytes were also present, localized to the periductal and periacinar compartments.

Immunomodulation is recognized as a driver of IR-induced pneumonitis and pulmonary fibrosis [102,104]. During the acute phase, myeloid- and lymphoid-derived immune cells infiltrate lung tissue, leading to inflammation and the release of cytokines and chemokines [102].

In the chronic phase, interactions between IR-damaged tissue-resident cells, recruited immune cells and the microenvironment activate signaling pathways that promote immunomodulation, myofibroblast activation and fibrosis [102]. In IR-induced pulmonary fibrosis, CD4+ T cells shift from pro-inflammatory (TH1 and TH17) during the pneumonitic phase to anti-inflammatory (TH2 and T_{REG}) during the fibrotic phase [102,104]. In addition to TH2 and T_{REG} cells, resident innate lymphoid cells (ILCs) are important regulators of fibrosis [105–107]. Notably, a unique subset of ILCs has been described in mouse SMGs [108,109], although their potential contributions to IR-induced fibrosis of the salivary gland are yet to be investigated. Nonetheless, the recent findings in CH3 mice [54], highlight the potential for future research to investigate the role of salivary gland immune cells in IR-induced hyposalivation.

4. Bystander Effect: Potential Role for Purinergic Signaling

Ionizing radiation affects cells within the radiation field and indirectly on adjacent, non-irradiated cells and tissue. This phenomenon, called the bystander effect, has been described for multiple cancer models [110–114] and has been investigated in relation to the protection of non-irradiated tissue [115], therapeutic approaches to cancer progression [112,116] and secondary radiation-induced neoplasms [112,117]. The bystander effect can be initiated by the release of several signaling molecules from irradiated cells, including ROS, nitric oxide (NO) or cytokines such as TGF-β1 [111,118] and through direct intercellular interactions via gap junctions or membrane channels [119–121] (Figure 2). While sparing techniques in cancer therapies for RT have attempted to remove salivary glands from the radiation field and/or reduce the overall radiation dose delivered to the glands, bystander effects still persist, suggesting that other radioprotective and regenerative approaches are needed [122].

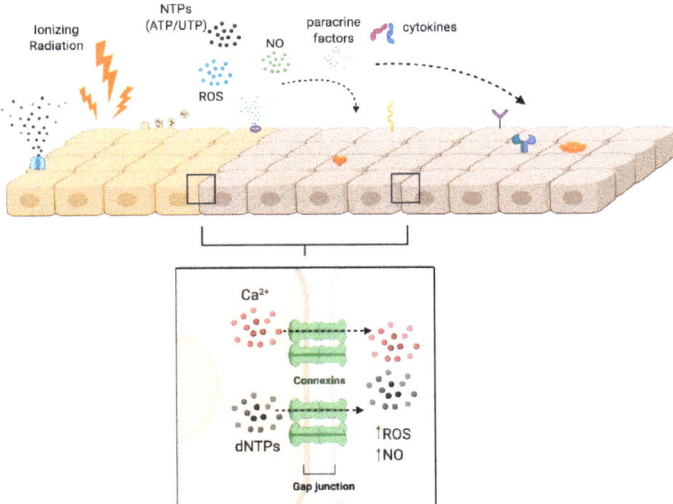

Figure 2. Radiation-Induced Bystander Effects. The bystander effect can be propagated by intercellular communication between adjacent cells via gap junctions or by autocrine or paracrine signaling processes whereby NTPs, nitric oxide (NO), reactive oxygen species (ROS), cytokines (e.g., TGF-β), or other second messengers elicit a response in non-irradiated cells. Created with Biorender.com.

In the past ten years, mounting evidence demonstrates that purinergic signaling can mediate the IR-induced bystander effect in adjacent, non-irradiated cells [110,122–128]. Extracellular nucleotides such as ATP (eATP), which are released into the extracellular space in response to cellular damage including ionizing radiation [124,128], act as autocrine or paracrine signaling molecules via activation of P2 receptors (P2Rs) on nearby cells [122–124,128–134]. In response to γ-irradiation, both human and murine cell lines have been shown to release ATP, thereby activating G protein-coupled P2Y [110,129,135] and ATP-gated ionotropic P2X receptors [126,136], which initiate purinergic signaling. Although no studies have yet investigated this bystander effect in IR-induced salivary gland dysfunction, we and others have reported on the expression of $P2Y_2$, P2X7 and P2X4 receptors in salivary gland epithelia of mice [137–139] and humans [139], suggesting that irradiated salivary glands in vivo should be highly sensitive to elevated levels of IR-induced eATP release. Mechanisms of P2 receptor signaling relevant to the bystander effect have been investigated in multiple tissues [110,122–128] and their potential roles in IR-induced salivary gland damage are summarized in Figure 3.

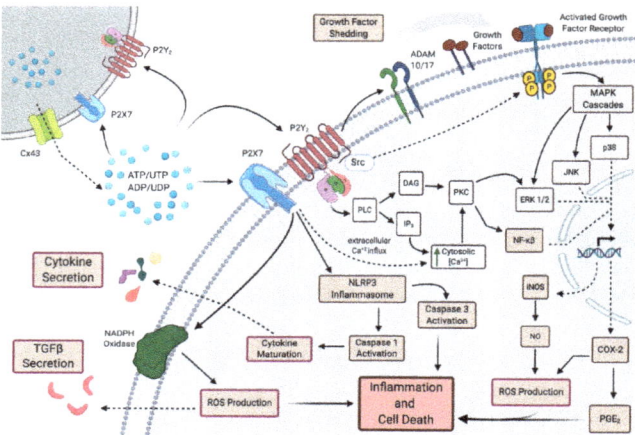

Figure 3. Purinergic Signaling in Bystander Effects. In response to elevated extracellular ATP (eATP) levels following irradiation, $P2Y_2R$ and P2X7R, which are expressed in murine and human salivary glands, may mediate a number of bystander effects. Through activation of the NLRP3 inflammasome, P2X7Rs promote ROS production, growth factor maturation (e.g., IL-1β) and subsequent release and apoptosis. Activation of either $P2Y_2R$ or P2X7R causes increased $[Ca^{2+}]_i$ and subsequent downstream signaling processes (e.g., ERK1/2 signaling, gene expression changes, inflammatory processes). $P2Y_2R$ activates phospholipase C (PLC) resulting in the production of inositol 1,4,5 trisphosphate (IP_3) and diacylglycerol (DAG), in turn mobilizing intracellular Ca^{2+} and activating protein kinase C (PKC), respectively, and subsequent downstream signaling. Through its C-terminal Src-homology 3 (SH3) domain, the $P2Y_2R$ is involved in Src-dependent activation of growth factor receptors (e.g., EGFR, VEGFR-2) and downstream MAPK signaling as well as transactivation of EGFRs through activation of metalloproteases, ADAM10 and ADAM17. $P2Y_2Rs$ may also contribute to the bystander effect by promoting latent TGF-β signaling. DAG: diacylglycerol; PLC: phospholipase C; PKC: protein kinase C; ERK: extracellular signal-regulated protein kinase; JNK: c-Jun N-terminal kinase; MAPK: mitogen-activated protein kinase; COX: cyclooxygenase; PGE_2: prostaglandin E_2; ADAM: A Disintegrin And Metalloprotease. Created with Biorender.com.

4.1. ATP Release

In addition to responding to elevated eATP, the P2X7 receptor (P2X7R) has been implicated in the IR-induced release of ATP. As previously described in B16 murine melanoma cells [124], we recently demonstrated that γ-irradiation of parotid epithelial cells induces release of eATP in a P2X7R-dependent manner [48]. One way that IR induces the release of eATP is through upregulation of connexin 43 (Cx43) [140], a gap junction hemichannel involved in intercellular communication [141], as well as eATP release [142,143]. The activation of P2X7R by eATP induces an increase in the cytoplasmic calcium concentration, $[Ca^{2+}]_i$, which promotes eATP release via Cx43 [128]. Indeed, Cx43-mediated release of ATP following irradiation of B16 melanoma cells is dependent on P2X7R [123]. As reported, IR-induced ATP release through Cx43 could be suppressed by blockade of P2X7R or downstream purinergic signaling pathways, including tyrosine kinase and Rho kinase activation, actin cytoskeletal rearrangements and increases in $[Ca^{2+}]_i$ and ROS production [123]. Together, these data demonstrate a role for P2X7R in mediating release of eATP following IR.

4.2. Dysregulated Calcium Signaling

Once released, eATP can then bind available P2 receptors, such as P2X7Rs or P2Y$_2$Rs, and promote a host of signaling processes. As we discussed earlier, a rapid increase in $[Ca^{2+}]_i$ is observed following irradiation of submandibular glands in mice via store-operated Ca^{2+} entry (SOCE), a response that was abrogated in TRMP2$^{-/-}$ mice [45]. Activation of either P2X7R or P2Y$_2$R by eATP leads to elevated $[Ca^{2+}]_i$ though by different mechanisms. Like TRPM2, P2Y$_2$Rs promote cytoplasmic entry of Ca^{2+} via SOCE [144], while P2X7Rs mediate extracellular Ca^{2+} influx [138]. Calcium signaling contributes to many of the signaling processes underlying bystander responses [145–147] that we will discuss in more detail below, including MAPK signaling [148], ROS production [146], NF-κB-mediated iNOS synthesis [149] and COX-2/PGE$_2$ signaling [149–152]. A rapid increase in $[Ca^{2+}]_i$ was observed in bystander cells that were exposed to conditioned medium (CM) from irradiated human keratinocytes [146], glioma and fibroblasts [148]. In human keratinocytes, the apoptosis observed in bystander cells following exposure to CM was blocked by treatment with the calcium chelator, EGTA, suggesting influx, not SOCE, was important for the observed bystander effect [146]. Because of the central role of Ca^{2+} signaling in mediating bystander effects, the contributions of P2 receptors to IR-induced increases in $[Ca^{2+}]_i$ following irradiation of the salivary gland should be further investigated.

4.3. MAPK Signaling

A number of groups have implicated MAPK signaling in propagating bystander effects in non-irradiated cells [146,147,153]. Using human B-lymphoblastoid cell lines, one group reported phosphorylation of ERK1/2, JNK and p38 in bystander cells exposed to CM from X-ray irradiated cells [153]. Additionally, bystander-induced caspase 3/7 activation could be diminished by treatment with ERK inhibitor U0126, JNK inhibitor SP600125 or p38 inhibitor SB203580. Human keratinocytes treated with conditioned medium (CM) from irradiated keratinocytes showed elevated ERK and JNK signaling [146]. CM-mediated apoptosis in bystander keratinocytes could be blocked by JNK inhibition, although ERK inhibition seemed to increase bystander-induced apoptosis in these cells [146].

G$_q$-coupled P2Y receptors (P2Y$_{1,2,4,6,11}$Rs) activate phospholipase C (PLC) resulting in the production of inositol 1,4,5-triphosphate (IP3) and diacylglycerol (DAG), in turn mobilizing intracellular Ca^{2+} and activating protein kinase C (PKC) and subsequent downstream signaling pathways [144], including ERK1/2 activation, that have been implicated in mediating the bystander effect [146,154]. Further, through its C-terminal Src homology 3 (SH3) domain, the P2Y$_2$R is involved in Src-dependent activation of growth factor receptors (e.g., EGFR, VEGFR-2), ERK1/2, and JNK [144]. P2Y$_2$R is also capable of transactivation of EGFRs by activating metalloproteases (i.e., ADAM10 and ADAM17) [155]. In turn, EGFR activation initiates MAPK signaling cascades. In this way, P2Y$_2$Rs are capable of mediating MAPK signaling through canonical G$_q$-coupled signaling or through activation of growth factor receptors such as EGFR.

Another potential role for P2Rs in mediating bystander effects involves PKC. We discussed above that knocking down PKCδ expression inhibits IR-induced apoptosis in irradiated murine parotid glands [63], while blocking PKCδ activity by administration of nanoparticles containing siRNA targeting PKCδ reduces apoptosis in irradiated mouse SMG [3]. Directly blocking c-Src with imatinib or dasatinib had a similar anti-apoptotic effect and enhanced saliva production [78]. P2R antagonists (DIDS, suramin and Cibacron Blue 3GA) increase phosphorylation of PKCδ in rat parotid acinar cells, confirming that P2 activity promotes PKCδ activation [156]. Together these data suggest that ATP-induced activation of P2Rs promotes apoptosis in bystander cells via PKCδ phosphorylation.

4.4. COX-2/Prostaglandin E_2 Signaling

The inflammatory cyclooxygenase-2 (COX-2) signaling pathway that is required for PGE_2 synthesis has been implicated in promoting bystander effects [149–152,157]. Most bystander studies involve the transfer of conditioned medium from irradiated cells to non-irradiated cells in vitro. Zhou et al. used a novel mylar strip culture dish to shield a portion of human fibroblasts from irradiation while remaining in the same culture vessel as irradiated cells [150]. Using this technique, bystander human fibroblasts showed overexpression of COX-2 [150]. Inhibition of COX-2 with NS-398 decreased the bystander effect in non-irradiated cells, as determined by the frequency of mutations in the hypoxanthine-guanine phosphoribosyltransferase (HPRT⁻) locus and the percent of surviving cells [150]. They also demonstrated that inhibition of ERK1/2, which lies upstream of COX-2, could diminish the bystander effects. More recently, this same group reported that NF-κB was important for mediating bystander effects in human fibroblasts, which could be attributed to NF-κB-mediated inducible NO synthase (iNOS) and COX-2 expression [149]. The NF-κB inhibitor, Bay 11-7082, and 2-(4-carboxyphenyl)-4,4,5,5-tetramethylimidazoline-1-oxyl-3-oxide, a scavenger of NO, decreased mutation frequency in bystander cells [149].

PGE_2 has also been suggested to mediate the bystander effect [147,157]. We have previously reported that PGE_2 levels are increased in parotid acinar cell culture supernatant 24–72 h post-IR [48]. We also reported reduced levels of PGE_2 release in mice lacking P2X7R [48]. In addition to these findings, P2X7Rs and P2Y$_2$Rs lie upstream of many of the signaling pathways resulting in expression of COX-2 (Figure 3). Together, these findings suggest that COX-2/PGE_2-mediated bystander effects are dependent on signaling through P2X7Rs or P2Y$_2$Rs.

4.5. DNA Damage Response

Elevated levels of γH2AX are an indicator of DNA damage, a well-documented response to ionizing radiation [59]. In irradiated A549 human lung cancer cells, elevated γH2AX levels were abrogated by pretreatment with the ectonucleotidase apyrase [158], a response that could be eliminated by the ectonucleotidase inhibitor ARL67156 or addition of ATP or UTP. Similar to our findings in primary murine parotid epithelial cells [48], ATP is released from A549 cells following γ-irradiation (2 Gy) in a P2X7R-dependent manner. The finding that antagonism of P2Y$_6$R, P2Y$_{12}$R or P2X7R blocked activation of DNA repair mechanisms led to the overall hypothesis that P2X7R-dependent release of ATP and subsequent autocrine activation of G protein-coupled P2Y receptors was responsible for the observed DNA damage response [158]. Additionally, downstream P2R signaling molecules, such as nitric oxide (NO), are important mediators of radiation-induced DNA damage in bystander cells [128,159].

4.6. Reactive Oxygen Species and TGF-β1

ROS and TGF-β1 are well-appreciated mediators of the bystander effect in multiple IR models [160], serving as second messengers in an autocrine or paracrine fashion. In response to ATP, P2X7Rs regulate production of ROS by NLRP3 inflammasome activation [161] and ROS promote TGF-β1 release [162]. P2Y$_2$Rs may also contribute to the bystander effect by promoting latent TGF-β signaling. TGF-β, latency activated protein (LAP) and latent TGF-β binding proteins (LTBP) form a covalently-bound large latent complex (LLC) that is secreted from cells, whereupon it binds to integrins (e.g., $\alpha_v\beta_5$, $\alpha_v\beta_6$, $\alpha_v\beta_3$ and $\alpha_v\beta_8$) in the extracellular matrix (ECM) through LAP interaction with RGD sequences. Latent activation of TGF-β signaling can occur through metalloprotease-dependent cleavage of LAP or LTBP or disruption of LAP-RGD interaction with integrins [163–166]. P2Y$_2$R activation also induces metalloprotease activity [167,168] and the P2Y$_2$R contains an extracellularly-oriented RGD sequence that enables its direct binding and activation of the $\alpha_v\beta_5$ integrin [167]. Through these mechanisms, activation of P2Y$_2$R or P2X7R could promote the TGF-β1 and ROS-mediated bystander effects.

4.7. Immunomodulation

There is currently insufficient research regarding the role of immunomodulation in IR-induced salivary gland dysfunction or in models of IR-induced bystander effects to fully define the role of P2 receptors. A T cell-mediated mechanism of long-distance effects on metastatic lesions following irradiation of primary tumors—coined the abscopal effect—has been described [169–171]. Most bystander effect studies are performed in vitro, making it difficult to ascertain the contributions of various immune cells that recapitulate in vivo conditions [172]. However, one study utilized an in vivo model of radiation-induced acute myeloid leukemia to investigate the bystander effect. They found that the long-term bystander consequences of irradiation in vivo were due to altered macrophage activity [172]. P2Y$_2$R signaling pathways are involved in the recruitment, migration and proliferation of immune cells [173–175], and thus activation of this receptor by elevated eATP levels following IR should mediate the modification of the immune landscape in the salivary gland.

In conclusion, the available data strongly support the notion that purinergic signaling plays a role in the IR-induced bystander effect in multiple models. In particular, the role of P2X7R, P2X4R, and P2Y$_2$R, given their reported expression in human and mouse salivary glands, should be further investigated for their potential as novel targets for the prevention of the bystander effects underlying IR-induced salivary hypofunction.

5. Therapeutics

As mentioned above, treatments for RT-induced hyposalivation are limited to sialagogues, such as pilocarpine and cevimeline, which induce saliva secretion from residual acinar cells, artificial saliva and the single FDA-approved radioprotective therapeutic, amifostine. There are also a number of salivary gland radiation sparing techniques that have been utilized to minimize IR-induced damage. Promising new radioprotective and regenerative approaches are being investigated in preclinical animal models. The next section summarizes current and promising therapeutic approaches to IR-induced salivary gland dysfunction.

5.1. Salivary Gland-Sparing Techniques

5.1.1. Dosing Strategies

Fractionated radiation is the primary method of radiotherapy for cancer patients, including for the treatment of HNC, but causes cell toxicity and other severe side effects. Fractionated radiation divides the total curative dose into a series of smaller doses, which allows the patient to better tolerate and maintain the treatment. Conventional fractionated radiotherapy for HNC patients is commonly prescribed as 2 Gy per day, five days per week, for multiple weeks, to a total dose of 70 Gy [18]. Multiple small radiation doses allow non-tumor cells to recover between IR exposures, while more severely damaging malignant cells due to their high proliferation rates. A meta-analysis, including 34 trials and 11,969 HNC patients (with primarily late-stage tumors of the oropharynx and larynx), comparing different subtypes of fractionated radiation found that hyper-fractionated radiation, where a patient receives the same total curative dose of radiation, but in two fractions per day (totaling 4 Gy/day), showed improved overall survival and progression-free survival when compared to conventional fractionation (2 Gy/day). However, these more intensive radiation schedules induced more severe side effects, including increased instances of mucositis, which caused RT patients to go on feeding tubes more frequently [176]. Overall, hyper-fractionated radiation was less feasible than conventional approaches due to the cost, scheduling difficulties and the increased severity of side effects. Other altered fractionation dosing schedules, including increasing the IR doses per day and shortening the total time to curative dose, were evaluated, but these treatments did not show improvement in disease outcomes or sparing organs at risk compared to conventional fractionation [176]. While fractionated therapies are more efficacious as cancer treatments, there is currently no evidence that hyper-fractionated radiotherapy or other altered fractionated dosing schedules have any effect on decreasing the incidence of xerostomia [19,176].

5.1.2. Intensity Modulated Radiation Therapy (IMRT)

IMRT is a form of radiotherapy for tumors with advanced precision and dosing control. IMRT utilizes three-dimensional (3D) imaging of tumors, typically by computerized tomography (CT) or magnetic resonance imaging (MRI), to design beam patterns with varying intensities to direct at the tumor with the goal of sparing non-malignant tissues, especially radiosensitive tissues, such as the brain, spinal cord and salivary glands [177]. These complex, variable RT patterns aim to keep the total dose to below 26 Gy for parotid glands [178,179] and 39 Gy for submandibular glands [180] to spare gland function without decreasing the dose to the tumor. Computer-calculated dosing and beam angles are defined with the 3D images and the beam is typically targeted at the tumor site with image guidance from CT or X-ray scans of the patient to deliver varying beam doses across the tumor in a fixed field. IMRT controls tumor growth better than or similarly to 3D-conformal radiotherapy (CRT). A study looking at tumor recurrence in 3D-CRT- versus IMRT-treated HNC patients found that those receiving IMRT following surgical resection of the primary tumor had improved tumor control two years post-treatment compared to patients receiving 3D-CRT; however, treatment modalities showed no difference in tumor recurrence following definitive radiotherapy [181]. Conversely, a meta-analysis of studies evaluating disease-free survival and overall survival in patients receiving 3D-CRT or IMRT found that there was no difference in outcomes [182]. Compared to conventional radiotherapy, IMRT is substantially more time-intensive, with the need for extensive planning and increased clinician and machine time [177]. However, IMRT reduces non-malignant tissue radiation exposure and improves the QoL for HNC survivors post-therapy [182]. The first study to evaluate differences in xerostomia rankings across patients receiving 3D-CRT versus IMRT found that patients who underwent IMRT, while still experiencing xerostomia, had significantly improved scores at all times during and following radiotherapy [183]. Despite the improvements in sparing salivary glands, IMRT still leads to hyposalivation and xerostomia and has been shown to alter saliva composition, including pH and electrolyte content; however, these patients have improved saliva output one year after ending treatment [184].

5.1.3. Volumetric Modulated Arc Therapy (VMAT)

VMAT, also known as Rapid Arc therapy, is a recently developed form of radiotherapy that continuously exposes the tumor to a radiation beam while rotating in an arc shape around the tumor. VMAT improves radiation targeting by more precisely controlling rotational speed, shape and dose rate, where radiation beams can be directed as a single or double beam towards the tumor site and can rotate in a full or half arc [185]. One major benefit of VMAT is the efficiency in delivering radiotherapy and the reduction in machine time, when compared to IMRT; however, extensive planning for targeting radiation arcs to the tumor is a limitation [185]. Radiation dosing measurements between VMAT and IMRT were compared and IMRT offered greater homogeneity while VMAT had increased conformity, although both therapies used similar dosing strategies for planning target volume and VMAT showed reduced radiation exposure to organs at risk, including salivary glands, brain stem, spinal cord and the oral cavity [186]. These results were supported by a more recent study that slightly favored VMAT, particularly in the context of increasing the patient's QoL [187]. Although VMAT is a relatively recent development in radiotherapy [185], there have been studies over the last decade offering improvements in VMAT, such as auto-planning to precisely target tumors while conserving organs at risk. Manual contouring around organs at risk is a standard planning objective of VMAT to avoid radiation exposure to non-malignant regions, but this is time and labor intensive. Auto-contouring, accomplished with a computer system, has been combined with simplified contouring, which uses simple drawn structures of organs at risk to develop VMAT plans with acceptable dosing strategies for organs, specifically salivary glands, that can be completed in a more efficient time as compared to manual contouring (2 min for auto-planning VMAT versus 7 min for manual) [188]. In auto-planning VMAT, computer calculated dosing strategies are generated with input on planning target volume as well as contours of organs at risk that require minimal radiation exposure. Computational plans can then be manually edited by clinicians to better define therapy components. Auto-planning VMAT shows similar or improved dosing characteristics for tumors, reduces exposure to organs at risk and requires less clinician time, when compared to manual planning [189]. These studies show the continuous improvements being made in radiotherapy techniques, with VMAT becoming a more accessible and efficient treatment option for HNC patients, especially in areas with limited medical resources.

5.1.4. Proton Beam Radiotherapy (PBRT)

PBRT is a relatively new and alternative form of radiotherapy that focuses protons in a beam to target a tumor site. Compared to photons, protons have unique physical characteristics and decelerate very quickly as they travel through matter, exhibiting a phenomenon referred to as the Bragg peak [190]. This difference allows for more precise targeting of protons to the malignancy and reduces potential damage to organs at risk, such as salivary glands. In a recent study comparing the development of secondary tumors following 3D-CRT, IMRT or PBRT, 3D-CRT and IMRT had similar rates of cancer recurrence, whereas PBRT showed reduced recurrence across cancer types [191]. Unfortunately, proton therapy is currently expensive and understudied, making it a less ideal option for most clinicians and patients [192]. More research evaluating the differences in tumor control and damage to organs at risk with PBRT versus IMRT or VMAT should be conducted to further validate the efficacy of this alternative type of radiotherapy.

5.1.5. Intraoral Stents and Temporary Submandibular Gland (SMG) Transplantation

Two additional non-pharmacological salivary gland-sparing interventions have been utilized, i.e., intraoral stents and temporary submandibular gland transplantation. Intraoral stents are personalized medical devices designed to position and stabilize the oral cavity to prevent unnecessary irradiation of adjacent tissues. These devices are easy to manufacture [193] and have been demonstrated to efficiently reduce irradiation of off-target tissues [194–196]. Salivary glands can be protected from irradiation by temporarily relocating them further away from the field of irradiation in a procedure known as temporary SMG transplantation. This surgical alternative has been shown to be safe and cost effective and involves releasing the SMG from surrounding tissues and temporarily repositioning it in the submental space over the digastric muscle, thereby removing it from the radiation field [197]. Pathak et al. showed that in patients receiving RT, those that underwent temporary SMG transplantation had no significant differences in salivary flow rates before RT compared to those who did not undergo transplantation [168]. After RT, 73% of the group that received the transplantation had a preserved mean salivary flow rate, compared to 27% of the group that did not receive transplantation [198]. Despite its success, due to the risks of co-transplantation of malignant tissues and subsequent relapse or secondary metastases, SMG transplantation is only used in RT for specific types of head and neck cancers.

Recently, novel salivary glands have been identified in humans, dubbed the tubarial glands due to their proximity to the torus tubarius [199], in a retrospective analysis of PET/CT scans of 100 prostate or para-urethral gland cancer patients using radiolabeled ligands that bind prostate-specific membrane antigen (PSMA), which is highly expressed in all major and minor salivary glands [199,200]. The tubarial glands were described as predominantly mucous gland tissue with multiple draining ducts located in the dorsolateral pharyngeal wall. The sparing techniques we describe in this review have not taken into consideration these glands and none of the current targeted techniques avoid these structures that lie posterior to the nasopharynx [199]. The effect of RT dose on tubarial glands was further investigated with the incidence of xerostomia and dysphagia found to be correlated in 723 HNC patients at both 12- and 24-months after initial physician-rated xerostomia. This exciting discovery raises the question of whether modifying radiation fields to spare the tubarial glands will prevent RT-induced xerostomia. As of yet, these glands have not been identified in any preclinical animal models and it is noteworthy that mice lack the torus tubarius [201]. However, if similar glands are present in animal models, we anticipate that future studies will examine possible RT field modifications to optimize radioprotective therapies that preserve glandular function.

Radiation treatment plans for HNC are not one size fits all and depend on many factors, such as cancer type, location, stage and the patient's overall health. Comparisons of multiple types of radiotherapy plans for HNC have been performed and researchers found that there are benefits to certain planning methods, depending on the type and stage of HNC [202]. Furthermore, while there have been substantial improvements in RT techniques in recent years to reduce exposure to organs at risk, patients still exhibit side effects, such as hyposalivation and xerostomia, which can lead to multiple complications, as discussed earlier [1]. Further evaluation of mechanisms of radiation damage to salivary glands to develop novel radioprotective and/or regenerative approaches is, therefore, necessary to improve the quality of life for HNC survivors.

5.2. Symptom Relief

5.2.1. Artificial Saliva

Radiation-induced xerostomia is influenced by factors including the patient's salivary gland health and function prior to treatment, the magnitude of the treatment and the individual response of the patient. Current strategies to manage RT-induced xerostomia provide only short-term relief. Artificial saliva products have played a limited role in the treatment of xerostomia due to their extremely transient nature. Despite human saliva consisting of approximately 99.5% water, the proteins, lipids, ions and other biomolecules that compose the remaining 0.5% are essential and have yet to be efficiently mimicked artificially [41]. Spirk et al. conducted a small clinical study evaluating the three most utilized artificial saliva products, characterizing their physiochemical properties in comparison to unstimulated human saliva [42]. Their study demonstrated that these artificial saliva products differed significantly from human saliva in pH, osmolarity and/or electrical conductivity [42]. Their findings explain why the utility of artificial saliva or saliva substitutes is limited.

5.2.2. Sialagogues

Treatments to stimulate the function of remaining salivary gland tissue have had more success than artificial saliva. Systemic sialagogues stimulate saliva secretion from residual, functional salivary gland acinar cells to compensate somewhat for decreases in saliva flow due to RT and, thus, their effectiveness depends heavily on the number of surviving acinar cells [203]. Both pilocarpine and bethanechol are systemic sialagogues that activate muscarinic-cholinergic receptors. A phase III randomized clinical trial studying the effects of pilocarpine therapy after RT in HNC patients demonstrated that unstimulated saliva flow in the patients who received pilocarpine therapy was significantly higher than in those receiving a placebo [204]. The authors reported that this increase in saliva flow did not correlate with improved QoL scores and also concluded that pilocarpine therapy had no significant effect on the incidence of mucositis. These observations support previous clinical studies [205–207]. Cevimeline, a quinuclidine derivative of acetylcholine that selectively activates M3 muscarinic receptors, has obtained FDA approval for xerostomia treatment in Sjögren's syndrome patients, although its use for RT-induced xerostomia remains off-label [21,208]. In a prospective, single-arm study with 255 participants, cevimeline taken orally for 52 weeks improved symptoms in 59.2% of HNC patients who received RT [209]. The benefit of cevimeline over pilocarpine is that its half-life is much longer [210], offering prolonged benefit to patients. Similarly, bethanechol is a stable analogue of acetylcholine and, thus, its effects last longer, as it undergoes slower degradation by cholinesterases. Similar to pilocarpine, bethanechol stimulates the parasympathetic nervous system by activating muscarinic receptors. Although still only indicated for post-operative or postnatal urinary retention, studies by Epstein et al. and Gorsky et al. demonstrate that post-RT bethanechol therapy is just as effective as pilocarpine therapy [211,212]. Patients receiving either bethanechol or pilocarpine reported a 39% or 33% subjective increase in unstimulated saliva production, respectively [212]. Patients receiving a combination therapy of bethanechol and pilocarpine did not show statistically significant improvements over either monotherapy. The authors postulate that this is due to "parenchymal fatigue", hinting at a saturation limit of the remaining healthy tissues [212]. Jham et al. was one of the first studies to evaluate bethanechol therapy concomitant with receiving RT in regards to preventing rather than ameliorating xerostomia [213]. They observed that the use of bethanechol throughout the duration of RT led to a statistically significant increase in whole resting saliva secretion at the culmination of RT, compared to a control group receiving artificial saliva. Similarly, a double-blind randomized clinical study [214] evaluating the utility of bethanechol therapy concomitantly with or after RT demonstrated that patients receiving bethanechol reported improved xerostomia symptoms and had statistically significant increases in unstimulated and stimulated whole saliva flow [214]. Despite many promising studies with a diverse cohort of HNC patients, there is still a lack of longitudinal studies. A systemic meta-analysis assessing the effect of pharmacological interventions for RT-induced xerostomia found that there was insufficient data to support any effect of pilocarpine therapy on salivary gland function or QoL [215]. The authors noted that what data were available were of very low quality, supporting the need for additional studies. As the time of writing this review, there have been no clinical studies evaluating treatment outcomes utilizing muscarinic receptor agonists beyond a few months post-RT. Given the lifelong presentation of post-RT xerostomia, therapies need to be effective over an extended period of time. Additionally, because of the transient effect of artificial saliva and sialagogues, these treatment options present a significant financial burden [12].

5.3. Radioprotection

5.3.1. Amifostine

While drugs such as pilocarpine and cevimeline have been approved by the FDA to treat xerostomia, amifostine was the first and currently the only FDA-approved radioprotective drug to prevent xerostomia following RT. The radioprotective effects of amifostine are thought to be due to its ability to scavenge free radicals [216] (Figure 4). In an open-label phase III clinical trial, Wasserman et al. showed that 2 years post-RT HNC patients who received both RT and amifostine presented with a lower incidence of xerostomia, compared to those receiving RT alone [190]. Additionally, the amifostine group had significantly reduced mouth dryness scores and a significant number of these patients exhibited meaningful unstimulated saliva production. Moreover, amifostine administration with RT did not significantly alter progression-free survival and overall survival rates compared to RT alone [217], a finding supported by a meta-analysis [218]. This is important, given that two major criticisms of amifostine therapy are its toxicity and the possibility that it could reduce the efficacy of RT by protecting cancer cells. In contrast to these promising findings, a randomized double-blind trial reported that amifostine did not affect the incidence of acute or late RT-induced xerostomia (grade ≥ 2) over placebo in HNC patients [219]. A 2017 meta-analysis concluded that there is little evidence that amifostine provides any benefit, and no evidence that reported benefits last longer than 12 months [215]. Additionally, a phase III clinical study by Rades et al. reported that adverse effects of amifostine therapy in combination with RT were responsible for a statistically significant percentage (41%) of patients in the study group discontinuing treatment [220]. The reported clinical benefit of amifostine is questionable and, due to toxicity concerns, amifostine is not widely used [17].

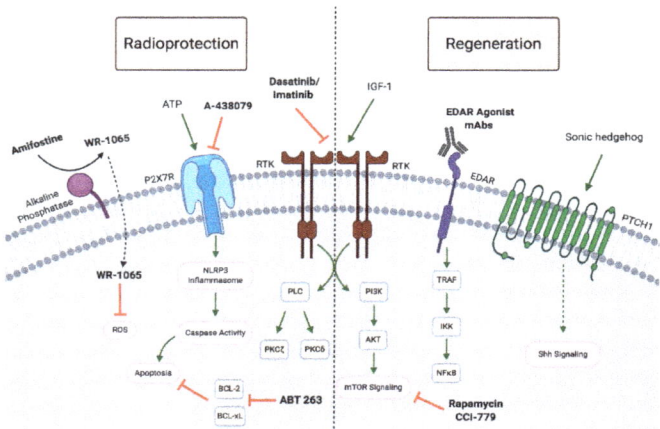

Figure 4. Pharmacological Approaches to Salivary Gland Radioprotection and Regeneration. Amifostine is currently the only radioprotective therapeutic approved for the prevention of RT-induced hyposalivation. The membrane-bound alkaline phosphatase converts Amifostine to WR-1065 that is then taken up by the cell. WR-1065 is thought to promote radioprotection by scavenging reactive species in turn affecting gene expression, apoptosis, chromatin stability, DNA damage repair and enzymatic activity [221,222]. Other promising radioprotective therapeutics being investigated in preclinical animal models include the P2X7R antagonist, A-438079 [48], and the tyrosine kinase inhibitors, dasatinib and imatinib [77,78]. Pharmacological approaches to regeneration studied in animal models post-IR target a number of signaling pathways. IGF-1 treatment 4–7 days post-IR restored saliva production in a PKCζ-dependent manner [55]. mTOR signaling is another target that has been investigated by several groups to promote salivary gland regeneration [88,223]. Administration of the rapamycin analog, CCI-779, following IR improved saliva flow rates at 30 days post-IR [88]. Transient upregulation of Shh signaling by either overexpressing a Shh transgene or by administering a smoothened agonist, restored stimulated saliva flow [224]. EDAR agonists, such as monoclonal antibodies that promote EDAR signaling, are essential for salivary gland development and have shown promise in restoring salivary gland function in mice [65]. The senolytic agent, ABT263, which depletes senescent cells by inhibiting BCL-2 and BCL-xL, has been shown to promote salivary gland regeneration and self-renewal capabilities of residual salivary gland stem cells [68]. RTK: receptor tyrosine kinase; PLC: phospholipase C; PKC: protein kinase C; BCL: B-cell lymphoma; TRAF: tumor necrosis factor receptor-associated factor; IKK: IkB kinase; AKT: protein kinase B; EDAR: ectodysplasin A-1 receptor; PTCH: patched receptor. Created with Biorender.com.

5.3.2. Promising Preclinical Studies

Although there is currently only one FDA-approved radioprotective therapy, there are promising preclinical studies investigating potential radioprotective approaches (Figure 4). We recently reported that antagonism of the ATP-gated ionotropic P2X7 receptor (P2X7R) by i.p. injection of A-438079 in FVB mice provided significant radioprotection and maintained carbachol-induced saliva flow rates similar to non-irradiated mice [48]. P2X7R is highly expressed in mouse salivary glands, where its activation induces pro-inflammatory responses, including membrane blebbing, caspase activation, IL-1β release, recruitment of immune cells and NLRP3 inflammasome assembly [161,225,226]. We also have previously reported that A-438079 attenuates lymphocytic infiltration of SMGs and increases saliva secretion in a mouse model of the autoimmune disease Sjögren's syndrome [161,227]. Another promising pharmacological approach is the use of tyrosine kinase inhibitors (TKIs). Delivery of TKIs, dasatinib or imatinib, protect the mouse salivary gland from IR-induced damage and loss of function without affecting xenograft tumor growth [78]. This response was due to reduced activation of PKCδ, an important regulator of apoptosis in salivary gland acinar cells [63,77,228–230].

Introduction of human neurotrophic factor neurturin (NRTN) using an adeno-associated virus serotype 2 (AAV2) vector prior to IR, but not post-IR, was radioprotective, preventing hyposalivation in both murine and porcine models [54]. NRTN is essential for proper innervation of the salivary glands, which is required for salivary secretory function. RNA sequencing analysis revealed a reduction in expression of fibrotic genes and both innate and humoral immune responses in mice and minipigs receiving AAV2-NRTN [54]. While additional studies are warranted to further investigate immune responses and the duration of improvement of saliva secretion in the IR-treated porcine model, these exciting findings in the highly translational Yucatan minipig model [57,231] are promising for future clinical trials.

5.4. Regeneration

There are currently no FDA-approved therapeutics available to patients to restore salivary function after RT. Stem cell therapies to repair or regenerate damaged salivary gland tissue and gene therapy approaches are being studied in preclinical animal models [232]. Additionally, there are two active clinical trials that are testing the efficacy of delivering human aquaporin-1 (hAQP1) to IR-damaged salivary glands to improve secretory function.

5.4.1. Gene Therapy

There are currently two clinical trials investigating the delivery of aquaporin-1 (AQP1) via adeno-associated viral vector 2 (AAV2) to treat IR-induced salivary hypofunction (ClinicalTrials.gov NCT02446249 and NCT04043104). AQP1 is a constitutively active water channel that facilitates secretion of fluid along an osmotic gradient [233]. AQP1 is expressed in the myoepithelial and endothelial cells of the human [234–236] and mouse [237] salivary glands and is limited to endothelial cells in the rat SMG [238]. Adenoviral delivery of human AQP1 (AdhAQP1) to rat SMGs by retrograde ductal instillation 3–4 months following IR (17.5 or 21 Gy) resulted in a 2- to 3-fold increase in salivary fluid secretion compared to controls [233]. The minipig closely replicates the structural and functional responses of the human salivary gland to irradiation [57,231] and, thus, is a highly translational model for evaluating novel therapies to prevent or reverse IR-induced salivary gland damage in humans. After determining an 85–90% decrease in saliva flow in minipigs at 16 weeks post-IR (20 Gy), AAV2-hAQP1 was delivered directly to the parotid gland via the Stensen's duct at 17 weeks post-IR [239]. In contrast to minipigs receiving control vector or saline that continued to exhibit diminished salivary output, minipigs receiving AAV2-hAQP1 had a consistent improvement in saliva secretory volume up to 35% of pre-IR levels by 8 weeks following AAV2-hAQP1 administration. As anticipated, the water channel hAQP1 did not reverse changes in saliva composition induced by IR [239]. Adenoviral delivery of hAQP1 in a phase I clinical trial in patients experiencing RT-induced xerostomia resulted in both short- and long-term improvement of parotid salivary flow and sustained symptomatic relief for 2–3 years [240,241]. In contrast to delivery of exogenous AQP1, forced expression of native AQP1 in human cells, including salivary gland cell lines and primary human salivary progenitor cells, has been achieved by delivery of guide RNAs targeting the promoter region of human AQP1 [242,243].

5.4.2. Stem Cell Therapies

As discussed above, progenitor and/or stem cell populations are essential for regeneration of functional salivary glands in mice [2,55,85,86]. Regeneration of salivary glands using stem cell therapies is a promising approach to ameliorate IR-induced salivary gland dysfunction. Isolation of Sca-1-, c-Kit- and Musashi-1-expressing mouse salivary gland stem cells has been achieved by in vitro culture in 3D salispheres followed by enrichment of stem cells with FACS using c-Kit as a marker [86]. These c-Kit+ cells were capable of differentiating into functional amylase-producing acinar cells. This same group then investigated the effect of transplanting salisphere cultures in salivary glands of irradiated (15 Gy) female mice. Ninety days after salisphere transplantation, IR-damaged salivary glands in mice showed similar morphology to non-irradiated glands, with restored acinar cell populations and improved saliva production compared to irradiated, untreated glands [86]. Perhaps most impressive was the number of cells required for restoration, i.e., as few as 300 c-Kit$^+$ progenitor cells were capable of restoring salivary gland function [86]. Additional populations of murine salivary stem and/or progenitor cells have been identified that are capable of regenerating salivary gland tissue and rescuing IR-induced hyposalivation in mouse models. As few as 100 CD24$^+$c-Kit$^+$Sca1$^+$ progenitor cells from adult murine SMGs were capable of restoring saliva secretion and functional acini in vivo [244]. Isolated CD24^{hi}/Cd29^{hi} adult murine salivary gland progenitor cells were capable of multi-lineage differentiation in vitro and restored salivary function in vivo [245]. While less is known about adult human salivary gland stem cells, a similar c-Kit$^+$ stem cell population has been identified [246] that is capable of self-renewal and restoring salivary gland function following irradiation in a murine xenotransplantation model [247]. A number of groups are testing novel biomaterials approaches harnessing the regenerative potential of isolated stem or progenitor cells to engineer implantable tissue [248]. Additionally, one group is using primary murine SMG cells—rather than isolated stem cells—to build cell sheets for salivary gland regeneration [249].

Rather than delivering progenitor cells to IR-damaged glands, other groups are investigating signaling pathways that may restore progenitor cell populations lost in RT (Figure 4). Transient overexpression of Shh restored IR-induced hyposalivation in mice by maintaining salivary stem/progenitor cells [224]. Shh signaling has been shown to be essential for SMG development in mice [250,251] and is activated during regeneration [252]. Activation of the Shh pathway also preserves normal parasympathetic innervation of the SMG [224]. Recently, another group found that depleting senescent salivary gland cells following IR by treatment with the senolytic agent, ABT263, an inhibitor of BCL-2 and BCL-xL that selectively induces apoptosis in senescent cells, at either 8 or 11 weeks post-IR (15 Gy) led to regeneration of aquaporin-5-expressing acinar cells and improved salivary gland function in C57BL/6 mice [68]. Using an in vitro organoid culture model, this group demonstrated that elimination of IR-induced senescent cells enhanced the self-renewal potential of remaining salivary gland stem cells [68]. Another pharmacological approach for preventing IR-induced progenitor cell damage involves administration of insulin-like growth factor 1 (IGF-1). Chibly et al. demonstrated that IGF-1 delivered 4–7 days following irradiation improved saliva production in a PKCζ-dependent manner [55]. Finally, Emmerson et al. identified a SOX2$^+$ adult human salivary gland progenitor cell population in all three major salivary glands (submandibular, sublingual and parotid glands) that was capable of differentiating into acinar, but not ductal cells [24]. They demonstrated that SOX2 was essential for salivary gland regeneration following a single 10 Gy dose of γ-radiation to the murine sublingual gland. Using an ex vivo model, SOX2$^+$ cells were capable of repopulating the irradiated murine sublingual gland. Furthermore, in human SMG cells, SOX2 expression as well as both acinar and ductal markers were maintained by muscarinic activation [24], suggesting that future studies should target muscarinic signaling as a means to restore residual progenitor cell function after RT.

5.4.3. Pharmacological Approaches

In addition to gene and stem cell therapies, some groups are taking a pharmacological approach to salivary gland regeneration (Figure 4). Rapamycin, an inhibitor of mTOR signaling, is one such agent [88,223]. As discussed earlier, treating FVB mice with the rapamycin analog, CCI-779, on days 4–8 following IR reduced proliferation rates and improved saliva flow rates 30 days post-IR [88]. CCI-779 is an FDA-approved therapy for the treatment of renal cell carcinoma and mantle cell lymphoma [253] and both CCI-779 and rapamycin are currently being investigated in clinical trials for several other cancer types and amyotrophic lateral sclerosis (ALS) (clinicaltrials.gov). Minipigs receiving i.p. injection of rapamycin 1 h prior to RT had improved saliva flow rates 12 weeks post-IR [223], suggesting that targeting mTOR signaling may be beneficial as either a radioprotective or regenerative therapeutic approach. Another potential pharmacological intervention to promote salivary gland regeneration is the post-irradiation delivery of EDAR agonist monoclonal antibodies. EDAR signaling is involved in salivary gland development and transient activation of EDAR signaling post-IR (5 Gy) restores salivary gland function and amylase levels through 90 days in mice [65]. In conclusion, although still in the developmental phase, pharmacological approaches as well as gene and stem cell therapies provide promising new avenues for restoring salivary gland function in HNC patients who have undergone RT.

6. Summary

Whether as a result of direct radiation exposure or due to bystander effects, radiotherapy of the head and neck region results in damage to salivary glands that often leads to permanent dysfunction and associated complications, such as increased oral infections, functional impairments in speaking, swallowing, and eating and diminished quality of life. The mechanisms of acute and chronic dysfunction have been investigated using multiple animal models. In the present review, we discussed the available data describing the mechanisms of acute and chronic IR-induced salivary gland dysfunction. In animal models of RT, acute salivary gland dysfunction involves DNA damage and insufficient repair, aberrant calcium signaling, acinar cell apoptosis and ROS production. While these mechanisms contribute to long-term loss of function, sustained salivary dysfunction is further influenced by inflammatory responses, neuronal and vascular changes, loss of epithelial polarity, compensatory proliferation, impaired stem or progenitor cell populations, cytoskeletal rearrangements and fibrosis. One area that deserves further investigation is the contribution of immune cells to IR-induced salivary gland dysfunction. IR-induced immunomodulation is a well-appreciated driver of damage in other models of IR, both with regard to direct IR exposure as well as influencing bystander effects. Further, our overall understanding of bystander effects in the salivary glands following irradiation is inadequate. Building on research performed in other IR-induced damage models, we propose that purinergic signaling through P2 receptors in the salivary gland may be a critical mediator of bystander effects in IR-induced salivary gland dysfunction. At present, artificial saliva and sialagogues provide inadequate and temporary symptom relief in RT. The therapeutic benefit of amifostine, the only FDA-approved radioprotective treatment, is questionable due to toxicity concerns. The need for additional preventative and regenerative approaches is essential. Here, we discussed current and future therapeutic approaches for the treatment or prevention of RT-induced salivary gland damage, including a number of promising radioprotective and regenerative therapies being investigated in preclinical animal models and clinical trials. Radioprotective approaches currently being investigated target many of the signaling pathways discussed in this review, while regenerative approaches include gene therapy, pharmacological interventions and stem cell transplantation.

Author Contributions: K.J.J., K.E.G. and K.M.F. reviewed available literature and wrote the manuscript. G.A.W. and K.H.L. critically revised the manuscript. All authors have read and agreed to the published version of the manuscript.

Funding: This work was supported by National Institute of Dental and Craniofacial Research grants R01DE007389 (G.A.W.), R01DE023534 (K.H.L.), R01DE029166 (K.H.L.), F31DE028737 (K.E.G.) and R01DE023342 (G.A.W. and K.H.L.) and a Sjögrens Syndrome Foundation grant (K.J.J.). K.M.F. is supported by a University of Missouri Life Sciences Fellowship and a fellowship from the Wayne L. Ryan Foundation.

Conflicts of Interest: The authors declare no conflict of interest.

References

1. Grundmann, O.; Mitchell, G.; Limesand, K. Sensitivity of Salivary Glands to Radiation: From Animal Models to Therapies. *J. Dent. Res.* **2009**, *88*, 894–903. [CrossRef]
2. Konings, A.W.; Coppes, R.P.; Vissink, A. On the mechanism of salivary gland radiosensitivity. *Int. J. Radiat. Oncol.* **2005**, *62*, 1187–1194. [CrossRef]
3. Arany, S.; Benoit, D.S.W.; Dewhurst, S.; Ovitt, C.E. Nanoparticle-mediated Gene Silencing Confers Radioprotection to Salivary Glands In Vivo. *Mol. Ther.* **2013**, *21*, 1182–1194. [CrossRef]

4. Avila, J.L.; Grundmann, O.; Burd, R.; Limesand, K.H. Radiation-Induced Salivary Gland Dysfunction Results From p53-Dependent Apoptosis. *Int. J. Radiat. Oncol.* **2009**, *73*, 523–529. [CrossRef]
5. Limesand, K.H.; Said, S.; Anderson, S.M. Suppression of Radiation-Induced Salivary Gland Dysfunction by IGF-1. *PLoS ONE* **2009**, *4*, e4663. [CrossRef]
6. Limesand, K.H.; Schwertfeger, K.L.; Anderson, S.M. MDM2 Is Required for Suppression of Apoptosis by Activated Akt1 in Salivary Acinar Cells. *Mol. Cell. Biol.* **2006**, *26*, 8840–8856. [CrossRef]
7. Stramandinoli-Zanicotti, R.T.; Sassi, L.M.; Schussel, J.L.; Torres, M.F.; Funchal, M.; Smaniotto, G.H.; Dissenha, J.L.; Carvalho, A.L. Effect of fractionated radiotherapy on the parotid gland: An experimental study in Brazilian minipigs. *Int. Arch. Otorhinolaryngol.* **2013**, *17*, 163–167.
8. Coppes, R.P.; Meter, A.; Latumalea, S.P.; Roffel, A.F.; Kampinga, H.H. Defects in muscarinic receptor-coupled signal transduction in isolated parotid gland cells after in vivo irradiation: Evidence for a non-DNA target of radiation. *Br. J. Cancer* **2005**, *92*, 539–546. [CrossRef]
9. Jensen, S.B.; Vissink, A.; Limesand, K.H.; Reyland, M. Salivary Gland Hypofunction and Xerostomia in Head and Neck Radiation Patients. *J. Natl. Cancer Inst. Monogr.* **2019**, *2019*. [CrossRef]
10. Atkinson, J.C.; Grisius, M.; Massey, W. Salivary Hypofunction and Xerostomia: Diagnosis and Treatment. *Dent. Clin. N. Am.* **2005**, *49*, 309–326. [CrossRef]
11. Khaw, A.; Logan, R.; Keefe, D.; Bartold, M. Radiation-induced oral mucositis and periodontitis-proposal for an inter-relationship. *Oral Dis.* **2014**, *20*, e7–e18. [CrossRef]
12. Jensen, S.B.; Pedersen, A.M.L.; Vissink, A.; Andersen, E.; Brown, C.G.; Davies, A.N.; Dutilh, J.; Fulton, J.S.; Jankovic, L.; Lopes, N.N.F.; et al. A systematic review of salivary gland hypofunction and xerostomia induced by cancer therapies: Prevalence, severity and impact on quality of life. *Support. Care Cancer* **2010**, *18*, 1039–1060. [CrossRef]
13. Wijers, O.B.; Levendag, P.C.; Braaksma, M.M.J.; Boonzaaijer, M.; Visch, L.L.; Schmitz, P.I.M. Patients with head and neck cancer cured by radiation therapy: A survey of the dry mouth syndrome in long-term survivors. *Head Neck* **2002**, *24*, 737–747. [CrossRef]
14. Li, Y.; Taylor, J.M.G.; Haken, R.K.T.; Eisbruch, A. The impact of dose on parotid salivary recovery in head and neck cancer patients treated with radiation therapy. *Int. J. Radiat. Oncol.* **2007**, *67*, 660–669. [CrossRef]
15. Fox, P.C. Salivary Enhancement Therapies. *Caries Res.* **2004**, *38*, 241–246. [CrossRef]
16. Brizel, D.M.; Wasserman, T.H.; Henke, M.; Strnad, V.; Rudat, V.; Monnier, A.; Eschwege, F.; Zhang, J.; Russell, L.; Oster, W.; et al. Phase III randomized trial of amifostine as a radioprotector in head and neck cancer. *J. Clin. Oncol.* **2000**, *18*, 3339–3345. [CrossRef]
17. King, M.; Joseph, S.; Albert, A.; Thomas, T.V.; Nittala, M.R.; Woods, W.C.; Vijayakumar, S.; Packianathan, S. Use of Amifostine for Cytoprotection during Radiation Therapy: A Review. *Oncology* **2019**, *98*, 61–80. [CrossRef]
18. Cramer, J.D.; Burtness, B.; Le, Q.T.; Ferris, R.L. The changing therapeutic landscape of head and neck cancer. *Nat. Rev. Clin. Oncol.* **2019**, *16*, 669–683. [CrossRef]
19. Dirix, P.; Nuyts, S.; Van den Bogaert, W. Radiation-induced xerostomia in patients with head and neck cancer: A literature review. *Cancer* **2006**, *107*, 2525–2534. [CrossRef]
20. Dirix, P.; Nuyts, S.; Vander Poorten, V.; Delaere, P.; Van den Bogaert, W. The influence of xerostomia after radiotherapy on quality of life: Results of a questionnaire in head and neck cancer. *Support Care Cancer* **2008**, *16*, 171–179. [CrossRef]
21. Pinna, R.; Campus, G.; Cumbo, E.; Mura, I.; Milia, E. Xerostomia induced by radiotherapy: An overview of the physiopathology, clinical evidence, and management of the oral damage. *Ther. Clin. Risk Manag.* **2015**, *11*, 171–188. [CrossRef]
22. Meirovitz, A.; Murdoch-Kinch, C.A.; Schipper, M.; Pan, C.; Eisbruch, A. Grading xerostomia by physicians or by patients after intensity-modulated radiotherapy of head-and-neck cancer. *Int. J. Radiat. Oncol.* **2006**, *66*, 445–453. [CrossRef]
23. Redman, R.S. On approaches to the functional restoration of salivary glands damaged by radiation therapy for head and neck cancer, with a review of related aspects of salivary gland morphology and development. *Biotech. Histochem.* **2008**, *83*, 103–130. [CrossRef]
24. Emmerson, E.; May, A.J.; Berthoin, L.; Cruz-Pacheco, N.; Nathan, S.; Mattingly, A.J.; Chang, J.L.; Ryan, W.R.; Tward, A.D.; Knox, S.M. Salivary glands regenerate after radiation injury through SOX2-mediated secretory cell replacement. *EMBO Mol. Med.* **2018**, *10*, e8051. [CrossRef]

25. Maria, O.M.; Eliopoulos, N.; Muanza, T. Radiation-Induced Oral Mucositis. *Front. Oncol.* **2017**, *7*, 89. [CrossRef]
26. Trotti, A.; Bellm, L.; Epstein, J.B.; Frame, D.; Fuchs, H.J.; Gwede, C.K.; Komaroff, E.; Nalysnyk, L.; Zilberberg, M.D. Mucositis incidence, severity and associated outcomes in patients with head and neck cancer receiving radiotherapy with or without chemotherapy: A systematic literature review. *Radiother. Oncol.* **2003**, *66*, 253–262. [CrossRef]
27. Funegard, U.; Franzen, L.; Ericson, T.; Henriksson, R. Parotid saliva composition during and after irradiation of head and neck cancer. *Eur. J. Cancer B Oral Oncol.* **1994**, *30B*, 230–233. [CrossRef]
28. Wu, V.W.C.; Leung, K.Y. A Review on the Assessment of Radiation Induced Salivary Gland Damage after Radiotherapy. *Front. Oncol.* **2019**, *9*, 1090. [CrossRef]
29. Makkonen, T.A.; Tenovuo, J.; Vilja, P.; Heimdahl, A. Changes in the protein composition of whole saliva during radiotherapy in patients with oral or pharyngeal cancer. *Oral Surg. Oral Med. Oral Pathol.* **1986**, *62*, 270–275. [CrossRef]
30. Vesty, A.; Gear, K.; Boutell, S.; Taylor, M.W.; Douglas, R.G.; Biswas, K. Randomised, double-blind, placebo-controlled trial of oral probiotic Streptococcus salivarius M18 on head and neck cancer patients post-radiotherapy: A pilot study. *Sci. Rep.* **2020**, *10*, 13201. [CrossRef]
31. Epstein, J.B.; Thariat, J.; Bensadoun, R.J.; Barasch, A.; Murphy, B.A.; Kolnick, L.; Popplewell, L.; Maghami, E. Oral complications of cancer and cancer therapy: From cancer treatment to survivorship. *CA Cancer J. Clin.* **2012**, *62*, 400–422. [CrossRef] [PubMed]
32. Cheng, S.C.H.; Wu, V.W.C.; Kwong, D.L.W.; Ying, M.T.C. Assessment of post-radiotherapy salivary glands. *Br. J. Radiol.* **2011**, *84*, 393–402. [CrossRef] [PubMed]
33. Teymoortash, A.; Simolka, N.; Schrader, C.; Tiemann, M.; Werner, J. Lymphocyte subsets in irradiation-induced sialadenitis of the submandibular gland. *Histopathology* **2005**, *47*, 493–500. [CrossRef] [PubMed]
34. Dreyer, J.O.; Sakuma, Y.; Seifert, G. Radiation-induced sialadenitis. Stage classification and immunohistology. *Pathologist* **1989**, *10*, 165–170.
35. Sullivan, C.A.; Haddad, R.I.; Tishler, R.B.; Mahadevan, A.; Krane, J.F. Chemoradiation-Induced Cell Loss in Human Submandibular Glands. *Laryngoscope* **2005**, *115*, 958–964. [CrossRef]
36. Luitje, M.E.; Israel, A.-K.; Cummings, M.A.; Giampoli, E.J.; Allen, P.D.; Newlands, S.D.; Ovitt, C.E. Long-Term Maintenance of Acinar Cells in Human Submandibular Glands After Radiation Therapy. *Int. J. Radiat. Oncol.* **2020**, *S0360–3016(20)*, 34483–34487. [CrossRef]
37. Van Der Laan, H.P.; Bijl, H.P.; Steenbakkers, R.J.; Van Der Schaaf, A.; Chouvalova, O.; Hoek, J.G.V.-V.D.; Gawryszuk, A.; Van Der Laan, B.F.; Oosting, S.F.; Roodenburg, J.L.; et al. Acute symptoms during the course of head and neck radiotherapy or chemoradiation are strong predictors of late dysphagia. *Radiother. Oncol.* **2015**, *115*, 56–62. [CrossRef]
38. Denham, J.W.; Peters, L.J.; Johansen, J.; Poulsen, M.; Lamb, D.S.; Hindley, A.; O'brien, P.C.; Spry, N.A.; Penniment, M.; Krawitz, H.; et al. Do acute mucosal reactions lead to consequential late reactions in patients with head and neck cancer? *Radiother. Oncol.* **1999**, *52*, 157–164. [CrossRef]
39. Pal, M.; Gupta, N.; Rawat, S.; Grewal, M.S.; Garg, H.; Chauhan, D.; Ahlawat, P.; Tandon, S.; Khurana, R.; Pahuja, A.K.; et al. Radiation-induced dental caries, prevention and treatment–A systematic review. *Natl. J. Maxillofac. Surg.* **2015**, *6*, 160–166. [CrossRef]
40. Sroussi, H.Y.; Epstein, J.B.; Bensadoun, R.-J.; Saunders, D.P.; Lalla, R.V.; Migliorati, C.A.; Heaivilin, N.; Zumsteg, Z.S. Common oral complications of head and neck cancer radiation therapy: Mucositis, infections, saliva change, fibrosis, sensory dysfunctions, dental caries, periodontal disease, and osteoradionecrosis. *Cancer Med.* **2017**, *6*, 2918–2931. [CrossRef]
41. Roblegg, E.; Coughran, A.; Sirjani, D. Saliva: An all-rounder of our body. *Eur. J. Pharm. Biopharm.* **2019**, *142*, 133–141. [CrossRef]
42. Spirk, C.; Hartl, S.; Pritz, E.; Gugatschka, M.; Kolb-Lenz, D.; Leitinger, G.; Roblegg, E. Comprehensive investigation of saliva replacement liquids for the treatment of xerostomia. *Int. J. Pharm.* **2019**, *571*, 118759. [CrossRef] [PubMed]
43. Ambudkar, I.S. Calcium signaling defects underlying salivary gland dysfunction. *Biochim. et Biophys. Acta (BBA) Bioenerg.* **2018**, *1865*, 1771–1777. [CrossRef]
44. Liu, X.; Ong, H.L.; Ambudkar, I.S. TRP Channel Involvement in Salivary Glands—Some Good, Some Bad. *Cells* **2018**, *7*, 74. [CrossRef] [PubMed]

45. Liu, X.; Gong, B.; De Souza, L.B.; Ong, H.L.; Subedi, K.P.; Cheng, K.T.; Swaim, W.; Zheng, C.; Mori, Y.; Ambudkar, I.S. Radiation inhibits salivary gland function by promoting STIM1 cleavage by caspase-3 and loss of SOCE through a TRPM2-dependent pathway. *Sci. Signal.* **2017**, *10*, eaal4064. [CrossRef] [PubMed]
46. Liu, X.; Cotrim, A.P.; Teos, L.Y.; Zheng, C.; Swaim, W.D.; Mitchell, J.B.; Mori, Y.; Ambudkar, I.S. Loss of TRPM2 function protects against irradiation-induced salivary gland dysfunction. *Nat. Commun.* **2013**, *4*, 1515. [CrossRef] [PubMed]
47. Mitchell, G.C.; Fillinger, J.L.; Sittadjody, S.; Avila, J.L.; Burd, R.; Limesand, K.H. IGF1 activates cell cycle arrest following irradiation by reducing binding of DeltaNp63 to the p21 promoter. *Cell Death Dis.* **2010**, *1*, e50. [CrossRef]
48. Gilman, K.E.; Camden, J.M.; Klein, R.R.; Zhang, Q.; Weisman, G.A.; Limesand, K.H. P2X7 receptor deletion suppresses gamma-radiation-induced hyposalivation. *Am. J. Physiol. Regul. Integr. Comp. Physiol.* **2019**, *316*, R687–R696. [CrossRef]
49. Muhvic-Urek, M.; Bralic, M.; Curic, S.; Pezelj-Ribaric, S.; Borcic, J.; Tomac, J. Imbalance between apoptosis and proliferation causes late radiation damage of salivary gland in mouse. *Physiol. Res.* **2005**, *55*, 89–95.
50. Wong, W.Y.; Pier, M.; Limesand, K.H. Persistent disruption of lateral junctional complexes and actin cytoskeleton in parotid salivary glands following radiation treatment. *Am. J. Physiol. Integr. Comp. Physiol.* **2018**, *315*, R656–R667. [CrossRef]
51. Coppes, R.P.; Zeilstra, L.J.W.; Kampinga, H.H.; Konings, A.W.T. Early to late sparing of radiation damage to the parotid gland by adrenergic and muscarinic receptor agonists. *Br. J. Cancer* **2001**, *85*, 1055–1063. [CrossRef] [PubMed]
52. Hu, L.; Zhu, Z.; Hai, B.; Chang, S.; Ma, L.; Xu, Y.; Li, X.; Feng, X.; Wu, X.; Zhao, Q.; et al. Intragland Shh gene delivery mitigated irradiation-induced hyposalivation in a miniature pig model. *Theranostics* **2018**, *8*, 4321–4331. [CrossRef] [PubMed]
53. Knox, S.M.; Lombaert, I.M.A.; Haddox, C.L.; Abrams, S.R.; Cotrim, A.P.; Wilson, A.J.; Hoffman, M.P. Parasympathetic stimulation improves epithelial organ regeneration. *Nat. Commun.* **2013**, *4*, 1494. [CrossRef] [PubMed]
54. Lombaert, I.M.; Patel, V.N.; Jones, C.E.; Villier, D.C.; Canada, A.E.; Moore, M.R.; Berenstein, E.; Zheng, C.; Goldsmith, C.M.; Chorini, J.A.; et al. CERE-120 Prevents Irradiation-Induced Hypofunction and Restores Immune Homeostasis in Porcine Salivary Glands. *Mol. Ther. Methods Clin. Dev.* **2020**, *18*, 839–855. [CrossRef]
55. Chibly, A.M.; Wong, W.Y.; Pier, M.; Cheng, H.; Mu, Y.; Chen, J.; Ghosh, S.; Limesand, K.H. aPKCζ-dependent repression of Yap is necessary for functional restoration of irradiated salivary glands with IGF-1. *Sci. Rep.* **2018**, *8*, 6347. [CrossRef]
56. Morgan-Bathke, M.; Hill, G.A.; Harris, Z.I.; Lin, H.H.; Chibly, A.M.; Klein, R.R.; Burd, R.S.; Ann, D.K.; Limesand, K.H. Autophagy Correlates with Maintenance of Salivary Gland Function Following Radiation. *Sci. Rep.* **2015**, *4*, 5206. [CrossRef] [PubMed]
57. Radfar, L.; Sirois, D. Structural and functional injury in minipig salivary glands following fractionated exposure to 70 Gy of ionizing radiation: An animal model for human radiation-induced salivary gland injury. *Oral Surg. Oral Med. Oral Pathol. Oral Radiol. Endodontol.* **2003**, *96*, 267–274. [CrossRef]
58. Kim, J.H.; Kim, K.M.; Jung, M.H.; Jung, J.H.; Kang, K.M.; Jeong, B.K.; Park, J.J.; Woo, S.H.; Kim, J.P. Protective effects of alpha lipoic acid on radiation-induced salivary gland injury in rats. *Oncotarget* **2016**, *7*, 29143–29153. [CrossRef]
59. Meyer, S.; Chibly, A.; Burd, R.; Limesand, K. Insulin-Like Growth Factor-1–Mediated DNA Repair in Irradiated Salivary Glands Is Sirtuin-1 Dependent. *J. Dent. Res.* **2016**, *96*, 225–232. [CrossRef]
60. Hai, B.; Zhao, Q.; Deveau, M.A.; Liu, F. Delivery of Sonic Hedgehog Gene Repressed Irradiation-induced Cellular Senescence in Salivary Glands by Promoting DNA Repair and Reducing Oxidative Stress. *Theranostics* **2018**, *8*, 1159–1167.
61. Akyuz, M.; Taysi, S.; Baysal, E.; Demir, E.; Alkis, H.; Akan, M.; Binici, H.; Karatas, Z.A. Radioprotective effect of thymoquinone on salivary gland of rats exposed to total cranial irradiation. *Head Neck* **2017**, *39*, 2027–2035. [CrossRef] [PubMed]
62. Wong, W.Y.; Allie, S.; Limesand, K.H. PKCζ and JNK signaling regulate radiation-induced compensatory proliferation in parotid salivary glands. *PLoS ONE* **2019**, *14*, e0219572. [CrossRef] [PubMed]

63. Humphries, M.J.; Limesand, K.H.; Schneider, J.C.; Nakayama, K.I.; Anderson, S.M.; Reyland, M.E. Suppression of apoptosis in the protein kinase c-δ null mouse in vivo. *J. Biol. Chem.* **2006**, *281*, 9728–9737. [CrossRef] [PubMed]
64. Wong, W.Y.; Gilman, K.; Limesand, K.H. Yap activation in irradiated parotid salivary glands is regulated by ROCK activity. *PLoS ONE* **2020**, *15*, e0232921. [CrossRef]
65. Hill, G.; Headon, D.; Harris, Z.I.; Huttner, K.; Limesand, K.H. Pharmacological Activation of the EDA/EDAR Signaling Pathway Restores Salivary Gland Function following Radiation-Induced Damage. *PLoS ONE* **2014**, *9*, e112840. [CrossRef]
66. Grundmann, O.; Fillinger, J.L.; Victory, K.R.; Burd, R.; Limesand, K.H. Restoration of radiation therapy-induced salivary gland dysfunction in mice by post therapy IGF-1 administration. *BMC Cancer* **2010**, *10*, 417. [CrossRef]
67. Marmary, Y.; Adar, R.; Gaska, S.; Wygoda, A.; Maly, A.; Cohen, J.; Eliashar, R.; Mizrachi, L.; Orfaig-Geva, C.; Baum, B.J.; et al. Radiation-induced loss of salivary gland function is driven by cellular senescence and prevented by IL6 modulation. *Cancer Res.* **2016**, *76*, 1170–1180. [CrossRef]
68. Peng, X.; Wu, Y.; Brouwer, U.; Van Vliet, T.; Wang, B.; DeMaria, M.; Barazzuol, L.; Coppes, R.P. Cellular senescence contributes to radiation-induced hyposalivation by affecting the stem/progenitor cell niche. *Cell Death Dis.* **2020**, *11*, 854. [CrossRef]
69. Yokoyama, M.; Narita, T.; Sakurai, H.; Katsumata-Kato, O.; Sugiya, H.; Fujita-Yoshigaki, J. Maintenance of claudin-3 expression and the barrier functions of intercellular junctions in parotid acinar cells via the inhibition of Src signaling. *Arch. Oral Biol.* **2017**, *81*, 141–150. [CrossRef]
70. Kim, J.H.; Jeong, B.K.; Jang, S.J.; Yun, J.W.; Jung, M.H.; Kang, K.M.; Kim, T.; Woo, S.H. Alpha-Lipoic Acid Ameliorates Radiation-Induced Salivary Gland Injury by Preserving Parasympathetic Innervation in Rats. *Int. J. Mol. Sci.* **2020**, *21*, 2260. [CrossRef]
71. De La Cal, C.; Fernández-Solari, J.; Mohn, C.; Prestifilippo, J.P.; Pugnaloni, A.; Medina, V.; Elverdin, J. Radiation Produces Irreversible Chronic Dysfunction in the Submandibular Glands of the Rat. *Open Dent. J.* **2012**, *6*, 8–13. [CrossRef] [PubMed]
72. Martin, K.L.; Hill, G.A.; Klein, R.R.; Arnett, D.G.; Burd, R.; Limesand, K.H. Prevention of Radiation-Induced Salivary Gland Dysfunction Utilizing a CDK Inhibitor in a Mouse Model. *PLoS ONE* **2012**, *7*, e51363. [CrossRef] [PubMed]
73. Shin, H.-S.; Lee, S.; Kim, Y.M.; Lim, J. Hypoxia-Activated Adipose Mesenchymal Stem Cells Prevents Irradiation-Induced Salivary Hypofunction by Enhanced Paracrine Effect Through Fibroblast Growth Factor 10. *Stem Cells* **2018**, *36*, 1020–1032. [CrossRef] [PubMed]
74. Limesand, K.H.; Avila, J.L.; Victory, K.; Chang, H.H.; Shin, Y.J.; Grundmann, O.; Klein, R.R. IGF-1 preserves salivary gland function following fractionated radiation. *Int. J. Radiat. Oncol. Biol. Phys.* **2010**, *78*, 579–586. [CrossRef]
75. Choi, J.-S.; Shin, H.-S.; An, H.-Y.; Kim, Y.-M.; Lim, J.-Y. Radioprotective effects of Keratinocyte Growth Factor-1 against irradiation-induced salivary gland hypofunction. *Oncotarget* **2017**, *8*, 13496–13508. [CrossRef]
76. Lamas, D.J.M.; Carabajal, E.; Prestifilippo, J.P.; Rossi, L.; Elverdín, J.C.; Merani, S.; Bergoc, R.M.; Rivera, E.S.; Medina, V. Protection of Radiation-Induced Damage to the Hematopoietic System, Small Intestine and Salivary Glands in Rats by JNJ7777120 Compound, a Histamine H4 Ligand. *PLoS ONE* **2013**, *8*, e69106.
77. Wie, S.M.; Adwan, T.S.; DeGregori, J.; Anderson, S.M.; Reyland, M.E. Inhibiting Tyrosine Phosphorylation of Protein Kinase Cδ (PKCδ) Protects the Salivary Gland from Radiation Damage. *J. Biol. Chem.* **2014**, *289*, 10900–10908. [CrossRef]
78. Wie, S.M.; Wellberg, E.; Karam, S.D.; Reyland, M.E. Tyrosine Kinase Inhibitors Protect the Salivary Gland from Radiation Damage by Inhibiting Activation of Protein Kinase C-δ. *Mol. Cancer Ther.* **2017**, *16*, 1989–1998. [CrossRef]
79. Heuckeroth, R.O.; Enomoto, H.; Grider, J.R.; Golden, J.P.; Hanke, J.; Jackman, A.; Molliver, D.C.; Bardgett, M.E.; Snider, W.D.; Johnson, E.M.; et al. Gene targeting reveals a critical role for neurturin in the development and maintenance of enteric, sensory, and parasympathetic neurons. *Neuron* **1999**, *22*, 253–263. [CrossRef]
80. Rossi, J.; Luukko, K.; Poteryaev, D.; Laurikainen, A.; Sun, Y.F.; Laakso, T.; Eerikainen, S.; Tuominen, R.; Lakso, M.; Rauvala, H.; et al. Retarded growth and deficits in the enteric and parasympathetic nervous system in mice lacking GFR alpha2, a functional neurturin receptor. *Neuron* **1999**, *22*, 243–252. [CrossRef]

81. Ferreira, J.N.; Zheng, C.; Lombaert, I.M.; Goldsmith, C.M.; Cotrim, A.P.; Symonds, J.M.; Patel, V.N.; Hoffman, M.P. Neurturin Gene Therapy Protects Parasympathetic Function to Prevent Irradiation-Induced Murine Salivary Gland Hypofunction. *Mol. Ther. Methods Clin. Dev.* **2018**, *9*, 172–180. [CrossRef] [PubMed]
82. Mizrachi, A.; Cotrim, A.P.; Katabi, N.; Mitchell, J.B.; Verheij, M.; Haimovitz-Friedman, A. Radiation-Induced Microvascular Injury as a Mechanism of Salivary Gland Hypofunction and Potential Target for Radioprotectors. *Radiat. Res.* **2016**, *186*, 189–195. [CrossRef] [PubMed]
83. Lombaert, I.M.A.; Brunsting, J.F.; Wierenga, P.K.; Kampinga, H.H.; De Haan, G.; Coppes, R.P. Cytokine Treatment Improves Parenchymal and Vascular Damage of Salivary Glands after Irradiation. *Clin. Cancer Res.* **2008**, *14*, 7741–7750. [CrossRef]
84. Van Luijk, P.; Pringle, S.; Deasy, J.O.; Moiseenko, V.V.; Faber, H.; Hovan, A.; Baanstra, M.; Laan, H.P.; Kierkels, R.G.; Schaaf, A.; et al. Sparing the region of the salivary gland containing stem cells preserves saliva production after radiotherapy for head and neck cancer. *Sci. Transl. Med.* **2015**, *7*, 305ra147. [CrossRef]
85. Aure, M.H.; Konieczny, S.F.; Ovitt, C.E. Salivary Gland Homeostasis Is Maintained through Acinar Cell Self-Duplication. *Dev. Cell* **2015**, *33*, 231–237. [CrossRef]
86. Lombaert, I.M.A.; Brunsting, J.F.; Wierenga, P.K.; Faber, H.; Stokman, M.A.; Kok, T.; Visser, W.H.; Kampinga, H.H.; De Haan, G.; Coppes, R.P. Rescue of Salivary Gland Function after Stem Cell Transplantation in Irradiated Glands. *PLoS ONE* **2008**, *3*, e2063. [CrossRef]
87. Weng, P.-L.; Aure, M.H.; Maruyama, T.; Ovitt, C.E. Limited Regeneration of Adult Salivary Glands after Severe Injury Involves Cellular Plasticity. *Cell Rep.* **2018**, *24*, 1464–1470.e3. [CrossRef] [PubMed]
88. Morgan-Bathke, M.; Harris, Z.I.; Arnett, D.G.; Klein, R.R.; Burd, R.; Ann, D.K.; Limesand, K.H. The Rapalogue, CCI-779, Improves Salivary Gland Function following Radiation. *PLoS ONE* **2014**, *9*, e113183. [CrossRef]
89. O'Keefe, K.; DeSantis, K.; Altrieth, A.; Nelson, D.; Taroc, E.; Stabell, A.; Pham, M.; Larsen, M. Regional Differences following Partial Salivary Gland Resection. *J. Dent. Res.* **2019**, *99*, 79–88. [CrossRef] [PubMed]
90. Cooper, J.S.; Fu, K.; Marks, J.; Silverman, S. Late effects of radiation therapy in the head and neck region. *Int. J. Radiat. Oncol.* **1995**, *31*, 1141–1164. [CrossRef]
91. Gyorfi, A.H.; Matei, A.E.; Distler, J.H.W. Targeting TGF-beta signaling for the treatment of fibrosis. *Matrix Biol.* **2018**, *68–69*, 8–27. [CrossRef] [PubMed]
92. Wynn, T.A. Cellular and molecular mechanisms of fibrosis. *J. Pathol.* **2008**, *214*, 199–210. [CrossRef] [PubMed]
93. Ignotz, R.A.; Massague, J. Transforming growth factor-beta stimulates the expression of fibronectin and collagen and their incorporation into the extracellular matrix. *J. Biol. Chem.* **1986**, *261*, 4337–4345. [PubMed]
94. Meng, X.M.; Huang, X.R.; Xiao, J.; Chen, H.Y.; Zhong, X.; Chung, A.C.; Lan, H.Y. Diverse roles of TGF-beta receptor II in renal fibrosis and inflammation in vivo and in vitro. *J. Pathol.* **2012**, *227*, 175–188. [CrossRef]
95. Hakim, S.G.; Ribbat, J.; Berndt, A.; Richter, P.; Kosmehl, H.; Benedek, G.A.; Jacobsen, H.C.; Trenkle, T.; Sieg, P.; Rades, D.; et al. Expression of Wnt-1, TGF-beta and related cell-cell adhesion components following radiotherapy in salivary glands of patients with manifested radiogenic xerostomia. *Radiother. Oncol.* **2011**, *101*, 93–99. [CrossRef]
96. Spiegelberg, L.; Swagemakers, S.M.; Van Ijcken, W.F.; Oole, E.; Wolvius, E.B.; Essers, J.; Braks, J.A.M. Gene expression analysis reveals inhibition of radiation-induced TGFbeta-signaling by hyperbaric oxygen therapy in mouse salivary glands. *Mol. Med.* **2014**, *20*, 257–269. [CrossRef]
97. Woods, L.T.; Camden, J.M.; El-Sayed, F.G.; Khalafalla, M.G.; Petris, M.J.; Erb, L.; Weisman, G.A. Increased expression of TGF-beta signaling components in a mouse model of fibrosis induced by submandibular gland duct ligation. *PLoS ONE* **2015**, *10*, e0123641. [CrossRef]
98. Park, S.H.; Kim, J.Y.; Kim, J.M.; Yoo, B.R.; Han, S.Y.; Jung, Y.J.; Bae, H.; Cho, J. PM014 attenuates radiation-induced pulmonary fibrosis via regulating NF-kB and TGF-b1/NOX4 pathways. *Sci. Rep.* **2020**, *10*, 16112. [CrossRef]
99. Flechsig, P.; Dadrich, M.; Bickelhaupt, S.; Jenne, J.; Hauser, K.; Timke, C.; Peschke, P.; Hahn, E.W.; Gröne, H.; Yingling, J.; et al. LY2109761 attenuates radiation-induced pulmonary murine fibrosis via reversal of TGF-beta and BMP-associated proinflammatory and proangiogenic signals. *Clin. Cancer Res.* **2012**, *18*, 3616–3627. [CrossRef]
100. Liu, Y.; Kudo, K.; Abe, Y.; Hu, D.-L.; Kijima, H.; Nakane, A.; Ono, K. Inhibition of transforming growth factor-beta, hypoxia-inducible factor-1alpha and vascular endothelial growth factor reduced late rectal injury induced by irradiation. *J. Radiat. Res.* **2009**, *50*, 233–239. [CrossRef]

101. Campbell, A.M.; Decker, R.H. Harnessing the immunomodulatory effects of radiation therapy. *Oncology* **2018**, *32*, 370–374.
102. Wirsdörfer, F.; Jendrossek, V. The Role of Lymphocytes in Radiotherapy-Induced Adverse Late Effects in the Lung. *Front. Immunol.* **2016**, *7*, 591.
103. Daguenet, E.; Louati, S.; Wozny, A.-S.; Vial, N.; Gras, M.; Guy, J.-B.; Vallard, A.; Rodriguez-Lafrasse, C.; Magné, N. Radiation-induced bystander and abscopal effects: Important lessons from preclinical models. *Br. J. Cancer* **2020**, *123*, 339–348. [CrossRef]
104. Tsuda, E.; Kawanishi, G.; Ueda, M.; Masuda, S.; Sasaki, R. The role of carbohydrate in recombinant human erythropoietin. *JBIC J. Biol. Inorg. Chem.* **1990**, *188*, 405–411. [CrossRef]
105. Horsburgh, S.; Todryk, S.M.; Ramming, A.; Distler, J.H.; O'Reilly, S. Innate lymphoid cells and fibrotic regulation. *Immunol. Lett.* **2018**, *195*, 38–44. [CrossRef]
106. Mikami, Y.; Takada, Y.; Hagihara, Y.; Kanai, T. Innate lymphoid cells in organ fibrosis. *Cytokine Growth Factor Rev.* **2018**, *42*, 27–36. [CrossRef]
107. Zhang, Y.; Tang, J.; Tian, Z.; Van Velkinburgh, J.C.; Song, J.; Wu, Y.; Ni, B. Innate Lymphoid Cells: A Promising New Regulator in Fibrotic Diseases. *Int. Rev. Immunol.* **2015**, *35*, 399–414. [CrossRef]
108. Cortez, V.S.; Cervantes-Barragan, L.; Robinette, M.L.; Bando, J.K.; Wang, Y.; Geiger, T.L.; Gilfillan, S.; Fuchs, A.; Vivier, E.; Sun, J.C.; et al. Transforming growth factor-beta signaling guides the differentiation of innate lymphoid cells in salivary glands. *Immunity* **2016**, *44*, 1127–1139. [CrossRef] [PubMed]
109. Cortez, V.S.; Fuchs, A.; Cella, M.; Gilfillan, S.; Colonna, M. Cutting edge: Salivary gland NK cells develop independently of Nfil3 in steady-state. *J. Immunol.* **2014**, *192*, 4487–4491. [CrossRef] [PubMed]
110. Tsukimoto, M.; Homma, T.; Ohshima, Y.; Kojima, S. Involvement of purinergic signaling in cellular response to gamma radiation. *Radiat. Res.* **2010**, *173*, 298–309. [CrossRef]
111. Hamada, N.; Maeda, M.; Otsuka, K.; Tomita, M. Signaling pathways underpinning the manifestations of ionizing radiation-induced bystander effects. *Curr. Mol. Pharmacol.* **2011**, *4*, 79–95. [CrossRef]
112. Heeran, A.B.; Berrigan, H.P.; O'Sullivan, J.N. The Radiation-Induced Bystander Effect (RIBE) and its Connections with the Hallmarks of Cancer. *Radiat. Res.* **2019**, *192*, 668–679. [CrossRef]
113. Christen, O.; Regad, C.; Neroni, M.; Thoenen, S.; Holz, J. [Substitute model of an in-vitro biological trials. I. Standardized method using human pulp cells]. *J. Boil. Buccale* **1989**, *17*, 275–284.
114. Prise, K.M.; O'Sullivan, J.M. Radiation-induced bystander signalling in cancer therapy. *Nat. Rev. Cancer* **2009**, *9*, 351–360. [CrossRef]
115. Kirolikar, S.; Prasannan, P.; Raghuram, G.V.; Pancholi, N.; Saha, T.; Tidke, P.; Chaudhari, P.; Shaikh, A.; Rane, B.; Pandey, R.; et al. Prevention of radiation-induced bystander effects by agents that inactivate cell-free chromatin released from irradiated dying cells. *Cell Death Dis.* **2018**, *9*, 1142. [CrossRef]
116. Klammer, H.; Mladenov, E.; Li, F.; Iliakis, G. Bystander effects as manifestation of intercellular communication of DNA damage and of the cellular oxidative status. *Cancer Lett.* **2015**, *356*, 58–71. [CrossRef]
117. Najafi, M.; Fardid, R.; Hadadi, G.; Fardid, M. The mechanisms of radiation-induced bystander effect. *J. Biomed. Phys. Eng.* **2014**, *4*, 163–172.
118. Matsumoto, H.; Hayashi, S.; Hatashita, M.; Ohnishi, K.; Shioura, H.; Ohtsubo, T.; Kitai, R.; Ohnishi, T.; Kano, E. Induction of radioresistance by a nitric oxide-mediated bystander effect. *Radiat. Res.* **2001**, *155*, 387–396. [CrossRef]
119. Azzam, E.I.; de Toledo, S.M.; Little, J.B. Direct evidence for the participation of gap junction-mediated intercellular communication in the transmission of damage signals from alpha -particle irradiated to nonirradiated cells. *Proc. Natl. Acad. Sci. USA* **2001**, *98*, 473–478. [CrossRef]
120. Zhou, H.; Randers-Pehrson, G.; Waldren, C.A.; Vannais, D.; Hall, E.J.; Hei, T.K. Induction of a bystander mutagenic effect of alpha particles in mammalian cells. *Proc. Natl. Acad. Sci. USA* **2000**, *97*, 2099–2104. [CrossRef]
121. Azzam, E.I.; de Toledo, S.M.; Gooding, T.; Little, J.B. Intercellular communication is involved in the bystander regulation of gene expression in human cells exposed to very low fluences of alpha particles. *Radiat. Res.* **1998**, *150*, 497–504. [CrossRef]
122. Tsukimoto, M. Purinergic signaling is a novel mechanism of the cellular response to ionizing radiation. *Biol. Pharm. Bull.* **2015**, *38*, 951–959. [CrossRef] [PubMed]
123. Ohshima, Y.; Tsukimoto, M.; Harada, H.; Kojima, S. Involvement of connexin43 hemichannel in ATP release after gamma-irradiation. *J. Radiat. Res.* **2012**, *53*, 551–557. [CrossRef] [PubMed]

124. Ohshima, Y.; Tsukimoto, M.; Takenouchi, T.; Harada, H.; Suzuki, A.; Sato, M.; Kitani, H.; Kojima, S. Gamma-Irradiation induces P2X(7) receptor-dependent ATP release from B16 melanoma cells. *Biochim. Biophys. Acta* **2010**, *1800*, 40–46. [CrossRef] [PubMed]
125. Kojima, S.; Ohshima, Y.; Nakatsukasa, H.; Tsukimoto, M. Role of ATP as a key signaling molecule mediating radiation-induced biological effects. *Dose Response* **2017**, *15*, 1559325817690638. [CrossRef]
126. Tanamachi, K.; Nishino, K.; Mori, N.; Suzuki, T.; Tanuma, S.I.; Abe, R.; Tsukimoti, M. Radiosensitizing effect of P2X7 receptor antagonist on melanoma in vitro and in vivo. *Biol. Pharm. Bull.* **2017**, *40*, 878–887. [CrossRef]
127. Bill, M.A.; Srivastava, K.; Breen, C.; Butterworth, K.T.; McMahon, S.J.; Prise, K.M.; McCloskey, K. Dual effects of radiation bystander signaling in urothelial cancer: Purinergic-activation of apoptosis attenuates survival of urothelial cancer and normal urothelial cells. *Oncotarget* **2017**, *8*, 97331–97343. [CrossRef]
128. Hoorelbeke, D.; Decrock, E.; De Smet, M.; De Bock, M.; Descamps, B.; Van Haver, V.; Delvaeye, T.; Krysko, D.; Vanhove, C.; Bultynck, G.; et al. Cx43 channels and signaling via IP3/Ca(2+), ATP, and ROS/NO propagate radiation-induced DNA damage to non-irradiated brain microvascular endothelial cells. *Cell Death Dis.* **2020**, *11*, 194. [CrossRef]
129. Ohshima, Y.; Kitami, A.; Kawano, A.; Tsukimoto, M.; Kojima, S. Induction of extracellular ATP mediates increase in intracellular thioredoxin in RAW264.7 cells exposed to low-dose gamma-rays. *Free Radic. Biol. Med.* **2011**, *51*, 1240–1248. [CrossRef]
130. Savio, L.E.B.; de Andrade Mello, P.; da Silva, C.G.; Coutinho-Silva, R. The P2X7 receptor in inflammatory diseases: Angel or demon? *Front. Pharmacol.* **2018**, *9*, 52. [CrossRef]
131. Di Virgilio, F.; Dal Ben, D.; Sarti, A.C.; Giuliani, A.L.; Falzoni, S. The P2X7 receptor in infection and inflammation. *Immunity* **2017**, *47*, 15–31. [CrossRef] [PubMed]
132. Erb, L.; Woods, L.T.; Khalafalla, M.G.; Weisman, G.A. Purinergic signaling in Alzheimer's disease. *Brain Res. Bull.* **2019**, *151*, 25–37. [CrossRef] [PubMed]
133. Ahn, J.S.; Camden, J.M.; Schrader, A.M.; Redman, R.S.; Turner, J.T. Reversible regulation of P2Y(2) nucleotide receptor expression in the duct-ligated rat submandibular gland. *Am. J. Physiol. Cell Physiol.* **2000**, *279*, C286–C294. [CrossRef] [PubMed]
134. Schrader, A.M.; Camden, J.M.; Weisman, G.A. P2Y2 nucleotide receptor up-regulation in submandibular gland cells from the NOD.B10 mouse model of Sjogren's syndrome. *Arch. Oral Biol.* **2005**, *50*, 533–540. [CrossRef]
135. Tamaishi, N.; Tsukimoto, M.; Kitami, A.; Kojima, S. P2Y6 receptors and ADAM17 mediate low-dose gamma-ray-induced focus formation (activation) of EGF receptor. *Radiat. Res.* **2011**, *175*, 193–200. [CrossRef]
136. Xu, P.; Xu, Y.; Hu, B.; Wang, J.; Pan, R.; Murugan, M.; Wu, L.; Tang, Y. Extracellular ATP enhances radiation-induced brain injury through microglial activation and paracrine signaling via P2X7 receptor. *Brain Behav. Immun.* **2015**, *50*, 87–100. [CrossRef]
137. Ishibashi, K.; Okamura, K.; Yamazaki, J. Involvement of apical P2Y2 receptor-regulated CFTR activity in muscarinic stimulation of Cl(-) reabsorption in rat submandibular gland. *Am. J. Physiol. Regul. Integr. Comp. Physiol.* **2008**, *294*, R1729–R1736. [CrossRef]
138. Nakamoto, T.; Brown, D.A.; Catalan, M.A.; Gonzalez-Begne, M.; Romanenko, V.G.; Melvin, J.E. Purinergic P2X7 receptors mediate ATP-induced saliva secretion by the mouse submandibular gland. *J. Biol. Chem.* **2009**, *284*, 4815–4822. [CrossRef]
139. Khalafalla, M.G.; Woods, L.T.; Jasmer, K.J.; Forti, K.M.; Camden, J.M.; Jensen, J.L.; Limesand, K.H.; Galtung, H.K.; Weisman, G.A. P2 receptors as therapeutic targets in the salivary gland: From physiology to dysfunction. *Front. Pharmacol.* **2020**, *11*, 222. [CrossRef]
140. Ramadan, R.; Vromans, E.; Anang, D.C.; Decrock, E.; Mysara, M.; Monsieurs, P.; Baatout, S.; Leybaert, L.; Aerts, A. Single and fractionated ionizing radiation induce alterations in endothelial connexin expression and channel function. *Sci. Rep.* **2019**, *9*, 4643.
141. Zhang, Q.; Bai, X.; Liu, Y.; Wang, K.; Shen, B.; Sun, X. Current concepts and perspectives on connexin43: A Mini Review. *Curr. Protein. Pept. Sci.* **2018**, *19*, 1049–1057. [CrossRef] [PubMed]
142. De Vuyst, E.; Wang, N.; Decrock, E.; De Bock, M.; Vinken, M.; Van Moorhem, M.; Lai, C.; Culot, M.; Rogiers, V.; Cecchelli, R.; et al. Ca(2+) regulation of connexin 43 hemichannels in C6 glioma and glial cells. *Cell Calcium.* **2009**, *46*, 176–187. [CrossRef] [PubMed]

143. Alvarez, A.; Lagos-Cabre, R.; Kong, M.; Cardenas, A.; Burgos-Bravo, F.; Schneider, P.; Quest, A.; Leyton, L. Integrin-mediated transactivation of P2X7R via hemichannel-dependent ATP release stimulates astrocyte migration. *Biochim. Biophys. Acta* **2016**, *1863*, 2175–2188. [CrossRef] [PubMed]
144. Erb, L.; Weisman, G.A. Coupling of P2Y receptors to G proteins and other signaling pathways. *Wiley Interdiscip. Rev. Membr. Transp. Signal.* **2012**, *1*, 789–803. [CrossRef] [PubMed]
145. Decrock, E.; Hoorelbeke, D.; Ramadan, R.; Delvaeye, T.; De Bock, M.; Wang, N.; Krysko, D.; Baatout, S.; Bultynck, G.; Aerts, A.; et al. Calcium, oxidative stress and connexin channels, a harmonious orchestra directing the response to radiotherapy treatment? *Biochim. Biophys. Acta Mol. Cell Res.* **2017**, *1864*, 1099–1120. [CrossRef]
146. Lyng, F.M.; Maguire, P.; McClean, B.; Seymour, C.; Mothersill, C. The involvement of calcium and MAP kinase signaling pathways in the production of radiation-induced bystander effects. *Radiat. Res.* **2006**, *165*, 400–409.
147. Hei, T.K.; Zhou, H.; Chai, Y.; Ponnaiya, B.; Ivanov, V.N. Radiation induced non-targeted response: Mechanism and potential clinical implications. *Curr. Mol. Pharmacol.* **2011**, *4*, 96–105. [CrossRef]
148. Shao, C.; Lyng, F.M.; Folkard, M.; Prise, K.M. Calcium fluxes modulate the radiation-induced bystander responses in targeted glioma and fibroblast cells. *Radiat. Res.* **2006**, *166*, 479–487. [CrossRef]
149. Zhou, H.; Ivanov, V.N.; Lien, Y.C.; Davidson, M.; Hei, T.K. Mitochondrial function and nuclear factor-kappaB-mediated signaling in radiation-induced bystander effects. *Cancer Res.* **2008**, *68*, 2233–2240. [CrossRef]
150. Zhou, H.; Ivanov, V.N.; Gillespie, J.; Geard, C.R.; Amundson, S.A.; Brenner, D.J.; Yu, Z.; Lieberman, H.B.; Hei, T.K. Mechanism of radiation-induced bystander effect: Role of the cyclooxygenase-2 signaling pathway. *Proc. Natl. Acad. Sci. USA* **2005**, *102*, 14641–14646. [CrossRef]
151. Hei, T.K. Cyclooxygenase-2 as a signaling molecule in radiation-induced bystander effect. *Mol. Carcinog.* **2006**, *45*, 455–460. [CrossRef] [PubMed]
152. Hei, T.K.; Zhou, H.; Ivanov, V.N.; Hong, M.; Lieberman, H.B.; Brenner, D.J.; Amundson, S.A.; Geard, C.R. Mechanism of radiation-induced bystander effects: A unifying model. *J. Pharm. Pharmacol.* **2008**, *60*, 943–950. [CrossRef] [PubMed]
153. Asur, R.; Balasubramaniam, M.; Marples, B.; Thomas, R.A.; Tucker, J.D. Involvement of MAPK proteins in bystander effects induced by chemicals and ionizing radiation. *Mutat. Res.* **2010**, *686*, 15–29. [CrossRef] [PubMed]
154. Azzam, E.I.; De Toledo, S.M.; Spitz, D.R.; Little, J.B. Oxidative metabolism modulates signal transduction and micronucleus formation in bystander cells from alpha-particle-irradiated normal human fibroblast cultures. *Cancer Res.* **2002**, *62*, 5436–5442.
155. Ratchford, A.M.; Baker, O.J.; Camden, J.M.; Rikka, S.; Petris, M.J.; Seye, C.I.; Erb, L.; Weisman, G.A. P2Y2 nucleotide receptors mediate metalloprotease-dependent phosphorylation of epidermal growth factor receptor and ErbB3 in human salivary gland cells. *J. Biol. Chem.* **2010**, *285*, 7545–7555. [CrossRef] [PubMed]
156. Hedden, L.; Benes, C.H.; Soltoff, S.P. P2X(7) receptor antagonists display agonist-like effects on cell signaling proteins. *Biochim. Biophys. Acta* **2011**, *1810*, 532–542. [CrossRef] [PubMed]
157. Chai, Y.; Calaf, G.M.; Zhou, H.; Ghandhi, S.A.; Elliston, C.D.; Wen, G.; Nohmi, T.; Amundson, S.A.; Hei, T.K. Radiation induced COX-2 expression and mutagenesis at non-targeted lung tissues of gpt delta transgenic mice. *Br. J. Cancer* **2013**, *108*, 91–98. [CrossRef] [PubMed]
158. Nishimaki, N.; Tsukimoto, M.; Kitami, A.; Kojima, S. Autocrine regulation of gamma-irradiation-induced DNA damage response via extracellular nucleotides-mediated activation of P2Y6 and P2Y12 receptors. *DNA Repair* **2012**, *11*, 657–665. [CrossRef]
159. Han, W.; Wu, L.; Chen, S.; Bao, L.; Zhang, L.; Jiang, E.; Zhao, Y.; Xu, A.; Hei, T.K.; Yu, Z. Constitutive nitric oxide acting as a possible intercellular signaling molecule in the initiation of radiation-induced DNA double strand breaks in non-irradiated bystander cells. *Oncogene* **2007**, *26*, 2330–2339. [CrossRef]
160. Shao, C.; Folkard, M.; Prise, K.M. Role of TGF-beta1 and nitric oxide in the bystander response of irradiated glioma cells. *Oncogene* **2008**, *27*, 434–440. [CrossRef]
161. Khalafalla, M.G.; Woods, L.T.; Camden, J.M.; Khan, A.A.; Limesand, K.H.; Petris, M.J.; Erb, L.; Weisman, G.A. P2X7 receptor antagonism prevents IL-1beta release from salivary epithelial cells and reduces inflammation in a mouse model of autoimmune exocrinopathy. *J. Biol. Chem.* **2017**, *292*, 16626–16637. [CrossRef] [PubMed]

162. Liu, R.M.; Desai, L.P. Reciprocal regulation of TGF-beta and reactive oxygen species: A perverse cycle for fibrosis. *Redox Biol.* **2015**, *6*, 565–577. [CrossRef] [PubMed]
163. Murphy-Ullrich, J.E.; Poczatek, M. Activation of latent TGF-beta by thrombospondin-1: Mechanisms and physiology. *Cytokine Growth Factor Rev.* **2000**, *11*, 59–69. [CrossRef]
164. Yu, Q.; Stamenkovic, I. Cell surface-localized matrix metalloproteinase-9 proteolytically activates TGF-beta and promotes tumor invasion and angiogenesis. *Genes Dev.* **2000**, *14*, 163–176. [PubMed]
165. Munger, J.S.; Huang, X.; Kawakatsu, H.; Griffiths, M.J.; Dalton, S.L.; Wu, J.; Pittet, J.F.; Kaminski, N.; Garat, C.; Matthay, M.A.; et al. The integrin alpha v beta 6 binds and activates latent TGF beta 1: A mechanism for regulating pulmonary inflammation and fibrosis. *Cell* **1999**, *96*, 319–328. [CrossRef]
166. Wipff, P.J.; Rifkin, D.B.; Meister, J.J.; Hinz, B. Myofibroblast contraction activates latent TGF-beta1 from the extracellular matrix. *J. Cell. Biol.* **2007**, *179*, 1311–1323. [CrossRef]
167. Erb, L.; Liu, J.; Ockerhausen, J.; Kong, Q.; Garrad, R.C.; Griffin, K.; Neal, C.; Krugh, B.; Santiago-Pérez, L.I.; González, F.A.; et al. An RGD sequence in the P2Y(2) receptor interacts with alphaVbeta3 integrins and is required for G(o)-mediated signal transduction. *J. Cell. Biol.* **2001**, *153*, 491–501. [CrossRef]
168. Camden, J.M.; Schrader, A.M.; Camden, R.E.; Gonzalez, F.A.; Erb, L.; Seye, C.I.; Weisman, G.A. P2Y2 nucleotide receptors enhance alpha-secretase-dependent amyloid precursor protein processing. *J. Biol. Chem.* **2005**, *280*, 18696–18702. [CrossRef]
169. Dewan, M.Z.; Galloway, A.E.; Kawashima, N.; Dewyngaert, J.K.; Babb, J.S.; Formenti, S.C.; Demaria, S. Fractionated but not single-dose radiotherapy induces an immune-mediated abscopal effect when combined with anti-CTLA-4 antibody. *Clin. Cancer Res.* **2009**, *15*, 5379–5388. [CrossRef]
170. Demaria, S.; Ng, B.; Devitt, M.L.; Babb, J.S.; Kawashima, N.; Liebes, L.; Formenti, S.C. Ionizing radiation inhibition of distant untreated tumors (abscopal effect) is immune mediated. *Int. J. Radiat. Oncol. Biol. Phys.* **2004**, *58*, 862–870. [CrossRef]
171. Rodriguez-Ruiz, M.E.; Vanpouille-Box, C.; Melero, I.; Formenti, S.C.; Demaria, S. Immunological mechanisms responsible for radiation-induced abscopal effect. *Trends Immunol.* **2018**, *39*, 644–655. [CrossRef] [PubMed]
172. Coates, P.J.; Robinson, J.I.; Lorimore, S.A.; Wright, E.G. Ongoing activation of p53 pathway responses is a long-term consequence of radiation exposure in vivo and associates with altered macrophage activities. *J. Pathol.* **2008**, *214*, 610–616. [CrossRef] [PubMed]
173. Elliott, M.R.; Chekeni, F.B.; Trampont, P.C.; Lazarowski, E.R.; Kadl, A.; Walk, S.F.; Park, D.; Woodson, R.I.; Ostankovich, M.; Sharma, P.; et al. Nucleotides released by apoptotic cells act as a find-me signal to promote phagocytic clearance. *Nature* **2009**, *461*, 282–286. [CrossRef] [PubMed]
174. Eun, S.Y.; Park, S.W.; Lee, J.H.; Chang, K.C.; Kim, H.J. P2Y2R activation by nucleotides released from oxLDL-treated endothelial cells (ECs) mediates the interaction between ECs and immune cells through RAGE expression and reactive oxygen species production. *Free Radic. Biol. Med.* **2014**, *69*, 157–166. [CrossRef]
175. Chen, Y.; Corriden, R.; Inoue, Y.; Yip, L.; Hashiguchi, N.; Zinkernagel, A.; Nizet, V.; Insel, P.; Junger, W. ATP release guides neutrophil chemotaxis via P2Y2 and A3 receptors. *Science* **2006**, *314*, 1792–1795. [CrossRef]
176. Lacas, B.; Bourhis, J.; Overgaard, J.; Zhang, Q.; Grégoire, V.; Nankivell, M.; Zackrisson, B.; Szutkowski, Z.; Suwiński, R.; Poulsen, M.; et al. Role of radiotherapy fractionation in head and neck cancers (MARCH): An updated meta-analysis. *Lancet Oncol.* **2017**, *18*, 1221–1237. [CrossRef]
177. Taylor, A.; Powell, M.E.B. Intensity-modulated radiotherapy—What is it? *Cancer Imaging* **2004**, *4*, 68–73. [CrossRef]
178. Deasy, J.O.; Moiseenko, V.; Marks, L.; Chao, K.S.; Nam, J.; Eisbruch, A. Radiotherapy dose-volume effects on salivary gland function. *Int. J. Radiat. Oncol. Biol. Phys.* **2010**, *76* (Suppl. 3), S58–S63. [CrossRef]
179. Eisbruch, A.; Ten Haken, R.K.; Kim, H.M.; Marsh, L.H.; Ship, J.A. Dose, volume, and function relationships in parotid salivary glands following conformal and intensity-modulated irradiation of head and neck cancer. *Int. J. Radiat. Oncol. Biol. Phys.* **1999**, *45*, 577–587. [CrossRef]
180. Murdoch-Kinch, C.A.; Kim, H.M.; Vineberg, K.A.; Ship, J.A.; Eisbruch, A. Dose-effect relationships for the submandibular salivary glands and implications for their sparing by intensity modulated radiotherapy. *Int. J. Radiat. Oncol. Biol. Phys.* **2008**, *72*, 373–382. [CrossRef]
181. Ghosh, G.; Gupta, G.; Malviya, A.; Saroj, D. Comparison three-dimensional conformal radiotherapy versus intensity modulated radiation therapy in local control of head and neck cancer. *J. Cancer Res. Ther.* **2018**, *14*, 1412–1417. [CrossRef] [PubMed]

182. Alterio, D.; Gugliandolo, S.G.; Augugliaro, M.; Marvaso, G.; Gandini, S.; Bellerba, F.; Russell-Edu, S.W.; Simone, I.D.; Cinquini, M.; Starzyńska, A.; et al. IMRT vs 2D/3D conformal RT in oropharyngeal cancer: A review of the literature and meta-analysis. *Oral Dis.* **2020**. [CrossRef]
183. Nutting, C.M.; Morden, J.P.; Harrington, K.J.; Urbano, T.G.; Bhide, S.A.; Clark, C.; Miles, E.A.; Miah, A.B.; Newbold, K.; Tanay, M.; et al. Parotid-sparing intensity modulated versus conventional radiotherapy in head and neck cancer (PARSPORT): A phase 3 multicentre randomised controlled trial. *Lancet Oncol.* **2011**, *12*, 127–136. [CrossRef]
184. Lan, X.; Chan, J.Y.K.; Pu, J.J.; Qiao, W.; Pang, S.; Yang, W.F.; Wong, K.C.W.; Kwong, D.L.W.; Su, Y.X. Saliva electrolyte analysis and xerostomia-related quality of life in nasopharyngeal carcinoma patients following intensity-modulated radiation therapy. *Radiother. Oncol.* **2020**, *150*, 97–103. [CrossRef]
185. Teoh, M.; Clark, C.H.; Wood, K.; Whitaker, S.; Nisbet, A. Volumetric modulated arc therapy: A review of current literature and clinical use in practice. *Br. J. Radiol.* **2011**, *84*, 967–996. [CrossRef] [PubMed]
186. Mashhour, K.; Kamaleldin, M.; Hashem, W. RapidArc vs conventional IMRT for head and neck cancer irradiation: Is faster necessarily better? *Asian Pac. J. Cancer Prev.* **2018**, *19*, 207–211. [PubMed]
187. Nagarajan, M.; Banu, R.; Sathya, B.; Sundaram, T.; Chellapandian, T.P. Dosimetric evaluation and comparison between volumetric modulated arc therapy (VMAT) and intensity modulated radiation therapy (IMRT) plan in head and neck cancers. *Gulf J. Oncolog.* **2020**, *1*, 45–50.
188. Delaney, A.R.; Dahele, M.; Slotman, B.J.; Verbakel, W. Is accurate contouring of salivary and swallowing structures necessary to spare them in head and neck VMAT plans? *Radiother. Oncol.* **2018**, *127*, 190–196. [CrossRef]
189. Ouyang, Z.; Liu Shen, Z.; Murray, E.; Kolar, M.; LaHurd, D.; Yu, N.; Joshi, N.; Koyfman, S.; Bzdusek, K.; Xia, P. Evaluation of auto-planning in IMRT and VMAT for head and neck cancer. *J. Appl. Clin. Med. Phys.* **2019**, *20*, 39–47. [CrossRef]
190. Holliday, E.B.; Frank, S.J. Proton radiation therapy for head and neck cancer: A review of the clinical experience to date. *Int. J. Radiat. Oncol. Biol. Phys.* **2014**, *89*, 292–302. [CrossRef]
191. Xiang, M.; Chang, D.T.; Pollom, E.L. Second cancer risk after primary cancer treatment with three-dimensional conformal, intensity-modulated, or proton beam radiation therapy. *Cancer* **2020**, *126*, 3560–3568. [CrossRef] [PubMed]
192. Lukens, J.N.; Lin, A.; Hahn, S.M. Proton therapy for head and neck cancer. *Curr. Opin. Oncol.* **2015**, *27*, 165–171. [CrossRef] [PubMed]
193. Feng, Z.; Wang, P.; Gong, L.; Xu, L.; Zhang, J.; Zheng, J.; Zhang, D.; Tian, T.; Wang, P. Construction and clinical evaluation of a new customized bite block used in radiotherapy of head and neck cancer. *Cancer Radiother.* **2019**, *23*, 125–131. [CrossRef] [PubMed]
194. Stieb, S.; Perez-Martinez, I.; Mohamed, A.S.R.; Rock, S.; Bajaj, N.; Deshpande, T.S.; Zaid, M.; Garden, A.S.; Goepfert, R.P.; Cardoso, R.; et al. The impact of tongue-deviating and tongue-depressing oral stents on long-term radiation-associated symptoms in oropharyngeal cancer survivors. *Clin. Transl. Radiat. Oncol.* **2020**, *24*, 71–78. [CrossRef] [PubMed]
195. Verrone, J.R.; Alves, F.A.; Prado, J.D.; Marcicano, A.; de Assis Pellizzon, A.C.; Damascena, A.S.; Jaguar, G.C. Benefits of an intraoral stent in decreasing the irradiation dose to oral healthy tissue: Dosimetric and clinical features. *Oral Surg. Oral Med. Oral Pathol. Oral Radiol. Endodontol.* **2014**, *118*, 573–578. [CrossRef] [PubMed]
196. Appendino, P.; Della Ferrera, F.; Nassisi, D.; Blandino, G.; Gino, E.; Solla, S.D.; Redda, M.G.R. Are intraoral customized stents still necessary in the era of highly conformal radiotherapy for head & neck cancer? Case series and literature review. *Rep. Pract. Oncol. Radiother.* **2019**, *24*, 491–498.
197. Jha, N.; Seikaly, H.; Harris, J.; Williams, D.; Liu, R.; McGaw, T.; Hofmann, H.; Robinson, D.; Hanson, J.; Barnaby, P. Prevention of radiation induced xerostomia by surgical transfer of submandibular salivary gland into the submental space. *Radiother. Oncol.* **2003**, *66*, 283–289. [CrossRef]
198. Pathak, K.A.; Bhalavat, R.L.; Mistry, R.C.; Deshpande, M.S.; Bhalla, V.; Desai, S.B.; Malpini, B.L. Upfront submandibular salivary gland transfer in pharyngeal cancers. *Oral Oncol.* **2004**, *40*, 960–963. [CrossRef]
199. Valstar, M.H.; de Bakker, B.S.; Steenbakkers, R.; de Jong, K.H.; Smit, L.A.; Klein Nulent, T.J.W.; van Es, R.J.J.; Hofland, I.; de Keizer, B.; Jasperse, B.; et al. The tubarial salivary glands: A potential new organ at risk for radiotherapy. *Radiother. Oncol.* **2020**. [CrossRef]

200. Troyer, J.K.; Beckett, M.L.; Wright, G.L., Jr. Detection and characterization of the prostate-specific membrane antigen (PSMA) in tissue extracts and body fluids. *Int. J. Cancer* **1995**, *62*, 552–558.
201. Harkema, J.R.C.S.; Wagner, J.G.; Dintzis, S.M.; Liggitt, D. Nose, Sinus, Pharynx, and Larynx. In *Comparative Anatomy and Histology*; Elsevier: London, UK, 2018.
202. Leung, W.S.; Wu, V.W.C.; Liu, C.Y.W.; Cheng, A.C.K. A dosimetric comparison of the use of equally spaced beam (ESB), beam angle optimization (BAO), and volumetric modulated arc therapy (VMAT) in head and neck cancers treated by intensity modulated radiotherapy. *J. Appl. Clin. Med. Phys.* **2019**, *20*, 121–130. [CrossRef] [PubMed]
203. Roesink, J.M.; Moerland, M.A.; Hoekstra, A.; Van Rijk, P.P.; Terhaard, C.H. Scintigraphic assessment of early and late parotid gland function after radiotherapy for head-and-neck cancer: A prospective study of dose-volume response relationships. *Int. J. Radiat. Oncol. Biol. Phys.* **2004**, *58*, 1451–1460. [CrossRef] [PubMed]
204. Scarantino, C.; LeVeque, F.; Swann, R.S.; White, R.; Schulsinger, A.; Hodson, D.I.; Meredith, R.; Foote, R.; Brachman, D.; Lee, N. Effect of pilocarpine during radiation therapy: Results of RTOG 97-09, a phase III randomized study in head and neck cancer patients. *J. Support Oncol.* **2006**, *4*, 252–258. [PubMed]
205. Rieke, J.W.; Hafermann, M.D.; Johnson, J.T.; LeVeque, F.G.; Iwamoto, R.; Steiger, B.W.; Muscoplat, C.; Gallagher, S.C. Oral pilocarpine for radiation-induced xerostomia: Integrated efficacy and safety results from two prospective randomized clinical trials. *Int. J. Radiat. Oncol. Biol. Phys.* **1995**, *31*, 661–669. [CrossRef]
206. Zimmerman, R.P.; Mark, R.J.; Tran, L.M.; Juillard, G.F. Concomitant pilocarpine during head and neck irradiation is associated with decreased posttreatment xerostomia. *Int. J. Radiat. Oncol. Biol. Phys.* **1997**, *37*, 571–575. [CrossRef]
207. Nyarady, Z.; Nemeth, A.; Ban, A.; Mukics, A.; Nyarady, J.; Ember, I.; Olasz, L. A randomized study to assess the effectiveness of orally administered pilocarpine during and after radiotherapy of head and neck cancer. *Anticancer Res.* **2006**, *26*, 1557–1562.
208. Chambers, M.S.; Posner, M.; Jones, C.U.; Biel, M.A.; Hodge, K.M.; Vitti, R.; Armstrong, I.; Yen, C.; Weber, R.S. Cevimeline for the treatment of postirradiation xerostomia in patients with head and neck cancer. *Int. J. Radiat. Oncol. Biol. Phys.* **2007**, *68*, 1102–1109. [CrossRef]
209. Chambers, M.S.; Jones, C.U.; Biel, M.A.; Weber, R.S.; Hodge, K.M.; Chen, Y.; Holland, J.M.; Ship, J.A.; Vitti, R.; Armstrong, I.; et al. Open-label, long-term safety study of cevimeline in the treatment of postirradiation xerostomia. *Int. J. Radiat. Oncol. Biol. Phys.* **2007**, *69*, 1369–1376. [CrossRef]
210. Masunaga, H.; Ogawa, H.; Uematsu, Y.; Tomizuka, T.; Yasuda, H.; Takeshita, Y. Long-lasting salivation induced by a novel muscarinic receptor agonist SNI-2011 in rats and dogs. *Eur. J. Pharmacol.* **1997**, *339*, 1–9. [CrossRef]
211. Epstein, J.B.; Burchell, J.L.; Emerton, S.; Le, N.D.; Silverman, S., Jr. A clinical trial of bethanechol in patients with xerostomia after radiation therapy. A pilot study. *Oral Surg. Oral Med. Oral Pathol.* **1994**, *77*, 610–614. [CrossRef]
212. Gorsky, M.; Epstein, J.B.; Parry, J.; Epstein, M.S.; Le, N.D.; Silverman, S., Jr. The efficacy of pilocarpine and bethanechol upon saliva production in cancer patients with hyposalivation following radiation therapy. *Oral Surg. Oral Med. Oral Pathol. Oral Radiol. Endodontol.* **2004**, *97*, 190–195. [CrossRef] [PubMed]
213. Jham, B.C.; Teixeira, I.V.; Aboud, C.G.; Carvalho, A.L.; Coelho Mde, M.; Freire, A.R. A randomized phase III prospective trial of bethanechol to prevent radiotherapy-induced salivary gland damage in patients with head and neck cancer. *Oral Oncol.* **2007**, *43*, 137–142. [CrossRef] [PubMed]
214. Jaguar, G.C.; Lima, E.N.; Kowalski, L.P.; Pellizzon, A.C.; Carvalho, A.L.; Boccaletti, K.W.; Alves, F.A. Double blind randomized prospective trial of bethanechol in the prevention of radiation-induced salivary gland dysfunction in head and neck cancer patients. *Radiother. Oncol.* **2015**, *115*, 253–256. [CrossRef] [PubMed]
215. Riley, P.; Glenny, A.M.; Hua, F.; Worthington, H.V. Pharmacological interventions for preventing dry mouth and salivary gland dysfunction following radiotherapy. *Cochrane Database Syst. Rev.* **2017**, *7*, CD012744. [PubMed]
216. Kouvaris, J.R.; Kouloulias, V.E.; Vlahos, L.J. Amifostine: The first selective-target and broad-spectrum radioprotector. *Oncologist* **2007**, *12*, 738–747. [CrossRef]

217. Wasserman, T.H.; Brizel, D.M.; Henke, M.; Monnier, A.; Eschwege, F.; Sauer, R.; Strnad, V. Influence of intravenous amifostine on xerostomia, tumor control, and survival after radiotherapy for head-and-neck cancer: 2-year follow-up of a prospective, randomized, phase III trial. *Int. J. Radiat. Oncol. Biol. Phys.* **2005**, *63*, 985–990. [CrossRef]
218. Bourhis, J.; Blanchard, P.; Maillard, E.; Brizel, D.M.; Movsas, B.; Buentzel, J.; Langendijk, J.A.; Komaki, R.; Leong, S.S.; Levendag, P.; et al. Effect of amifostine on survival among patients treated with radiotherapy: A meta-analysis of individual patient data. *J. Clin. Oncol.* **2011**, *29*, 2590–2597. [CrossRef]
219. Lee, M.G.; Freeman, A.R.; Roos, D.E.; Milner, A.D.; Borg, M.F. Randomized double-blind trial of amifostine versus placebo for radiation-induced xerostomia in patients with head and neck cancer. *J. Med. Imaging Radiat. Oncol.* **2019**, *63*, 142–150. [CrossRef]
220. Rades, D.; Fehlauer, F.; Bajrovic, A.; Mahlmann, B.; Richter, E.; Alberti, W. Serious adverse effects of amifostine during radiotherapy in head and neck cancer patients. *Radiother. Oncol.* **2004**, *70*, 261–264. [CrossRef]
221. Singh, V.K.; Seed, T.M. The efficacy and safety of amifostine for the acute radiation syndrome. *Expert Opin. Drug Saf.* **2019**, *18*, 1077–1090. [CrossRef]
222. Grdina, D.J.; Kataoka, Y.; Murley, J.S. Amifostine: Mechanisms of action underlying cytoprotection and chemoprevention. *Drug Metabol. Drug Interact.* **2000**, *16*, 237–279. [CrossRef] [PubMed]
223. Zhu, Z.; Pang, B.; Iglesias-Bartolome, R.; Wu, X.; Hu, L.; Zhang, C.; Wang, J.; Gutkind, J.S.; Wang, S. Prevention of irradiation-induced salivary hypofunction by rapamycin in swine parotid glands. *Oncotarget* **2016**, *7*, 20271–20281. [CrossRef] [PubMed]
224. Hai, B.; Qin, L.; Yang, Z.; Zhao, Q.; Shangguan, L.; Ti, X.; Zhao, Y.; Kim, S.; Rangaraj, D.; Liu, F. Transient activation of hedgehog pathway rescued irradiation-induced hyposalivation by preserving salivary stem/progenitor cells and parasympathetic innervation. *Clin. Cancer Res.* **2014**, *20*, 140–150. [CrossRef] [PubMed]
225. Lister, M.F.; Sharkey, J.; Sawatzky, D.A.; Hodgkiss, J.P.; Davidson, D.J.; Rossi, A.G.; Finlayson, K. The role of the purinergic P2X7 receptor in inflammation. *J. Inflamm.* **2007**, *4*, 5. [CrossRef]
226. Di Virgilio, F. Liaisons dangereuses: P2X(7) and the inflammasome. *Trends Pharmacol. Sci.* **2007**, *28*, 465–472. [CrossRef]
227. Woods, L.T.; Camden, J.M.; Batek, J.M.; Petris, M.J.; Erb, L.; Weisman, G.A. P2X7 receptor activation induces inflammatory responses in salivary gland epithelium. *Am. J. Physiol. Cell Physiol.* **2012**, *303*, C790–C801. [CrossRef]
228. DeVries, T.A.; Neville, M.C.; Reyland, M.E. Nuclear import of PKCdelta is required for apoptosis: Identification of a novel nuclear import sequence. *EMBO J.* **2002**, *21*, 6050–6060. [CrossRef]
229. Leitges, M.; Mayr, M.; Braun, U.; Mayr, U.; Li, C.; Pfister, G.; Ghaffari-Tabrizi, N.; Baier, G.; Hu, Y.; Xu, Q. Exacerbated vein graft arteriosclerosis in protein kinase Cdelta-null mice. *J. Clin. Investig.* **2001**, *108*, 1505–1512. [CrossRef]
230. Allen-Petersen, B.L.; Miller, M.R.; Neville, M.C.; Anderson, S.M.; Nakayama, K.I.; Reyland, M.E. Loss of protein kinase C delta alters mammary gland development and apoptosis. *Cell Death Dis.* **2010**, *1*, e17. [CrossRef]
231. Li, J.; Shan, Z.; Ou, G.; Liu, X.; Zhang, C.; Baum, B.J.; Wang, S. Structural and functional characteristics of irradiation damage to parotid glands in the miniature pig. *Int. J. Radiat. Oncol. Biol. Phys.* **2005**, *62*, 1510–1516. [CrossRef]
232. Lombaert, I.; Movahednia, M.M.; Adine, C.; Ferreira, J.N. Concise Review: Salivary gland regeneration: Therapeutic approaches from stem cells to tissue organoids. *Stem Cells* **2017**, *35*, 97–105. [CrossRef] [PubMed]
233. Baum, B.J.; Zheng, C.; Cotrim, A.P.; McCullagh, L.; Goldsmith, C.M.; Brahim, J.S.; Atkinson, J.C.; Turner, R.J.; Liu, S.; Nikolov, N.; et al. Aquaporin-1 gene transfer to correct radiation-induced salivary hypofunction. *Handb. Exp. Pharmacol.* **2009**, *190*, 403–418.
234. Mobasheri, A.; Marples, D. Expression of the AQP-1 water channel in normal human tissues: A semiquantitative study using tissue microarray technology. *Am. J. Physiol. Cell Physiol.* **2004**, *286*, C529–C537. [CrossRef] [PubMed]
235. Wang, W.; Hart, P.S.; Piesco, N.P.; Lu, X.; Gorry, M.C.; Hart, T.C. Aquaporin expression in developing human teeth and selected orofacial tissues. *Calcif. Tissue Int.* **2003**, *72*, 222–227. [CrossRef] [PubMed]

236. Gresz, V.; Kwon, T.H.; Hurley, P.T.; Varga, G.; Zelles, T.; Nielsen, S.; Case, R.M.; Steward, M.C. Identification and localization of aquaporin water channels in human salivary glands. *Am. J. Physiol. Gastrointest. Liver Physiol.* **2001**, *281*, G247–G254. [CrossRef] [PubMed]
237. Nakamura, M.; Saga, T.; Watanabe, K.; Takahashi, N.; Tabira, Y.; Kusukawa, J.; Yamaki, K.I. An immunohistochemistry-based study on aquaporin (AQP)-1, 3, 4, 5 and 8 in the parotid glands, submandibular glands and sublingual glands of Sjogren's syndrome mouse models chronically administered cevimeline. *Kurume Med. J.* **2013**, *60*, 7–19. [CrossRef]
238. Akamatsu, T.; Parvin, M.N.; Murdiastuti, K.; Kosugi-Tanaka, C.; Yao, C.; Miki, O.; Kanamori, N.; Hosoi, K. Expression and localization of aquaporins, members of the water channel family, during development of the rat submandibular gland. *Pflugers Arch.* **2003**, *446*, 641–651. [CrossRef]
239. Gao, R.; Yan, X.; Zheng, C.; Goldsmith, C.M.; Afione, S.; Hai, B.; Xu, J.; Zhou, J.; Chiorini, J.A.; Baum, B.J.; et al. AAV2-mediated transfer of the human aquaporin-1 cDNA restores fluid secretion from irradiated miniature pig parotid glands. *Gene Ther.* **2011**, *18*, 38–42. [CrossRef]
240. Alevizos, I.; Zheng, C.; Cotrim, A.P.; Liu, S.; McCullagh, L.; Billings, M.E.; Goldsmith, C.M.; Tandon, M.; Helmerhorst, E.J.; Catalan, M.A.; et al. Late responses to adenoviral-mediated transfer of the aquaporin-1 gene for radiation-induced salivary hypofunction. *Gene Ther.* **2017**, *24*, 176–186. [CrossRef]
241. Baum, B.J.; Alevizos, I.; Zheng, C.; Cotrim, A.P.; Liu, S.; McCullagh, L.; Goldsmith, C.M.; Burbelo, P.D.; Citrin, D.E.; Mitchell, J.B.; et al. Early responses to adenoviral-mediated transfer of the aquaporin-1 cDNA for radiation-induced salivary hypofunction. *Proc. Natl. Acad. Sci. USA* **2012**, *109*, 19403–19407. [CrossRef]
242. Wang, Z.; Pradhan-Bhatt, S.; Farach-Carson, M.C.; Passineau, M.J. Artificial induction of native aquaporin-1 expression in human salivary cells. *J. Dent. Res.* **2017**, *96*, 444–449. [CrossRef]
243. Wang, Z.; Wang, Y.; Wang, S.; Zhang, L.R.; Zhang, N.; Cheng, Z.; Liu, Q.; Shields, K.J.; Hu, B.; Passineau, M.J. CRISPR-Cas9 HDR system enhances AQP1 gene expression. *Oncotarget* **2017**, *8*, 111683–111696. [CrossRef] [PubMed]
244. Xiao, N.; Lin, Y.; Cao, H.; Sirjani, D.; Giaccia, A.J.; Koong, A.C.; Kong, C.S.; Diehn, M.; Le, Q.T. Neurotrophic factor GDNF promotes survival of salivary stem cells. *J. Clin. Investig.* **2014**, *124*, 3364–3377. [CrossRef] [PubMed]
245. Nanduri, L.S.; Baanstra, M.; Faber, H.; Rocchi, C.; Zwart, E.; de Haan, G.; van Os, R.; Coppes, R.P. Purification and ex vivo expansion of fully functional salivary gland stem cells. *Stem Cell Rep.* **2014**, *3*, 957–964. [CrossRef] [PubMed]
246. Feng, J.; van der Zwaag, M.; Stokman, M.A.; van Os, R.; Coppes, R.P. Isolation and characterization of human salivary gland cells for stem cell transplantation to reduce radiation-induced hyposalivation. *Radiother. Oncol.* **2009**, *92*, 466–471. [CrossRef] [PubMed]
247. Pringle, S.; Maimets, M.; van der Zwaag, M.; Stokman, M.A.; van Gosliga, D.; Zwart, E.; Witjes, M.J.H.; de Haan, G.; van Os, R.; Coppes, R.P. Human salivary gland stem cells functionally restore radiation damaged salivary glands. *Stem Cells* **2016**, *34*, 640–652. [CrossRef] [PubMed]
248. Ozdemir, T.; Fowler, E.W.; Hao, Y.; Ravikrishnan, A.; Harrington, D.A.; Witt, R.L.; Farach-Carson, M.C.; Pradhan-Bhatt, S.; Jia, X. Biomaterials-based strategies for salivary gland tissue regeneration. *Biomater Sci.* **2016**, *4*, 592–604. [CrossRef]
249. Nam, K.; Kim, K.; Dean, S.M.; Brown, C.T.; Davis, R.S.; Okano, T.; Baker, O.J. Using cell sheets to regenerate mouse submandibular glands. *NPJ Regen. Med.* **2019**, *4*, 16. [CrossRef]
250. Haara, O.; Fujimori, S.; Schmidt-Ullrich, R.; Hartmann, C.; Thesleff, I.; Mikkola, M.L. Ectodysplasin and Wnt pathways are required for salivary gland branching morphogenesis. *Development* **2011**, *138*, 2681–2691. [CrossRef]
251. Fiaschi, M.; Kolterud, A.; Nilsson, M.; Toftgard, R.; Rozell, B. Targeted expression of GLI1 in the salivary glands results in an altered differentiation program and hyperplasia. *Am. J. Pathol.* **2011**, *179*, 2569–2579. [CrossRef]
252. Hai, B.; Yang, Z.; Millar, S.E.; Choi, Y.S.; Taketo, M.M.; Nagy, A.; Liu, F. Wnt/beta-catenin signaling regulates postnatal development and regeneration of the salivary gland. *Stem Cells Dev.* **2010**, *19*, 1793–1801. [CrossRef] [PubMed]

253. Gera, J.; Lichtenstein, A. The mammalian target of rapamycin pathway as a therapeutic target in multiple myeloma. *Leuk. Lymphoma* **2011**, *52*, 1857–1866. [CrossRef] [PubMed]

Publisher's Note: MDPI stays neutral with regard to jurisdictional claims in published maps and institutional affiliations.

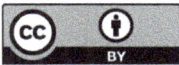

© 2020 by the authors. Licensee MDPI, Basel, Switzerland. This article is an open access article distributed under the terms and conditions of the Creative Commons Attribution (CC BY) license (http://creativecommons.org/licenses/by/4.0/).

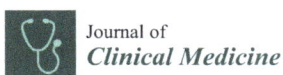

Review

Candida Infection Associated with Salivary Gland—A Narrative Review

Soo-Min Ok [1,2,3], Donald Ho [3], Tyler Lynd [3], Yong-Woo Ahn [1,2], Hye-Min Ju [1,2], Sung-Hee Jeong [1,2] and Kyounga Cheon [3,*]

[1] Department of Oral Medicine, Dental and Life Science Institute, Pusan National University, Yangsan 50612, Korea; oksoomin@pusan.ac.kr (S.-m.O.); ahnyongw@pusan.ac.kr (Y.-W.A.); hyungtaejoa@naver.com (H.-M.J.); drcookie@pusan.ac.kr (S.-H.J.)
[2] Dental Research Institute, Pusan National University Dental Hospital, Yangsan 50612, Korea
[3] Department of Pediatric Dentistry, University of Alabama at Birmingham, Birmingham, AL 35294, USA; donaldho@uab.edu (D.H.); tlynd@uab.edu (T.L.)
* Correspondence: kcheon@uab.edu

Received: 29 November 2020; Accepted: 26 December 2020; Published: 30 December 2020

Abstract: *Candida* species are common global opportunistic pathogens that could repeatedly and chronically cause oral mucosa infection and create an inflammatory environment, leading to organ dysfunction. Oral *Candida* infections may cause temporary or permanent damage to salivary glands, resulting in the destruction of acinar cells and the formation of scar tissue. Restricted function of the salivary glands leads to discomfort and diseases of the oral mucosa, such as dry mouth and associated infection. This narrative review attempts to summarize the anatomy and function of salivary glands, the associations between *Candida* and saliva, the effects of *Candida* infection on salivary glands, and the treatment strategies. Overall, clinicians should proactively manage *Candida* infections by educating patients on oral hygiene management for vulnerable populations, conducting frequent checks for a timely diagnosis, and providing an effective treatment plan.

Keywords: oral candidiasis; salivary gland; saliva; treatment

1. Introduction

Salivary glands, an essential component to maintaining oral health, are susceptible to a variety of pathologies, including candidiasis. The salivary glands are commonly classified as either major or minor salivary glands based on their sizes, distributions, and functional characteristics [1]. The major salivary glands consist of the parotid, submandibular, and sublingual glands [2], which produce and secrete saliva, moisturize intraoral mucosa and teeth, maintain oral hygiene, and facilitate taste, swallowing, speech, and mastication [3]. The minor salivary glands are distributed throughout oral mucosa surfaces, producing mucous saliva with organic substances, even at night, and protect oral mucosa from injury [4–6]. Notably, salivary glands produce high concentrations of the secretory immunoglobulin (Ig) A, which prevents other Igs from being broken down by proteolytic enzymes from microbes [7,8]. These critical functions of saliva are repressed when the salivary glands are damaged by *Candida* infections.

Candida is a genus of yeast and major human fungal pathogens [9]. *Candida* species are opportunistic pathogens that could repeatedly and chronically cause oral mucosa infections [10,11]. The most prevalent species found in oral *Candida* infection is *Candida albicans*, due to its cell adherence properties and great pathogenic potential [12]. *C. albicans* is isolated from more than 80% of oral *Candida* lesions [13]. Other clinically relevant species include *Candida glabrata*, *Candida* tropicalis, *Candida* parapsilosis, *Candida kefyr*, *Candida* dubliniensis, *Candida* lusitaniae, *Candida* krusei, and Candida guilliermondii [14]. It has been reported that 30–45% of healthy adults carry oral *Candida* organisms, and 25–80% of adults develop oral candidiasis under the condition of using antibiotics, steroids, or immunosuppressants; impaired salivary gland function; improperly fitted dentures; poor oral hygiene; and a high carbohydrate diet. Additionally, 49–54% of healthy infants carry oral *Candida* organisms, and 5–7% of infants develop oral candidiasis [15,16]. In general, the most commonly affected populations are middle-aged to elderly people. Prevalence rates as high as 70% have been reported in nursing-home residents [17]. Denture-associated oral candidiasis is frequent and occurs globally. Additionally, females are affected slightly more frequently than males [17]. Oral candidiasis also occurs in immunocompromised patients, with an estimated prevalence of 9–31% of acquired immunodeficiency syndrome (AIDS) patients and 20% of cancer patients [18].

Host inflammatory reaction to *Candida* infection may negatively affect salivary gland tissue and function. During *Candida* infection, epithelial leukocyte penetration and subepithelial inflammation are observed in histological examinations [19]. The inflammatory mediators, such as chemokines and cytokines (TNF-α, IL-6, and IL1β), are secreted from oral epithelial cells and phagocytic cells, including neutrophils, macrophages, and dendritic cells [19]. The inflammatory reaction could damage salivary glands in the form of sialectasis, ductal ectasia, and progressive acinar destruction. The sublingual and minor salivary glands are located in the superficial layer of the oral mucosa and may be more vulnerable to inflammatory-mediated damage.

Based on clinical observation and pathological evidence from the literature, this review article discusses the anatomy and function of the salivary gland, the association between *Candida* and saliva, the effects of oral *Candida* infection on salivary glands, and treatment strategies to combat *Candida* infection.

2. Anatomy and Function of the Salivary Glands

To understand the implications of *Candida* infection and how it affects salivary glands, the anatomy and function of normal salivary gland are described. As shown in Figure 1, there are three major salivary glands: parotid, submandibular, and sublingual glands in the oral cavity. The paired parotid glands are the largest of the major salivary gland; they are encapsulated and located lateral to the ramus of the mandible [20]. The parotid gland consists mainly of serous acini, secreting α-amylase-rich saliva. Saliva α-amylase is known to play a secondary role in preventing bacterial attachment to the oral surface and removing bacteria from the oral cavity [21]. The paired submandibular glands are the second largest salivary gland, located in the submandibular triangle, consisting of anterior and posterior digastric muscles, and lower border of the mandible, making up the posterior part of the floor of the mouth, above the mylohyoid muscle. The submandibular glands are composed of mixed acini populations with mucous and serous function [20]. The sublingual glands are the smallest major salivary gland and are located right under the mucous membrane at the floor of the mouth [22]. Unlike the parotid and submandibular glands, the sublingual glands are not encapsulated and spread throughout the sublingual space. The sublingual space is just below the floor of mouth and above the mylohyoid muscles. The sublingual glands secrete mucous saliva, a viscous solution rich in mucins. While the parotid and submandibular glands have long branched ducts containing all the ductal segments (excretory, intercalated, and striated), the sublingual glands lack striated ducts. The three main salivary glands account for more than 90% of secreted saliva by volume.

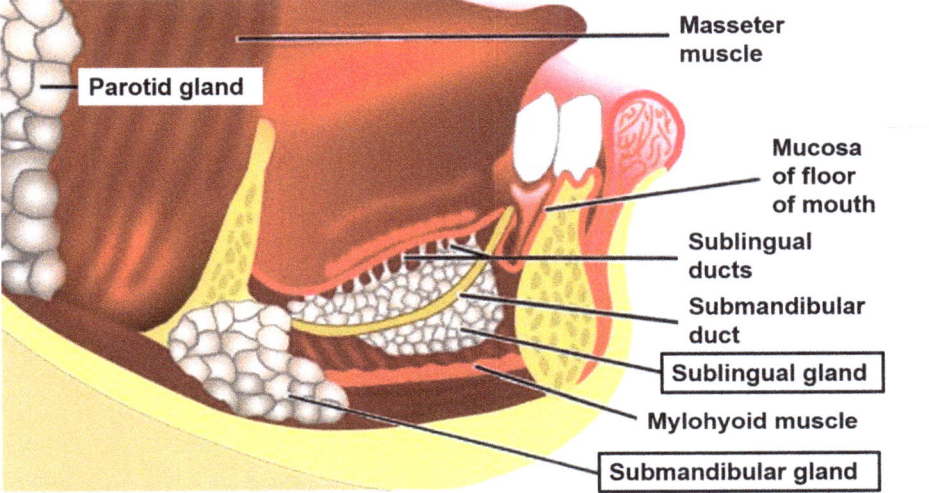

Figure 1. Drawing shows the location of the major salivary glands and its ducts. Note: Sublingual gland is located below the oral epithelium of the floor of the mouth. Adapted with permission of Radiological Society of North America, from "Imaging the Floor of the Mouth and the Sublingual Space", 31, 5, 2011 [23]; permission conveyed through Copyright Clearance Center, Inc.

Minor salivary glands are located in the submucosa, where they are surrounded by connective tissue, or embedded between muscle fibers (Figure 2). Between 600 and 1000 minor salivary glands are scattered throughout the oral mucosa except for the gingiva, the anterior dorsal aspect of the tongue, the midline and anterior part of the hard palate. Minor salivary glands consist of small secretory cell clusters with short excretory ducts that convey saliva products to the mucosal surface [4]. Minor salivary glands have a diameter of 1–5 mm and no actual capsule like the sublingual gland. Most of the minor salivary glands secrete mucus saliva; however, Von Ebner glands secrete serous or mixed saliva. The Von Ebner glands are adjacent to the foliate and circumvallate papillae in the dorsum and posterior tongue [4]. Although minor salivary glands produce about 10% of the total saliva volume [24], the minor salivary glands are widely distributed throughout the oral submucosa and secrete an abundance of salivary mucins, which acts as a lubricant. Mucin is important component of saliva, to avoid the subjective sensation of oral dryness [6]. By secretion of salivary mucins from the minor salivary glands, the formation of a lubricating film on the oral surfaces contributes to mucosal wetting and protection [5]. Meanwhile, researchers demonstrated that the flow rate of the minor salivary glands is a critical factor for dry-mouth assessment [25,26]. Since subjective feelings from dry mouth are associated with decreased flow rates of the minor salivary gland, the minor salivary gland flow rate could be used a xerostomia-assessment tool [25,26]. Furthermore, minor salivary glands produce saliva during sleep. It appears that a reduced minor salivary gland flow rate could account for dry mouth at night [27]. By secretion of salivary mucins from the minor salivary glands, the formation of a lubricating film on the oral surfaces contributes to mucosal wetting and protection [5]. Minor salivary glands also secrete high concentrations of antibacterial components, such as IgA, to protect the oral mucosa [28]. More than a third of secretory IgA is secreted from the minor salivary glands in whole saliva [29]. Secretory IgA enhances the antibacterial activity of mucin, lactoferrin, peroxidase, and aglutinin [30].

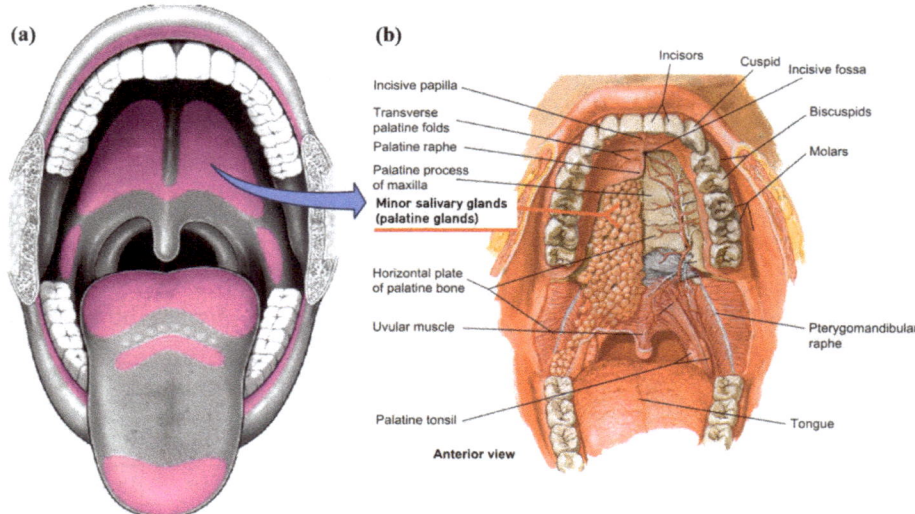

Figure 2. (**a**) Minor salivary gland distribution in the oral cavity (shown as purple shade). Adapted with permission of Wolters Kluwer Medknow Publications from Review of the Major and Minor Salivary Glands, Part 1: Anatomy, Infectious, and Inflammatory Processes, 8, 1, 2018 [31]. (**b**) Minor salivary gland are located just below the oral epithelium (Adapted with permission of Elsevier Science and Technology Books from *Comparative Anatomy and Histology: A Mouse, Rat, and Human Atlas*, 2017 [32]). (**a**,**b**) Permission conveyed through Copyright Clearance Center, Inc.

Whole saliva secreted by both major and minor salivary glands is an essential fluid for oral maintenance and function. Saliva initiates the digestive process with digestive enzymes, while simultaneously lubricating the solid diet, to assist with passage through the esophagus. Saliva plays an important role in pronunciation and taste by moisturizing the tongue and other tissues in the mouth. Saliva maintains the acid–base balance of the oral cavity, to protect teeth and soft tissues from prolonged acid exposure due to diet and gastroesophageal reflux [33,34]. Additionally, whole saliva contains several signaling molecules essential for the regeneration of oral and esophageal mucosa, including epidermal growth factor, fibroblast growth factor, nerve growth factor, and transforming growth factor alpha. Furthermore, lactoferrin, saliva's Ig, and lysozyme inhibit the progression of oral bacterial or fungal infections [33]. Due to their location directly below the mucosa, the sublingual gland and the minor salivary glands are susceptible to mucosal infection. Therefore, saliva from the major and minor salivary glands prevents oral mucosal diseases, maintains oral hygiene, and lubricates the oral cavity.

3. Pathology of Salivary Glands

3.1. Infectious Diseases Involving Virus, Bacteria, and Fungi

3.1.1. Viral and Bacterial Infectious Diseases

Salivary gland tissue may become infected with numerous viruses and bacteria, thus increasing the susceptibility of candidiasis. Epidemic parotitis is caused by the *Paramyxovirus* (mumps is the most common infection) and develops parotid edema with systemic symptoms, including fever, anorexia, malaise, and headache [35]. HIV infects the parotid gland and can lead to the formation of benign lymphoepithelial cystic lesions. *Coxsackie* virus and Hepatitis C virus are RNA-bound viruses that can infect the salivary glands and damage host tissues, causing dry mouth [35]. *Cytomegalovirus* (CMV) is a widespread virus with symptoms ranging from asymptomatic to severe-end organ dysfunction. Human CMV infection, usually affecting salivary glands, could be asymptomatic in healthy people, or it could be a life-threatening viral infection to immunocompromised individuals [36]. Recent evidence suggests that salivary glands are a potential target of severe acute respiratory syndrome coronavirus 2 (SARS-CoV-2) infection [37]. The study explains that SARS-CoV-2 infection was found in the salivary glands by identifying the presence of angiotensin I–converting enzyme 2 and cellular protease transmembrane serine protease 2 in the salivary glands [38]. Furthermore, many researchers reported sialadenitis by SARS-CoV-2 infection and the importance of saliva as a diagnostic tool [39–41]. In minor salivary glands, various viral infections also have been reported, such as Epstein–Barr virus, HIV, and human T-lymphotropic virus [42–44].

Bacterial infections are comparatively rare to viral infections. These infections are caused by either a ductal obstruction or a retrograde spread of infection up the duct secondary to decreased salivary flow. Salivary gland bacterial infections develop in patients who have existing conditions, including postoperative recovery, diabetes or immunodeficiency. Radiation therapy or antidepressant medication could reduce salivary flow and consequently induce staphylococcal and streptococcal strains associated with the biofilm on oral mucosa to infect the salivary gland [20]. Untreated bacterial infections could spread beyond the glandular borders and extend between the neck muscles, leading to serious complications, such as sepsis. In attempt to combat bacterial infection, immune cells infiltrate into the salivary gland and may destroy the secretory system resulting in dry mouth, local pain, and edema [45]. Mycoplasma infection affecting the minor salivary glands has been reported to damage the ductal epithelium, disrupt acinar structures, and cause mucus outflow into connective tissue [46]. Salivary gland dysfunction and destruction caused by various viral and bacterial infection can create a vulnerable condition that causes *Candida* infection in the oral mucosa and even in the salivary glands.

3.1.2. Infectious Diseases with *Candida*

A study reported that *Candida* infection of the parotid gland among healthy adults was caused by deep wounds from dentures [47]. Importantly, dentures were found to disrupt the epithelial barrier and induce *Candida* infection, infiltrating below the mucous membrane. Although fungal infection is reported less frequently, *C. albicans*, *Histoplasma capsulatum*, and *Cryptococcus neoformans* are the most common causes of sialadenitis, salivary gland inflammation [48–54]. Signs and symptoms of sialadenitis by *C. albicans* are low grade fever (37.4–37.8 °C), painful inflammatory-mediated swelling, and salivary gland duct discharge [10]. Histopathologically, the pus from the parotid gland demonstrated budding yeast cells. The yeast-like cells were between 2 and 4 µm in length within the intra- and extra-cellular space of macrophages [10]. Mostly, salivary gland infection with *Candida* occurs in individuals with impaired immunity, including persons impacted by HIV/AIDS [55]. Additionally, diabetic patients were reported to have increased susceptibility to *Candida* associated parotitis [10,48].

3.2. Non-Infectious Inflammatory Disease

Sjögren's syndrome is an autoimmune disorder that causes chronic inflammation and fibrosis of the salivary glands. The primary presenting symptoms of Sjögren's syndrome are dry eyes and mouth. A study reported that Sjögren's syndrome is associated with the IgG4 spectrum of disease [46]. As the disease progresses and becomes chronic, salivary glands show atrophy, parenchymal calcification, fat replacement, cystic destruction, or multiple lymphocyte cysts [47]. Chronic Sjögren's sialadenitis demonstrates ductal stenosis and swelling using sialography [56]. Chronic sclerosis sialadenitis, also known as Küttner's tumor, indicates chronic enlargement of the salivary glands caused by immune-mediated infiltration of lymphoplasmacytic cells [57]. Remarkably, recent works in the literature have shown strong associations with IgG4-related plasma cell infiltration in over 90% of patients with chronic sclerosing sialadenitis [58]. Mikulicz disease's cause is unknown, but it is believed to be autoimmune. The disease resembles Sjögren's syndrome except the fact that salivary and lacrimal secretion is less than that of Sjögren's syndrome [20]. Sarcoidosis is an autoimmune disease of unknown etiology and can affect multiple systems of the body. Large granulomas can develop in the salivary glands. The granulomas appear as masses with several non-cavity characteristics [45]. The loss of salivary function associated with these inflammatory diseases may cause consequent *Candida* infection.

3.3. Secondary Candida Infection with Salivary Gland Tumors

Salivary gland tumors are often manifested as painless, slow growing, and benign. However, 20% of salivary gland tumors are diagnosed as malignant tumor. Salivary gland tumors are indicated to be benign in 85% of tumors affecting the parotid, 60% of tumors affecting the submandibular, 50% of tumors affecting the minor glands, and only 10% of tumors affecting the sublingual glands [59]. Several studies have reported the association between Epstein–Barr virus infection and salivary gland neoplasm. Epstein–Barr virus may be a major factor in its etiology or pathogenesis [55,60–62]. HIV infection was also found to increase the risk of salivary gland cancers. Salivary gland neoplasms, such as adenoid cystic carcinoma, Kaposi sarcoma, and lymphoma, are reported in HIV infection [63].

Candida infection associated with salivary gland neoplasm has been rarely reported. However, *Candida* infection in the development of squamous cell carcinoma has been suspected for years. Common sites for oral squamous cell carcinoma to develop are on the tongue, lips, and floor of the mouth, where minor salivary glands and sublingual and submandibular glands are distributed. *Candida* species are more prevalent in potentially malignant oral mucosa diseases and cancerous oral mucosa lesions than in mucosa with the non-cancerous diseases [64,65]. With *Candida* infection, the rate of malignant transformation in leukoplakia is higher than in leukoplakia without candidiasis. The susceptibility to *Candida* infection often relies on an imbalance between *Candida* virulence factors and the host's defensive immune system [66]. In order for *C. albicans* to penetrate into mucosa, cell surface proteins, called adhesins, must recognize host molecules and adhere to the host cell. After they adhere to the cell surface, the cellular phenotype converts from yeast form to hyphae form by two mechanisms. The first mechanism is the secretion of a protease, a degrading enzyme that can digest epithelial cell surface components. This, in turn, allows physical migration into/between epithelial host cells. The second mechanism is the epithelial cell endocytosis of *C. albicans*. During this process, *Candida* can damage the host epithelium and the host's immune system [19,66,67]. Furthermore, *Candida* can produce carcinogenic compounds, nitrosamines, N-nitrosobenzylmethylamine. Strains with high nitrosamines were isolated from lesions with advanced precancerous changes. In such cases, the yeast cells expand from the mucosal surface toward epithelial cells that exhibit the ability to transport and deposit precursors, nitrosamines, into the deep layer, leading to epithelial dysplasia [65]. An in vivo study reported the carcinogenic susceptibility of salivary glands to nitrosamine [68]. It has also been reported that the workers exposed to nitrosamine have a higher mortality rate from salivary gland carcinoma [69].

4. *Candida* Infection and Salivary Gland Function

4.1. Candida Infection Affecting Salivation

In the early stages of oral candidiasis, *Candida* attaches to the oral mucosa and begins to multiply [64,70]. Several proteins, such as secretory IgA, lactoferrin, histatins, and defensins, downregulate adhesion and multiplication of *Candida* [10,71–73]. Among the proteins, histatins and defensins are particularly effective as antifungal factors, which are produced in epithelial cells and salivary glands [74]. Histatins 1, 3, and 5 are present within saliva, accounting for about 80% of total salivary histatins [75]. Human β-defensin-1 was isolated from both the major and minor salivary glands, especially from ductal cells and not acinar cells [76]. Therefore, when salivation or the antifungal agent levels of saliva are reduced, oral microbial hyperproliferation is permitted and oral candidiasis can more easily manifest [73].

Salivary flow showed a significantly negative correlation between stimulated salivary flow rates and *Candida* colony-forming units (CFUs) in the patients with xerostomia [77]. This trend also appeared in patients with reduced salivation after radiation therapy [78]. Antifungal therapy for candidiasis patients can expect to relieve pain, redness, and oral mucosa atrophy. Notably, antifungal therapy often increases the amount of saliva by removing *Candida*. A clinical study investigated the effects of *Candida* elimination on stimulating whole salivary flow rate [79]. The patients with successful elimination of *Candida* showed significantly increased stimulated whole salivary flow rate, whereas patients with unsuccessful elimination of *Candida* did not show increased stimulated whole salivary flow rate. Sympathetic stimuli, like acute pain and stress from *Candida* infection, can reduce salivary flow rate. In other words, parasympathetic stimuli result in increased saliva flow rate; on the other hand, sympathetic stimuli result in more viscous saliva secretions [24,80]. On the basis of this evidence, researchers have suggested that the increased stimulated whole salivary flow rate after treatment was the result of reduced sympathetic stimulation by oral pain reduction [79]. The study states that a decrease in sympathetic stimulation could lead to changed watery salivary secretion. However, 13.5% of the patients with successful elimination of *Candida* did not show increased stimulated whole salivary flow rate [79]. The unrestored salivary flow rate may be a result of salivary gland destruction from the *Candida* infection, and the salivary glands could not restore function even after successful *Candida* treatment [20,62].

4.2. Candida Infection and Host Immune Response

Oral *Candida* infection on salivary glands causes host immune responses by activation of T lymphocytes. The T cells mediate inflammation by stimulating the production of inflammatory cytokines, such as TNF-α, IL-1ß, and IL-6. These T cells also stimulate the production of inflammatory chemokines and recruit neutrophils and macrophages. The rapid and localized induction of these cytokines form the first line of defense that limits the transmission of invading *Candida*. However, recurrent or chronic infections can provide an elevated inflammatory environment, leading to organ dysfunction [81]. TNF-α and IL-1ß play well-known roles in the pathogenesis of chronic inflammatory diseases. These cytokines may affect salivary gland damage [82–84]. The role of these cytokines in the etiology has been determined experimentally in Sjögren's syndrome with dry mouth [85]. TNF-α suppresses the transcription of Aquaporin-5 and destroys human salivary gland acinar cells. Aquaporin-5 is critical for saliva production and a specific channel protein found in the acinar cells that allows for rapid transcellular migration of water in response to an hydrostatic/osmotic pressure gradient [86,87]. There is a cycle of destruction where *Candida* causes immune mediated salivary gland destruction, following reduced salivary flow and consequent *Candida* infection.

5. Diagnosis of Oral Candidiasis

5.1. Tentative Diagnosis Using Clinical Features and Characteristics

The diagnosis of oral candidiasis can usually be made through a complete medical history and physical examination [88]. Most commonly, candidiasis demonstrates as acute pseudomembranous candidiasis, acute atrophic candidiasis, chronic atrophic candidiasis, chronic hyperplastic candidiasis, angular cheilitis, or median rhomboid glossitis (Figure 3) [89]. (a) Pseudomembranous candidiasis accounts for approximately 35% of oral candidiasis cases. In these cases, the pseudomembrane can be easily removed, revealing underlying mucosa, with minimal bleeding. The pseudomembranous white matter consists of debris, fibrin, and exfoliated epithelium invaded by *Candida* and its hyphae. Acute pseudomembranous candidiasis can be chronic, either intermittently or constantly affecting the patient. The condition may occur in infants, immune-compromised patients (leukemia and AIDS), or patients taking medication such as antibiotics, immunosuppressants, or topical corticosteroids [18,90,91]. (b) Acute atrophic candidiasis, also known as erythema candidiasis, is usually associated with a burning sensation in oral mucosa. It presents as a raw-looking red lesion and occurs prior to the formation of the pseudomembrane or appears after the removal of the pseudomembrane. Acute atrophic candidiasis usually occurs on the dorsal surface of tongue and is characterized by absent papilla due to the use of topical antibiotics or systemic long-term corticosteroids or antibiotics [18,90,91]. (c) Chronic atrophic candidiasis, referred to AS "denture stomatitis", is usually associated with wearing dentures and inhibited salivary flow. It appears as erythematous inflammation and edema in denture occluded areas. These lesions are caused by dentures rubbing against the oral mucosa, creating a moist and warm environment that is ideal for the growth of *Candida*. Chronic atrophic candidiasis can be symptomatic, causing soreness and burning, or asymptomatic and only found on routine examination [92,93]. (d) Chronic hyperplastic candidiasis is a rare type of oral candidiasis and appears as a rough or nodular lesion, which complicates the diagnosis by differentiating from oral cancer. It typically appears as white patches on the commissures of the oral mucosa. The main cause of chronic hyperplastic candidiasis is *C. albicans*, but other systemic co-factors, such as vitamin deficiency and generalized immune suppression, may contribute. Clinically, the lesions are asymptomatic and regress after proper antifungal treatment and correction of underlying nutritional deficiencies or other co-factors. If the lesion is not treated, it can develop into dysplasia or carcinoma [94]. (e) *Candida*-associated angular cheilitis is inflammatory fissures that emanate from the commissure of the mouth. Angular cheilitis is frequently found in the clinic, including cases involving a combination of *Candida* and bacterial organisms. Signs and symptoms may include bleeding, blisters, cracks, crusts, itchiness, pain, redness, and swelling. Predisposing factors can be loss of vertical height in the denture wearer, habitual lip licking, mouth breathing, or nutritional deficiencies, particularly with vitamin B12 or iron [95]. (f) Median rhomboid glossitis is a term used to describe the area of a smooth, red, flat, or raised nodule in the middle of the dorsal surface of the tongue. The affected area of the tongue usually does not have a normal coating of filiform papilla covering the entire upper surface of the tongue. High levels of *Candida* can be discovered from these lesions, which are associated with the frequent use of steroid inhalers or cigarettes [18,90,91].

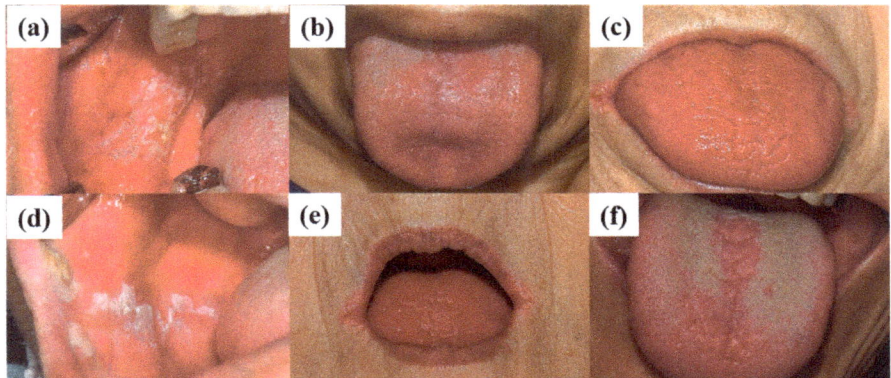

Figure 3. Clinical manifestations of oral candidiasis: (**a**) acute pseudomembranous candidiasis, (**b**) acute atrophic candidiasis, (**c**) chronic atrophic candidiasis, (**d**) chronic hyperplastic candidiasis, (**e**) angular cheilitis, and (**f**) median rhomboid glossitis. Clinical photographs were taken under patients' informed-consent agreement, with approved Institutional Review Board, PNUDH-2017-026, from the Pusan National University Dental Hospital.

5.2. Definite Diagnosis Using Cytology and Culture

Diagnosis can be confirmed by smear, oral rinse sample, whole saliva sample, culture, or oral biopsy [88]. Specimens for cytology can be obtained by scraping the lesion with a tongue blade. PAS staining of specimens reveals the existence of *Candida* hyphae and budding yeast. Moreover, 10% potassium hydroxide (KOH), gram, and methylene blue staining can be used instead of PAS. The sensitivity of smear is 51.6%, which is less than that of sample (oral rinse or whole saliva sample) culture. *Candida* species at a low concentration of 200 to 500 cells per milliliter of saliva could be detected using cell culture method rather than cytology method. Of the asymptomatic healthy population carry *Candida* in the oral cavity. Therefore, it is necessary to identify a threshold amount of *Candida* species (>270 CFU/mL), to distinguish oral candidiasis from oral carriage [96]. A definitive diagnosis of candidiasis requires the confirmation of tissue invasion by *Candida*, using biopsy with PAS staining. Biopsies are always required in hyperplastic candidiasis in order to discard the existence of epithelial dysplasia [97].

6. Prevention and Treatments of Oral Candidiasis

6.1. Prevention

Clinicians should notice that patients with immunocompromised disease, such as AIDS and diabetes, or individuals who have the risk factors of usage of medication (antibiotics, steroids, or immunosuppressants), impaired salivary gland function, dentures, poor oral hygiene, or a high-carbohydrate diet can develop candidiasis easily. Therefore, periodical oral examinations, oral hygiene instruction, and periodic prophylaxis could prevent oral candidiasis. Oral hygiene includes cleaning the tongue with a tongue cleaner, cleaning teeth and dentures with a toothbrush [98], and rinsing oral mucosa with chlorhexidine. In addition, dentures should be removed at night and meticulously washed and soaked in a disinfectant solution, such as chlorhexidine and sodium hypochlorite (1%) [15,99]. To reduce the destruction of salivary glands due to repetitive candidiasis, periodical oral examinations with prophylaxis and proper oral hygiene instruction should be recommended and practiced.

6.2. Treatments of Candida Infection

The treatment of oral candidiasis is based on four basic principles [98,100]: Assess the *Candida* infection type, diagnose the infection early and accurately, correct the predisposing factor or underlying disease, and administer antifungal agents appropriately. In order to select the proper medications, studies consider factors including local or systematic approach, type of *Candida*, clinical findings [90], and medication efficacy and toxicity [101]. Commonly used antifungal medications are included in Table 1.

Table 1. Summary of the antifungal medications and their side effects.

Drug	Formulation	Dose	Side Effect
Amphotericin B	Infusion 50 mg	100–200 mg/6 h	Renal, cardiovascular, spinal, and neurological
Nystatin	Suspension 60 mL	4–6 mL/6 h	Well tolerated
	Ointment 30 g	2–4 times/day	
	Tablets	2 every 8 h	Uncommon nausea, vomiting, and gastrointestinal effects
Clotrimazole	Gel 1%	3 times/day	Occasionally skin irritation and burning sensation.
	Tablets 10 mg	5 times/day	
Miconazole	Gel	100 mg/6 h	Uncommon burning, irritation, nausea, and diarrhea.
Ketoconazole	Gel 2%	3 times/day	Nausea, vomiting
	Tablets	200 mg, 1–2/day	abdominal pain.
	Suspension 30 mL		
Fluconazole	Tablets	50–100 mg/day	Nausea, vomiting, diarrhea, and abdominal pain.
	Suspension	10 mg/mL	
Itraconazole	Capsule	100–200 mg/day	Nausea, vomiting, diarrhea, and abdominal pain.

Table was adapted with permission of CEDRO, Centro Espanol de Derechos Reprograficos, from "Current treatment of oral candidiasis: A literature review", 6, 5, 2014 [98]); permission conveyed through Copyright Clearance Center, Inc. (Danvers, MA, USA).

Based on the histopathological information via microscopic examination and fungal culture, clinicians should choose the most appropriate antifungal medication. Polyene was the first broad spectrum antifungal agent discovered in the 1940s and 1950s [102]. Polyenes, such as nystatin and amphotericin B, bind to and weaken ergosterols in fungal cell membranes that can initiate the leakage of K+ and Na+ ions, thus contributing to fungal cell death. Polyenes are considered fungicidal and have broad activity against most fungal organisms. Amphotericin B is an antifungal drug used for serious fungal infections and nystatin is used to treat *Candida* infections of the skin, vagina, mouth, and esophagus [102,103]. Although resistance to polyene medication is rare, some fungal species exhibit intrinsic resistance to polyenes [104,105]. Nystatin is only effective topically, and amphotericin B, which is effective orally and intravenously, is well-known for its severe and potentially lethal side effects such as high fever, kidney damage, and multiple-organ damage. The search for antifungal agents with an acceptable toxicity profile first led to the discovery of azole. Therefore the first azoles were discovered in 1944, but were not approved for use in humans until the early 1960s [102]. Azoles inhibit 14-α-sterol demethylase, a cytochrome P-450 enzyme involved in ergosterol synthesis [106], resulting in the accumulation of toxic sterol intermediaries and loss of membrane integrity. Most azoles are fungistatic and have a broad spectrum against filamentous fungi and yeasts [107,108]. The search for azole antifungal agents with an acceptable toxicity profile led to the discovery of the first ketoconazole. Later, the triazoles fluconazole and itraconazole were developed with an improved safety profile and comparatively broader range of antifungal activity. Analogs have been developed to overcome limitations, such as a suboptimal spectra of activity, need to develop resistance, unfavorable pharmacokinetics, drug–drug interactions, and toxicity [109]. *Candida* species resistance to the azole medications (e.g., itraconazole, clotrimazole, and fluconazole), including *Candida glabrata*, *Candida tropicalis*, or *Candida parapsilosis* are susceptible to polyene medication. Polyene medications are not well absorbed from the gastrointestinal tract but are effective for topical application [89]. Topical antifungal therapy is recommended as the primary treatment option for mild cases of *Candida* infection. If the lesion is refractory to topical treatment or recurs frequently, systemic antifungal therapy is suggested. However, systemic antifungal therapy must be considered as the primary treatment for patients with immunocompromised conditions due to the risk of candidemia [103].

The removal of *Candida* biofilm is necessary, in combination with appropriate medication. Successful treatment of candidiasis depends upon biofilm control, using daily oral hygiene and professional prophylaxis. The *Candida* biofilm is a thick extracellular polymeric substances layer with a dense network of yeasts, pseudohyphae, and hyphae [110]. The biofilm allows *Candida* to easily attach between cells and other surfaces, such as dentures. The biofilm provides barriers between *Candida* and the surrounding environment, thus protecting *Candida* from antifungal medications [90]. Therefore, the removal of *Candida* biofilm from the dentures, as well as from all sides of the oral cavity, contributes to lowering the failure rate of antifungal treatment; it is essential for the effective treatment of *Candida* infection.

6.3. Treatments of Salivary Gland Dysfunction

6.3.1. Symptomatic Management

Hyposalivation is symptomatically managed with methods such as lifestyle changes, synthetic saliva supplementation, salivary gland stimulants, and the use of sialagogues (e.g., muscarinic receptor agonists, pilocarpine, and sevimeline) to elevate the flow rate of saliva [111,112]. Among the sialagogue treatment options, pilocarpine is the most commonly selected medication to increase saliva secretion by stimulating the salivary gland. However, pilocarpine's effect is temporary and causes side effects, including excessive sweating and tearing, chills, dizziness, flushing, nasal congestion, vocal changes, nervousness, tremors, and diarrhea [113,114]. To improve the side effects of pilocarpine, consistent and controlled release of pilocarpine in the salivary glands was considered [115]. Controlled drug-release systems have been developed and are expected to deliver therapeutic agents directly to salivary glands using novel biomedical approaches, such as hydrogels [116], polymer-based microchips [117], nanoshells [118], and microfluidics technology [119]. For example, polymer hydrogels for controlling pilocarpine release have already been clinically tested in patients with Sjögren's syndrome [115]. However, the polymer hydrogel and associated medication could not improve the discomfort of patients who had completely destroyed acinar cells. Since the severity of salivary dysfunction may vary from patient to patient [115], the literature suggests that the most effective therapy depends on the evaluation of salivary glands damage.

6.3.2. Gene Therapy and Cellular Stimulation

Gene delivery therapy could be applied to salivary gland cells to ameliorate salivary gland function. Loss of functional water channels in salivary gland epithelia is often considered one of the hallmarks of salivary gland dysfunction, and recent advances are aimed at restoring the permeability in an attempt to increase saliva production. Gene therapy was attempted to deliver the human aquaporin 1 (AQP1) gene to the salivary gland via recombinant adenovirus delivery (AdhAQP1) in rats [120]. The result suggests that AQP1 gene transfer may have potential as an approach for the treatment of salivary hypofunction. In the human study, five of 11 patients experienced elevated salivary flow 3–4.7 years after the AdhAQP1 vector delivery treatment [121]. Clinically, gene delivery to salivary glands offers the accessibility of transfer vectors in a less invasive manner [122]. The administration of bioactive components, cells, and genes directly into the salivary gland is a promising therapeutic option, when salivary-gland cells are intact. Systemic and local delivery was performed to administer a multitude of reagents, including adenoviral vectors, primary cells, growth factors, antioxidant compounds, and cytokines [123–129]. In addition, bone-marrow-derived cell (BMC) recruitment by cytokine stimulation has been reported for recovery of salivary gland cells in vivo [130,131]. Studies demonstrate that subcutaneous injection of granulocyte colony stimulating factor mobilized BMC into the bloodstream and induced migration of BMC to the damaged salivary gland, resulting in improvement of morphology and function of the submandibular salivary gland [130].

6.3.3. Stem Cell Therapy

Among the stem cell approaches, a majority of research relies on mesenchymal stem cells (MSCs) [132, 133]. In the MSC salivary transplant in vivo studies, MSCs have been acquired from bone marrow, adipose tissue, or umbilical cord blood [132,134,135]. MSCs are able to be harvested in a non-invasive manner, with relative abundance. Although the differentiation of MSCs into salivary gland acinar cells has been observed in vitro, the actual contribution to differentiation in vivo is unclear and controversial. Their beneficial action can occur primarily through paracrine pro-survival/proliferative effects on the remaining local stem/progenitor cells and cells of the surrounding environment [136,137]. However, MSCs have primary safety concerns, including unknown long-term report, tumorigenic, and metastatic potential. In addition, donor-dependent efficacy and heterogeneous properties of MSCs pose critical obstacles [138]. Therefore, autologous stem cells are preferred to repair salivary gland function. Transplantation of pluripotent salivary gland-specific epithelial stem/progenitor cells has been shown to morphologically and functionally repair salivary gland tissues. Multi-level of potency from the salivary gland cells could be applied to repair compartments of the salivary gland, recover the secretory compartment conditions, and maintain the secretory compartment [139,140]. Permanently differentiated and post-mitotic acinar cells may be able to self-duplicate after damage in post-chronic sialadenitis [141], post-duct ligation [142], partial salivary gland excision [143], and post-radiation therapy. In fact, most patients requiring autologous cell therapy are elderly and do not have enough stem/progenitor cells [144,145]. Although the number of stem/progenitor cells was increased by using heparin sulfate–stimulated growth factors [146] or Aldehyde dehydrogenase-3 activator [147], the absolute number of stem/progenitor cells required for functional regeneration of the human gland has not been clearly defined.

6.3.4. Tissue Engineering

In cases of full destruction of salivary glands, it is insufficient to restore part of the damaged salivary glands and their function. To achieve a complete functional replacement of lost or damaged tissue, tissue-engineered organoids to reconstruct fully functional organs has been proposed [148,149]. In vitro tissue-engineered organoids, using three-dimensional biomaterials loaded with salivary gland cells and/or bioactive cues, can be embedded in extracellular matrix to connect with remaining tissue residues. This approach, called the "organ germ method", has been evaluated for the regeneration of fully functional salivary glands in mice, which has been induced by mutual epithelial and mesenchymal interactions [149]. The bioengineered salivary gland responded to pilocarpine administration and taste stimulation by producing saliva. To be utilized in clinical practice, an appropriate cell source needs to be clearly identified. Recently, induced pluripotent stem cells or embryonic stem cells have been studied in salivary-gland tissue engineering [150].

Although notable progress in the treatment of hypofunctional salivary gland has been attempted over the last decades, no definitive treatment has been confirmed. Limitations of in vivo studies for translation to human trial are present due to the biological differences between human and rodent salivary glands and require further study [140]. In addition, potential differences in the development and/or regeneration strategies between different glands (e.g., parotid, submandibular, and sublingual) should be considered for future translation.

7. Conclusions

A mutual vicious cycle presents itself between the salivary gland and *Candida* infection: A decrease in the saliva flow rate creates conditions that encourage *Candida* infections, and then the *Candida* infection damages salivary glands, leading to a further decrease in saliva secretion. This pathological malfunction could result in temporary or permanent destruction of the salivary glands and may cause various intraoral symptoms, including dry mouth, speech and swallowing difficulties, and oral infections. Oral candidiasis should be detected early and treated correspondently, using an antifungal agent like nystatin and fluconazole to prevent the development of chronic salivary gland dysfunction. Correction of the underlying disease, biofilm control by using tongue cleaners, and chlorhexidine rinses must be accompanied. Limitation of current treatment options of salivary gland dysfunction are symptomatic management with medication with their side effects. Therefore, scientists have made an effort to regenerate salivary glands, using various sources to overcome the limitations of current treatments. Regeneration of salivary glands has been attempted by the activation of remaining cells with growth factors, genes, cytokines, and the transplantation of progenitor cells and mesenchymal stem cells. However, these technologies are still limited in clinical application and are in a stage that requires further research. Therefore, the clinician's role in the early detection and proper treatment of vulnerable populations who could be exposed to *Candida*-mediated salivary gland dysfunction is important.

Author Contributions: Conceptualization, Y.-W.A., H.-M.J., S.-H.J., S.-M.O., and K.C.; methodology, Y.-W.A., H.-M.J., S.-H.J., S.-M.O., and K.C.; writing—original draft preparation, D.H., T.L., S.-M.O., and K.C.; writing—review and editing, Y.-W.A., H.-M.J., S.-H.J., D.H., T.L., S.-M.O., and K.C.; supervision, K.C.; project administration, S.-M.O. and K.C. All authors have read and agreed to the published version of the manuscript.

Funding: This work was supported by the National Research Foundation of Korea (NRF) grant funded by the Korea government (MSIT) (NRF-2020R1F1A1049150).

Conflicts of Interest: The authors declare no conflict of interest.

References

1. Hellquist, H.; Skalova, A. *Histopathology of the Salivary Glands*; Springer: Berlin/Heidelberg, Germany, 2014.
2. Aframian, D.J.; Keshet, N.; Nadler, C.; Zadik, Y.; Vered, M. Minor salivary glands: Clinical, histological and immunohistochemical features of common and less common pathologies. *Acta Histochem.* **2019**, *121*, 151451. [CrossRef] [PubMed]
3. Amano, O.; Mizobe, K.; Bando, Y.; Sakiyama, K. Anatomy and histology of rodent and human major salivary glands: -Overview of the Japan salivary gland society-sponsored workshop-. *Acta Histochem. Cytochem.* **2012**, *45*, 241–250. [CrossRef] [PubMed]
4. Hand, A.R.; Pathmanathan, D.; Field, R.B. Morphological features of the minor salivary glands. *Arch. Oral Biol.* **1999**, *44* (Suppl. S1), S3–S10. [CrossRef]
5. Won, S.; Kho, H.; Kim, Y.; Chung, S.; Lee, S. Analysis of residual saliva and minor salivary gland secretions. *Arch. Oral Biol.* **2001**, *46*, 619–624. [CrossRef]
6. Rayment, S.A.; Liu, B.; Offner, G.D.; Oppenheim, F.G.; Troxler, R.F. Immunoquantification of human salivary mucins MG1 and MG2 in stimulated whole saliva: Factors influencing mucin levels. *J. Dent. Res.* **2000**, *79*, 1765–1772.
7. Smith, D.J.; Joshipura, K.; Kent, R.; Taubman, M.A. Effect of age on immunoglobulin content and volume of human labial gland saliva. *J. Dent. Res.* **1992**, *71*, 1891–1894. [CrossRef]

8. Rudney, J.D.; Krig, M.A.; Neuvar, E.K.; Soberay, A.H.; Iverson, L. Antimicrobial proteins in human unstimulated whole saliva in relation to each other, and to measures of health status, dental plaque accumulation and composition. *Arch. Oral Biol.* **1991**, *36*, 497–506. [CrossRef]
9. Skinner, C.E.; Fletcher, D.W. A review of the genus candida. *Bacteriol. Rev.* **1960**, *24*, 397–416. [CrossRef]
10. Enache-Angoulvant, A.; Torti, F.; Tassart, M.; Poirot, J.-L.; Jafari, A.; Roux, P.; Hennequin, C. Candidal abscess of the parotid gland due to Candida glabrata: Report of a case and literature review. *Med. Mycol.* **2010**, *48*, 402–405. [CrossRef]
11. Edgerton, M.; Koshlukova, S.E. Salivary histatin 5 and its similarities to the other antimicrobial proteins in human saliva. *Adv. Dent Res.* **2000**, *14*, 16–21. [CrossRef]
12. Tsui, C.; Kong, E.F.; Jabra-Rizk, M.A. Pathogenesis of Candida albicans biofilm. *Pathog. Dis.* **2016**, *74*, ftw018. [CrossRef] [PubMed]
13. Reichart, P.A.; Samaranayake, L.P.; Philipsen, H.P. Pathology and clinical correlates in oral candidiasis and its variants: A review. *Oral Dis.* **2000**, *6*, 85–91. [CrossRef] [PubMed]
14. Muadcheingka, T.; Tantivitayakul, P. Distribution of Candida albicans and non-albicans Candida species in oral candidiasis patients: Correlation between cell surface hydrophobicity and biofilm forming activities. *Arch. Oral Biol.* **2015**, *60*, 894–901. [CrossRef] [PubMed]
15. Akpan, A.; Morgan, R. Oral candidiasis. *Postgrad. Med. J.* **2002**, *78*, 455–459. [CrossRef] [PubMed]
16. Barnett, J.A. A history of research on yeasts 12: Medical yeasts part 1, Candida albicans. *Yeast* **2008**, *25*, 385–417. [CrossRef] [PubMed]
17. Scully, C. *Oral and Maxillofacial Medicine: The Basis of Diagnosis and Treatment*, 2nd ed.; Elsevier: Philadelphia, PA, USA, 2008; pp. 191–200.
18. Lalla, R.V.; Patton, L.L.; Dongari-Bagtzoglou, A. Oral candidiasis: Pathogenesis, clinical presentation, diagnosis and treatment strategies. *J. Calif. Dent. Assoc.* **2013**, *41*, 263–268.
19. Vila, T.; Sultan, A.S.; Montelongo-Jauregui, D.; Jabra-Rizk, M.A. Oral candidiasis: A disease of opportunity. *J. Fungi* **2020**, *6*, 15. [CrossRef]
20. Ogle, O.E. Salivary Gland Diseases. *Dent. Clin. N. Am.* **2020**, *64*, 87–104. [CrossRef]
21. Ochiai, A.; Harada, K.; Hashimoto, K.; Shibata, K.; Ishiyama, Y.; Mitsui, T.; Tanaka, T.; Taniguchi, M. α-Amylase is a potential growth inhibitor of Porphyromonas gingivalis, a periodontal pathogenic bacterium. *J. Periodontal Res.* **2014**, *49*, 62–68. [CrossRef]
22. Kondo, Y.; Nakamoto, T.; Jaramillo, Y.; Choi, S.; Catalan, M.A.; Melvin, J.E. Functional differences in the acinar cells of the murine major salivary glands. *J. Dent. Res.* **2015**, *94*, 715–721. [CrossRef]
23. La'porte, S.J.; Juttla, J.K.; Lingam, R.K. Imaging the floor of the mouth and the sublingual space. *Radiographics* **2011**, *31*, 1215–1230. [CrossRef] [PubMed]
24. Iorgulescu, G. Saliva between normal and pathological. Important factors in determining systemic and oral health. *J. Med. Life* **2009**, *2*, 303–307.
25. Eliasson, L.; Birkhed, D.; Carlén, A. Feeling of dry mouth in relation to whole and minor gland saliva secretion rate. *Arch. Oral Biol.* **2009**, *54*, 263–267. [CrossRef] [PubMed]
26. Bretz, W.A.; Loesche, W.J.; Chen, Y.M.; Schork, M.A.; Dominguez, B.L.; Grossman, N. Minor salivary gland secretion in the elderly. *Oral Surg. Oral Med. Oral Pathol. Oral Radiol. Endod.* **2000**, *89*, 696–701. [CrossRef] [PubMed]
27. Dijkema, T.; Raaijmakers, C.P.J.; Braam, P.M.; Roesink, J.M.; Monninkhof, E.M.; Terhaard, C.H.J. Xerostomia: A day and night difference. *Radiother. Oncol.* **2012**, *104*, 219–223. [CrossRef] [PubMed]
28. Eliasson, L.; Carlén, A. An update on minor salivary gland secretions. *Eur. J. Oral Sci.* **2010**, *118*, 435–442. [CrossRef] [PubMed]
29. Shern, R.J.; Fox, P.C.; Cain, J.L.; Li, S.H. A method for measuring the flow of saliva from the minor salivary glands. *J. Dent. Res.* **1990**, *69*, 1146–1149. [CrossRef] [PubMed]
30. Marcotte, H.; Lavoie, M.C. Oral microbial ecology and the role of salivary immunoglobulin A. *Microbiol. Mol. Biol. Rev.* **1998**, *62*, 71–109. [CrossRef]

31. Kessler, A.T.; Bhatt, A.A. Review of the major and minor salivary glands, part 1: Anatomy, infectious, and inflammatory processes. *J. Clin. Imaging Sci.* **2018**, *8*, 47. [CrossRef]
32. Treuting, P.M.; Morton, T.H. Oral cavity and teeth. In *Comparative Anatomy and Histology*; Elsevier: Amsterdam, The Netherlands, 2012; pp. 95–110.
33. Matsuo, R. Role of saliva in the maintenance of taste sensitivity. *Crit. Rev. Oral Biol. Med.* **2000**, *11*, 216–229. [CrossRef]
34. Yoshikawa, H.; Furuta, K.; Ueno, M.; Egawa, M.; Yoshino, A.; Kondo, S.; Nariai, Y.; Ishibashi, H.; Kinoshita, Y.; Sekine, J. Oral symptoms including dental erosion in gastroesophageal reflux disease are associated with decreased salivary flow volume and swallowing function. *J. Gastroenterol.* **2012**, *47*, 412–420. [CrossRef] [PubMed]
35. Hviid, A.; Rubin, S.; Mühlemann, K. Mumps. *Lancet* **2008**, *371*, 932–944. [CrossRef]
36. Gupta, M.; Shorman, M. Cytomegalovirus. In *StatPearls*; StatPearls Publishing: Treasure Island, FL, USA, 2020.
37. Xu, J.; Li, Y.; Gan, F.; Du, Y.; Yao, Y. Salivary Glands: Potential Reservoirs for COVID-19 Asymptomatic Infection. *J. Dent. Res.* **2020**, *99*, 989. [CrossRef]
38. Pascolo, L.; Zupin, L.; Melato, M.; Tricarico, P.M.; Crovella, S. TMPRSS2 and ACE2 Coexpression in SARS-CoV-2 Salivary Glands Infection. *J. Dent. Res.* **2020**, *99*, 1120–1121. [CrossRef]
39. Fisher, J.; Monette, D.L.; Patel, K.R.; Kelley, B.P.; Kennedy, M. COVID-19 associated parotitis: A case report. *Am. J. Emerg. Med.* **2020**. [CrossRef]
40. Chern, A.; Famuyide, A.O.; Moonis, G.; Lalwani, A.K. Sialadenitis: A Possible Early Manifestation of COVID-19. *Laryngoscope* **2020**, *130*, 2595–2597. [CrossRef]
41. Lechien, J.R.; Chetrit, A.; Chekkoury-Idrissi, Y.; Distinguin, L.; Circiu, M.; Saussez, S.; Berradja, N.; Edjlali, M.; Hans, S.; Carlier, R. Parotitis-Like Symptoms Associated with COVID-19, France, March-April 2020. *Emerg. Infect. Dis.* **2020**, *26*, 2270. [CrossRef]
42. Mariette, X.; Gozlan, J.; Clerc, D.; Bisson, M.; Morinet, F. Detection of Epstein-Barr virus DNA by in situ hybridization and polymerase chain reaction in salivary gland biopsy specimens from patients with Sjögren's syndrome. *Am. J. Med.* **1991**, *90*, 286–294. [CrossRef]
43. Rivera, H.; Nikitakis, N.G.; Castillo, S.; Siavash, H.; Papadimitriou, J.C.; Sauk, J.J. Histopathological analysis and demonstration of EBV and HIV p-24 antigen but not CMV expression in labial minor salivary glands of HIV patients affected by diffuse infiltrative lymphocytosis syndrome. *J. Oral Pathol. Med.* **2003**, *32*, 431–437. [CrossRef]
44. Mariette, X.; Agbalika, F.; Zucker-Franklin, D.; Clerc, D.; Janin, A.; Cherot, P.; Brouet, J.C. Detection of the tax gene of HTLV-I in labial salivary glands from patients with Sjögren's syndrome and other diseases of the oral cavity. *Clin. Exp. Rheumatol.* **2000**, *18*, 341–347.
45. Ugga, L.; Ravanelli, M.; Pallottino, A.A.; Farina, D.; Maroldi, R. Diagnostic work-up in obstructive and inflammatory salivary gland disorders. *Acta Otorhinolaryngol. Ital.* **2017**, *37*, 83–93. [PubMed]
46. Wray, W.; Scully, C.; Rennie, J.; Mason, D.K.; Love, W.C. Major and minor salivary gland swelling in Mycoplasma pneumoniae infection. *Br. Med. J.* **1980**, *280*, 1421. [CrossRef] [PubMed]
47. De Gomes, P.S.; Juodzbalys, G.; Fernandes, M.H.; Guobis, Z. Diagnostic Approaches to Sjögren's syndrome: A Literature Review and Own Clinical Experience. *J. Oral Maxillofac. Res.* **2012**, *3*, e3. [CrossRef] [PubMed]
48. Even-Tov, E.; Niv, A.; Kraus, M.; Nash, M. Candida parotitis with abscess formation. *Acta Otolaryngol.* **2006**, *126*, 334–336. [CrossRef]
49. Kantarcioğlu, A.S.; Gulenc, M.; Yücel, A.; Uzun, N.; Taskin, T.; Sakiz, D.; Altas, K. Cryptococcal parotid involvement: An uncommon localization of Cryptococcus neoformans. *Med. Mycol.* **2006**, *44*, 279–283. [CrossRef]
50. Marioni, G.; Rinaldi, R.; de Filippis, C.; Gaio, E.; Staffieri, A. Candidal abscess of the parotid gland associated with facial nerve paralysis. *Acta Otolaryngol.* **2003**, *123*, 661–663. [CrossRef]
51. Namiq, A.L.; Tollefson, T.; Fan, F. Cryptococcal parotitis presenting as a cystic parotid mass: Report of a case diagnosed by fine-needle aspiration cytology. *Diagn. Cytopathol.* **2005**, *33*, 36–38. [CrossRef]
52. Stefanopoulos, P.K.; Karakassis, D.T.; Triantafyllidou, A. Stensen's duct obstruction by foreign body and subsequent candidal infection of the parotid gland. *J. Laryngol. Otol.* **2003**, *117*, 662–665. [CrossRef]

53. Vargas, P.A.; Mauad, T.; Böhm, G.M.; Saldiva, P.H.N.; Almeida, O.P. Parotid gland involvement in advanced AIDS. *Oral Dis.* **2003**, *9*, 55–61. [CrossRef]
54. Souza Filho, F.J.; Lopes, M.; Almeida, O.P.; Scully, C. Mucocutaneous histoplasmosis in AIDS. *Br. J. Dermatol.* **1995**, *133*, 472–474. [CrossRef]
55. De Repentigny, L.; Lewandowski, D.; Jolicoeur, P. Immunopathogenesis of oropharyngeal candidiasis in human immunodeficiency virus infection. *Clin. Microbiol. Rev.* **2004**, *17*, 729–759. [CrossRef]
56. Liang, Y.; Yang, Z.; Qin, B.; Zhong, R. Primary Sjogren's syndrome and malignancy risk: A systematic review and meta-analysis. *Ann. Rheum. Dis.* **2014**, *73*, 1151–1156. [CrossRef]
57. Wei, T.-W.; Lien, C.-F.; Hsu, T.-Y.; He, H.-L. Chronic sclerosing sialadenitis of the submandibular gland: An entity of IgG4-related sclerosing disease. *Int. J. Clin. Exp. Pathol.* **2015**, *8*, 8628–8631.
58. Geyer, J.T.; Ferry, J.A.; Harris, N.L.; Stone, J.H.; Zukerberg, L.R.; Lauwers, G.Y.; Pilch, B.Z.; Deshpande, V. Chronic sclerosing sialadenitis (Küttner tumor) is an IgG4-associated disease. *Am. J. Surg. Pathol.* **2010**, *34*, 202–210. [CrossRef]
59. Speight, P.M.; Barrett, A.W. Salivary gland tumours. *Oral Dis.* **2002**, *8*, 229–240. [CrossRef]
60. Venkateswaran, L.; Gan, Y.J.; Sixbey, J.W.; Santana, V.M. Epstein-Barr virus infection in salivary gland tumors in children and young adults. *Cancer* **2000**, *89*, 463–466. [CrossRef]
61. Mozaffari, H.R.; Ramezani, M.; Janbakhsh, A.; Sadeghi, M. Malignant Salivary Gland Tumors and Epstein-Barr Virus (EBV) Infection: A Systematic Review and Meta-Analysis. *Asian Pac. J. Cancer Prev.* **2017**, *18*, 1201–1206.
62. Raab-Traub, N.; Rajadurai, P.; Flynn, K.; Lanier, A.P. Epstein-Barr virus infection in carcinoma of the salivary gland. *J. Virol.* **1991**, *65*, 7032–7036. [CrossRef]
63. Sujatha, D.; Babitha, K.; Prasad, R.S.; Pai, A. Parotid lymphoepithelial cysts in human immunodeficiency virus: A review. *J. Laryngol. Otol.* **2013**, *127*, 1046–1049. [CrossRef]
64. Nagao, Y.; Hashimoto, K.; Sata, M. Candidiasis and other oral mucosal lesions during and after interferon therapy for HCV-related chronic liver diseases. *BMC Gastroenterol.* **2012**, *12*, 155. [CrossRef]
65. Sankari, S.L.; Gayathri, K.; Balachander, N.; Malathi, L. Candida in potentially malignant oral disorders. *J. Pharm. Bioallied Sci.* **2015**, *7*, S162–S164.
66. Archambault, L.S.; Trzilova, D.; Gonia, S.; Gale, C.; Wheeler, R.T. Intravital Imaging Reveals Divergent Cytokine and Cellular Immune Responses to Candida albicans and Candida parapsilosis. *MBio* **2019**, *10*. [CrossRef]
67. Ohta, H.; Tanimoto, M.; Taniai, M.; Taniguchi, M.; Ariyasu, T.; Arai, S.; Ohta, T.; Fukuda, S. Regulation of Candida albicans morphogenesis by tumor necrosis factor-alpha and potential for treatment of oral candidiasis. *In Vivo* **2007**, *21*, 25–32.
68. Okamura, M.; Moto, M.; Kashida, Y.; Machida, N.; Mitsumori, K. Carcinogenic susceptibility to N-bis(2-hydroxypropyl)nitrosamine (DHPN) in rasH2 mice. *Toxicol. Pathol.* **2004**, *32*, 474–481. [CrossRef]
69. Kim, D.; Hwang, Y.-I.; Choi, S.; Park, C.; Lee, N.; Kim, E.-A. A case of tracheal adenoid cystic carcinoma in a worker exposed to rubber fumes. *Ann. Occup. Environ. Med.* **2013**, *25*, 22. [CrossRef]
70. Murtaugh, L.C.; Keefe, M.D. Regeneration and repair of the exocrine pancreas. *Annu. Rev. Physiol.* **2015**, *77*, 229–249. [CrossRef]
71. Mahalakshmi, S.; Kandula, S.; Shilpa, P.; Kokila, G. Chronic Recurrent Non-specific Parotitis: A Case Report and Review. *Ethiop. J. Health Sci.* **2017**, *27*, 95–100. [CrossRef]
72. Tanida, T.; Okamoto, T.; Okamoto, A.; Wang, H.; Hamada, T.; Ueta, E.; Osaki, T. Decreased excretion of antimicrobial proteins and peptides in saliva of patients with oral candidiasis. *J. Oral Pathol. Med.* **2003**, *32*, 586–594. [CrossRef]
73. Lynge Pedersen, A.M.; Belstrøm, D. The role of natural salivary defences in maintaining a healthy oral microbiota. *J. Dent.* **2019**, *80* (Suppl. S1), S3–S12. [CrossRef]
74. Ciociola, T.; Giovati, L.; Conti, S.; Magliani, W.; Santinoli, C.; Polonelli, L. Natural and synthetic peptides with antifungal activity. *Future Med. Chem.* **2016**, *8*, 1413–1433. [CrossRef]
75. Edgerton, M.; Koshlukova, S.E.; Araujo, M.W.; Patel, R.C.; Dong, J.; Bruenn, J.A. Salivary histatin 5 and human neutrophil defensin 1 kill Candida albicans via shared pathways. *Antimicrob. Agents Chemother.* **2000**, *44*, 3310–3316. [CrossRef]

76. Sahasrabudhe, K.S.; Kimball, J.R.; Morton, T.H.; Weinberg, A.; Dale, B.A. Expression of the antimicrobial peptide, human beta-defensin 1, in duct cells of minor salivary glands and detection in saliva. *J. Dent. Res.* **2000**, *79*, 1669–1674. [CrossRef]
77. Nadig, S.D.; Ashwathappa, D.T.; Manjunath, M.; Krishna, S.; Annaji, A.G.; Shivaprakash, P.K. A relationship between salivary flow rates and Candida counts in patients with xerostomia. *J. Oral Maxillofac. Pathol.* **2017**, *21*, 316. [CrossRef]
78. Karbach, J.; Walter, C.; Al-Nawas, B. Evaluation of saliva flow rates, Candida colonization and susceptibility of Candida strains after head and neck radiation. *Clin. Oral Investig.* **2012**, *16*, 1305–1312. [CrossRef]
79. Ohga, N.; Yamazaki, Y.; Sato, J.; Asaka, T.; Morimoto, M.; Hata, H.; Satoh, C.; Kitagawa, Y. Elimination of oral candidiasis may increase stimulated whole salivary flow rate. *Arch. Oral Biol.* **2016**, *71*, 129–133. [CrossRef]
80. Porcheri, C.; Mitsiadis, T.A. Physiology, pathology and regeneration of salivary glands. *Cells* **2019**, *8*, 976. [CrossRef]
81. Deshmukh, U.S.; Nandula, S.R.; Thimmalapura, P.-R.; Scindia, Y.M.; Bagavant, H. Activation of innate immune responses through Toll-like receptor 3 causes a rapid loss of salivary gland function. *J. Oral Pathol. Med.* **2009**, *38*, 42–47. [CrossRef]
82. Ferretti, S.; Bonneau, O.; Dubois, G.R.; Jones, C.E.; Trifilieff, A. IL-17, produced by lymphocytes and neutrophils, is necessary for lipopolysaccharide-induced airway neutrophilia: IL-15 as a possible trigger. *J. Immunol.* **2003**, *170*, 2106–2112. [CrossRef]
83. Kany, S.; Vollrath, J.T.; Relja, B. Cytokines in inflammatory disease. *Int. J. Mol. Sci.* **2019**, *20*, 6008. [CrossRef]
84. Festa, A.; D'Agostino, R.; Howard, G.; Mykkänen, L.; Tracy, R.P.; Haffner, S.M. Chronic subclinical inflammation as part of the insulin resistance syndrome: The Insulin Resistance Atherosclerosis Study (IRAS). *Circulation* **2000**, *102*, 42–47. [CrossRef]
85. Ohyama, Y.; Carroll, V.A.; Deshmukh, U.; Gaskin, F.; Brown, M.G.; Fu, S.M. Severe focal sialadenitis and dacryoadenitis in NZM2328 mice induced by MCMV: A novel model for human Sjögren's syndrome. *J. Immunol.* **2006**, *177*, 7391–7397. [CrossRef] [PubMed]
86. King, L.S.; Yasui, M. Aquaporins and disease: Lessons from mice to humans. *Trends Endocrinol. Metab.* **2002**, *13*, 355–360. [CrossRef]
87. Yamamura, Y.; Motegi, K.; Kani, K.; Takano, H.; Momota, Y.; Aota, K.; Yamanoi, T.; Azuma, M. TNF-α inhibits aquaporin 5 expression in human salivary gland acinar cells via suppression of histone H4 acetylation. *J. Cell Mol. Med.* **2012**, *16*, 1766–1775. [CrossRef] [PubMed]
88. Williams, D.W.; Lewis, M.A.O. Oral Microbiology: Isolation and identification of candida from the oral cavity. *Oral Dis.* **2008**, *6*, 3–11. [CrossRef]
89. Hellstein, J.W.; Marek, C.L. Candidiasis: Red and white manifestations in the oral cavity. *Head Neck Pathol.* **2019**, *13*, 25–32. [CrossRef]
90. Williams, D.; Lewis, M. Pathogenesis and treatment of oral candidosis. *J. Oral Microbiol.* **2011**, *3*, 3. [CrossRef]
91. Reamy, B.V.; Derby, R.; Bunt, C.W. Common tongue conditions in primary care. *Am. Fam. Physician* **2010**, *81*, 627–634.
92. Khan, T.S.; Muddebihal, F.; Koshy, A. Chronic atrophic candidiasis: A case report and review of literature. *Univ. Res. J. Dent.* **2015**, *5*, 123. [CrossRef]
93. Aoun, G.; Berberi, A. Prevalence of Chronic Erythematous Candidiasis in Lebanese Denture Wearers: A Clinico-microbiological Study. *Mater. Sociomed.* **2017**, *29*, 26–29. [CrossRef]
94. Sitheeque, M.A.M.; Samaranayake, L.P. Chronic hyperplastic candidosis/candidiasis (candidal leukoplakia). *Crit. Rev. Oral Biol. Med.* **2003**, *14*, 253–267. [CrossRef]
95. Sharon, V.; Fazel, N. Oral candidiasis and angular cheilitis. *Dermatol. Ther.* **2010**, *23*, 230–242. [CrossRef] [PubMed]
96. Zhou, P.R.; Hua, H.; Liu, X.S. Quantity of candida colonies in saliva: A diagnostic evaluation for oral candidiasis. *Chin. J. Dent. Res.* **2017**, *20*, 27–32. [PubMed]
97. Coronado-Castellote, L.; Jiménez-Soriano, Y. Clinical and microbiological diagnosis of oral candidiasis. *J. Clin. Exp. Dent.* **2013**, *5*, e279–e286. [CrossRef] [PubMed]

98. Garcia-Cuesta, C.; Sarrion-Pérez, M.-G.; Bagán, J.V. Current treatment of oral candidiasis: A literature review. *J. Clin. Exp. Dent.* **2014**, *6*, e576–e582. [CrossRef]
99. Vigneswaran, N.; Muller, S. Pharmacologic management of oral mucosal inflammatory and ulcerative diseases. In *Contemporary Dental Pharmacology: Evidence-Based Considerations*; Jeske, A.H., Ed.; Springer International Publishing: Cham, Switzerland, 2019; pp. 91–108.
100. Aguirre Urizar, J.M. Oral candidiasis. *Rev. Iberoam Micol.* **2002**, *19*, 17–21.
101. Martínez-Beneyto, Y.; López-Jornet, P.; Velandrino-Nicolás, A.; Jornet-García, V. Use of antifungal agents for oral candidiasis: Results of a national survey. *Int. J. Dent. Hyg.* **2010**, *8*, 47–52. [CrossRef]
102. Odds, F.C.; Brown, A.J.P.; Gow, N.A.R. Antifungal agents: Mechanisms of action. *Trends Microbiol.* **2003**, *11*, 272–279. [CrossRef]
103. Lombardi, A.; Ouanounou, A. Fungal infections in dentistry: Clinical presentations, diagnosis, and treatment alternatives. *Oral Surg. Oral Med. Oral Pathol. Oral Radiol.* **2020**, *130*, 533–546. [CrossRef]
104. Parente-Rocha, J.A.; Bailão, A.M.; Amaral, A.C.; Taborda, C.P.; Paccez, J.D.; Borges, C.L.; Pereira, M. Antifungal Resistance, Metabolic Routes as Drug Targets, and New Antifungal Agents: An Overview about Endemic Dimorphic Fungi. *Mediators Inflamm.* **2017**, *2017*, 9870679. [CrossRef]
105. Cowen, L.E.; Sanglard, D.; Howard, S.J.; Rogers, P.D.; Perlin, D.S. Mechanisms of Antifungal Drug Resistance. *Cold Spring Harb. Perspect. Med.* **2014**, *5*, a019752. [CrossRef]
106. Whaley, S.G.; Berkow, E.L.; Rybak, J.M.; Nishimoto, A.T.; Barker, K.S.; Rogers, P.D. Azole Antifungal Resistance in Candida albicans and Emerging Non-albicans Candida Species. *Front. Microbiol.* **2016**, *7*, 2173. [CrossRef] [PubMed]
107. Chang, Y.-L.; Yu, S.-J.; Heitman, J.; Wellington, M.; Chen, Y.-L. New facets of antifungal therapy. *Virulence* **2017**, *8*, 222–236. [CrossRef] [PubMed]
108. Pianalto, K.; Alspaugh, J. New horizons in antifungal therapy. *J. Fungi* **2016**, *2*, 26. [CrossRef] [PubMed]
109. Ghannoum, M.A.; Rice, L.B. Antifungal agents: Mode of action, mechanisms of resistance, and correlation of these mechanisms with bacterial resistance. *Clin. Microbiol. Rev.* **1999**, *12*, 501–517. [CrossRef]
110. Kumamoto, C.A. Candida biofilms. *Curr. Opin. Microbiol.* **2002**, *5*, 608–611. [CrossRef]
111. Vissink, A.; Mitchell, J.B.; Baum, B.J.; Limesand, K.H.; Jensen, S.B.; Fox, P.C.; Elting, L.S.; Langendijk, J.A.; Coppes, R.P.; Reyland, M.E. Clinical management of salivary gland hypofunction and xerostomia in head-and-neck cancer patients: Successes and barriers. *Int. J. Radiat. Oncol. Biol. Phys.* **2010**, *78*, 983–991. [CrossRef]
112. Silvestre, F.J.; Minguez, M.P.; Suñe-Negre, J.M. Clinical evaluation of a new artificial saliva in spray form for patients with dry mouth. *Med. Oral Patol. Oral Cir. Bucal* **2009**, *14*, E8–E11.
113. Jansma, J.; Vissink, A.; Spijkervet, F.K.; Roodenburg, J.L.; Panders, A.K.; Vermey, A.; Szabó, B.G.; Gravenmade, E.J. Protocol for the prevention and treatment of oral sequelae resulting from head and neck radiation therapy. *Cancer* **1992**, *70*, 2171–2180. [CrossRef]
114. Jellema, A.P.; Slotman, B.J.; Doornaert, P.; Leemans, C.R.; Langendijk, J.A. Impact of radiation-induced xerostomia on quality of life after primary radiotherapy among patients with head and neck cancer. *Int. J. Radiat. Oncol. Biol. Phys.* **2007**, *69*, 751–760. [CrossRef]
115. Gibson, J.; Halliday, J.A.; Ewert, K.; Robertson, S. A controlled release pilocarpine buccal insert in the treatment of Sjögren's syndrome. *Br. Dent. J.* **2007**, *202*, E17. [CrossRef]
116. Tabata, Y. Tissue regeneration based on growth factor release. *Tissue Eng.* **2003**, *9* (Suppl. S1), S5–S15. [CrossRef]
117. Richards Grayson, A.C.; Choi, I.S.; Tyler, B.M.; Wang, P.P.; Brem, H.; Cima, M.J.; Langer, R. Multi-pulse drug delivery from a resorbable polymeric microchip device. *Nat. Mater.* **2003**, *2*, 767–772. [CrossRef] [PubMed]
118. Hirsch, L.R.; Gobin, A.M.; Lowery, A.R.; Tam, F.; Drezek, R.A.; Halas, N.J.; West, J.L. Metal nanoshells. *Ann. Biomed. Eng.* **2006**, *34*, 15–22. [CrossRef] [PubMed]
119. Sershen, S.R.; Mensing, G.A.; Ng, M.; Halas, N.J.; Beebe, D.J.; West, J.L. Independent Optical Control of Microfluidic Valves Formed from Optomechanically Responsive Nanocomposite Hydrogels. *Adv. Mater. Weinheim* **2005**, *17*, 1366–1368. [CrossRef]

120. Delporte, C.; O'Connell, B.C.; He, X.; Lancaster, H.E.; O'Connell, A.C.; Agre, P.; Baum, B.J. Increased fluid secretion after adenoviral-mediated transfer of the aquaporin-1 cDNA to irradiated rat salivary glands. *Proc. Natl. Acad. Sci. USA* **1997**, *94*, 3268–3273. [CrossRef] [PubMed]
121. Alevizos, I.; Zheng, C.; Cotrim, A.P.; Liu, S.; McCullagh, L.; Billings, M.E.; Goldsmith, C.M.; Tandon, M.; Helmerhorst, E.J.; Catalán, M.A.; et al. Late responses to adenoviral-mediated transfer of the aquaporin-1 gene for radiation-induced salivary hypofunction. *Gene Ther.* **2017**, *24*, 176–186. [CrossRef]
122. Samuni, Y.; Baum, B.J. Gene delivery in salivary glands: From the bench to the clinic. *Biochim. Biophys. Acta* **2011**, *1812*, 1515–1521. [CrossRef]
123. Varghese, J.J.; Schmale, I.L.; Wang, Y.; Hansen, M.E.; Newlands, S.D.; Ovitt, C.E.; Benoit, D.S.W. Retroductal nanoparticle injection to the murine submandibular gland. *J. Vis. Exp.* **2018**, *135*, e57521. [CrossRef]
124. Shan, Z.; Li, J.; Zheng, C.; Liu, X.; Fan, Z.; Zhang, C.; Goldsmith, C.M.; Wellner, R.B.; Baum, B.J.; Wang, S. Increased fluid secretion after adenoviral-mediated transfer of the human aquaporin-1 cDNA to irradiated miniature pig parotid glands. *Mol. Ther.* **2005**, *11*, 444–451. [CrossRef]
125. Redman, R.S.; Ball, W.D.; Mezey, E.; Key, S. Dispersed donor salivary gland cells are widely distributed in the recipient gland when infused up the ductal tree. *Biotech. Histochem.* **2009**, *84*, 253–260. [CrossRef]
126. Grundmann, O.; Fillinger, J.L.; Victory, K.R.; Burd, R.; Limesand, K.H. Restoration of radiation therapy-induced salivary gland dysfunction in mice by post therapy IGF-1 administration. *BMC Cancer* **2010**, *10*, 417. [CrossRef] [PubMed]
127. Okazaki, Y.; Kagami, H.; Hattori, T.; Hishida, S.; Shigetomi, T.; Ueda, M. Acceleration of rat salivary gland tissue repair by basic fibroblast growth factor. *Arch. Oral Biol.* **2000**, *45*, 911–919. [CrossRef]
128. Zheng, C.; Cotrim, A.P.; Rowzee, A.; Swaim, W.; Sowers, A.; Mitchell, J.B.; Baum, B.J. Prevention of radiation-induced salivary hypofunction following hKGF gene delivery to murine submandibular glands. *Clin. Cancer Res.* **2011**, *17*, 2842–2851. [CrossRef] [PubMed]
129. Marmary, Y.; Adar, R.; Gaska, S.; Wygoda, A.; Maly, A.; Cohen, J.; Eliashar, R.; Mizrachi, L.; Orfaig-Geva, C.; Baum, B.J.; et al. Radiation-Induced Loss of Salivary Gland Function Is Driven by Cellular Senescence and Prevented by IL6 Modulation. *Cancer Res.* **2016**, *76*, 1170–1180. [CrossRef]
130. Lombaert, I.M.A.; Wierenga, P.K.; Kok, T.; Kampinga, H.H.; de Haan, G.; Coppes, R.P. Mobilization of bone marrow stem cells by granulocyte colony-stimulating factor ameliorates radiation-induced damage to salivary glands. *Clin. Cancer Res.* **2006**, *12*, 1804–1812. [CrossRef] [PubMed]
131. Lombaert, I.M.A.; Brunsting, J.F.; Wierenga, P.K.; Kampinga, H.H.; de Haan, G.; Coppes, R.P. Cytokine treatment improves parenchymal and vascular damage of salivary glands after irradiation. *Clin. Cancer Res.* **2008**, *14*, 7741–7750. [CrossRef]
132. Rocchi, C.; Emmerson, E. Mouth-Watering Results: Clinical Need, Current Approaches, and Future Directions for Salivary Gland Regeneration. *Trends Mol. Med.* **2020**, *26*, 649–669. [CrossRef]
133. Jensen, D.H.; Oliveri, R.S.; Trojahn Kølle, S.-F.; Fischer-Nielsen, A.; Specht, L.; Bardow, A.; Buchwald, C. Mesenchymal stem cell therapy for salivary gland dysfunction and xerostomia: A systematic review of preclinical studies. *Oral Surg. Oral Med. Oral Pathol. Oral Radiol.* **2014**, *117*, 335–342.e1. [CrossRef]
134. Lim, J.-Y.; Yi, T.; Choi, J.-S.; Jang, Y.H.; Lee, S.; Kim, H.J.; Song, S.U.; Kim, Y.-M. Intraglandular transplantation of bone marrow-derived clonal mesenchymal stem cells for amelioration of post-irradiation salivary gland damage. *Oral Oncol.* **2013**, *49*, 136–143. [CrossRef] [PubMed]
135. Kojima, T.; Kanemaru, S.-I.; Hirano, S.; Tateya, I.; Ohno, S.; Nakamura, T.; Ito, J. Regeneration of radiation damaged salivary glands with adipose-derived stromal cells. *Laryngoscope* **2011**, *121*, 1864–1869. [CrossRef] [PubMed]
136. Grønhøj, C.; Jensen, D.H.; Glovinski, P.V.; Jensen, S.B.; Bardow, A.; Oliveri, R.S.; Specht, L.; Thomsen, C.; Darkner, S.; Kiss, K.; et al. First-in-man mesenchymal stem cells for radiation-induced xerostomia (MESRIX): Study protocol for a randomized controlled trial. *Trials* **2017**, *18*, 108. [CrossRef] [PubMed]
137. Grønhøj, C.; Jensen, D.H.; Vester-Glowinski, P.; Jensen, S.B.; Bardow, A.; Oliveri, R.S.; Fog, L.M.; Specht, L.; Thomsen, C.; Darkner, S.; et al. Safety and Efficacy of Mesenchymal Stem Cells for Radiation-Induced Xerostomia:

A Randomized, Placebo-Controlled Phase 1/2 Trial (MESRIX). *Int. J. Radiat. Oncol. Biol. Phys.* **2018**, *101*, 581–592. [CrossRef] [PubMed]
138. Barkholt, L.; Flory, E.; Jekerle, V.; Lucas-Samuel, S.; Ahnert, P.; Bisset, L.; Büscher, D.; Fibbe, W.; Foussat, A.; Kwa, M.; et al. Risk of tumorigenicity in mesenchymal stromal cell-based therapies–bridging scientific observations and regulatory viewpoints. *Cytotherapy* **2013**, *15*, 753–759. [CrossRef]
139. Van Luijk, P.; Pringle, S.; Deasy, J.O.; Moiseenko, V.V.; Faber, H.; Hovan, A.; Baanstra, M.; van der Laan, H.P.; Kierkels, R.G.J.; van der Schaaf, A.; et al. Sparing the region of the salivary gland containing stem cells preserves saliva production after radiotherapy for head and neck cancer. *Sci. Transl. Med.* **2015**, *7*, 305ra147. [CrossRef]
140. Pringle, S.; Maimets, M.; van der Zwaag, M.; Stokman, M.A.; van Gosliga, D.; Zwart, E.; Witjes, M.J.H.; de Haan, G.; van Os, R.; Coppes, R.P. Human salivary gland stem cells functionally restore radiation damaged salivary glands. *Stem Cells* **2016**, *34*, 640–652. [CrossRef]
141. Ihrler, S.; Blasenbreu-Vogt, S.; Sendelhofert, A.; Rössle, M.; Harrison, J.D.; Löhrs, U. Regeneration in chronic sialadenitis: An analysis of proliferation and apoptosis based on double immunohistochemical labelling. *Virchows Arch.* **2004**, *444*, 356–361. [CrossRef]
142. Aure, M.H.; Konieczny, S.F.; Ovitt, C.E. Salivary gland homeostasis is maintained through acinar cell self-duplication. *Dev. Cell* **2015**, *33*, 231–237. [CrossRef]
143. Boshell, J.L.; Pennington, C. Histological observations on the effects of isoproterenol on regenerating submandibular glands of the rat. *Cell Tissue Res.* **1980**, *213*, 411–416. [CrossRef]
144. Maimets, M.; Bron, R.; de Haan, G.; van Os, R.; Coppes, R.P. Similar ex vivo expansion and post-irradiation regenerative potential of juvenile and aged salivary gland stem cells. *Radiother. Oncol.* **2015**, *116*, 443–448. [CrossRef]
145. Feng, J.; van der Zwaag, M.; Stokman, M.A.; van Os, R.; Coppes, R.P. Isolation and characterization of human salivary gland cells for stem cell transplantation to reduce radiation-induced hyposalivation. *Radiother. Oncol.* **2009**, *92*, 466–471. [CrossRef]
146. Patel, V.N.; Lombaert, I.M.A.; Cowherd, S.N.; Shworak, N.W.; Xu, Y.; Liu, J.; Hoffman, M.P. Hs3st3-modified heparan sulfate controls KIT+ progenitor expansion by regulating 3-O-sulfotransferases. *Dev. Cell* **2014**, *29*, 662–673. [CrossRef] [PubMed]
147. Banh, A.; Xiao, N.; Cao, H.; Chen, C.-H.; Kuo, P.; Krakow, T.; Bavan, B.; Khong, B.; Yao, M.; Ha, C.; et al. A novel aldehyde dehydrogenase-3 activator leads to adult salivary stem cell enrichment in vivo. *Clin. Cancer Res.* **2011**, *17*, 7265–7272. [CrossRef] [PubMed]
148. Nakao, K.; Morita, R.; Saji, Y.; Ishida, K.; Tomita, Y.; Ogawa, M.; Saitoh, M.; Tomooka, Y.; Tsuji, T. The development of a bioengineered organ germ method. *Nat. Methods* **2007**, *4*, 227–230. [CrossRef] [PubMed]
149. Ogawa, M.; Oshima, M.; Imamura, A.; Sekine, Y.; Ishida, K.; Yamashita, K.; Nakajima, K.; Hirayama, M.; Tachikawa, T.; Tsuji, T. Functional salivary gland regeneration by transplantation of a bioengineered organ germ. *Nat. Commun.* **2013**, *4*, 2498. [CrossRef]
150. Hirayama, M.; Oshima, M.; Tsuji, T. Development and prospects of organ replacement regenerative therapy. *Cornea* **2013**, *32* (Suppl. S1), S13–S21. [CrossRef]

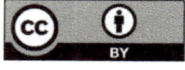

© 2020 by the authors. Licensee MDPI, Basel, Switzerland. This article is an open access article distributed under the terms and conditions of the Creative Commons Attribution (CC BY) license (http://creativecommons.org/licenses/by/4.0/).

MDPI
St. Alban-Anlage 66
4052 Basel
Switzerland
Tel. +41 61 683 77 34
Fax +41 61 302 89 18
www.mdpi.com

Journal of Clinical Medicine Editorial Office
E-mail: jcm@mdpi.com
www.mdpi.com/journal/jcm

www.ingramcontent.com/pod-product-compliance
Lightning Source LLC
LaVergne TN
LVHW070202100526
838202LV00015B/1987